Design and Analysis of Clinical Trials with Time-to-Event Endpoints

Chapman & Hall/CRC Biostatistics Series

Chapman & Hall/CRC Biostatistics Series

Published Titles

Chapman & Hall/CRC Biostatistics Series

Design and Analysis of Clinical Trials with Time-to-Event Endpoints

Edited by
Karl E. Peace

Jiann-Ping Hsu College of Public Health
Georgia Southern University
Statesboro, U. S. A.

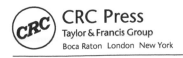

CRC Press
Taylor & Francis Group
Boca Raton London New York

CRC Press is an imprint of the
Taylor & Francis Group, an **informa** business

A CHAPMAN & HALL BOOK

CRC Press
Taylor & Francis Group
6000 Broken Sound Parkway NW, Suite 300
Boca Raton, FL 33487-2742

First issued in paperback 2019

© 2009 by Taylor & Francis Group, LLC
CRC Press is an imprint of Taylor & Francis Group, an Informa business

No claim to original U.S. Government works

ISBN-13: 978-1-4200-6639-5 (hbk)
ISBN-13: 978-1-138-37266-5 (pbk)

Library of Congress Cataloging-in-Publication Data

Design and analysis of clinical trials with time-to-event endpoints / editor, Karl
  E. Peace.
       p. ; cm. -- (Chapman & Hall/CRC biostatistics series ; 31)
    Includes bibliographical references and index.
    ISBN 978-1-4200-6639-5 (hardcover : alk. paper)
    1. Clinical trials. I. Peace, Karl E., 1941- II. Series: Chapman & Hall/CRC
  biostatistics series ; 31.
       [DNLM: 1. Clinical Trials as Topic. QV 771 D4571 2009]

  R853.C55D465 2009
  610.72'4--dc22   2009007293

Visit the Taylor & Francis Web site at
http://www.taylorandfrancis.com

and the CRC Press Web site at
http://www.crcpress.com

Dedication

To the memory of my mother,

Elsie Mae Cloud Peace, and to

my wife, Jiann-Ping Hsu,

and my son, Christopher K. Peace.

Contents

Preface

In many clinical trials and other experimental settings, the primary endpoint is some critical event. In analgesic studies such as postdental-extraction pain or postpartum pain, the event is relief of pain. In an anti-infective study such as chronic urinary tract infection, the event is microbiological cure or abatement of clinical signs and symptoms of the infection. In oncology studies such as carcinoma of the breast, head and neck cancer, liver cancer, colorectal cancer, etc., the primary event is death. However, if the primary treatment is surgery, which leaves the patient with no evidence of disease, another important event in patient follow-up is evidence of disease or recurrence. In a study of bladder tumors, e.g., important events in patient follow-up are remission or progression. In transplantation studies involving renal allografts, although death is "primary," rejection may be the primary event reflecting the experimental objective. Similarly, in long-term chronic toxicity studies of rodents, tumor development may directly reflect the experimental objective more than death.

In such studies, participants are usually monitored for a specified length of time. The frequency of follow-up may vary depending on the disease being studied, e.g., daily, weekly, monthly, quarterly, biannually, or over unequally spaced intervals. Seldom, if ever, would follow-up be less frequent than quarterly. Follow-up on each participant permits the recording of the observed occurrence or nonoccurrence of the event during the monitoring period. If the event is not observed to occur, it could be that the observation time was censored due to the subject's withdrawal prior to the end of the study (moved away from the area, died from causes unrelated to disease or treatment under study, adverse event unrelated to study conditions that prevented subject's continued study participation, etc.) or due to the study coming to an end.

Analyses of data from such studies include an analysis of the proportions of participants on whom the event was observed. This was essentially the only analysis prior to the 1950s. Criticisms of this analysis are (1) the time at which the event was observed to have occurred is ignored, and (2) the indecisive or inappropriate use of the information on participants censored prior to the end of the study. During the last half century there has been increasing use —fueled in a major way by the publications of Kaplan–Meier, Gehan, Zelan, and Cox in particular—of analysis methodology that is not subject to these criticisms. This methodology has been most often applied in studies where the primary endpoint is death. Consequently, this methodology has come to be known as survival analysis methodology. More generally, it is a time-to-event analysis methodology. Use of this methodology requires careful definition of the event, the censored observation, the provision of adequate follow-up, the number of events, and independence or "noninformativeness" of the censoring mechanisms relative to the event.

This book consists of 22 chapters. Chapter 1 provides an an overview of time-to-event endpoint methodology; Chapter 2 presents a thorough exposition of issues and methods in the design and monitoring of clinical trials with time-to-event endpoints. Phase 0 clinical trials are also covered in Chapter 2. This is followed by six chapters on inferential analysis methods. The first four (Chapters 3 through 6) span the types of inferential methods appropriate for analyzing time-to-event endpoints: parametric methodology, semiparametric methodology, categorical methodology, and Bayesian methodology. The remaining two (Chapters 7 and 8) covering special inferential cases complete the treatise on inferential methods. One provides an alternative to the Cox model for small time-to-event trials. The other covers estimation and testing for change in hazard.

Chapter 9 provides descriptive and graphical methods useful in analyzing time-to-event endpoints. A variety of clinical trials in which time-to-event endpoints are collected and analyzed are covered in the next nine chapters (Chapters 10 through 18): analgesic trials with and without paired time-to-event endpoints; antibiotic trials, cardiovascular prevention trials, antiviral trials, prostate cancer trials in which time-to-cure is of interest; cancer prevention trials, cancer prevention trials in which nonfatal competing risks and death from cancer are of interest; and astrocytoma brain tumor and chronic myelogonous leukemia trials that utilize the least absolute shrinkage and selection operator (LASSO) method for variable selection.

Two chapters that span all areas of drug development and medical practice in which time-to-some critical event is of interest are included. Chapter 19 presents methods for selecting optimal treatments based on predictive factors and Chapter 20 presents new methodology utilizing time-to-adverse event in the assessment of safety in clinical trials.

The final two chapters of the book provide a thorough presentation of design and analysis of clinical trials in animals required by the Food and Drug Administration (FDA) in the review of new drug applications for carcinogenic potential. Chapter 21 provides the frequentist approach to chronic carcinogenicity studies in rodents and Chapter 22 provides a Bayesian framework for the analysis of time-to-tumor response in such studies.

I would like to thank and express my gratitude to many individuals. First, I thank all contributing authors for their excellent work in developing their chapters and for their perseverance in meeting deadlines. The authors are truly world-class statisticians, reflecting collaboration among academia, the pharmaceutical industry, and governmental agencies such as the National Cancer Institute (NCI) and FDA. From Taylor & Francis, I would like to thank David Grubbs for his interest in the book, and Amy Blalock for her editorial assistance. Thanks also go to the Georgia Cancer Coalition whose grant in selecting me as one of their distinguished cancer scholars supported, in part, my time in developing the book. Finally, from the Jiann-Ping Hsu College of Public Health at Georgia Southern University, I thank Ruth Whitworth for her IT support, Dean Charlie Hardy for his support and encouragement to finish the project, Lee T. Mitchell for her jocularity and good cheer that brighten our entire college, and Benjamin Maligalig, my graduate assistant, for his assistance in proofing the format of the chapters.

Editor

Dr. Karl E. Peace is the Georgia Cancer Coalition Distinguished Cancer Scholar, senior research scientist, and professor of biostatistics in the Jiann-Ping Hsu College of Public Health (JPHCOPH) at Georgia Southern University (GSU). He was responsible for establishing the JPHCOPH—the first college of public health in the University System of Georgia. He is the architect of the Master of Public Health (MPH) in biostatistics and founding director of the Karl E. Peace Center for Biostatistics in the JPHCOPH. Dr. Peace holds a PhD in biostatistics from the Medical College of Virginia, an MS in mathematics from Clemson University, a BS in chemistry from Georgia Southern College, and a health science certificate from Vanderbilt University.

Dr. Peace started his career as a teacher and researcher at the university level. He previously taught mathematics at Georgia Southern College, Clemson University, Virginia Commonwealth University, and Randolph-Macon College, where he was a tenured professor. He holds or has held numerous adjunct professorships at the Medical College of Virginia, the University of Michigan, Temple University, the University of North Carolina, and Duke University.

Later in his career, Dr. Peace was involved in research, technical support, and management in the pharmaceutical industry. He held the positions of senior statistician at Burroughs-Wellcome; manager of clinical statistics at A.H. Robins; director of research statistics at SmithKline and French Labs; senior director of GI clinical studies, data management and analysis at G.D. Searle; and vice president of worldwide technical operations at Warner Lambert/Parke-Davis. He then founded Biopharmaceutical Research Consultants Inc. (BRCI), where he held the positions of president, chief executive officer, and chief scientific officer.

Dr. Peace is or has been a member of several professional and honorary societies, including the Drug Information Association (DIA), the Regulatory Affairs Professional Society (RAPS), the Biometric Society, Technometrics, the American Society for Quality Control (ASQC), Biometrika, the American Statistical Association (ASA), and Kappa Phi Kappa (KPK). He is a past member of the Committee on Applied and Theoretical Statistics, National Research Council, National Academy of Science. He is or has been chair of the biostatistics subsection of the Pharmaceutical Manufacturers Association (PMA), the biopharmaceutical section of the ASA, the training committee of the PMA biostatistics subsection, and is the founder of the Biopharmaceutical Applied Statistics Symposium (BASS).

Dr. Peace has received numerous citations and awards including (1) Georgia Cancer Coalition Distinguished Cancer Scholar; (2) Fellow of the ASA; (3) the Distinguished Service Award of the DIA; (4) Star and Featured Alumnus, School of Basic Sciences, and Founder's Society Medal from the Medical College of Virginia; (5) College of Science and Technology Alumnus of the year, Alumnus of the Year in private enterprise, Presidential Fellowship Award, JPHCOPH Researcher of the year award, GSU researcher of the year award, and the first recipient of the prestigious President's Medal for outstanding service and extraordinary contributions, all from GSU; (6) the 2007 APHA Statistics Section Award; (7) the 2008 Deen Day Smith Humanitarian Award; (8) the 2008 Shining Star recognition by GA House of Representatives; (9) the subject of the 2008 GA HR Resolution #2118; and (10) several meritorious service awards from the ASQC, BASS, the Georgia Cancer Coalition, and the Southwest Georgia Cancer Coalition.

Dr. Peace is a renowned philanthropist, having created 21 endowments at GSU, the Medical College of Virginia, the University of California at Berkeley, Randolph-Macon College, and the International Chinese Statistical Association. The endowments have established the Jiann-Ping Hsu College of Public Health, 3 eminent scholar chairs, 1 professorship, and 16 student scholarship funds, including 5 for students from his native Baker County, Georgia.

Contributors

Rafia Bhore
Division of Biostatistics
Department of Clinical Sciences
University of Texas Southwestern
  Medical Center
Dallas, Texas

Jianwen Cai
Department of Biostatistics
University of North Carolina
  at Chapel Hill
Chapel Hill, North Carolina

Ming-Hui Chen
Department of Statistics
University of Connecticut
Storrs, Connecticut

Lynn P. Dix
GlaxoSmithKline
Research Triangle Park, North Carolina

Laura H. Gunn
Karl E. Peace Center for Biostatistics
Jiann-Ping Hsu College of Public Health
Georgia Southern University
Statesboro, Georgia

Mohammad Huque
Division of Biometrics
Center for Drug Evaluation
  and Research
Food and Drug Administration
Silver Spring, Maryland

Sungduk Kim
Division of Epidemiology, Statistics &
  Prevention Research
National Institute of Child Health and
  Human Development
Bethesda, Maryland

Karl K. Lin
Division of Biometrics
Center for Drug Evaluation
  and Research
Food and Drug Administration
Silver Spring, Maryland

Michelle McNabb
Eli Lilly and Company
Indianapolis, Indiana

Devan V. Mehrotra
Merck Research Laboratories
North Wales, Pennsylvania

Surya Mohanty
Biometrics and Clinical Informatics
Johnson & Johnson Product Research
  and Development LLC
Titusville, New Jersey

Kelly L. Moore
Division of Biostatistics, School of
  Public Health
University of California at Berkeley
Berkeley, California

Hon Keung Tony Ng
Department of Statistical Science
Southern Methodist University
Dallas, Texas

Michael O'Connell
Insightful Corporation
Durham, North Carolina

Akiko Okamoto
Biometrics and Clinical Informatics
Johnson & Johnson Product Research
    and Development LLC
Titusville, New Jersey

Karl E. Peace
Jiann-Ping Hsu College of Public Health
Georgia Southern University
Statesboro, Georgia

Dennis Pearl
Department of Statistics
The Ohio State University
Columbus, Ohio

Eric C. Polley
Division of Biostatistics, School of
    Public Health
University of California at Berkeley
Berkeley, California

Mohammad Atiar Rahman
Division of Biometrics
Center for Drug and Evaluation
    Research
Food and Drug Administration
Silver Spring, Maryland

Arthur J. Roth
Pfizer Inc.
Ann Arbor, Michigan

Larry Rubinstein
Biometric Research Branch
Division of Cancer Treatment and
    Diagnosis
National Cancer Institute
Bethesda, Maryland

Andreas Sashegyi
Eli Lilly and Company
Indianapolis, Indiana

Anthony C. Segreti
ASG Inc.
Cary, North Carolina

Jennifer B. Shannon
GlaxoSmithKline
Research Triangle Park, North Carolina

Michael W. Sill
Department of Biostatistics
State University of New York at Buffalo

and

Gynecologic Oncology Group Statistical
    and Data Center
Roswell Park Cancer Institute
Buffalo, New York

Eric V. Slud
Mathematics Department
University of Maryland
College Park, Maryland

Matthew C. Somerville
GlaxoSmithKline
Research Triangle Park, North Carolina

Peter F. Thall
Department of Biostatistics
The University of Texas M.D. Anderson
    Cancer Center
Houston, Texas

Steve Thomson
Division of Biometrics
Center for Drug Evaluation
    and Research
Food and Drug Administration
Silver Spring, Maryland

Bob Treder
Department of Biostatistics
University of North Carolina
    at Chapel Hill
Chapel Hill, North Carolina

Kao-Tai Tsai
Global Biometric Sciences
Bristol-Myers Squibb Company
Plainsboro, New Jersey

Mark J. van der Laan
Jiann-Ping Hsu/Karl E. Peace
    Endowed Chair in Biostatistics
University of California at Berkeley
Berkeley, California

Julia Wang
Biometrics and Clinical Informatics
Johnson & Johnson Product Research
    and Development LLC
Raritan, New Jersey

Xuemei Wang
Department of Biostatistics
The University of Texas M.D. Anderson
    Cancer Center
Houston, Texas

Zhu Wang
Department of Internal Medicine
Yale University
New Haven, Connecticut

Timothy H. Wilson
GlaxoSmithKline
Research Triangle Park, North Carolina

Lili Yu
Jiann-Ping Hsu College of
    Public Health
Georgia Southern University
Statesboro, Georgia

Donglin Zeng
Department of Biostatistics
University of North Carolina
    at Chapel Hill
Chapel Hill, North Carolina

Chapter 1

Overview of Time-to-Event Endpoint Methodology

Karl E. Peace

Contents

1.1 Introduction

In many clinical trials and other experimental settings, the primary endpoint is some critical event. In analgesic studies such as postdental extraction pain [1] or postpartum pain, the event is relief of pain. In an anti-infective study such as chronic urinary tract infection [2], the event is microbiological cure or abatement of clinical signs and symptoms of the infection. In oncology studies such as carcinoma of the breast [3], head and neck cancer [4], liver cancer [5], colorectal cancer [6], etc., the primary event is death. However, if the primary treatment is surgery which leaves the patient with no evidence of disease, another important event in patient follow-up is evidence of disease or recurrence [7]. In the study of bladder tumors, for example, important events in patient follow-up are remission or progression [8]. In transplantation studies involving renal allografts [9], although death is "primary," rejection may be the primary event reflecting the experimental objective. Similarly, in long-term chronic toxicity studies of rodents, tumor development may directly reflect the experimental objective more so than death.

In studies such as these, participants are usually followed for a specified length of time. Depending on the disease being studied, the frequency of follow-up may vary; e.g., daily, weekly, monthly, quarterly, biannually, or over unequally spaced intervals. Seldom if ever would follow-up be less frequent than quarterly. Follow-up on each participant permits the recording of the observed occurrence of the event or nonoccurrence of the event during the opportunity to observe. If the event is not observed to occur, it could be that the observation time was censored due to subject withdrawal prior to the end of the study (moved away from the area, died from causes unrelated to disease or treatment under study, adverse event unrelated to study conditions that prevented subject's continued study participation, etc.) or due to the study ending.

Figure 1.1 illustrates nine patients who entered a clinical trial where the event was observed on five patients and the event was censored on four patients. The left portion of the line for each patient represents the beginning of the observation time (time of randomization or time of beginning the treatment intervention) and the right endpoint represents the last time the status (event or censored) of the patient was known. Time 0 represents the calendar time the study started (with entry of the first patient). The fact that the left endpoints of the lines are staggered reflects that patients usually enter a clinical trial at different calendar times. Time-to-event data from Figure 1.1 available for analysis are the lengths of the patient lines and the event status. This effectively scales event times for all patients back to the origin.

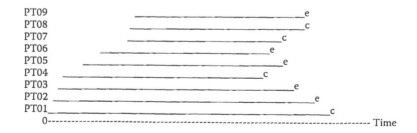

FIGURE 1.1: Observed event times. e, event was observed; c, event was censored.

Analyses of data from such studies include an analysis of the proportions of participants on whom the event was observed. This was essentially the only analysis prior to the 1950s. Criticisms of this analysis are (1) the time at which the event was observed to occur is ignored and (2) indecisive or inappropriate use of the information on participants censored prior to the end of the study. During the last half century there has been increasing use—fueled in a major way by the publications of Kaplan-Meier [10], Gehan [11], Zelen [12], and Cox [13] in particular—of analysis methodology that is not subject to these criticisms. This methodology has been most often applied in studies where the primary endpoint is death. Consequently, the methodology has become known as survival analysis methodology. More generally it is time-to-event analysis methodology. Use of the methodology requires careful definition of the event, the censored observation, the provision of adequate follow-up, the number of events, and independence or "noninformativeness" of the censoring mechanisms relative to the event.

1.2 Overview of General Methods

As a broad outline of this book, design and monitoring methods appropriate for clinical trials with time-to-event endpoints appear first (Chapter 2). Then several chapters follow that deal with inferential methods for analyzing time-to-event endpoints. Inferential methodology may be parametric (Chapter 3), semi- or quasi-parametric (Chapter 4), or nonparametric (Chapter 5). Prognostic (concomitant, covariate, or regressor) information may be incorporated into the methodology. The methodology is directed at parameter estimation, confidence intervals on parameters, and tests of hypotheses on parameters.

1.3 Design and Monitoring

A thorough treatment of design issues and attendant methodology for Phase II and Phase III clinical trials with time-to-event endpoints is presented in Chapter 2. Phase II studies include historically controlled and randomized studies, selection designs [14–16], screening designs [17], as well as factorial studies.

Procedures for determining the requisite number of deaths (and the number of patients to be entered) for specified Type I and Type II error levels under exponentially distributed times-to-event and under proportional hazards are provided for Phase III equivalency and factorial studies. Attention is also paid to determining the length of such studies, in addition to designing Phase III studies for the assessment of significant cure rates.

Several procedures useful in monitoring clinical trials with time-to-event endpoints are presented. These include group sequential procedures for the early termination of Phase III trials based on efficacy; e.g., Pocock's method [18], O'Brien and Fleming's method [19], Lan and DeMets' alpha-spending method [20], and repeated confidence interval methods; e.g., Jennison and Turnbull's method [21]. Methods for early termination based on stochastic curtailment [22,23] or futility [24,25] are also discussed.

Chapter 2 concludes with a section on Phase 0 trials. Issues are identified, methodology for design and analysis are presented, and the strengths and weaknesses are discussed. The potential utility of such trials is illuminated with a presentation of the NCI PARP Inhibitor Trial as an example [26].

1.4   Inferential Methods

Parametric-based inferential methods for commonly used models: exponential [12], Weibull [27], Rayleigh [28], Gompertz [29], and lognormal [30–32] are presented in Chapter 3. Semiparametric inferential methods based on the Cox proportional hazards model [13] and reflecting conditional likelihood [33,34], partial likelihood [35], and marginal likelihood [36] appear in Chapter 4.

Chapter 5 provides a thorough treatment of categorical data-based inferential methods as well as applications. Methods considered are contingency table methods with an ordered index for time-to-event categories; regression-type methods using a generalized linear model formulation; estimation and prediction from mixed-effect models; methods for handling dropouts including general estimating equations (GEEs); and goodness-of-fit assessment. Applications include an example illustrating the connection between polytomous logistic regression and the discrete-time Cox model [37–39]; an example illustrating model building for Poisson regression with time-dependent covariates using data from a study involving basal cell carcinoma counts; an example involving a discrete-time model with time-dependent hazard effects and dropouts; and an example involving mixed-effect general linear model (GLM) and goodness-of-fit assessments.

An overview of Bayesian inferential methods [40–42] appropriate for clinical trials with time-to-event endpoints appears in Chapter 6. Prior specification and posterior sampling are discussed. Both parametric and semiparametric survival models are presented. The chapter ends with application of Bayesian methods for clinical trial design.

An efficient alternative to the Cox proportional hazards model for small time-to-event clinical trials [43] is presented in Chapter 7.

Since a crucial assumption underlying the Cox proportional hazards model when comparing two groups, is that the ratio of the hazards for the two groups is constant over the time interval determined by the range of event times, methods are needed for estimating the time at which the hazard ratio changes [44,45]. These methods are presented in Chapter 8, along with procedures for testing the statistical significance of estimated departures from constancy.

1.5   Descriptive and Graphical Methods

Every inferential analysis is bolstered by the presence of tabular and graphical descriptive displays of the data being analyzed [46]. Such displays provide a summary of results that are informative about the trial design and data behavior over the course of the study. They may also provide a visual check of whether assumptions underlying the inferential methodology reasonably hold for the data. Chapter 9 presents an overview of descriptive and graphical methods appropriate for time-to-event data.

1.6   Clinical Trials in Specific Areas

The main focus of this book is the analysis of clinical trials with time-to-event endpoints from a variety of drug research and clinical development areas: analgesia, antibiotic, cardiovascular, oncology, antiviral, assignment of treatments based on predictive factors, and safety assessment. In addition, two chapters containing applications in preclinical drug development are included.

1.6.1   Analgesic Clinical Trials

Analgesic trials with nonpaired time-to-event endpoints are covered in Chapter 10. For completeness, traditional endpoints reflecting pain assessment are covered in this chapter. However, of particular interest is the discussion that time-to-rescue acts as a full surrogate endpoint [47,48] to the longitudinally collected pain relief/intensity scores in a properly designed study. Therefore, the authors argue for the use of time-to-rescue medication as a primary endpoint in analgesic clinical trials.

Methodology for analyzing paired time-to-event endpoints [49], occurring in analgesia studies, are presented in Chapter 11. The methods are applied to data on HL-A matching in the treatment of burned patients with skin allografts [50].

1.6.2   Antibiotic Clinical Trial

An application [2] of time-to-event methods in a clinical trial assessing the effectiveness of an antibiotic drug in the treatment of chronic urinary tract infections appears in Chapter 12. Specifically, the event is either time-to-microbiological cure or time-to-clinical cure. The methodology enables one to estimate the onset of cure. An interesting feature of this example is that cure cannot be determined prospectively, since in most antibiotic studies, defining clinical cure for example requires the abatement of clinical signs and symptoms of the infection at a point during the treatment period and at a posttreatment follow-up period.

1.6.3   Cardiovascular Prevention Trials

A very lucid and detailed exposition of the challenges in the design and conduct of prevention trials and cardiovascular prevention trials with time-to-event endpoints, in particular, appear in Chapter 13. The Raloxifene Use for The Heart (RUTH) Clinical Trial [51] is presented as a case study for illustration.

1.6.4   Antiviral Clinical Trials

Chapter 14 addresses the design and analysis of clinical trials pertinent to the clinical development of antiviral drugs. Whereas the discussion is relevant to the development of all antiviral drugs, the focus is on diseases caused by the human immunodeficiency virus (HIV), the hepatitis B virus, and the hepatitis C virus. Since the development and marketing of zidovudine (AZT) for the treatment of patients with AIDS and AIDS-related complex [52], viral diseases have been studied extensively and have generated the largest body of clinical and statistical research. Since they are chronic diseases, the assessment of their potential therapies requires the use of time-to-event endpoints.

1.6.5   Cure Rate Models in Prostate Cancer

Over the last half century, various authors have attempted to estimate the proportion of a population of cancer patients following some intervention that may be considered as cured of the disease. Boag [32] considered survival followed a lognormal model and used the method of maximum likelihood to facilitate estimating the proportion of patients with carcinoma of the breast that was cured following surgical intervention. Berkson and Gage [53] used the method of least squares to estimate the proportion of patients with cancer of the stomach cured following gastric resection.

More recently various methods, including Bayesian-based ones, have been applied in estimating the proportion cured in many areas of cancer research and has spawned a literature on cure rate models. Chapter 15 presents a thorough treatment of the Bayesian approach to cure rate models with applications to melanoma and prostate cancer.

1.6.6   Analysis of Nonfatal Competing Risks and Death in Cancer

In many clinical trials, and in particular cancer clinical trials, one or more intermediate events may precede the primary event; e.g., death. Generally the intermediate events and the primary event are not independent, and the occurrence of one event may preclude the others; i.e., the events may reflect competing risks. This is the case considered in Chapter 16. A multivariate parametric model for the times to the nonfatal events, the residual survival times following the events, and the time to death without any preceding intermediate event is described. The model is illustrated by fitting it to data on patients with acute myelogenous leukemia (AML) or myelodyplastic syndrome (MDS) that includes times to two intermediate events, one desirable and the other undesirable, as well as overall survival time. The model structure and statistical analyses are similar to those of Shen and Thall [54] and Estey et al. [55].

1.6.7 Cancer Prevention Trials

A thorough discussion of the design, summarization, analysis, and interpretation issues inherent in cancer prevention trials is presented in Chapter 17. Design issues include specifying the objective, selecting the population, specifying the interventions—including duration and follow-up, identifying the endpoints, statistical design requirements: sample size and power, randomization and blinding, and monitoring procedures. Summarization issues include accounting for withdrawals, and presentation of the primary endpoint and other variables of interest in cancer studies. Analysis issues considered are the basis for inference, statistical tests and estimates of treatment effects, and the number of studies. Interpretation issues considered are the impact of interim analysis results, efficacy as a multivariate response, compliance and competing risks, sensitivity analyses to address the robustness of inference, and the assessment of interaction.

The REduction of DUtasteride in Cancer Events (REDUCE) trial [56] is presented as a case study to illustrate issues and methods described in the chapter. The REDUCE trial was designed to assess the effectiveness of dutasteride in reducing prostate cancer risk.

1.6.8 LASSO Method in Chronic Myelogenous Leukemia Trials

The least absolute shrinkage and selection operator (LASSO) method [57,58] in covariable selection for right censored time-to-event endpoints within the context of the linear model with right censored data is discussed in Chapter 18. Methods extending the random-sieve likelihood approach for right censored data [59] are developed, and applied to survival times and covariate data on astrocytoma brain tumor patients [60–62] and on chronic myelogenous leukemia patients [63].

1.6.9 Selecting Optimal Treatments Based on Predictive Factors

The regulatory approval of new drugs, biologics, or devices for the treatment of a specific disease or medical condition, is based on demonstrating that the intervention is effective (as compared to a control) and that it has an acceptable benefit-to-risk ratio in a population that has been diagnosed with the disease or condition. Conclusions regarding effectiveness and acceptable benefit-to-risk derive from comparing intervention groups in terms of efficacy and risk measures defined on patients in the groups. Therefore, they provide no inference of effectiveness or acceptable risk of the intervention for the individual patient who might be prescribed the intervention in the future. Although the labeling of the intervention reflects characteristics of the patient population in whom the intervention may be prescribed, the characteristics mainly derive from descriptive summaries of the intervention groups studied.

A particular intervention may be successful in treating one patient, but not in another. This may be due to patients being different in terms of many factors: demographic characteristics, pharmacokinetic characteristics, pharmacodynamic characteristics, genetic characteristics, other biological characteristics, or other known risk factors. Some of the guesswork in choosing what intervention (and at what dose) to prescribe to the individual patient, would be reduced if the treating physician had a model or algorithm that would use individual patient characteristics to predict the likelihood that the intervention would be effective in that patient (individualized medicine). The Gail [64] model has helped in this regard in the treatment of breast cancer, and has been used extensively over the last two decades.

With interest in and demand for individualized medicine increasing, the need for robust statistical methods that can be used to predict optimal treatment assignment based on patient characteristics is compelling. Methodology, based on the super learner algorithm [65], for predicting optimal treatment is developed in Chapter 19. Use of the methodology is demonstrated via simulation and then by using data from a Phase III clinical trial in neuro-oncology.

1.6.10   Time-to-Event Methods in the Assessment of Safety in Clinical Trials

The assessment of safety of drugs based on adverse experience (AE) data from clinical trials has never been more important than it is today. The media has had a field day being critical of the pharmaceutical industry and the Food and Drug Administration (FDA) over the development and regulatory approval of drugs that later are pulled from the market due to safety issues (e.g., witness the press coverage received over Vioxx).

Prior to the mid-1980s, crude rates were used exclusively as the measure for summarization and analysis of AEs. This measure ignores the time at which the AE occurred, and consequently does not factor in the exposure to the drug. An AE occurring after one dose, 1 week of treatment, or 6 months of treatment would contribute the same information in the crude rate. Since O'Neill's [66] publication 20 years ago, analysis of AEs using time-to-event methods has increased.

Time-to-event methods are improvements over crude rate methods for observed events. Since clinical trials are designed to address efficacy, they are underpowered to address questions about safety, particularly for rare AEs [67]. It is clear that additional methodology is needed; methodology which incorporates the fact that failure to observe AEs does not mean that they will not occur upon use of the drug in larger populations.

Chapter 20 presents methodology that may be helpful in this regard. A method for increasing estimation efficiency helps to address the issue that randomized controlled clinical trials (RCTs) prior to market approval are not powered for safety. Using covariate information may be helpful in detecting AEs that may have gone undetected with the crude rate analysis. In addition, time-to-AE analysis methods that factor in their time-dependent nature can provide more efficient estimates for the effect of treatment on AE occurrence. A method for covariate adjustment, that utilizes targeted maximum likelihood [68] for estimating the effect of treatment on AEs failing to occur by a fixed time point in RCTs, is presented in Chapter 20.

1.6.11 Time-to-Event Methods in Preclinical Trials

Both short-term and long-term studies in animals are required by the FDA for new drugs in order to assess their carcinogenic potential. The last two chapters of the book cover long-term preclinical trials in animals in which time-to-event methods are used to assess carcinogenic risk.

1.6.11.1 Design and Analysis of Chronic Carcinogenicity Studies in Rodents

An extensive and detailed exposition of time-to-tumor response studies rodents is presented in Chapter 21. Topics covered include experimental design and collection of data, definition of endpoints, tumor count data and tumor classification, and statistical analysis methods for mortality and tumor data. Statistical analysis methods include logistic regression, the Cochran–Armitage regression test, the Armitage analysis of variance test, the Peto method, the prevalence method for incidental tumors, the death rate method for fatal tumors, the exact Peto test, the poly-K test, incorporating historical controls, and multiplicity issues and methods to address multiplicity. Analysis methods are largely from the traditional, frequentist approach.

In addition, carcinogenicity studies using transgenic mice, interpretation of study results, statistical review and evaluation generally followed in the FDA, and presentation of data and results to the FDA are discussed.

1.6.11.2 Design and Analysis of Time-to-Tumor Response in Animal Studies: A Bayesian Perspective

Design and analysis of rodent carcinogenicity studies, in which time-to-tumor response is the primary endpoint, are presented in Chapter 22. Topics covered include the design of such studies, Bayesian estimation and hypothesis testing, Bayes estimates, quadratic loss versus absolute loss, general decision theory, Bayes factors versus posterior probabilities, strengths and weaknesses of the Bayesian approach, and statistical analysis methods.

Statistical analysis methods of mortality data, models for tumorigenicity, logistic regression, incorporating prior information, methods for dealing with multiplicities, hierarchical models, a tumor process model, and a Bayesian version of Dunson's model for Tg.AC mice are presented in detail. In addition, some analysis software is included.

References

[1] Hill M, Sindet-Pederson S, Seymour R, Hawkesford II J, Coulthard P, Lamey P, Cowan CG, Wickens M, Jeppsson L, and Dean A (2006): Analgesic efficacy of the cyclooxygenase-inhibiting nitric oxide donor AZD3582 in postoperative dental pain: Comparison with naproxen and rofecoxib in two

randomized, double-blind, placebo-controlled studies. *Clinical Therapeutics*, 28(9): 1279–1295.

[2] Peace KE (2007): A survival analysis instead of an endpoint analysis for antibiotic data. *The Philippine Statistician*, 56(1–2): 9–18.

[3] Romond EH, Perez EA, Bryant J, Suman VJ, Geyer CE Jr, Davidson NE, Tan-Chiu E, et al. (2005): Trastuzumab plus adjuvant chemotherapy for operable HER2-positive breast cancer. *The New England Journal of Medicine*, 353: 1673–1684.

[4] Posner MR (2005): Paradigm shift in the treatment of head and neck cancer: The role of neoadjuvant chemotherapy. *The Oncologist*, 10(3): 11–19.

[5] Cheng B-Q, Jia CQ, Liu C-T, Fan W, Wang Q-L, Zhang Z-L, and Yi C-H (2008): Chemoembolization combined with radiofrequency ablation for patients with hepatocellular carcinoma larger than 3 cm. *Journal of the American Medical Association*, 299(14): 1669–1677.

[6] Ogata Y, Mori S, Ishibashi N, Akagi Y, Ushijima M, Murakami H, Fukushima T, and Shirouzu K (2007): Metronomic chemotherapy using weekly low-dosage CPT-11 and UFT as postoperative adjuvant therapy in colorectal cancer at high risk to recurrence. *Journal of Experimental & Clinical Cancer Research*, 26(4): 475–482.

[7] Peace KE (2005): National Cancer Institute: Herceptin combined with chemotherapy improves disease-free survival for patients with early-stage breast cancer. http://www.cancer.gov/newscenter/pressreleases/HerceptinCombination

[8] Fornari D, Steven K, Hansen A, Jepsen J, Poulsen A, Vibits H, and Horn T (2003): Transitional cell bladder tumor: Predicting recurrence and progression by analysis of microsatellite loss of heterozygosity in urine sediment and tumor tissue. *Cancer Genetics and Cytogenetics*, 167(1): 15–19.

[9] Thomas F, Thomas J, Flora R, Mendez-Picon G, Peace KE, and Lee HM (1977): Effect of antilymphocyte globulin potency on survival of cadaver renal transplants. *The Lancet*, 2: 671–674.

[10] Kaplan EL and Meier P (1958): Nonparametric estimation from incomplete observations. *Journal of American Statistical Association*, 53: 457–481.

[11] Gehan EA (1965): A generalized Wilcoxon test for comparing arbitrarily singly-censored samples. *Biometrika*, 52(1–2): 203–223.

[12] Zelen M (1966): Applications of exponential models to problems in cancer research. *Journal of the Royal Statistical Society, Series A*, 129, 368–398.

[13] Cox DR (1972): Regression models and life tables. *Journal of Royal Statistical Society, Series B*, 34: 187–220.

[14] Simon R, Wittes RE, and Ellenberg SS (1985): Randomized phase II clinical trials. *Cancer Treatment Reports*, 69(12): 1375–1381.

[15] Thall PF, Simon R, and Ellenberg SS (1988): Two-stage selection and testing designs for comparative clinical trials. *Biometrika*, 75: 303–310.

[16] Thall PF, Simon R, and Ellenberg SS (1989): A two-stage design for choosing among several experimental treatments and a control in clinical trials. *Biometrics*, 45: 537–547.

[17] Rubinstein LV, Korn EL, Freidlin B, Hunsberger S, Ivy SP, and Smith MA (2005): Design issues of randomized phase II trials and a proposal for phase II screening trials. *Journal of Clinical Oncology*, 23(28): 7199–7206.

[18] Pocock SJ (1977): Group sequential methods in the design and analysis of clinical trials. *Biometrika*, 64(2): 191–199.

[19] O'Brien PC and Fleming TR (1979): A multiple testing procedure for clinical trials. *Biometrics*, 35: 549–559.

[20] Lan KKG and DeMets DL (1983): Discrete sequential boundaries for clinical trials. *Biometrika*, 70(3), 659–663.

[21] Jennison C and Turnbull B (1985): Repeated confidence intervals for the median survival time. *Biometrika*, 72(3): 619–625.

[22] Lan KKG, Simon R, and Halperin M (1982): Stochastically curtailed tests in long-term clinical trials. *Sequential Analysis*, 1: 207–219.

[23] Emerson SS, Kittelson JM, and Gillen DL (2004): On the use of stochastic curtailment in group sequential clinical trials. UW Biostatistics Working Paper Series. http://www.bepress.com/uwbiostat

[24] Lachin JM (2005): A review of methods for futility stopping based on conditional power. *Statistics in Medicine*, 24(18): 2747–2764.

[25] Snapinn S, Chen MG, Jiang O, and Koutsoukos T (2006): Assessment of futility in clinical trials. *Pharmaceutical Statistics*, 5(4): 273–281.

[26] Kinders R, Parchment RE, Ji J, Kummar S, Murgo AJ, Gutierrez M, Collins J, et al. (2007): Phase 0 clinical trials in cancer drug development: From FDA guidance to clinical practice. *Molecular Interventions*, 7: 325–334.

[27] Cohen AC (1965): Maximum likelihood estimation in the Weibull distribution based on complete and censored samples. *Technometrics*, 5: 579–588.

[28] Bain L (1974): Analysis for the linear failure-rate life testing distribution. *Technometrics*, 15(4): 551–559.

[29] Garg ML, Rao BR, and Redmond CK (1970): Maximum-likelihood estimation of the parameters of the Gompertz survival function. *Applied Statistics*, 19(2): 152–159.

[30] Boag JW (1948): The presentation and analysis of the results of radiotherapy. Part I. Introduction. *British Journal of Radiology*, 21: 128–138.

[31] Boag JW (1948): The presentation and analysis of the results of radiotherapy. Part II. Mathematical theory. *British Journal of Radiology*, 21: 189–203.

[32] Boag JW (1949): Maximum likelihood estimates of the proportion of patients cured by cancer therapy. *Journal of the Royal Statistical Society (Series B)*, 11: 15–53.

[33] Cox DR and Reid N (1987): Parameter orthogonality and approximate conditional inference (with discussion). *Journal of the Royal Statistical Society B*, 49: 1–39.

[34] Ferguson H (1992): Asymptotic properties of a conditional maximum-likelihood estimator. *Canadian Journal of Statistics*, 20: 63–75.

[35] Cox DR (1975): Partial likelihood. *Biometrika*, 62: 269–276.

[36] Qin J and Zhang B (2005): Marginal likelihood, conditional likelihood and empirical likelihood: Connections and applications. *Biometrika*, 92(2): 251–270.

[37] Prentice RL and Gloeckler LA (1978): Regression analysis of grouped survival data with application to breast cancer data. *Biometrika*, 34: 57–67.

[38] Thompson WA Jr (1977): On the treatment of grouped observations life statistics. *Biometrika*, 33: 463–470.

[39] Yanagimoto T and Kamakura T (1984): The maximum full and partial likelihood estimators in the proportional hazard model. *Annals of the Institute of Statistical Mathematics*, 36: 363–373.

[40] Ironey TZ and Simon R (2005): Application of Bayesian methods to medical device trials. In: Becker KM and White JJ (eds.) *Clinical Evaluation of Medical Devices: Principles and Case Studies*, 2nd edn. Totowa, NJ: Humana Press Inc., pp. 99–116.

[41] Gelman A, Carlin JB, Stern HS, and Rubin DB (2003): *Bayesian Data Analysis*, 2nd edn. Boca Raton, FL: Chapman & Hall/CRC.

[42] Berry DA and Stangl DK (1996): Bayesian methods in health-related research. In: Berry DA and Stangl DK (eds.) *Bayesian Biostatistics*. New York: Marcel Dekker, Inc., pp. 3–66.

[43] Mehrotra D (2003): An efficient alternative to the Cox model for small time-to-event trials. FDA/Industry Statistics Workshop, Bethesda, MD, September 18.

[44] Pham DT and Nguyen HT (1990): Strong consistency of the maximum likelihood estimators in the change-point hazard rate model. *Statistics*, 21: 203–216.

[45] Pham DT and Nguyen HT (1993): Bootstrapping the change-point of a hazard rate. *Annals of the Institute of Statistical Mathematics*, 45: 331–340.

[46] Pocock SJ, Clayton TC, and Altman DG (2002): Survival plots of time-to-event outcomes in clinical trials: Good practice and pitfalls. *The Lancet*, 359: 1686–1689.

[47] Prentice RL (1989): Surrogate endpoints in clinical trials: Definition and operational criteria. *Statistics in Medicine*, 8: 431–440.

[48] Lin DY, Fleming TR, and De Gruttola V (1997): Estimating the proportion of treatment effect explained by a surrogate marker. *Statistics in Medicine*, 16: 1515–1527.

[49] Wang Z and Ng HKT (2006): A comparative study of tests for paired lifetime data. *Lifetime Data Analysis*, 12: 505–522.

[50] Batchelor JR and Hackett M (1970): HL-A matching in treatment of burned patients with skin allografts. *Lancet*, 2: 581–583.

[51] Mosca L, Barrett-Connor E, Wenger NK, Collins P, Grady D, Kornitzer M, Moscarelli E, et al. (2001): Design and methods of the Raloxifene Use for The Heart (RUTH) study. *American Journal of Cardiology*, 88(4): 392–395.

[52] Fischl MA, Richman DD, Grieco MH, Gottlieb MS, Volberding PA, Laskin OL, Leedom JM, et al. (1987): The efficacy of azidothymidine (AZT) in the treatment of patients with AIDS and AIDS-related complex. A double-blind, placebo-controlled trial. *New England Journal of Medicine*, 317(4): 185–191.

[53] Berkson J and Gage RP (1952): Survival curve for cancer patients following treatment. *Journal of the American Statistical Association*, 47: 501–515.

[54] Shen Y and Thall PF (1998): Parametric likelihoods for multiple non-fatal competing risks and death. *Statistics in Medicine*, 17: 999–1016.

[55] Estey EH, Shen Y, and Thall PF (2000): Effect of time to complete remission on subsequent survival and disease-free survival time in AML, RAEB-t, RAEB. *Blood*, 95: 72–77.

[56] Andriole G, Bostwick D, Brawley O, Gomela L, Marberger M, Tindal D, Breed S, Somerville M, Rittmaster R, et al. (2004): Chemoprevention of prostate cancer in men at high risk: Rationale and design of the reduction by dutasteride of prostate cancer events (REDUCE) trial. *Journal of Urology*, 172: 1314–1317.

[57] Tibshirani R (1996): Regression shrinkage and selection via the LASSO. *Journal of the Royal Statistical Society Series B-Methodological*, 58(1): 267–288.

[58] Tibshirani R (1997): The LASSO method for variable selection in the Cox model. *Statistics in Medicine*, 16(4): 385–395.

[59] Shen XT, Shi J, and Wong WH (1999): Random sieve likelihood and general regression models. *Journal of the American Statistical Association*, 94(447): 835–846.

[60] Sung CC, Pearl DK, Coons SW, Scheithauer BW, Johnson PC, Yates AJ, et al. (1994): Gangliosides as diagnostic markers of human astrocytomas and primitive neuroectodermal tumors. *Cancer*, 74(11): 3010–3022.

[61] Sung CC, Pearl DK, Coons SW, Scheithauer BW, Johnson PC, Zheng M, Yates AJ, et al. (1995): Correlation of ganglioside patterns of primary brain-tumors with survival. *Cancer*, 75(3): 851–859.

[62] Singh LPK, Pearl DK, Franklin TK, Spring PM, Scheithauer BW, Coons SW, Johnson PC, et al. (1994): Neutral glycolipid composition of primary human brain-tumors. *Molecular and Chemical Neuropathology*, 21(2–3): 241–257.

[63] McGlave PB, Shu XO, Wen W, Anasetti C, Nademanee A, Champlin R, Antin JH, Kernan NA, King R, Weisdorf DJ, et al. (2000): Unrelated donor marrow transplantation for chronic myelogenous leukemia: 9 years' experience of the national marrow donor program. *Blood*, 95(7): 2219–2225.

[64] Gail MH, Brinton LA, Byar DP, Corle DK, Green SB, Schairer C, Mulvihill JJ, et al. (1989): Projecting individualized probabilities of developing breast cancer for white females who are being examined annually. *Journal of the National Cancer Institute*, 81: 1879–1886.

[65] van der Laan MJ, Polley EC, and Hubbard AE (2007): Super learner. *Statistical Applications in Genetics and Molecular Biology*, 6(1): Article 25.

[66] O'Neill RT (1988): The assessment of safety. In: Peace KE (ed.) *Biopharmaceutical Statistics for Drug Development* (Chapter 13). New York: Marcel Dekker.

[67] Peace KE (1987): Design, monitoring and analysis issues relative to adverse events. *Drug Information Journal*, 21: 21–28.

[68] van der Laan MJ and Rubin D (2006): Targeted maximum likelihood learning. *The International Journal of Biostatistics*, 2(1): Article 11.

Chapter 2

Design (and Monitoring) of Clinical Trials with Time-to-Event Endpoints

Michael W. Sill and Larry Rubinstein

Contents

2.1   General Introduction to Clinical Trials with Time-to-Event Endpoints—Phase II, Phase III, and Phase 0

The current clinical pathway for the development and establishment of safety and efficacy for therapeutic agents and regimens, particularly in oncology, has been set since approximately 1960. First, phase I trials of approximately 15–30 patients are used to determine a safe dose for further testing, either the maximal tolerated dose or, in the case of agents with little toxicity (molecularly targeted or biologic agents), a biologically effective dose. These studies are generally done in broadly defined patient populations with sufficiently advanced disease to have few other appropriate treatment options. Then phase II studies of approximately 30–100 patients are used to initially indicate the presence or absence of promising clinical effect, often compared to historical controls. These studies are generally done in more narrowly defined patient populations, for which the agent or regimen is expected to show promise. Finally, randomized phase III trials of hundreds or thousands of patients are done to definitively establish whether or not the agent or regimen is superior to what is currently available for a particular patient population. These studies are generally done in patient populations defined by specific disease, stage of disease, and sometimes other prognostic factors, so that the control treatment is generally uniform. General reviews of the statistical issues involving cancer clinical trials are given, in brief, by Rubinstein [1] and, in more detail, by Simon [2]. Very recently, a new form of study, the phase 0 trial, has been added to the beginning of the clinical trials sequence [3]. Phase 0 studies of approximately 15 patients are used to determine whether a particular agent has the anticipated specific biologic effect, which is generally measured by a pharmacodynamic assay. These studies may be done in broadly defined patient populations, with varying disease and disease stage. They are useful in very quickly discovering ineffective agents or in prioritizing among agents designed to affect the same molecular target.

The endpoints used in phase III trials of agents or regimens designed to address serious diseases, particularly in oncology, are almost always time-to-event endpoints.

This is because the outcome of primary interest is usually either overall survival (OS) or progression-free survival (PFS—the minimum of time-to-death or time-to-disease progression). While these endpoints are occasionally measured in binomial fashion, as the percentage of patients who survive, or survive progression-free, at a particular point in time (for example, 1 year or 5 years), this is generally not done, since comparisons by means of the logrank test are much more statistically efficient. In Section 2.3, we discuss, in detail, issues concerning the logrank test, its statistical derivation, and the characteristics of its various uses in clinical trials design, analysis, and monitoring. Those readers who are unfamiliar with the logrank test may wish to read quickly through Section 2.3.1.1 to better understand some of the references to the logrank test in Section 2.2.

The endpoint used in phase II trials, in oncology, has been primarily the rate of objective tumor response across patients, until recently. With the advent of molecularly targeted agents, many of which are anticipated to prolong the time-to-disease progression, rather than cause outright tumor shrinkage, this is beginning to change, and randomized phase II trials using the logrank test to compare the time-to-event endpoint of PFS across patients are beginning to be used. In Section 2.2, we discuss randomized phase II studies using the logrank test, as well as other forms of phase II studies, to put the former in context and make it clear what role they have in the wider phase II setting. We do not discuss phase I studies at all in this chapter, since the endpoints have not been time-to-event variables, nor is there any expectation that they will be in the foreseeable future. Readers who wish to learn more about phase I trials for the purpose of rounding out their understanding of the clinical trials process are referred to the chapters cited above [1,2].

In Section 2.4 we briefly discuss the statistical issues concerning phase 0 trials. It is likely, in the immediate future, that the endpoints in phase 0 trials will remain as pharmacodynamic assays taken at a particular time, rather than time-to-event endpoints based on a progression of such assays, but this restriction may disappear soon. At any rate, phase 0 trials promise to be an important emerging tool, so we felt it important, in this introductory chapter, to discuss them and place them in the context of the larger clinical trials process.

Both authors of this chapter have worked primarily in oncology clinical trials, as have many biostatisticians involved in the development, refinement, and application of time-to-event statistical methodology. The structure, emphases, and examples in this chapter reflect that. However, we feel that the material certainly applies to clinical trials, in general.

2.2   Phase II Studies (with Time-to-Event Endpoints—PFS or OS)

Some phase II studies are beginning to be done with PFS endpoints, rather than tumor response endpoints, for reasons given below. Occasionally, for diseases with very short median OS, or where PFS cannot be reliably measured, OS is the endpoint. Such trials can be one-armed studies, with PFS or OS, measured at a particular time point, compared to that of historical controls, or they can be randomized studies, utilizing the logrank test. We will discuss the statistical issues concerning the use of PFS or OS as the phase II endpoint and we will put such trial designs in the context of phase II trials, in general.

2.2.1   Introduction and Statement of the Problem—How to Measure Efficacy in a Preliminary Fashion When Objective Response Is either Not Expected or Not Meaningful

Until recently, the phase II trial in oncology generally took the form of the Simon "optimal" two-stage design [4], for which the endpoint was objective tumor response, defined as shrinkage by at least 30% unidimensionally by the response evaluation criteria in solid tumor (RECIST) guidelines [5]. A Simon design is constructed to distinguish between an unfavorable (null hypothesis) response rate across patients (often 5%) and a favorable (alternative hypothesis) response rate across patients (often 20%) with type I and type II error rates of .10. The design has two stages to enable early termination if the first stage results are particularly discouraging. It is optimal in the sense that it has minimum expected sample size, under the null hypothesis, among two-stage designs with type I and type II error rates of .10 to distinguish between the null and alternative hypothesis response rates. The optimality criterion was defined thus because in 1989, when this design was published, the phase II trial in oncology was primarily a tool for screening out ineffective agents. It was felt that an agent that could not produce a tumor response rate of 20% (or, for some diseases with minimally effective therapy already in place, 30% or 40%) was not likely to produce a clinically meaningful OS or PFS benefit.

Now, 20 years later, the situation is a bit different in oncology. Many phase II trials are now designed to assess preliminarily the benefit of a molecularly targeted agent, given either alone or in combination with another regimen. It is not always anticipated that such agents are likely to produce or improve tumor response rates. Also, it is often anticipated that such agents will improve PFS or OS. In addition, for certain diseases, such as lung cancer, tumor response has failed to predict for a survival benefit, and for other diseases, such as glioblastoma and prostate cancer, tumor response has proven difficult to measure. For such diseases, phase II trials are also conducted with a PFS or OS endpoint.

2.2.2   Historically Controlled Studies: Advantages, Disadvantages, How to Appropriately Calculate Sample Size, and How to Adjust for Prognostic Factors

While objective tumor response is felt to be a result of treatment, not generally affected by prognostic factors which may vary between experimental and historical control patient samples, PFS and OS are felt to be affected by potential imbalances in these factors, sometimes to a substantial degree. For this reason, phase II trials with time-to-event endpoints (PFS or OS) are often randomized. However, there are also strong reasons why clinicians sometimes resist the use of randomized control groups in phase II trials. Perhaps the strongest reason is statistical efficiency. If there is confidence that the historical data concerning PFS or OS fairly represents what would be expected of the experimental group treated in the standard manner, then evaluating the results with an experimental agent or regimen can be done with half the patients or less, by using historical controls rather than randomizing against a control group. This is true even if there is not access to individual patient historical data, but only the median survival, or if the number of patients in the historic series is limited. Brookmyer and Crowley [6] give methodology for comparing against historic data, and calculating the required sample size, when only the median survival is available. Rubinstein et al. [7] give methodology for calculating the required sample size for randomized studies. Korn and Freidlin [8] show how this approach can be extended to one-armed studies compared against historical controls, if the patient data is available. They demonstrate that the power of the logrank test to detect a prespecified treatment effect (defined as the hazard ratio (HR) of treated versus control patients or, equivalently, as the ratio of median survival times), when experimental data are compared to historical controls, is identical to the power of the logrank test to detect that treatment effect in a randomized study, with the same number of patients in each arm. Use of the logrank test is valid even when experimental data are compared to historical controls, since the test requires only that the censorship is independent of outcome (survival), not that it is independent of treatment arm. The following example illustrates the above points.

Example 2.2.2

Assume that a consortium of investigators wish to evaluate a new treatment in a phase II study in a patient population for which a relatively large number of historical controls have a median PFS of 6 months. They anticipate accrual of approximately 100 patients per year and wish to have 90% power to detect a 50% increase (HR of control to treatment equal to 1.5) in median PFS (9 vs. 6 months), at the one-sided .10 significance level, with 6 months of follow-up subsequent to accrual termination. By the methodology of Brookmyer and Crowley [6], this would require approximately 96 patients, accrued over 1 year, if they conduct a one-armed study, using the 6 month median survival for the historical controls as a fixed value. If, instead, the investigators have individual patient data on a smaller number of historical controls, they may compare the data from a one-armed study of the experimental treatment to that of the historical controls, by means of the logrank test, thus accounting for the inherent variability in the controls. If there are approximately 200 control patients, by the methodology of Rubinstein et al. [7] and Korn and Freidlin [8], it can be calculated that approximately 96 patients, accrued over 1 year, are required to detect a 50% increase in median PFS with 90% power, as above. The superior statistical efficiency of the logrank test, as compared to the test based on median PFS, compensates for the inherent variability of the control patient data. Finally, if the investigators choose to conduct a randomized study, approximately 205 patients, accrued over 2.15 years, are required to detect a 50% increase in median PFS with 90% power, as above.

The most significant concern with using historical controls to assess PFS or OS in a one-armed phase II trial of an experimental treatment is that the historical controls may not fairly represent the expected outcome of the experimental patients, if given standard treatment. In other words, the historical control patients may be inherently inferior or superior in terms of expected PFS or OS, due to differences with respect to prognostic factors. If the important prognostic factors associated with clinical outcome in the patient population can be identified, this problem may be addressed, as demonstrated by Korn et al. [9]. Using a large meta-analysis of melanoma patients treated on phase II studies, they identify the important prognostic variables and their contributions to 1 year OS and 6 month PFS rates, as well as to the survival distributions for either time-to-event endpoint. This allows them to construct tests of the observed 1 year OS and 6 month PFS rates, or of the respective observed survival distributions, associated with a one-armed test of an experimental regimen, adjusting for the particular mix of prognostic factors in the experimental population. It should be noted, however, that this approach was more successful for OS than for PFS, where it was found that the prognostic factors did not adequately explain the variation across trials in the meta-analysis.

2.2.3   Dual-Endpoint (PFS and Objective Response) Historically Controlled Studies

A current common problem in phase II trial design in oncology is that a new agent is anticipated to yield prolonged PFS and not objective tumor response, but would be considered promising for either result. The investigators wish to use a trial design that accommodates either promising outcome explicitly and prospectively. There have been related dual-endpoint trial designs proposed in the past [10,11] that simultaneously evaluated objective tumor response and early progressive disease rates. These designs were meant primarily to enable trial termination at the first stage of a two-stage study for either discouragingly low response rates or discouragingly high early progressive disease rates. They did not meet the converse need for designs that yielded positive outcomes for either promising response rates or promising PFS rates at a predefined time point.

Sill [12] determined that such designs could be constructed by combining two separate single endpoint two-stage designs, one with a binomial tumor response rate endpoint and the other with a PFS endpoint, evaluated as a binomial endpoint at a prespecified time. The two separate designs share common stage 1 and stage 2 sample sizes, to allow for combination in a single study. Each separate design has 90% power to detect the targeted promising outcome (alternative hypothesis) with respect to its endpoint. The separate type 1 error rates, calculated for the two unfavorable outcomes (null hypotheses) separately, are designed to add to .10, the standard phase II significance level. Each separate design has an associated rule for termination at stage 1, and the trial is terminated only if the rules for both endpoints are satisfied. Each separate design has an associated rule for declaring the outcome positive after stage 2, and the overall study is declared positive if either rule is satisfied.

For such designs, the statistical operating characteristics of the overall study can be derived as follows. The power of the study to detect either the targeted response rate, or the targeted PFS rate, is 90%, independent of the outcome of the other. In other words, the power to detect the targeted alternative hypothesis rate, for either endpoint, is 90%, even if the other endpoint is totally unresponsive to treatment. The overall significance level of the study, under the overall null hypothesis that both separate null hypotheses hold, is no more than the sum of the separate type 1 error rates. Since the two endpoints are likely to be positively correlated, the actual significance level of the overall study is somewhere between this sum and the largest of the two separate type 1 error rates. Likewise, the probability of early termination under the overall null hypothesis is equal to the product of the two early termination probabilities calculated for the two endpoints separately, under the assumption that the two endpoints are uncorrelated. Since the two endpoints are likely to be positively correlated, the actual early termination probability under the overall null hypothesis is somewhere between this product and the smallest of the two separate early termination probabilities. These calculations arise from the fact that if the two endpoints are positively correlated then the separate negative outcome spaces will have greater overlap, in terms of probability, than if they were uncorrelated, with the extreme being that the larger space, in terms of probability, will always encompass the smaller. One of the attractive characteristics of these designs is that the dual-endpoint trial usually requires only modestly more patients than the larger of the two Simon optimal designs that would be used for the two endpoints assessed separately. The following example illustrates these points.

Example 2.2.3

Assume that a consortium of investigators wish to evaluate a new treatment in a phase II study, and they wish to simultaneously distinguish between true response rates of 20% vs. 5% across patients and true 4 month PFS rates of 60% vs. 40% (corresponding to median PFS of 5.5 vs. 3 months, with ratio of 1.8). They wish to have 90% power to detect either a 20% tumor response rate or a 60% 4 month PFS rate. They wish to have approximately .10 probability of a false positive outcome in case the true response rate is only 5% and the true 4 month PFS rate is only 40%, and they wish to have at least .5 probability of early stopping if such is the case. The Simon optimal designs to discriminate between such response rates or such PFS rates would require 37 and 46 patients, respectively. They can accomplish both objectives simultaneously with a trial of 50 patients. The new treatment would be considered promising if at least 6 of the 50 patients (12%) responded or at least 25 (50%) survived 4 months progression-free. The study would be terminated early and the new treatment considered not promising if no more than 1 patient of the initial 25 (4%) responded and no more than 11 (44%) survived 4 months progression-free. The study has 94% power to detect a true 20% response rate and 89% power to detect a true 60% 4 month PFS rate. The probability of a false positive result is .03 for a response rate of 5% and .08 for a 4 month PFS rate of 40%, with early termination probabilities of .64 and .73 for these two cases, respectively. Therefore, assuming that the two endpoints are uncorrelated, the overall study has .11 probability of a false positive outcome under the combined null hypothesis of 5% response rate and 40% 4 month PFS rate, and it has .47 probability of early termination for that case.

2.2.4   Randomized Studies—Advantages and Disadvantages of Various Designs

For several decades, there has been increased interest in randomized designs for phase II studies in oncology. This arises from two reasons, primarily. First, an increasing number of new agents are biologic or molecularly targeted, and thus are anticipated to yield increased PFS or OS but not necessarily tumor shrinkage. PFS or OS is affected by patient characteristics which may vary between a one-armed experimental sample and the historical control patients, so that it is often difficult to derive from the historical controls the expected PFS or OS for the experimental patients. A related reason is that an increasing number of phase II studies involve assessing the addition of a new agent to a standard chemotherapeutic regimen. It is often difficult to assess the contribution of the new agent by comparing outcome to that of the standard regimen, especially, as is often the case, if the new agent is expected to increase PFS or OS but not necessarily increase tumor shrinkage. As we have discussed in Section 2.2.2, randomized designs generally require at least twice as many patients as one-armed studies, compared to historical controls, with similar statistical operating characteristics. Therefore, there has been a series of attempts to develop randomized designs that offer some protection against the uncertainties and potential biases of one-armed studies, while retaining some of the statistical efficiency.

One early attempt by Herson and Carter [13] involved randomizing to a small reference arm. The experimental arm would not be compared to the reference arm; it would be analyzed against historical controls as if it were a one-armed study. The reference arm would only act as a check on the similarity of the current patients to the historical controls with respect to clinical outcome when given the standard treatment. The disadvantages of this sort of approach are that the reference arm is too small for its outcome to truly assure comparability for the experimental group, since there is little power to reliably detect moderate but clinically meaningful lack of comparability, and, if the reference arm has outcome substantially different from the historical controls, it is often difficult to interpret the outcome of the experimental arm. If the reference arm does very poorly compared to controls, an apparently negative outcome for the experimental arm may be due to inferior prognosis for the patients. Conversely, if the reference arm does very well compared to controls, an apparently positive outcome for the experimental arm may be due to superior prognosis for the patients. This is a generic problem with attempting to incorporate a randomized control arm into a phase II trial that is not large enough to allow for direct comparison, to reduce the associated cost in increased sample size.

A second early attempt by Ellenberg and Eisenberger [14] involved incorporating a randomized phase II trial as the initial stage in a phase III protocol. The proposal was to terminate the phase III study only if the experimental arm demonstrated inferior tumor response rate to that of the control arm in the phase II stage, and to make the phase II sample size sufficiently large so that there was only .05 probability that this would happen if the true experimental response rate was superior by some predefined amount. The disadvantage of this approach is that if the experimental treatment offers no true increase in tumor response rate, the phase III trial will still proceed beyond the initial phase II stage with .50 probability. In other words, the initial phase II stage is operating at the .50 significance level. This is a generic problem with randomized phase II/III designs; it is very difficult to operate at appropriate type 1 and type 2 error rates without having high sample size for the phase II portion. This sort of design is appropriate if the investigators are already reasonably certain that the experimental treatment is sufficiently promising to justify a phase III trial, but wish to build into the trial a check on that assumption.

2.2.4.1   Selection Design of Simon et al.

There is one context in which the use of a randomized phase II design can achieve its statistical objectives while maintaining a relatively small sample size, and that is in directly comparing two experimental regimens, primarily for the purpose of prioritizing between the two. Simon et al. [15] formalized such pick-the-winner selection designs, where the regimen with superior observed response rate (by any amount) is chosen, among the two, for further testing. The original designs were constructed to yield 90% power to detect the superior regimen if the true difference between the response rates was 15% (in absolute terms). The weakness in the original design is that it does not assure that the (sometimes nominally) superior experimental regimen is superior to standard therapy. It was occasionally argued that an ineffective experimental regimen could act as a control arm for the other regimen, but the design was not constructed to be used in this way, since, as designed, one of the two experimental regimens would always be chosen to go forward, even if neither was superior to standard treatment. To address this, in practice, each arm of the selection design is generally constructed as a two-stage Simon optimal trial, to be compared separately against an historically defined response rate. However, that approach requires that it be possible to compare the experimental regimens to historical controls; this, as we have argued above, is not always the case.

Where the randomized phase II selection design is appropriate, it can be conducted with modest sample size. For example, Simon et al. demonstrate that only 29–37 patients per arm will yield 90% power to detect the regimen that has response rate superior by 15%, in a two armed study. This approach can be adapted to randomized phase II trials with time-to-event endpoints, where the logrank test is used to choose between the two regimens, with dramatic results. We show, in Section 2.3 of this chapter (Equation 2.4), that the required sample size for such trials is proportional to $(z_\alpha + z_\beta)^2$ where z_α and z_β are the standard normal values associated with the type I and type II error bounds, respectively. This means that if the type I error is set to .5 ($z_\alpha = 0$), as it is for the selection design, then, compared to a randomized study with $z_\alpha = z_\beta$ (which is standard for phase II designs) with the same targeted an HR, the sample size is reduced by a factor of 4. This means that selection designs constructed to detect an HR of 1.5 with 90% power are generally similar in size to the original selection designs constructed to detect a response rate difference of 15% with 90% power. The following example illustrates this point.

Example 2.2.4
Assume that a consortium of investigators wish to compare two new treatments in a randomized phase II selection study in a patient population for which historical

controls have a median PFS of 6 months. They anticipate accrual of approximately 100 patients per year and wish to have 90% power to detect a 50% difference (HR equal to 1.5) in median PFS (9 vs. 6 months), with 6 months of follow-up subsequent to accrual termination. By the methodology of Rubinstein et al. [7], this would require a total of approximately 65 patients (accrued over .65 years). If, instead, they wished to detect a 33% difference (HR equal to 1.33) in median PFS (9 vs. 6 months), with the same power and follow-up, this would require approximately 120 patients (over 1.2 years).

2.2.4.2   Screening Design of Rubinstein et al.

None of the randomized phase II designs described above fully address the problem outlined in the beginning of Section 2.2.4—the increasing need in oncology to evaluate agents that are anticipated to increase PFS, but not objective tumor response, and to evaluate combinations with such agents added to standard regimens, where comparison to historical controls may be problematic. The reference arm and phase II/III designs have serious disadvantages, as outlined, and the selection design is meant for the limited situation where experimental regimens are to be compared for prioritization purposes, but, in general, each must also prove itself against historical controls. For this reason, Rubinstein et al. [16], building on previous work by Simon et al. [17] and Korn et al. [18], formalized the randomized phase II screening design. The intention was to define randomized phase II designs that yielded statistical properties and sample sizes appropriate to phase II studies. They were meant to enable preliminary comparisons of an experimental treatment regimen, generally composed of a standard regimen with an experimental agent added, to an appropriate control, generally the standard regimen.

Table 2.1 illustrates the statistical properties of such designs when the endpoint is PFS, and the logrank test is used. It gives the required numbers of failures for various type I and type II error rates appropriate to phase II, and for various targeted HRs. In general, it is expected that phase II studies will be conducted in patients with advanced disease, where most patients will progress within the trial period, so the required number of failures closely approximates the required number of patients. Table 2.1 could be extended to trials with endpoint OS, in which case it would give the required numbers of deaths. It can be noted that the usual limits for type I and

TABLE 2.1:   Approximate required numbers of observed (total) treatment failures for screening trials with PFS endpoints, using the logrank test.

Error Rates	HRs (Δ)			
	$\Delta = 1.3$	$\Delta = 1.4$	$\Delta = 1.5$	$\Delta = 1.75$
$(\alpha, \beta) = (10\%, 10\%)$	382	232	160	84
$(\alpha, \beta) = (10\%, 20\%)$ or $(20\%, 10\%)$	262	159	110	58
$(\alpha, \beta) = (20\%, 20\%)$	165	100	69	36

Note: Calculations were carried out using nQueryAdvisor 5.0 software (Statistical Solutions, Saugus, MA) based on methods given in Ref. [19] with one-sided α.

TABLE 2.2: Approximate required numbers of total patients for screening trials with PFS rate (at a specified time) endpoints, using the binomial test.

Error Rates	PFS Rates (at a Given Time Point)			
	20% vs. 35%	20% vs. 40%	40% vs. 55%	40% vs. 60%
$(\alpha, \beta) = (10\%, 10\%)$	256	156	316	182
$(\alpha, \beta) = (10\%, 20\%)$ or $(20\%, 10\%)$	184	112	224	132
$(\alpha, \beta) = (20\%, 20\%)$	126	78	150	90

Note: Calculations were carried out using nQueryAdvisor 5.0 software (Statistical Solutions, Saugus, MA) based on methods given in Ref. [20] with one-sided α.

type II errors are stretched; in fact, usage of type I error of .20 was discouraged. It can also be noted that restricting to a total sample size no greater than approximately 100 restricts the targeted HR to be at least 1.5.

Table 2.2 illustrates the statistical properties of such designs when the endpoint is PFS rate, measured at a prespecified time point, and the binomial proportion test is used. It gives the required numbers of patients for various type I and type II error rates and for various targeted PFS rate differences (with the equivalent HRs). The table reflects that the binomial proportion test, in general, is quite statistically inefficient in comparison to the logrank test. In fact, for the same targeted HR, the comparison of PFS rates at a particular time point requires approximately twice as many patients. Comparing PFS at a particular time point rather than across the entire survival curve means that restricting to a total sample size not greater than approximately 100 restricts the targeted HR to be at least 1.75. Nevertheless, comparing PFS at a prespecified time is often done since PFS is often considered to be an endpoint that is difficult to measure, potentially subject to investigator bias, or influenced by differential follow-up between the treatment arms.

2.2.4.3 Factorial Randomized Phase II Studies—Advantages and Caveats (Nonadditive Treatment Effects)

Factorial studies, especially 2×2 factorial studies designed to evaluate two experimental treatment approaches simultaneously, are often used in the context of phase III studies. For example, to evaluate the addition of agents A or B to standard treatment S, the four arms would be S, S + A, S + B, and S + A + B. (Another example might be the case of treatment B constituting an amplification of regimen S rather than an additional agent.) The study is designed not to compare the four arms individually, but rather to compare arms 1 + 3 to arms 2 + 4, to evaluate the addition of A, and to compare arms 1 + 2 to arms 3 + 4, to evaluate the addition of B. A positive treatment interaction (synergy) between agents A and B is not a problem, since it increases the likelihood that the addition of either agent will appear beneficial (which is probably desirable in this case). However, even a moderate negative treatment interaction (antagonism) between the two agents is a problem, since it decreases the likelihood that the addition of either agent will appear beneficial. Also, there is generally not adequate power to detect such a negative interaction.

It must be remembered that any effect that causes the addition of B to S + A to yield a lesser effect (HR) than that of the addition of B to S alone constitutes a negative treatment interaction.

If one can assume that such a negative treatment interaction is very unlikely, the increased efficiency of the factorial design is substantial. The kind of calculation made in Section 2.2.4.1, based on the fact that the required sample size is proportional to $(z_\alpha + z_\beta)^2$ where z_α and z_β are the standard normal values associated with the type I and type II error bounds, respectively, demonstrates that the factorial study, which addresses two treatment questions, requires only 18% more patients than a study addressing either question separately. This calculation is based on a type II error bound of .10 for either treatment question, and a type I error bound of .05 (two-sided) for either, which must be adjusted to .025 in the factorial study.

Factorial randomized phase II studies are similarly attractive. Again, one has to be concerned about the possibility of a negative treatment interaction. However, it may be argued that such effects are less likely in phase II studies, where the individual experimental approaches are more likely to have modest effect or no effect at all. Again, the increased efficiency is substantial. The kind of calculation made in Section 2.2.4.1, based on the fact that the required sample size is proportional to $(z_\alpha + z_\beta)^2$ demonstrates that the factorial phase II study requires only 30% more patients than a phase II study addressing either question separately. This calculation is based on a type II error bound of .10 for either treatment question, and a type I error bound of .10 (one-sided) for either, which must be adjusted to .05 in the factorial study.

2.2.5   Advantages and Disadvantages of Using PFS versus OS in Randomized Phase II Studies; Blinding and Use of Logrank Test versus Percent PFS at a Given Time

There are significant advantages to using PFS as the primary endpoint rather than OS in randomized phase II studies. Time-to-progression is shorter than time-to-death, sometimes substantially, so that the PFS endpoint yields more failures and thus greater power for the logrank test. HRs for PFS are generally greater than for OS, again yielding greater power for the logrank test. (Equation 2.4 indicates that the required sample size for a particular power is inversely proportional to the square of the log of the HR.) Finally, a positive phase II result based on PFS is less likely to complicate randomization to the definitive phase III study than a positive phase II result based on OS. There are also significant disadvantages to using PFS as the primary endpoint. Sometimes PFS is difficult to measure reliably. There may also be concern that evaluation of the endpoint is influenced by investigator treatment bias. Even if the determination of progression is unbiased, bias can arise from differential follow-up by treatment. If the control patients are followed more or less vigilantly, this may bias the observed time of progression. Sometimes the issues of bias can be addressed effectively by blinding the study. If this is not possible, at least the bias associated with differential follow-up can be addressed by using a comparison based on PFS rate at a prespecified time, rather than using the logrank test. However, as we have demonstrated in Section 2.2.4.2, this results in substantial loss of statistical efficiency. Freidlin et al. [21] address this problem by proposing a statistic based on comparing the two treatment arms at two prespecified time points. They demonstrate that this approach, which also promises to minimize bias due to differential treatment follow-up, recovers most of the efficiency lost in comparison to the logrank test.

2.3 Phase III Studies

2.3.1 Design

2.3.1.1 Logrank Test Statistic

Typically, comparisons of survival distributions between treatment groups are conducted with the logrank statistic, which is an asymptotically distribution-free, nonparametric test of equivalency of survival for g randomized treatment groups. Often, clinical trials are designed around the specific case where $g = 2$, and for ease of exposition, this simpler case will be considered exclusively here. Development of the test proceeds as follows: at each event time, t_i, the total number of patients at risk, n_i, and the total number of patients who experienced the event of concern, d_i, can be separated into two mutually exclusive groups by the patients' assigned treatment at registration according to Table 2.3.

Under the null hypothesis of no differences in survival by treatment group, H_0: $S_1(t) = S_0(t)$, the risk of experiencing the events is the same in each group. Therefore, the distribution of the d_i events over the two groups is expected to be a purely random process so that d_{1i}/n_{1i} tends to be proportional to d_i/n_i. More specifically, given d_i events in a total of n_i patients at risk with n_{1i} patients at risk in Group 1, the distribution of d_{1i} is hypergeometric according to the following probability mass function (pmf):

$$P(d_{1i} = d | n_{1i}, n_i, d_i) = \frac{\binom{n_{1i}}{d}\binom{n_{0i}}{d_i - d}}{\binom{n_i}{d_i}},$$

where $\max\{0, d_i - n_{0i}\} \le d \le \min\{d_i, n_{1i}\}$ and $\binom{x}{y}$ is the general binomial coefficient for 'x choose y'.

TABLE 2.3: At time t_i, d_{1i} patients experience the event out of a total of n_{1i} from Group 1, and d_{0i} patients experience the event out of a total of n_{0i} from Group 0.

	Randomized Treatment		
Event	Group 1	Group 0	Total
Yes	d_{1i}	d_{0i}	d_i
No	$n_{1i} - d_{1i}$	$n_{0i} - d_{0i}$	$n_i - d_i$
Total at risk	n_{1i}	n_{0i}	n_i

The logrank statistic can be developed heuristically as follows. It derives sensitivity to departures from the null hypothesis (such as H_A: $S_1(t) \neq S_0(t)$) by calculating the observed deviations from the expected values under H_0, e.g., $(d_{1i} - E[d_{1i}])$ and aggregating these differences over all of the times when the events are observed (i.e., $U_1 = \sum_{i=1}^{m}(d_{1i} - E[d_{1i}])$ where m is the total number of distinct event times. Under the null hypothesis, U_1 is statistically "close" to 0 because the observed number of events in Group 1, d_{1i}, tends to be close to its expected value. When the alternative hypothesis holds, on the other hand, U_1 tends to be statistically "distant" from 0 because the observed number of events are more likely to deviate from this expected value. The summation over all event times aggregates these effects. From Figure 2.1, we see example distributions of U_1 under different hypotheses. The solid curves shows a typical distribution of U_1 when the null hypothesis is true while the dashed curve demonstrates a distribution when an alternative hypothesis is true, yielding many observed values greater than their expected values. A rational method for rejecting the null hypothesis for this particular case, for example, is when the observed values of $U_1 > 5$ or $U_1 < -5$ (or alternatively, when $U_1^2 > 25$). Following a standard frequentist approach to decision making (e.g., the Neyman–Pearson lemma), the null hypothesis is rejected because the observed values of U_1 are unlikely, and a more likely, alternative hypothesis is accepted. In order to determine qualities such as "likely" and "unlikely" values of U_1, its distribution needs to be established more fully.

Distributional theory for hypergeometric distributions shows that the expected number of events at each event time in Group 1 is given by $E[d_{1i}] = n_{1i} \cdot d_i/n_i = n_{1i} \cdot P(\text{Event})$ with variance, $\text{Var}(d_{1i}) = n_{1i}n_{0i}d_i(n_i - d_i)/n_i^2(n_i - 1)$.

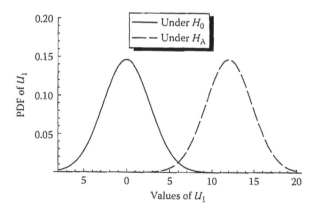

FIGURE 2.1: Distribution of U_1 under the null hypothesis (solid curve), which tends to be statistically "close" to zero, and under an alternative hypothesis (dashed curve) where the observed numbers of d_{1i} tend to be larger than expected when the null hypothesis is assumed. The distribution of U_1 under the alternative hypothesis has a tendency to be "distant" from zero. This forms the basis for distinguishing between the two hypotheses with the logrank test.

For the special case where $n_i = 1$, the $\text{Var}(d_{1i}) = 0$. The variance of U_1 is equal to the summation of the variances of d_{1i}, $\text{Var}(d_{1i})$, over all event times since the distribution of d_{1i} and d_{1j} are independent $\forall i \neq j$ under H_0. That is to say, $\text{Var}(U_1) = V_1 = \sum_{i=1}^{m} \text{Var}(d_{1i})$ Additionally, it can be shown (see Mantel-Haenszel [22] for details) that the following quantity tends toward a standard normal distribution:

$$Z = \frac{\sum_{i=1}^{m}(d_{1i} - E[d_{1i}])}{\sqrt{\sum_{i=1}^{m} \text{Var}(d_{1i})}} \to N(0, 1) \quad \text{as } m \to \infty$$

which provides the null distribution on which the logrank test is based. Often, the logrank test statistic is expressed as a square of the Z statistic, i.e., $W_L = Z^2 \sim \chi^2_{1df}$ (see DeGroot [23, pp. 384–385] for derivation). The statistic, W_L is useful for detecting deviations from the null hypothesis in favor of H_A: $S_1(t) \neq S_0(t)$ whereas Z is useful for one-sided alternatives such as H_A: $S_1(t) > S_0(t)$.

2.3.1.1.1 Example Calculating the Logrank Statistic and Assessing Its Significance

Consider a randomized phase III clinical trial designed to assess the effect of radiation therapy in addition to surgery (Group 1) to surgery alone (Group 0) in a cancer patient population whose prognosis is relatively good but in which a minority recur with distant metastases often leading to death. The origin time for each patient is the date of randomization. The endpoint for the study is the date of documented recurrence. The design of the study called for a targeted accrual of 300 patients (150 patients in each arm). The design also called for an analysis to begin after 30 patients recurred with a logrank test to be conducted at the 2.5% level of significance against a one-sided alternative hypothesis, H_A: $S_1(t) > S_0(t)$. Table 2.4 shows the event times (note that only the order of the event times are important). At each event time, the number of patients at risk and the number who had the event within each group are shown along with the calculated statistics for the variance and expected number of events in Group 1.

From Table 2.4, we see that the total number of events observed in Group 1 is 10. The expected total under the null hypothesis is about 15.4, suggesting the risk of having an event in Group 1 is less than in Group 0. To determine whether this difference, $U_1 = -5.416$, is "typical/likely" or "unusual/unlikely" requires an estimate of the variance for this statistic. This value is provided in the last row, $V_1 = 7.474$. The ratio, $Z = U_1/\sqrt{V_1} = -5.416/\sqrt{7.474} = -1.98$ is approximately normally distributed with $\mu = 0$ and $\sigma^2 = 1$ when the null hypothesis is true. When testing at the 2.5% level of significance, the null hypothesis would be rejected in favor of the alternative if $Z < -1.96$. Therefore, the study would conclude that patients in Group 1 survive longer than in Group 0.

2.3.1.1.2 Stratified Logrank Test

Many clinical trials use a related quantity called the stratified logrank test statistic to make survival comparisons between two (or more) treatments. The difficulty that leads to its use is the concern for systematic

TABLE 2.4: An example dataset used to illustrate the calculation of the logrank test statistic.

Event Time	d_{1i}	d_{0i}	n_{1i}	n_{0i}	d_i	n_i	$E[d_{1i}]$	$Var(d_{1i})$
1	0	1	151	148	1	299	0.50502	0.24997
2	1	0	151	147	1	298	0.50671	0.24995
3	0	1	150	147	1	297	0.50505	0.24997
4	1	2	150	146	3	296	1.52027	0.74478
5	0	1	149	144	1	293	0.50853	0.24993
6	1	1	149	143	2	292	1.02055	0.49807
7	1	0	148	142	1	290	0.51034	0.24989
8	0	2	147	142	2	289	1.01730	0.49811
9	0	1	147	140	1	287	0.51220	0.24985
10	1	0	147	139	1	286	0.51399	0.24980
11	0	3	146	139	3	285	1.53684	0.74427
12	1	1	146	136	2	282	1.03546	0.49759
13	1	0	145	135	1	280	0.51786	0.24968
14	0	1	144	135	1	279	0.51613	0.24974
15	0	1	144	134	1	278	0.51799	0.24968
16	0	1	144	133	1	277	0.51986	0.24961
17	2	0	144	132	2	276	1.04348	0.49724
18	0	1	142	132	1	274	0.51825	0.24967
19	0	1	142	131	1	273	0.52015	0.24959
20	0	2	142	130	2	272	1.04412	0.49719
21	1	0	142	128	1	270	0.52593	0.24933
Total	10	20			30		15.4160	7.47393

differences in survival by patient cofactors which could cause problems with confounding (such as Simpson's paradox). Examples of confounding variables are hospitals participating in a multi-institutional study, performance status (or a patient's ability to function), and classifications of disease aggressiveness. If there is a substantial lack of balance between the randomized treatment assignments and an important confounding variable, the data analysis could yield misleading results if it is not properly adjusted. For example, if the majority of the patients with poor functioning ability are randomized to Group 1 while the highly functioning patients are randomized mostly to Group 0, then an analysis of this data, ignoring this important confounder, would exaggerate the effectiveness of Group 0 relative to Group 1.

The stratified logrank test helps to counter this problem by essentially calculating separate logrank statistics, U_j for each stratum, $j = 1, 2, \ldots, s$, and aggregating the result over all the strata by summation, i.e., $U = \sum_{j=1}^{s} U_j$. Because it is acceptable to assume that patients in each strata act independently from those of other strata, the statistics, U_j are also independent. Therefore, the overall variance of U is found with $V = \sum_{j=1}^{s} V_j$ where V_j is the variance of U_j and is found in a similar manner to V_1 in

Section 2.3.1.1. Then the following ratio is well approximated by a standard normal distribution (Collett [19, p. 49]):

$$Z = \frac{\sum_{j=1}^{s} U_j}{\sqrt{\sum_{j=1}^{s} V_j}}$$

For the same reasons as listed in Section 2.3.1.1., $W_L = Z^2 \sim \chi^2_{1df}$. Additionally, the statistic is used to evaluate the null hypothesis in the same manner as in Section 2.3.1.1.

The nature of the strata in this test is conceptually one-dimensional, but factoring several potentially confounding variables (such as performance status and disease aggressiveness jointly) is generally not problematic if the primary interest remains in the comparison of the treatment effects since each multidimensional point can be mapped into a unique one-dimensional value. For example, two confounding variables that are dichotomized into "high risk" and "low risk" strata can be mapped jointly into four one-dimensional strata (i.e., H1H2 → strata 1, H1L2 → strata 2, L1H2 → strata 3, and L1L2 → strata 4 where H1L2 represents those patients with high risk on variable 1 and low risk on variable 2, etc.). The number of strata can escalate rather quickly when an increasing number of confounding variables are taken into account, especially if the number of strata within each variable is large. If we take for instance three factors with 4, 5, and 3 strata each, the total number of one-dimensional strata is 60. For cases like this, it is not unusual to have some of the levels of the factors (sometimes called cells) with only a few cases or actually be completely empty. However, the asymptotic behavior of the logrank statistic should not be adversely effected by this phenomenon since these cells contribute little or no variation to the overall distribution of U, so long as such cells are relatively uncommon. It is not possible to stratify in this manner on confounding variables that are continuous. Instead, these variables may be grouped into a finite set of categories and handled as shown above. If inclusion of a continuous variable without categorization was desired or if there was interest in drawing inferences about the effects of the confounding variables, then another approach to evaluating the equivalency of survival distributions would have to be considered such as a Cox proportional hazards (PH) model, e.g., Cox [24].

2.3.1.1.2.1 Blocked Randomization, Dynamic Allocation, and the Stratified Logrank Test   Proactive measures taken to counter the problem of confounding caused by unbalanced treatment allocation include blocked randomization and dynamic allocation. These procedures help to assure that certain risk factors known (or believed) to influence a patient's outcome are adequately balanced (or represented) across all of the randomized treatments being studied. Therefore, any treatment differences observed in the study are more likely to be the result of actual differences in treatment effect rather than chance variation and association with confounding variables. These procedures require the determination of the values of the risk factors in each patient before randomization. As a result, these methods are not helpful if a confounding variable is discovered after the study finishes accrual. In those cases, useful interpretation of the data may still be possible if the study incorporates the risk factor into the analysis such as listed in the previous paragraph, but in cases where the level of unbalance is particularly severe, even these corrections may not be able to reliably resolve the impact of each effect, rendering the study uninterpretable. The risk of such an occurrence is highest for relatively small studies, which is one reason why larger randomized studies have more influence on clinical practice. As the sample size increases, the risk factors (both known and unknown) have a tendency to balance across treatments naturally. Regardless of the expected size of the study at the completion of the study, most studies with known confounding variables attempt to balance them across assigned treatments. Some of the justifications include the possibility of early stopping of the study for toxicity or due to results from an early group sequential analysis (see Section 2.3.2 for additional details).

Blocked randomization balances risk factors across treatments by performing separate treatment allocations within each stratum. It also facilitates balance of treatment assignments over time by permuting treatment assignments in blocks of a particular size. Table 2.5 illustrates the use of blocked randomization to two treatment groups (Group 1 and Group 0) with a confounding variable categorized into three strata. When using a block size equal to two, the first low risk patient is assigned to Group 1. The next low risk patient is assigned to Group 0, and that completes the first block. The following low risk patient is assigned to Group 0, followed by Group 1, which completes the second block. If a block size of 4 was used, then the first medium risk patient is assigned to Group 1, followed by Group 1, then Group 0, and finally Group 0, which completes the first block of medium risk patients. As patients enter the trial, a determination of their risk group is assessed, and based on the order of entry for a particular risk group, a treatment assignment is made. Therefore, if the block size equal to 4 randomization scheme was used and the initial sequence of patients entering the trial was LMMHMLMLHH (where L = low

TABLE 2.5:   An example set of random numbers used to illustrate blocked randomization to two treatment groups (Group 0 and Group 1) by three strata (low, medium, and high risk patients) where the block size is either two or four.

Strata	Block Size 2
Low risk	10.01.01.10.10.10.01.01.01.10.10.01
Medium risk	01.01.10.01.10.01.10.01.10.10.01.01
High risk	10.01.01.10.10.10.01.01.01.01.10.01

	Block Size 4
Low risk	0110.1100.0101.0101.0011.1100.1010
Medium risk	1100.0011.1010.1001.0110.0011.1001
High risk	0110.1100.1100.0011.0110.1100.0011

TABLE 2.6:   Breakdown of treatment assignments by strata when 5 low risk patients, 25 medium risk patients, and 10 high risk patients entered the trial, using Table 2.5 to assign the treatment moving left to right.

Strata	Group 1	Group 0	Total
Low risk	3	2	5
Medium risk	13	12	25
High risk	6	4	10
Total	22	18	40

Note: Treatment assignments are fairly balanced within each stratum.

risk, M = medium risk, and H = high risk), then the random sequence of treatment assignments would be 0110010111.

If the procedure continued until 5 low risk patients, 25 medium risk patients, and 10 high risk patients entered the trial, then the breakdown of treatment assignments by strata would be provided in Table 2.6.

When the data are analyzed for differences of treatment effects, a stratified logrank testing procedure is often utilized with the same factors on which the randomization is balanced. However, since the risk factors are balanced across the treatments, the results are generally similar to that of the unstratified analysis. When the number of strata is large, it may be preferable to use Pocock–Simon [25] dynamic allocation to balance on the prognostic variables marginally, rather than within each stratum defined by the variables taken together, Pocock [25].

2.3.1.2   Evaluating the Distribution of the Logrank Statistic under the Alternative Hypothesis

The determination of the distribution of the logrank statistic under the alternative hypothesis for design considerations is just as important as the determination of the critical values is to the sound judgment of the plausibility of the null hypothesis. Often the goal of the analysis for the design is to establish the required number of patients that need to be accrued to a study in order to detect a clinically relevant difference between a control and an experimental therapy with high probability. Once the sample size is known, discussion of the feasibility of the study and the logistics of carrying it out can begin. As a general rule, the task of determining the distribution of a test statistic under the alternative hypothesis is often more difficult than under the null. In many cases, the null hypothesis simplifies the problem both mathematically and conceptually. For example the hypothesis, H_0: $S_1(t) = S_0(t)$ implies that d_i is distributed randomly across the treatment groups, which gives the distribution of d_{1i} a relatively simple distribution, and based on this distribution, the distribution of the logrank statistic, U_1, can be found fairly easily. No definitive or model based parametric connection between d_i, d_{1i}, $S_1(t)$, or $S_0(t)$ needs to be made in order to construct the test and carry it out, and the observation of unusual values of U_1 leading to rejection of the null hypothesis is legitimate. However in these cases, the acceptance of the alternative hypothesis is vague. The survival distributions are declared to be different, i.e., H_A: $S_1(t) \neq S_0(t)$. The questions then turn to: how different? Are they different early in the survival distribution, only later, or both? Do they deviate more as time goes on? Are all patients destined to have the event or are some cured? Can a confidence interval be placed on this difference?

Given all these possibilities in the alternative space, how does one begin to determine the distribution of the logrank statistic? What is the connection between U_1 and H_A: $S_1(t) \neq S_0(t)$?

2.3.1.2.1 Proportional Hazards Assumption One way to reduce the myriad of possibilities within the alternative hypothesis space and help gain a quantitative grasp on a reasonable set of distributions where $S_1(t) \neq S_0(t)$ is to make the simplifying assumption that the hazard function for patients being assigned to Group 1, $h_1(t)$ is proportional to the hazard function of those being in assigned to Group 0, $h_0(t)$, that is, $h_1(t) = \psi \cdot h_0(t)$ where ψ is the HR of Group 1 to Group 0 and is assumed to be constant $\forall t \in [0, \infty)$. The definition of the hazard function can be found in many texts and is reproduced below without reference:

$$h(t) \equiv \lim_{\Delta t \to 0} \frac{P(t \leq T < t + \Delta t | T \geq t)}{\Delta t}$$

where T is the random variable for the time until failure. In words, the hazard function is the instantaneous failure rate at time t, given that the patient has survived without failing to that time t. Because it is a rate, the value of the hazard function depends on the unit of time used to calculate its value. For example, an overall estimate of the hazard of cardiac-infarction for all people could be expressed as 0.2 incidents per decade, which is equivalent to 0.02 incidents per year or 0.00167 incidents per month. As would be expected, the hazard of such an event depends on the age of the individual so that the hazard for a 25 and 70 year old could be $h(2.5) = 0.006$ per decade and $h(7.0) = 0.8$ per decade. When the hazard rate is constant over time, the expected time until the event is experienced is provided with $E[T] = h(t)^{-1} = 1/h(t) = 1/h$ where h is the specific value. Therefore, assuming the risk of a cardiac infarction remained constant throughout the lifetimes of the people listed above, the 25 year old would expect to live another $1/0.006 = 167$ years before experiencing the event. Likewise, the 70 year old would expect to live another 12 years. The example with the 25 year old demonstrates some of the perils with making the constant hazard assumption but is none-the-less instructive in connecting a somewhat vague concept (the hazard function) with a more tangible idea (expected time until failure).

Specification of the hazard function enables complete specification of the survival distribution (Lawless [26, p. 9]):

$$S(t) = \exp\left\{ -\int_0^t h(u) du \right\} = \exp\{-H(t)\}$$

where $H(t)$ is commonly referred to as the cumulative hazard function. Therefore, the PH assumption enables the following relationships between Group 1 and Group 0 to be made:

$$S_1(t) = \exp\left\{-\int_0^t h_1(u)du\right\} = \exp\left\{-\psi\int_0^t h_0(u)du\right\}$$

$$= \left(\exp\left\{-\int_0^t h_0(u)du\right\}\right)^{\psi} = S_0(t)^{\psi}$$

When the HR is equal to 1, $\psi = 1$, that is to say, when the hazard functions are the same, the survival distributions are also the same (i.e., $S_1(t) = S_0(t)^1 = S_0(t)$). This is the null hypothesis. When the HR is equal to 2, which implies an incident rate in Group 1 twice that for Group 0, then the survival function for Group 1 is equal to the square of the survival function for Group 0, i.e., $S_1(t) = S_0(t)^2$. In this case, $S_1(t) < S_0(t)$. Specific values can be used to compare survivability. For example, when $S_0(t) = 0.6$, then $S_1(t) = 0.60^2 = 0.36$. Figure 2.2 shows survival functions for three groups that mutually follow a PH assumption. The middle curve is designated the Reference Group. Group 1 has a HR of one-half (compared to the Reference Group) whereas Group 2 has a HR of two. The HR of Group 2 to Group 1 is 4. From the figure, an inverse relationship can be seen between the hazard function and the

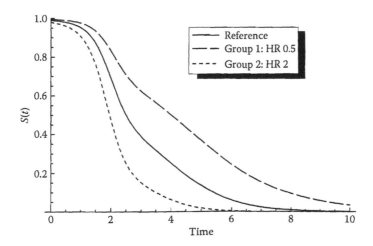

FIGURE 2.2: Plots of survival functions for a Reference Group (solid curve), Group 1 where the hazard function is one-half the hazard of the Reference Group (long dashed curve), and Group 2 where the hazard function is twice the hazard of the Reference Group (short dashed curve). These curves follow a proportional hazards assumption. The median survivals for the Reference Group, Group 1, and Group 2 are 2.5, 4.01, and 1.96, respectively.

survival function. Specifically, for a particular point in time, $S_1(t)$ decreases relative to $S_0(t)$ as ψ increases. Because $0 \leq S(t) \leq 1$, this result holds generally for survival distributions that follow the PH assumption (Bartle and Sherbert [27]).

2.3.1.2.2 Distribution of the Logrank Statistic under the Alternative Hypothesis (Proportional Hazards Assumption) When the PH assumption holds, it can be shown that the distribution of U_1 under the alternative hypothesis is approximately normal with mean θV_1 and variance V_1 where $\theta = \ln(\psi)$ when θ is small [19, 28]. Refer to Figure 2.3. This is an example of a typical analysis used to design a study. The distribution on the right that is centered on zero is the null distribution of U_1 where H_0: $S_1(t) = S_0(t)$. The alternative hypothesis is H_A: $S_1(t) \neq S_0(t)$. Values of U_1 that are statistically distant from zero lead the investigators to reject the null hypothesis. Depending on the desired level of significance for the test, α, critical values $-U_1^C$ and U_1^C are determined according to the following relationships:

$$P\left(U_1 < -U_1^C\right) = P\left(\frac{U_1}{\sqrt{V_1}} < \frac{-U_1^C}{\sqrt{V_1}}\right) = \Phi\left(\frac{-U_1^C}{\sqrt{V_1}}\right) = \frac{\alpha}{2}$$

where Φ and Φ^{-1} are the standard normal cumulative distribution function (cdf) and the probit function, respectively. Defining the upper pth quantile of the standard

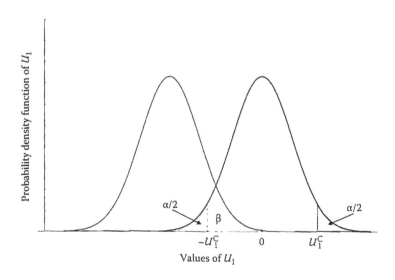

FIGURE 2.3: Distribution of U_1 under the null hypothesis (right density) and under the alternative hypothesis (left density) where the study is designed to reject the null hypothesis when $U_1 < -U_1^C$ or $U_1 > -U_1^C$. If the null hypothesis is true, then the total probability of rejecting it is P (type I error) $= \alpha$. If the alternative hypothesis is true, it is rejected in error if $-U_1^C < U_1 < U_1^C$. The probability of this kind of error is limited to P (type II error) $= \beta$.

normal distribution, z_p, as follows: $P(Z > z_p) = p \Rightarrow z_p = \Phi^{-1}(1-p)$, it can be seen that

$$\frac{-U_1^C}{\sqrt{V_1}} = \Phi^{-1}\left(\frac{\alpha}{2}\right) \Rightarrow U_1^C = -\sqrt{V_1} \cdot z_{1-\alpha/2} = \sqrt{V_1} \cdot z_{\alpha/2} \qquad (2.1)$$

When the alternative hypothesis is true, a type II error is committed if $-U_1^C < U_1 < U_1^C$ since this event leads to acceptance of the null hypothesis. Using the figure as a guide, the probability of this event can be expressed as

$$P\left(-U_1^C < U_1 < U_1^C\right) \approx P\left(U_1 > -U_1^C\right) = P\left(\frac{-U_1 - \theta_1 V_1}{\sqrt{V_1}} > \frac{-U_1^C - \theta_1 V_1}{\sqrt{V_1}}\right)$$

$$= 1 - \Phi\left[\frac{-U_1^C - \theta_1 V_1}{\sqrt{V_1}}\right]$$

It is desirable to limit this probability to β. Therefore,

$$1 - \Phi\left[\frac{-U_1^C - \theta_1 V_1}{\sqrt{V_1}}\right] = \beta \Rightarrow U_1^C = -\theta_1 V_1 - \sqrt{V_1} z_\beta \qquad (2.2)$$

The value of U_1^C was determined from Equation 2.1, so upon substitution into Equation 2.2, we get: $\sqrt{V_1} \cdot z_{\alpha/2} = -\theta_1 V_1 - \sqrt{V_1} z_\beta$, which yields the following quadratic-like form:

$$\sqrt{V_1} \cdot z_{\alpha/2} + \theta_1 V_1 + \sqrt{V_1} z_\beta = \sqrt{V_1}(z_{\alpha/2} + \theta_1 \sqrt{V_1} + z_\beta) = 0 \qquad (2.3)$$

It is noted that all of the variables are known except V_1. The Greek letter θ_1 is known and is often called a minimal but clinically significant improvement in the logarithm of the HR of the experimental therapy to the control therapy. Also the probabilities of type I and type II errors are specified as part of the operating characteristics of the design, so $z_{\alpha/2}$ and z_β are known. Now our goal is to "squeeze down" the variance of the logrank statistic so that both hypotheses can be distinguished with a sufficient level of significance (i.e., small α) and power (i.e., large $1 - \beta$). Solving the second factor of the equation gives

$$V_1 = \frac{(-z_{\alpha/2} - z_\beta)^2}{\theta_1^2} = \frac{(-1)^2(z_{\alpha/2} + z_\beta)^2}{\theta_1^2} = \frac{(z_{\alpha/2} + z_\beta)^2}{\theta_1^2}$$

It is noted that the variance of U_1 is provided with

$$V_1 = \sum_{i=1}^{m} \frac{n_{1i} n_{0i} d_i (n_i - d_i)}{n_i^2 (n_i - 1)} \approx \sum_{i=1}^{m} \frac{n_{1i} n_{0i} d_i}{n_i^2}$$

where the same notation applies as before with m being the number of distinct times where at least one individual experiences an event, etc. In many randomized clinical trials where the magnitude of θ is relatively small, the number of patients at risk in each arm at each event time tends to be proportional to the total number of patients accrued to the study arm, which is well approximated by the randomization scheme used for the study. So for example, if a study randomized patients to each arm in a 1:1 fashion, then $n_{1i} \approx n_{0i}$. Alternatively, if the randomization is done in a 2:1 scheme of experimental to control therapy, then $n_{1i} \approx 2 \cdot n_{0i}$. In general, assume that an $R{:}1$ randomization scheme is used so that $n_{1i} \approx R \cdot n_{0i}$. Then V_1 can be approximated with

$$V_1 \approx \sum_{i=1}^{m} \frac{R \cdot n_{0i}^2 \cdot d_i}{(R \cdot n_{0i} + n_{0i})^2} = \sum_{i=1}^{m} \frac{R \cdot d_i}{(R+1)^2} = \frac{R}{(R+1)^2} \sum_{i=1}^{m} d_i = \frac{R \cdot D}{(R+1)^2}$$

where D is the total number of events observed in the study. Rather than express the randomization as an odds ratio of being assigned to the experimental therapy, some investigators prefer to convey it as a probability of being assigned to the experimental therapy, π. Setting $R = \pi/(1-\pi)$, it can be shown that $V_1 = \pi(1-\pi)D$. As a result of these calculations, we see that the variance of U_1 is proportional to the number of events observed in the study. What is equally important with these designs is noting the fact that $E[U_1] = \theta V_1$ so even though the variance of U_1 is growing as the number of events increases (Figure 2.4), the expectation of U_1 is moving away from zero at a faster rate when $\theta \neq 0$ (Figure 2.5). The effect size for a particular study is given with

$$ES = \frac{\theta\pi(1-\pi)D}{\sqrt{\pi(1-\pi)D}} = \theta\sqrt{\pi(1-\pi)D}$$

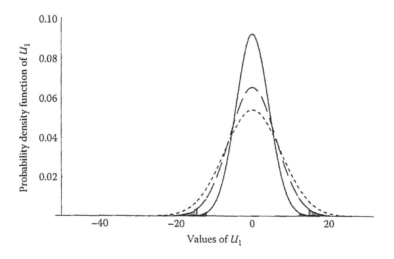

FIGURE 2.4:   Distribution of U_1 under the null hypothesis after 75 events (solid curve), 150 events (long dashed curve), and 219 events (short dashed curve) in a 1:1 randomized design. The probability of a type I error is held constant at 5% against a two-sided alternative. The value of U_1^C is 8.49, 12.00, and 14.50, respectively.

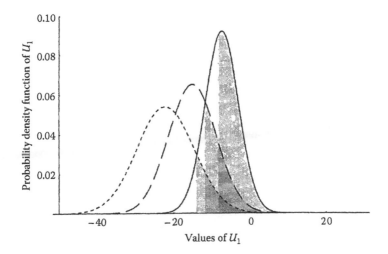

FIGURE 2.5:   Distribution of U_1 under the alternative hypothesis where $\theta = \ln$ (2/3) after 75 events (solid curve), 150 events (long dashed curve), and 219 events (short dashed curve) in a 1:1 randomized design. Although the distribution of U_1 is becoming more dispersed as the number of events increases, the expectation of U_1 is drifting away from 0 at a rate sufficient to reduce the probability of a type II error. The probabilities of type II errors are 58%, 30%, and 15%, respectively.

In order to find the number of observed events which are required to obtain a design with the desired operating characteristics, the variance of U_1 is substituted into Equation 2.3 and solved in terms of D:

$$D = \frac{(R+1)^2(z_{\alpha/2} + z_\beta)^2}{R \cdot \theta_1^2} = \frac{(z_{\alpha/2} + z_\beta)^2}{\pi(1-\pi)\theta_1^2} \tag{2.4}$$

2.3.1.2.3   Example   Suppose it is desired to conduct a 1:1 randomized study with a level of significance equal to 5% and power equal to 85%. Also, a reduction in the hazard by one-third is considered clinically significant. How many events are required to yield a study with these characteristics? If a 2:1 randomization scheme is used, how many events are required?

The level of significance is $\alpha = 5\% \Rightarrow \alpha/2 = 2.5\%$, so $z_{0.025} = 1.96$. With 85% power, $\beta = 0.15 \Rightarrow z_{0.15} = 1.04$. A reduction in the hazard by one-third is equivalent to a HR of $1 - 1/3 = 2/3 \Rightarrow \theta_1 = \ln(2/3) = -0.4055$. A 1:1 randomization scheme implies $R = 1$. Therefore, the required number of deaths is

$$D = \frac{(1+1)^2(1.96 + 1.04)^2}{1 \cdot (-0.4055)^2} = \frac{4 \cdot 9}{0.1644} = 218.97 \approx 219$$

If the study uses a 2:1 randomization, then the following would be obtained:

$$D = \frac{(2+1)^2(1.96+1.04)^2}{2 \cdot (-0.4055)^2} = \frac{9 \cdot 9}{2 \cdot 0.1644} = 246.35 \approx 247$$

2.3.1.2.4   Example   Obtain power as a function of the HR for a 1:1 randomized design with $\alpha = 2.5\%$ tested against a one-sided alternative $H_A: \psi < 1$ after 219 events are observed in the study.

The solution for the determination of the required number of events is particularly helpful in this instance since the derivation essentially made the simplifying assumption that the test was one-sided. In this case, $z_\alpha = z_{0.025} = 1.96$. It is better to start at a point in the derivation before $\sqrt{V_1}$ is squared. In particular with Equation 2.3 where $z_\alpha + \theta\sqrt{V_1} + z_\beta = 0 \Rightarrow z_\beta = -\theta\sqrt{V_1} - z_\alpha = -\ln(\psi)\sqrt{V_1} - z_\alpha$, so that:

$$z_\beta = -\ln(\psi)\sqrt{\pi(1-\pi)D} - z_\alpha$$

Applying the normal cdf function to the equation gives the general power function:

$$\Phi(z_\beta) = 1 - \beta = \text{Power} = \Phi\left[-\ln(\psi)\sqrt{\pi(1-\pi)D} - z_\alpha\right]$$

Substituting $D = 219$, $\pi = 0.5$, and $z_\alpha = 1.96$ gives power as a function of the HR. A plot of this function is provided in Figure 2.6.

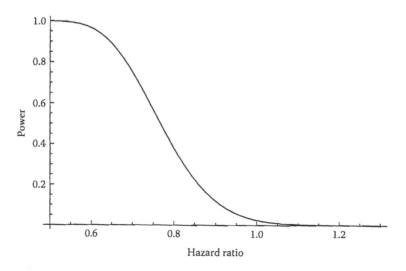

FIGURE 2.6:   Power as a function of the HR, ψ, for a design with $\alpha = 2.5\%$ testing $H_0: \psi \geq 1$ against $H_A: \psi < 1$ after 219 events are observed.

2.3.1.2.5 Alternative Formulas for the Number of Required Events Equation 2.4, derived by Schoenfeld [29], tends to slightly underestimate the required number of events in order to obtain a design with the desired operating characteristics due to the simplifying assumptions applied. An alternative formula provided by Freedman [30] tends to slightly overestimate the required number of events when a 1:1 randomization scheme is used. This method assures that a sufficient number of events have occurred before a final analysis is carried out when a 1:1 design is used. The general equation for an R:1 design is provided as follows:

$$D = \frac{(z_{\alpha/2} + z_\beta)^2(1 + R \cdot \psi)^2}{R \cdot (1 - \psi)^2} \qquad (2.5)$$

Figure 2.7 provides inflation factors as a function of the proportion of patients assigned to Group 1. For comparison, the inflation factor that was derived by the method of Schoenfeld is also provided.

When a 1:1 randomization is used, both methods yield approximately the same number of events in order to obtain a design with the desired operating characteristics with Freedman's approximation being slightly greater than Schoenfeld's. Simulation results indicate that Freedman's approximation mildly underestimates the desired power.

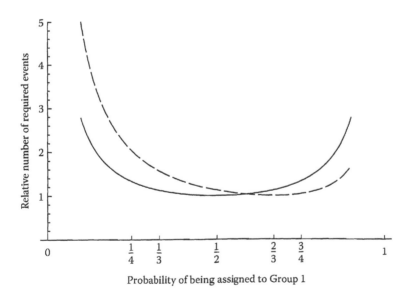

Probability of being assigned to Group 1

FIGURE 2.7: A comparison of the relative inflation factor for the method of Schoenfeld (solid curve) and Freedman (dashed curve). The inflation factor using Freedman's method depends on the value of ψ (unlike Schoenfeld). When $\psi \to 1$, the inflation factors are nearly identical, but as $|\psi - 1|$ increases, the inflation factors deviate. In the current plot, $\psi = 0.5$, indicating that a 2:1 design is slightly more efficient than a 1:1 design according to Freedman. Since both methods involve approximations, it would be incorrect to draw such definitive conclusions.

2.3.1.2.6   Using the Cox Model   Yet another approach uses the asymptotic distribution of the parameter associated with the treatment factor in Cox's PH model. To review the model note:

$$h_i(t) = h_0(t) \exp\{\beta_1 \cdot X_{1i}\}$$

where $h_i(t)$ is the hazard function associated with the ith patient on the study, and $h_0(t)$ is the baseline hazard function. If a patient is assigned to Group 1, then the covariate $X_{1i} = 1$. Else $X_{1i} = 0$. Therefore, the HR of being assigned to Group 1 to Group 0 is provided with

$$HR = \psi = \frac{h_0(t) \exp\{\beta_1 \cdot 1\}}{h_0(t) \exp\{\beta_1 \cdot 0\}} = \frac{h_0(t) \exp\{\beta_1\}}{h_0(t) \cdot 1} = \exp\{\beta_1\}$$

which implies that $\beta_1 = \theta = \ln(\psi)$ is the log of the HR. The coefficient, β_1, is commonly used with PH models. The maximum likelihood estimate (MLE) of β_1 is found by solving the following partial likelihood function:

$$PL = \prod_{i=1}^{n} \left[\frac{\exp\{\beta_1 X_{1i}\}}{\sum_{j=1}^{n} Y_{ij} \exp\{\beta_1 X_{1j}\}} \right]^{C_i}$$

where
  $Y_{ij} = 1$ if $t_j \geq t_i$
  $Y_{ij} = 0$ if $t_j < t_i$
  $C_i = 1$ if the ith case experienced an event, otherwise $C_i = 0$. See Collett [19]
    pp 63–67 for further elaboration.

The large sample behavior of the MLE, $\hat{\beta}_1$, follows typical properties of MLEs. In particular, it can be shown (Piantadosi [31, p. 169]) that

$$\hat{\beta}_1 \rightarrow N\left(\beta_1, \frac{1}{E[D_0]} + \frac{1}{E[D_1]}\right)$$

That is to say, $\hat{\beta}_1$ is asymptotically normal with mean β_1 and variance $E[D_0]^{-1} + E[D_1]^{-1}$ where D_0 and D_1 are the total number of deaths in the control group and experimental group, respectfully. Under the null hypothesis, $\beta_1 = \beta_{10}$ where β_{10} is often 0. Under the alternative hypothesis, $\beta_1 = \beta_{11}$ where β_{11} is the minimally clinically significant value. When the value of β_1 is relatively small, $E[D_0] \approx E[D_1]$, so $\sigma_{\hat{\beta}_1} \approx 2/\sqrt{D}$. Using these relationships to derive the total number of events required in order to obtain a design with α level of significance and power equal to $1 - \beta$ using a two sided alternative, it can be shown that

$$D = \frac{4(z_{\alpha/2} + z_\beta)^2}{\beta_{11}^2}$$

which is the same equation found in Ref. [29] when a 1:1 randomization design is used (i.e., Equation 2.4). Investigations into the similarity of Cox's PH model and the logrank test have shown that the Cox PH score test and the logrank test are equivalent when there are no tied event times (Collett [19, pp. 106–109]).

The PH model easily adapts to stratification by inclusion of additional covariates (i.e., potential confounders) into the model and can be used to jointly estimate the impact of all of the variables of interest. Because the treatment assignment is random, the method described above does not need to be adjusted for variance inflation factors (VIF) caused by confounding variables, Hsieh [32]. That is to say, the expected correlation between the treatment assignment variable and all of the confounding variables should be close to zero. As a matter of fact, inclusion of additional variables may increase the precision of the estimate of the effect of treatment on the HR, thereby increasing the sensitivity of the test, Hsieh [32]. Therefore, the method provided above can be considered to be a conservative approach.

For these reasons, it is not unusual for a study to be designed with the intention of using a Cox model to assess the significance of a new treatment instead of a logrank test (or another nonparametric approach such as Wilcoxon).

2.3.1.3   Evaluation of the Total Sample Size

From sections 2.3.1.2.2, 2.3.1.2.5, and 2.3.1.2.6, it is clear that the distributions of the test statistics are critically dependent on the number of events observed on the study, so calculating the number of events that are required in order to obtain the desired operating characteristics of the study is an important first step in the process of designing a study. The next question is to determine a sample size of patients that should be followed in order to observe the number of events in a reasonable amount of time. If the hazard rate is particularly high so that most patients experience the event in a relatively short period of time after entering the study, then an investigator may be tempted to let the sample size, $n = D$. That is to say, the investigator designs the study to enroll patients onto the trial with the expectation that all of the cases will be observed to fail before a final analysis is begun. This procedure certainly makes the analysis easier since the problem of censoring is no longer present, and the cost of administrating the trial may be reduced with a smaller sample of patients. However, this approach is almost never used in practice because the distribution of survival times, T, is often positively skewed, making outlying observations fairly likely. Therefore, the time until the final analysis for the entire study would be delayed for as long as the last patient remained event free. Given the practical problem of having patients lost to follow-up, strict adherence to such a procedure could delay the results indefinitely. As a result, the number of patients enrolled onto the study is almost always greater than the observed number of events.

To see more clearly the effects of having $n > D$, consider the simplified setting where all of the patients are entered simultaneously. Then the distribution of the time elapsed, t^*, until D events are observed when $n = D$ can be expressed as follows:

$$g(t^*) = D \cdot F(t^*)^{D-1} \cdot f(t^*)$$

where g, F, and f are the probability density function (pdf) of t^*, the underlying cdf, and the underlying pdf of the survival times for the population of patients under investigation, respectively. This equation is derived from the distribution of the maximum of D identically and independently distributed random variables. The time of data maturation occurs immediately following the last observed failure time $t^* = \max\{T_1, T_2, \ldots, T_D\}$ where T_i is the failure time of patient i.

On the other hand, if $n > D$, then the expression of the time elapsed until D events are observed can be expressed as follows:

$$g(t^*) = \binom{n}{D-1}(n - D + 1)F(t^*)^{D-1}S(t^*)^{n-D}f(t^*)$$

where the first expression inside the parentheses is the binomial coefficient (often read as "n choose $(D-1)$" and can be calculated with $n!/((D-1)!(n-D+1)!)$ where $x!$ is defined with the usual factorial function, i.e., $x! \equiv x \cdot (x-1)(x-2) \cdots 3 \cdot 2 \cdot 1$) This formula can be understood according to the following heuristic argument: Within a sample size of n patients, $D-1$ patients are observed to have failed before t^*. The total number of ways of selecting $D-1$ patients from a total of n is given by the binomial coefficient. The probability of observing a single patient failing before time t^* is given by $F(t^*)$, and because the patients are independent, the probability of observing $D-1$ failures before t^* is $F(t^*)$ to the $(D-1)$th power. There are $n - D + 1$ surviving patients from which one fails at exactly time t^*. The total number of ways of selecting $D-1$ patients to fail before t^* and one at exactly t^* is the product of the binomial coefficient and $n - D + 1$. The probability of one patient failing at exactly t^* is $f(t^*)$, which triggers the final analysis. Lastly, the probability of $n - D$ patients surviving beyond t^* is expressed through $S(t^*)$ raised to the power of $n - D$. Because of the assumption of independence, the probability of the event is the product of the individual events. This probability is a function of t^*, so now the distribution of t^* can be investigated.

Figure 2.8 provides an example of the distribution of t^* in two situations where the underlying distribution of survival times is exponential with median time to failure of two months (i.e., $f(t) = \lambda \exp(-\lambda t)$ where $\lambda = 0.3466$). The study is designed to mature at 219 events. If the investigator wishes to enroll only 219 patients and follow them until all have failed, then the distribution of the amount of time until maturation is provided by the dashed curve. The expected time of data maturation is 17 months with a standard deviation (SD) of 3.70. The probability that the study will take longer than 20 months to complete is 19%. On the other hand, if the investigator accrues just 11 more patients than the required 219, that is a total of 230 patients, then the distribution of t^* (time until 219 patients fail) is provided with the solid curve. The expected time of data maturation is 8.6 months with a SD of 0.83. This is a substantial savings in time with an impressive reduction in the variability in the timing of when the data mature, all obtained with only a 5% increase in the sample size. The reason for the dramatic shift in this important operational characteristic stems from the distribution of an extreme statistic, the last event time. By designing a

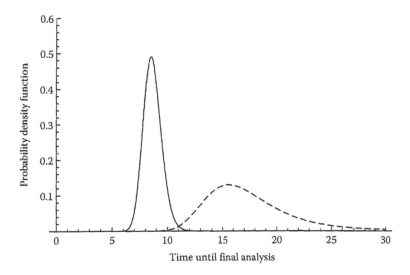

FIGURE 2.8:   Distribution of the length of time for a clinical trial to reach data maturation at 219 events with patients whose survival times are exponentially distributed with median times to failure equal to 2 months (hazard ratio assumed equal to 1 with all patients entering the study immediately after the trial opens). The dashed curve is a design with $n = 219$. The solid curve is a design with $n = 230$.

study to trigger after the observation of an order statistic that is less extreme (in this case, the approximately 95th percentile of the distribution), the investigator gains a substantial reduction in the time until the final analysis as well as greater predictability to the approximate time of the analysis.

This feature is almost entirely at the discretion of the investigators of the study. They can design the study to trigger at the 90th percentile of the distribution, the 80th percentile, or in some extreme cases, even at the 20th percentile with little harm done to the power of the study. Figure 2.9 shows the expected time of data maturation (at 219 events) as a function of the total sample size. The curve drops fairly quickly near $n = 220$ patients with the slope decreasing as n grows larger. Additional investigation shows the expected time of analysis can be taken arbitrarily close to zero by making n sufficiently large (a result of the simplifying assumption that all patients enter the study immediately). A similar effect can be seen in Figure 2.10 with an even more dramatic effect on the SD of the time until the final analysis. If the investigators wish to enroll only 219 patients then $\sigma_{t*} = 3.70$, but with 230 patients, $\sigma_{t*} = 0.829$, which is greater than a 75% reduction in the variability.

However, enrolling an additional 10 patients so that the total sample size is 240 yields $\sigma_{t*} = 0.594$ (or about a 30% reduction). Continuing with the example one step further, a sample size of 250 patients yields $\sigma_{t*} = 0.481$ (19% reduction relative to 240 patients). The benefit of adding additional patients to the expected time of the analysis and its SD becomes less and less. This is a typical example of

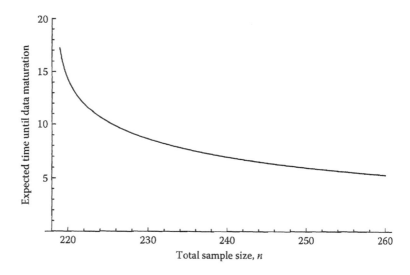

FIGURE 2.9:   Expected time until data maturation for a design requiring 219 events as a function of the total sample size. The population distribution of survival times is exponential with median time to failure equal to 2 months.

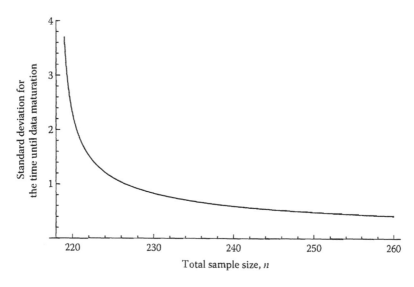

FIGURE 2.10:   SD of the time until data maturation for a design requiring 219 events as a function of the total sample size. Population parameters and design are the same as in Figure 2.8.

the law of diminishing returns. Meanwhile the cost of administering the trial tends to increase, at the very least, proportionally to the sample size. There are additional considerations to take into account such as the exposure of patients to potentially ineffective, less effective, or possibly harmful therapies (or therapies with side effects which do not justify treatment for the disease under consideration). Also, if there is interest in the effects of the treatment over a greater portion of the survival curve (for example interest in a benefit for patients with longer times until failure as well as those with shorter survival times), then it may be necessary to keep D/n relatively high. On the other hand, if the endpoint is relatively rare but the patient population fairly large (such as in chemoprevention trials), then by necessity of trial feasibility, the study may require a small D/n. Classic examples of such trials were the aspirin studies in the prevention of cardiac infarctions [33–35]. All of these criteria need to be carefully weighed, and in the end, the ultimate decision on the actual value of D/n is a bit subjective.

2.3.1.4   Staggered Entry

The assumption that all of the patients enroll onto the study immediately after the clinical trial opens is unrealistic. In practice, patients enter the study at a certain rate which is often beyond the control of the investigators. This rate is usually slower in the early stage of the accrual period and frequently increases to some constant value for the remainder of the study. As patients enter the trial during the course of time, their probability of being observed to fail tends to decrease since their maximum period of observation decreases (i.e., $t^* - t_{enter(i)}$ decreases where $t_{enter(i)}$ is the time of entry for the ith patient). If the accrual rate is particularly slow and the hazard rate relatively high, then patients entering the study early will likely fail during the study period. If the period of follow-up (i.e., the period of time from when a study closes to accrual until the observation of D events) is relatively small, then the duration of study time will be largely a function of the accrual rate, r. In particular, $t^* \approx n/r$. On the other hand, if the accrual rate is particularly brisk so that the accrual period, T, is fairly short with a fairly low hazard rate for the event of concern, then the majority of the time will be spent waiting for the events to occur. In that case, the methods provided in the last section may yield good approximations. Most often the accrual and hazard rates are in intermediate ranges requiring further analysis in order to produce more accurate design parameters and outcomes.

To review, the goal of the study is to expose a reasonable amount of patients, n, to the control or experimental therapy in order to obtain a sufficient number of events, D, to reliably detect a true deviation from the null hypothesis when $\theta = \theta_1$ with adequate power, $1 - \beta$, while limiting the type I error rate to α, all within a reasonable amount of time, t^*, until data maturation. Aspects of the design available to the investigators are the duration of the accrual time, T, and the follow-up period, τ. Critical parameters in the solution to these problems are the anticipated accrual rate, r, the survival function of the control treatment, $S_0(t)$, and the value of a clinically significant difference in the HR that is considered important to detect (i.e., $\psi = \psi_1$). A method that yields solutions to these problems as provided by Schoenfeld [36] and elaborated by Collett [19] is outlined in the paragraphs below:

In order to obtain the required number of events, n patients need to be exposed to the two therapies for an adequate period so that a sufficient proportion experience the event:

$$D = n \cdot P(d_i)$$

where $P(d_i)$ is the probability that a patient experiences the event during the observational period of the study. This probability is related to a function of the duration of accrual time and follow-up time, that is, $P(d_i) = f(T, \tau)$. Additionally, the total sample size is usually well approximated by $n = r \cdot T$, which assumes uniform accrual during the study's period of active accrual. Therefore, the relationship can be written as

$$D = r \cdot T \cdot f(T, \tau) \qquad (2.6)$$

Note that $f(T, \tau) = P(d_i) = \int P(d_i \cap t_{\text{enter}(i)}) = \int P(d_i | t_{\text{enter}(i)}) P(t_{\text{enter}(i)})$ where the integral marginalizes the joint probability over all $t_{\text{enter}(i)}$, and d_i in this context denotes the event that patient i is observed experiencing the event at some point during the entire study. The period of time when patients are being recruited into the study is from the opening of the clinical trial to patient entry (i.e., time $t = 0$) until termination of accrual (i.e., time $t = T$). Assuming uniform accrual over this interval, $[0, T]$, the pdf for one patient being recruited into the study over this interval is T^{-1}. Therefore:

$$P(d_i) = \int_0^T P(d_i | t_{\text{enter}(i)}) T^{-1} dt_{\text{enter}(i)} = 1 - \frac{1}{T} \int_0^T P\left(d_i^C | t_{\text{enter}(i)}\right) dt_{\text{enter}(i)}$$

where d_i^C is the event that patient i is observed surviving beyond the accrual and follow-up periods, $T + \tau$. Conditioned on time of entry at $t_{\text{enter}(i)}$, this probability can be expressed with the survival function, $S(T + \tau - t_{\text{enter}(i)})$. Note that a patient entering immediately after the trial opens (i.e., $t_{\text{enter}(i)} = 0$) has probability of surviving beyond t^* equal to $S(T + \tau)$ whereas the last patient (i.e., $t_{\text{enter}(i)} = T$) needs to survive only beyond the period of follow-up, which has probability $S(T + \tau - T) = S(\tau)$. The overall probability of a patient experiencing the event is given as

$$P(d_i) = 1 - \frac{1}{T} \int_0^T S(T + \tau - t_{\text{enter}(i)}) dt_{\text{enter}(i)} = 1 - \frac{1}{T} \int_\tau^{T+\tau} S(u) du \qquad (2.7)$$

For many designs, use of the exponential survival distribution to approximate the true survival distribution is sufficient (note that investigations into the robustness of the procedure were conducted, e.g., Rubinstein et al. [7]). With this assumption,

$S(t) = \exp(-\lambda_0 t)$ where λ_0 is the constant hazard rate on the control arm. An estimate of the hazard rate can be obtained from historical control data, usually using the median survival time. For example, if the median survival was 2 months, an estimate of the hazard rate can be provided by $\tilde{\lambda}_0 = -\ln(0.5)/2 = 0.35$, or about 0.35 events per month. In general, $\tilde{\lambda}_0 = -\ln(0.5)/t_{median}$ where t_{median} is an estimate of the median survival time. Under the alternative hypothesis with the PH assumption, the hazard rate for the experimental treatment would be given by $\lambda_1 = \psi \cdot \lambda_0 \approx \psi \cdot \tilde{\lambda}_0$. With a 1:1 randomization scheme, the overall hazard for any patient entering the study is roughly an average of λ_0 and λ_1, such as $\bar{\lambda} = (\lambda_0 + \lambda_1)/2 = \lambda_0(1+\psi)/2$, $G_\lambda = \sqrt{\lambda_0\lambda_1} = \lambda_0\sqrt{\psi}$, or $H_\lambda = 2/(1/\lambda_0 + 1/\lambda_1) = 2\lambda_0/(1+\psi^{-1})$ where G_λ and H_λ are the geometric and harmonic means. Using the geometric mean, the probability of observing a particular patient experiencing a failure during the study is

$$P(d_i) = 1 - \frac{1}{T}\int_\tau^{T+\tau} \exp(-G_\lambda u)du = 1 - \frac{\exp(-\tau \cdot G_\lambda) - \exp\{-(T+\tau)G_\lambda\}}{T \cdot G_\lambda} = f(T,\tau)$$

Placing $f(T, \tau)$ into Equation 2.6 and solving for τ in closed form gives the following required follow-up time in order to observe a total of D events:

$$\tau = G_\lambda^{-1}\ln\left(\frac{r - \exp\{-G_\lambda T\}r}{G_\lambda(r\cdot T - D)}\right) \tag{2.8}$$

Note that the lower bound on T is D/r which would yield the case where $n=D$. Additionally, the interpretation of values of $\tau < 0$ is one where the observation of the Dth event occurred while the trial is still accruing patients. Since the goal of the study is to obtain only D events for the final analysis, it is not necessary to expose additional patients to the experimental therapy after D events have occurred. Therefore a trial with an accrual time of T that gives $\tau < 0$ is too long. As a result, the upper bound of T is T_U such that $\tau = 0$. This value can be found through numerical or graphical methods.

2.3.1.4.1 Example Consider the design in Section 2.3.1.2.3 with the 1:1 randomization scheme. In that case, it was determined that 219 events needed to be observed in order to detect a one-third reduction in the hazard with 85% power while testing at the 5% level of significance. Suppose this trial is to be conducted in a population of patients in the control group with a median survival time of 2 months. If the expected accrual rate onto the trial is 10 patients per month, plot the time until final analysis as a function of T. Also look at the total sample size as a function of T. How does a median survival time of 12 months influence the operating characteristics of the study?

Note that $\tilde{\lambda}_0 = -\ln(0.5)/2 = 0.3466 \Rightarrow \lambda_1 = 0.3466 \cdot 2/3 = 0.2311 \Rightarrow G_\lambda = \sqrt{0.08010} = 0.2830$. The lower bound on T is $T_L = 219/10 = 21.9$ months. The upper bound can be found with software packages such as Mathematica, Wolfram [37], which yields the solution:

$$T_U = \frac{D \cdot G_\lambda + r + r \cdot \text{ProductLog}\left[-\exp\left\{-1 - (D \cdot G_\lambda/r)\right\}\right]}{r \cdot G_\lambda}$$

where ProductLog[z] gives the solution for w in the equation $z = w \cdot \exp\{w\}$. The numeric evaluation for the set of parameters given in the present problem yields $T_U = 25.43$. Looking at the range of valid values of T, it is fairly clear that the accrual rate is relatively slow in comparison to the hazard of the event under consideration, which yields the somewhat extreme case where $t^* \approx D/r$. Looking at Figure 2.11, we see that the trial duration could be excessive if the trial closed to patient entry before 22 months after opening. Based on these results, it appears that the study should remain open for at least 23 months (or approximately 230 patients enroll). Given that the window for study closure is narrow, making the sample size relatively static, the investigator of the study may wish to accrue patients until the Dth event is observed (minimizing the duration of the trial, e.g., see George and Desu [38]). Additional consideration needs to be made for the level of confidence in r. If patient entry is more brisk than expected, then this design strategy could yield undesirable characteristics.

The second part considers the case where the median survival time is 12 months $\Rightarrow \lambda_0 = -\ln(0.5)/12 = 0.05776 \Rightarrow \lambda_1 = 0.05776 \cdot 2/3 = 0.03851 \Rightarrow G_\lambda = \sqrt{0.002224} = 0.04716$. The lower bound on T is still $T_L = 219/10 = 21.9$ months; however, the upper bound is 39.87 months. This provides a much broader range of accrual periods to consider. Looking at the sample size of the study as a function of accrual time in Figure 2.12, we see that it can almost be doubled in value, depending on the length of the accrual period. However, the return in terms of saving time on t^* for terminating accrual after 39.87 months relative to 30 months is 39.87 vs. 44.5 months (or about a 10% savings in the duration of the trial). On the other hand, the sample size is increased from 300 to 400 patients (or about 33%). Given the small benefit, it is unlikely that an investigator would want to accrue patients for longer than 30 months.

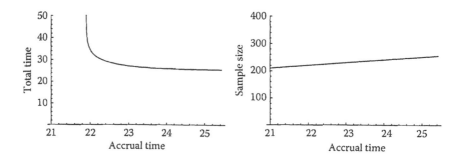

FIGURE 2.11:   Total time until data maturation (e.g., $T + \tau$) as a function of the accrual period, T (left graph), and the sample size, n as a function of the accrual period (right graph) for the first case in Section 2.3.1.4.1 where $t_{\text{median}} = 2$ months.

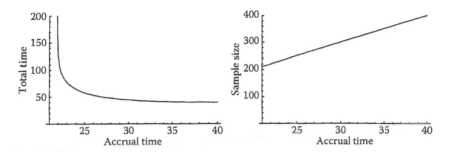

FIGURE 2.12: Total time until data maturation (e.g., $T+\tau$) as a function of the accrual period, T (left graph), and the sample size, n as a function of the accrual period (right graph) for the second case in Section 2.3.1.4.1 where $t_{median} = 12$ months.

2.3.1.4.2 General Survival Distributions It is certainly possible that use of the exponential survival distribution is inappropriate. In such cases, another estimate of the survival function for the control group is often available through a previous study. This estimate is usually provided as the Kaplan–Meier (KM) product limit estimate of $S_0(t)$ and is denoted symbolically as $\hat{S}_0(t)$. This historical function is sometimes used directly to provide important calculations for the design of the study. Schoenfeld [36] noted in particular that the integral in Equation 2.7 can be approximated with Simpson's rule where

$$\int_{\tau}^{T+\tau} S_0(u)du \approx \frac{T}{6}\left[\hat{S}_0(\tau) + 4 \cdot \hat{S}_0(0.5 \times T + \tau) + \hat{S}_0(T + \tau)\right]$$

So that the probability of a patient on the control arm experiencing an event at some point during the trial is given by

$$P(d_{0i}) \approx 1 - \frac{1}{6}\left[\hat{S}_0(\tau) + 4 \cdot \hat{S}_0(0.5 \times T + \tau) + \hat{S}_0(T + \tau)\right]$$

Assuming PH, the probability of a patient experiencing an event on the experimental therapy is given with

$$P(d_{1i}) = 1 - (1 - P(d_{0i}))^{\psi}$$

Then, the overall probability of a patient experiencing the event is given by

$$P(d_i) = \pi \cdot P(d_{1i}) + (1 - \pi)P(d_{0i})$$

where π is the probability of being assigned to Group 1 as stated earlier.

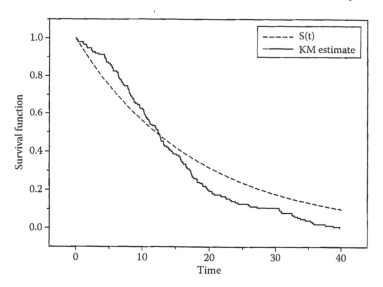

FIGURE 2.13: KM estimate of the survival function from a previous study that can be used to help design the subsequent study. The stepped curve provides the actual KM estimate of patients who received the control treatment for the current study under consideration. The smoothed, dashed curve provides the theoretical exponential survival distribution with median survival time of 12 months.

2.3.1.4.2.1 Example   An estimate of a survival distribution for a historical control is available and provided in Figure 2.13 with the dashed curve. Suppose this curve has some of the investigators concerned about whether the assumption of exponential survival will provide a reliable prediction of the power for the study. To investigate this, determine the power of a study designed in Section 2.3.1.4.1 for the case where the median survival time is 12 months, using the KM estimates. Assume 1:1 randomization with accrual for 30 months and follow-up for 14.5 months.

Note the following: $T = 30$ months and $\tau = 14.5$ months, so $\hat{S}(14.5) = 0.400$, $\hat{S}_0(0.5 \times 30 + 14.5) = \hat{S}_0(29.5) = 0.107$, and $\hat{S}_0(30 + 14.5) = \hat{S}_0(44.5) = 0$, which gives

$$P(d_{0i}) \approx 1 - \frac{1}{6}[0.4 + 4 \times 0.107 + 0] = 0.862$$

$$P(d_{1i}) = 1 - (1 - 0.862)^{0.66667} = 0.733$$

$$P(d_i) = 0.5 \times 0.862 + 0.5 \times 0.733 = 0.798$$

Therefore, $D = r \cdot T \cdot f(T, \tau) = 10 \times 30 \times 0.798 = 239.4$.   Under the alternative hypothesis, the following equation obtained (in part) from Section 2.3.1.2.4 gives a fairly accurate estimate of the power of the design:

$$\Phi(z_\beta) = 1 - \beta = \text{Power} = \Phi\left[-\ln(\psi)\sqrt{\pi(1 - \pi)D} - z_{\alpha/2}\right]$$

$$\text{Power} = \Phi\left[-\ln(2/3)\sqrt{0.25 \times 239.4} - 1.96\right] = \Phi[1.18] = 0.88$$

For the case under consideration, both methods (the exponential survival approximation and the KM survival estimates) yield essentially the same operating characteristics.

2.3.1.5   Problem of Loss to Follow-Up

A common problem with the practical administration of clinical trials is one where patients can no longer be followed after a certain period of time. Reasons for loss to follow-up include a patient moving to a different city (or state), patient desire to drop from the study or to switch to another physician not associated with the study, and noncompliance with study guidelines. These patients reduce the sensitivity of the analysis for a particular sample size, so the sample size must be adjusted to accommodate this loss, thereby requiring longer periods of accrual time in order to obtain the necessary total amount of follow-up.

It is important to note that differential losses to follow-up by treatment regimens can be a serious sign of problems with one of the treatments being administered. Like informative censoring, this situation can add considerable challenges to the analysis. On the other hand, if the losses can be assumed to be independent of treatment as well as independent of the timing of the primary endpoint of the study, then solutions to the problem are not intractable. Rubinstein et al. [7] incorporated loss to follow-up into the design under the assumption of an exponential survival distribution. The MLE of the logarithm of the HR, $\hat{\theta} = \ln(\hat{\lambda}_1/\hat{\lambda}_0)$, can be shown to be asymptotically normal with mean θ and variance $E[D_0]^{-1} + E[D_1]^{-1}$. Utilizing a similar procedure as outlined in sections 2.3.1.2.2 and 2.3.1.2.6, it can be shown that the following relationship holds for a one-sided alternative:

$$\frac{\ln(\psi)^2}{(Z_\alpha + Z_\beta)^2} = E[D_0]^{-1} + E[D_1]^{-1}$$

Substituting the expected number of events as a function of λ_0, λ_1, T, τ, and ϕ where ϕ is the constant hazard of a patient being lost to follow-up, a fundamental result is obtained:

$$\sum_{i \in \{0,1\}} \frac{2(\lambda_i + \phi_i)^2}{r\lambda_i[(\lambda_i + \phi_i)T - \exp\{-(\lambda_i + \phi_i)\tau\}(1 - \exp\{-(\lambda_i + \phi_i)T\})]} = \frac{\ln(\psi)^2}{(Z_\alpha + Z_\beta)^2}$$

$$(2.9)$$

For a particular value of τ, this equation can be solved numerically for T.

2.3.1.5.1   Example   Continuing with Sections 2.3.1.4.1 and 2.3.1.4.2.1 with the case where the median survival for the control group is 12 months, examine the impact of a loss to follow-up for $\phi_i = \lambda_0/4$ and $\phi_i = \lambda_0/2$ on the duration of accrual time.

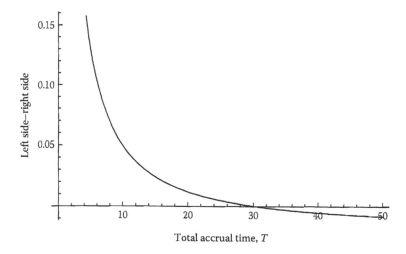

Total accrual time, T

FIGURE 2.14:   This is a plot of the left side of Equation 2.9 minus the right side of Equation 2.8 as a function of the total accrual time, T, when $\tau = 14.5$. The value of T where the curve is equal to 0 yields the solution to the equation, which is near 30 months.

First, we will examine the original case where $\phi_i = 0$ to consider the agreement between the method used in the previous examples and the one under consideration. We noted in the previous examples that a clinical trial that accrued patients for 30 months with an additional 14.5 months of follow-up yielded a fairly reasonable design. Since the procedure was developed under the conception of a one-sided test, the value of α is divided by two (e.g., see Rubinstein [7, p. 473]) so that $Z_{0.025} = 1.96$. Looking at Figure 2.14, we see that the solution for the total accrual time is about 30 months when $\tau = 14.5$ months. Solving for the solution using numerical methods gives $T = 30.232$ months. As expected, the method of this section agrees closely with Section 2.3.1.4.1 when there is no loss to follow-up.

In order to examine the case where $\phi_i = \lambda_0/4$, the following equation needs to be solved for T:

$$\sum_{i \in \{0,1\}} \frac{2(\lambda_i + \lambda_0/4)^2}{10 \cdot \lambda_i[(\lambda_i + \lambda_0/4)T - \exp\{-(\lambda_i + \lambda_0/4) \cdot 14.5\}(1 - \exp\{-(\lambda_i + \lambda_0/4)T\})]}$$
$$= \frac{\ln(2/3)^2}{(1.96 + 1.04)^2} \tag{2.10}$$

where (as before) $\lambda_0 = 0.05776$ and $\lambda_1 = 0.03851$. The solution for T in this case is 34.732 months. When $\phi_i = \lambda_0/2$, the solution for T is 39.796, or approximately 40 months.

If the problem of loss to follow-up was overlooked and the trial conducted with 30 months of accrual, then the study would never obtain the required number of events to achieve the desired power. This fact can be seen from Figure 2.15 where the difference

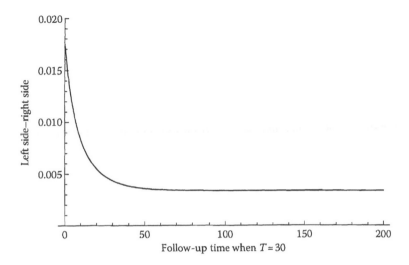

FIGURE 2.15: This is a plot of the left side of Equation 2.9 minus the right side of Equation 2.9 when $\phi_i = \lambda_0/2$ instead of $\lambda_0/4$ as a function of the follow-up time, τ, when $T = 30$. Since this quantity never equals 0, there is no value of τ which satisfies the equation.

between the right side and left side of the equation is plotted as a function of τ. Since the curve never passes through the τ-axis, there is no solution to the equation. In practical terms, the investigators would need to either open the study to additional patients or wait until the study had an acceptable number of events to conduct an analysis without the desired operating characteristics. If the investigators conducted the analysis with 14.5 months of follow-up time, then the study would have 73% power. After 24.5 months of follow-up (i.e., 40 months and 14.5 months), the study would have 76% power. No matter how long the investigators waited, they would never achieve more than 79% power unless they accrued more patients. This example highlights the importance of knowing the values of some of the parameters in planning a study. Inaccurate specifications can lead to incomplete or inadequate studies.

2.3.2 Clinical Trial Monitoring

Ethical considerations are an important part in the planning of clinical trials. For regimens with a concern for safety, careful periodic review of treatment toxicities are often conducted in the initial stages of the trial to assure the investigators the agents under examination are not causing adverse events that are unacceptably severe or too frequent. If the data indicate otherwise, the trial may be suspended or terminated early. Furthermore, if the new regimen is not sufficiently effective to justify continuing the exposure of additional patients to it (e.g., there may be statistically significant evidence to suggest that it performs worse than the standard of care), then the investigators should consider stopping the study early. Conversely, if the new treatment showed a dramatic improvement over the standard of care, it likely would not be appropriate to continue to randomized subjects to the inferior therapy. Instead, the investigators would need to consider sharing this important information with the public.

However, using early efficacy or toxicity data to make important decisions about the conduct of the remainder of the clinical trial carries the risk of making an error in the decision as well as biasing the final analysis. For example, a new agent that is better than the standard of care may be performing comparably to the standard in the early part of a clinical trial, and because of its lack of superior activity, it could be wrongfully rejected early in the study. Had the trial completed its accrual, this result may have become apparent and the new agent could have been detected as superior. A complement of this problem is a setting where an equally performing regimen is declared to be superior to the standard of care. It is well-known that when investigators take multiple looks at the data and test the null hypothesis, they are inflating their probability of type I error, α, above their advertised levels. Figure 2.16 shows a simulated example of the problem. Each of the traces shows the development of a standardized, normally distributed test statistic during the course of a clinical trial when the null hypothesis is true (that is to say, the true distribution of the test statistic is $Z \sim N(0, 1)$. If it is desired to test this hypothesis at the end of the trial with $\alpha = 0.05$ against a two sided alternative, then a decision rule such as $Z > 1.96$ or

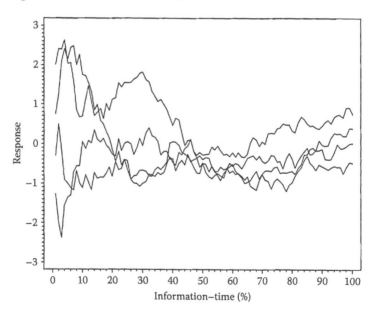

FIGURE 2.16: Traces of a normally distributed test statistic for four clinical trials during the course of study under the null hypothesis (i.e., each test statistic is distributed as $Z \sim N(0, 1)$). If these test statistics were used to test the null hypothesis against the alternative with $Z > 1.96$ or $Z < -1.96$ at the end of the trials (i.e., when time $= 100\%$), then all of these examples would lead to the correct conclusion. However, if the rule used $Z > 1.96$ or $Z < -1.96$ at any point in the trial, then three of the four examples would have falsely rejected the null hypothesis.

$Z < -1.96$ can be legitimately used to reject the null hypothesis. In the example provided, none of the test statistics meet this criterion when the information time is 100%, so all of the tests would yield the correct conclusion. However, if a clinical trial continually monitored the data so that the study would reject the null hypothesis if the test statistic was "significant" at any time, then this example shows that three of the four cases would falsely reject the null hypothesis. Two cases have $Z > 1.96$ at some point while another has $Z < -1.96$. This example shows that adjustments to the decision rules are required in order to maintain the operating characteristics of the study when the data are monitored continuously or periodically.

2.3.2.1 Group Sequential Testing Procedures

From a logistical perspective, it would be fairly difficult to monitor trials continuously. Data would have to be updated from all sources and evaluated for accuracy after each patient entered the study. Fortunately, it is not necessary to conduct continuous monitoring. Group sequential designs enable nearly the same benefits as continuous monitoring but with only several interim analyses performed during the course of the study. The basic idea behind these designs is to prospectively determine the number and timing of the interim analyses for a clinical trial using a particular method of evaluating the critical values for early stopping. Commonly used methods for evaluating the critical values include Pocock [39] and O'Brien and Fleming [40], which can have a distinctive effect on the characteristics of the study (to be discussed later). Once the critical values are established, the trial is generally conducted as follows:

Assuming that a maximum of m interim analyses are to be conducted, the test statistics, $Z_1, Z_2, \ldots, Z_m$, are to be computed at the prespecified times. With time-to-event analyses, these interim times are often given in terms of information time, which is a scale from 0 to 1, [0, 1]. In practical terms, information time is the ratio of the number of observed events at the time of the analysis to the maximum number of events required in order to obtain the desired characteristics of the study. For example, if there are 100 events observed in the study, and the required number of events is 219, then the information time is $100/219 = 0.4566 \approx 46\%$. At each analysis, the computed test statistic, Z_i, is compared to the prespecified critical value, say u_i or l_i, where $i = 1, 2, \ldots, m$. Assuming larger values of Z_i indicate that the new regimen is better than the standard of care, then sufficiently large values of $Z_i (Z_i > u_i)$ may dictate early closure of the study with rejection of the null hypothesis in favor of the new regimen. On the other hand, if one of the $Z_i (Z_i < l_i)$ is relatively small, then there may be a desire to close the study early and conclude that the drug is not superior. Otherwise, the study continues until the timing of the next interim analysis where the next interim test statistic is compared to the subsequent critical values. These decision rules can be summarized in the following table at interim level i:

Event	Action
$Z_i > u_i$	Stop and declare superior efficacy
$l_i \le Z_i \le u_i$	Continue to next interim analysis, or if $i = m$, accept H_0
$Z_i < l_i$	Stop and declare not superior

The key to maintaining the desired operating characteristics while allowing early stopping is to adjust the maximum sample size and critical values, which require numerical computations to solve. Therefore, computer software is generally used to determine the specific values of u_i and l_i.

2.3.2.1.1 Comparison of the Methods by Pocock and O'Brien and Fleming

Pocock's approach is to adjust the interim probabilities of type I errors, based on the number of interim analyses, to a common value (or critical value) so that the overall probability of a type I error is equal to the desired level, α. Mathematically, this is expressed as $\alpha_1 = \alpha_2 = \cdots = \alpha_m = \alpha'$ and $u_1 = u_2 = \cdots = u_m = u$. So for example, if the total number of interim analyses is 2, 3, and 4 (i.e., $m = 2, 3,$ or 4), then $\alpha' = 0.0294$, 0.0221, and 0.0182, respectively, corresponding to $u = 2.178, 2.289,$ and 2.361. These designs yield an overall $\alpha = 0.05$. O'Brien and Fleming's approach tends to yield relatively conservative critical values for early interim analyses while "spending" a greater proportion of α at later stages. See Table 2.7 for specific critical values and corresponding levels of significance (derived from Table 2.3 of Jennison and Turnbull [41]) for a standard normal distribution (overall $\alpha = 0.05$).

In practical terms, Pocock's method is more likely to yield early termination of the study when the new regimen is active than O'Brien-Fleming's method, but there is a greater risk of observing a nonsignificant test statistic at the end of the study that would have been significant if the single-stage approach was applied (i.e., if there were no interim analyses). This has the potential to lead to considerable investigator regret. Of the two methods, O'Brien–Fleming seems to be favored because it reserves most of the significance testing until the final analysis. This enables

TABLE 2.7: Critical values and corresponding levels of significance for group sequential designs that use either the method of O'Brien-Fleming or Pocock. $l_i = -u_i$.

m	Interim Analysis	O'Brien-Fleming u_i	p	Pocock u_i	p
2	1	2.796	0.0052	2.178	0.0294
	2	1.977	0.0480	2.178	0.0294
3	1	3.471	0.0005	2.289	0.0221
	2	2.454	0.0141	2.289	0.0221
	3	2.004	0.0451	2.289	0.0221
4	1	4.048	0.0001	2.361	0.0182
	2	2.862	0.0042	2.361	0.0182
	3	2.337	0.0194	2.361	0.0182
	4	2.024	0.0430	2.361	0.0182
5	1	4.562	~0	2.413	0.0158
	2	3.226	0.0013	2.413	0.0158
	3	2.634	0.0084	2.413	0.0158
	4	2.281	0.0226	2.413	0.0158
	5	2.040	0.0414	2.413	0.0158

investigators to gain the most precise information about the regimen under study while meeting the ethical obligation of stopping the study early in the event of overwhelming evidence in favor of the new regimen. Additionally, using the O'Brien–Fleming approach leads to designs with smaller maximum sample sizes, in some cases, with almost insignificant changes to the single stage design.

2.3.2.1.2 Alpha Spending Functions Lan and DeMets [42] introduced the concept of alpha spending functions. An alpha spending function relates the incremental expenditure of type I error to the information time of the analysis. For example, if the spending function is defined as $\alpha(t) = \alpha t^2$, then the first analysis can spend αt_1^2 error if it is performed at information time t_1. If $t_1 = 0.5$, then one-quarter of the error can be spent at that time. This procedure is carried out by solving $P(Z_1 > u_1 \mid H_0) = \alpha(t_1) \Rightarrow u_1 = \Phi^{-1}(1 - \alpha(t_1))$. If the study proceeds to the second group for analysis at time t_2, then the critical value u_2 is found by solving the following equation:

$$P(Z_1 \leq u_1, Z_2 > u_2 \mid H_0) = \alpha(t_2) - \alpha(t_1)$$

The process continues in the general manner for the kth analysis:

$$P(Z_1 \leq u_1, \ldots, Z_{k-1} \leq u_{k-1}, Z_k > u_k \mid H_0) = \alpha(t_k) - \alpha(t_{k-1})$$

One of the difficulties with applying the group sequential methods such as those listed in the Section 2.3.2.1.1 is that they require an analysis at exactly the planned information time. This rigidity makes it difficult to time the analysis to more convenient times such as a week before a scheduled meeting with the study's data monitoring committee. Lan and DeMets' procedures allow for more flexibility. Because the timing of the analysis can be taken as arbitrary, there is not a strict requirement to conduct the interim analyses at precisely the originally planned times.

There have been recommendations (e.g., Dmitrienko [43, pp. 184–185]) to design studies with the strict group sequential methods such as Pocock or O'Brien and Fleming but to use the alpha spending method in applying them. In order for this approach to yield valid conclusions, it is important to use alpha spending functions that coincide closely with the actual alpha spending function used by the group sequential design. Some spending functions follow below by Lan and DeMets [42] and Jennison and Turnbull [44]:

$$\alpha(t) = 2 - 2 \cdot \Phi(z_{\alpha/2}/\sqrt{t}) \quad \text{O'Brien–Fleming}$$
$$\alpha(t) = \alpha t^3 \quad \text{O'Brien–Fleming}$$
$$\alpha(t) = \alpha \ln(1 + [e - 1]) \quad \text{Pocock}$$
$$\alpha(t) = \alpha t \quad \text{Pocock}$$

2.3.2.1.3 Futility Bounds The lower bounds for the interim test statistics are sometimes called futility bounds since an observation such as $Z_i < l_i$ makes it highly unlikely that the new regimen would yield statistically significant results in its favor at the end of the study (even if the drug is as active as hypothesized under the alternative). Therefore, it can be argued that there is little point to continuing the trial. One approach to determining the critical values for futility is to use a method such as O'Brien and Fleming or Pocock under the alternative hypothesis and assess as a beta spending problem. This method has been criticized as being heavily dependent on the specified HR in the alternative space, thereby making the decision rules appear to be a bit arbitrary.

Another approach to the problem is with stochastic curtailment tests. Lan, Simon, and Halperin [45] look at conditional power of the final test statistic, Z_m, (under the assumption that the alternative hypothesis is true) after an interim value, Z_i, is computed at $d < D$ deaths. Mathematically, consideration is given to $P(Z_m > u_m \mid Z_i)$. Given a particular futility index, γ, if this probability is $(1 - \gamma)$ or less (i.e., if $P(Z_m > u_m \mid Z_i) \leq 1 - \gamma$), then the trial is terminated for futility. Typical values of γ are between 0.8 and 1.

Although the method may be perceived as yielding liberal decision rules, they are in fact quite conservative and often have a minimal impact on the operating characteristics of the design, which is one reason why they can be applied post hoc. The authors demonstrate that this method cannot reduce the power of the original design to less than $(1 - \gamma\beta)$, and in practice often effects the power to a lesser degree.

Weiand [46] proposed a simple interim futility rule after approximately half of the information time becomes available. If this interim test statistic, $Z_i < 0$, indicating that the new regimen is performing worse than the control, then the trial terminates. Under the alternative hypothesis, $P(Z_i < 0) \approx 0$, so using this decision rule does not disrupt the operating characteristics of the study in any severe way. In addition, if the drug is only performing equally to the control or is performing worse, then $P(Z_i < 0) \geq 0.5$.

2.4   Phase 0 Studies

The phase 0 trial is a new form, designed to be a first-in-man study of an agent, to assess effectiveness against a molecular target, by means of a pharmacokinetic (PD) assay, in a very small number (10–15) of patients. It could be argued that the phase 0 trial currently has little place in a book concerning clinical trials with time-to-event endpoints, since the PD assay endpoints used are not time-to-event variables. However, in the future phase 0 studies are likely to include those with time-to-event endpoints, and at that time it will likely be necessary to develop new statistical techniques to address the problem of assessing such endpoints with a certain amount of statistical rigor, despite the small sample size—the same challenge that exists now with the PD assay endpoints. Meanwhile, the phase 0 trial promises to become an increasingly important tool for facilitating and speeding the development of new therapeutic agents, particularly in oncology, and as such, we felt it important to include it in this review of the design of clinical studies.

2.4.1 Introduction and Statement of the Concept—Measuring Biological Effectiveness (with a PD Endpoint) As a Very Early Screening and Drug Development Tool

Currently only 10% of investigational new drug (IND) applications to the Food and Drug Administration (FDA) result in clinically approved agents, and in oncology it is only 5% [3,47]. This is a very serious problem, since the development of a new agent is a lengthy and expensive process and many of these agents fail relatively late in that process. The fact that an increasing proportion of IND agents are molecularly targeted suggests testing the agent for effectiveness against the target by means of a PD assay very early in the drug development process. This is particularly useful and important since the preclinical tests of such effectiveness are often misleading, yielding both false positive and false negative results. For this reason, the FDA issued a new exploratory IND (expIND) Guidance in 2006, to allow for such studies as small first-in-man trials, conducted at dose levels and administration schedules not expected to result in significant clinical toxicity, and generally restricted to at most a few weeks per patient. Conducting studies under this guidance requires substantially less preclinical toxicology work than is required for standard IND phase I studies. Therefore phase 0 studies can be administered while the toxicology studies preparatory to filing a standard IND are being conducted, and they will not postpone the time until the phase I trial can be initiated.

Phase 0 studies can be very effective tools for determining very early in the drug development process that an agent is not having the anticipated biologic effect. They can also be used to prioritize among analog agents or agents designed to have the same molecularly targeted effect. They are an opportunity for developing and validating clinical PD assays very early in the drug development process, to enable more reliable usage of such assays in phase I and phase II trials. Finally, they can contribute to better defining the appropriate dose range or administration schedule to take into phase I and phase II testing.

2.4.2 Statistical Design of a Phase 0 Trial

The challenge presented by the phase 0 study is to assess the change in the PD endpoint effected by the agent, with a very few patients, each treated over a short period of time, but to maintain a certain amount of statistical rigor. Kummar et al. [3] and Murgo et al. [47] give several statistical designs to address this challenge in different clinical contexts, two of which we present here. In general, the approach they take is to mimic the design of a phase II study, and to design the phase 0 study as a phase II study in miniature for each separate dose level. Thus, the first step is to define what is meant by a PD "response" for each individual patient, which is analogous to defining what constitutes an objective tumor response for a patient in a phase II trial. The second step is to define what constitutes a promising observed PD response rate for each dose level—in other words, how many patients must demonstrate a PD response for the dose level to be declared biologically effective.

This is analogous to setting a threshold for observed response rate in a phase II trial, in order that the agent be deemed sufficiently promising for further testing. Further details of the approach given in Kummar et al. [3] and Murgo et al. [47] are given in the sections below.

2.4.2.1   Determining Statistical Significance of a PD Effect at the Patient Level—Defining a PD Response

In oncology, generally, the PD endpoint is assessed both in tumor tissue and in an easily assayed surrogate tissue such as blood (peripheral blood mononuclear cells, PBMCs). The tumor tissue assay is considered to be more reliable with respect to reflecting the biological effect of the agent in what is generally the target tissue of interest. However, the number of tumor biopsies usually is severely limited for ethical reasons. Therefore, the PBMC assay, for example, is used as a surrogate, since multiple PBMC assays can be performed both pretreatment and posttreatment, thus allowing for assessment of both the pretreatment variability at the patient level and the posttreatment PD effect over time. Generally, there are only two tumor biopsies, one taken immediately before treatment with the agent, and one taken at the posttreatment time point of greatest interest, often when the PD effect is anticipated to be at its maximum. The measure of treatment effect for the tumor PD assay is the difference between the pretreatment and posttreatment values (often measured on the log scale rather than on the original). Generally, there are multiple PBMC assays both pretreatment and posttreatment. The primary measure of treatment effect for the PBMC assay is the one that corresponds in time to that of the tumor assay—the difference between the most immediately pretreatment PBMC assay and the post-treatment PBMC assay closest in time to that of the tumor biopsy. The other pretreatment PBMC assays should, ideally, cover a time span comparable to that of the pretreatment versus posttreatment biopsies. In that way, they provide a measure of the natural variation of the assay, for an individual patient, over that time span. The other posttreatment PBMC assays provide a means of assessing the posttreatment PD effect over time, as a secondary set of PD endpoints.

Defining a PD "response," both for the tumor assay and for the PBMC assay, involves both a biologic criterion and a statistical criterion for what is significant. The biologic criterion generally depends upon characteristics of the biologic target of the agent. For example, in the recent National Cancer Institute (NCI) phase 0 trial of ABT-888 [47,48], the criterion chosen was that the reduction in the assay value had to be at least twofold. The statistical criterion may be either 90% confidence or 95% confidence that the observed treatment effect is not a result of the sort of natural random variation in the assay, for an individual patient, that would be seen in the absence of a treatment effect. For the PBMC assay, this natural variation can be assessed by the pooled intrapatient SD of the pretreatment values. However, for the tumor assay, multiple pretreatment assays per patient will generally not be available. Therefore, the interpatient SD of the pretreatment values must be used instead. Details concerning the definition of a PD response are illustrated in Figure 2.17.

Defining PD response at the patient level

Calculate the baseline variance and standard deviation (SD) of the PD value
(In surrogate tissue, the baseline variance is the pooled intrapatient baseline
variance determined by calculating the baseline variances for each patient,
separately, and then averaging the separate variances across patients. In tumor
tissue, the baseline variance is the interpatient baseline variance calculated
across patients. In either case, the baseline SD is the square root of the baseline
variance.)

⇓

Measure PD effect as posttreatment value minus pretreatment value

⇓

If the PD effect is greater than 1.8 (2.3) times the baseline SD,
then it is statistically significant at the .10 (.05) significance level

⇓

A statistically significant PD effect, at the patient level,
is called a PD response

FIGURE 2.17: PD "response" for an individual patient. Multipliers of the baseline SD are derived from asymptotic normal distribution theory.

2.4.2.2 Determining Statistical Significance of a PD Effect for a Given Dose Level

For each dose level, the investigators may set a threshold for the number of patients, among the total, that must demonstrate a PD response, in order for the dose level to be judged as yielding a promising biologic effect. Since the false positive rate for a PD response, for an individual patient, has been determined (as given above), the false positive rate for declaring a dose level effective, for each assay separately and for the two combined, can be calculated from the binomial distribution. Likewise, for a targeted PD response rate, across patients, the power to declare the dose level effective, for each of the two assays, can be calculated. The investigators may employ a one-stage or two-stage design to assess the PD response rate at each dose level, just as in phase II studies, and the calculations of power and false positive rate are done in an identical fashion. Examples are given below of designs to target 80% or 60% PD response rates, across patients.

2.4.2.3 Two Trial Designs—One Design to Detect an 80% PD Response Rate across Patients and One to Detect a 60% PD Response Rate across Patients

To target an 80% PD response rate at each dose level, a one-stage design may be used. Three patients are accrued and the dose level is declared effective with respect to either PD assay if at least two of the patients demonstrate a PD response which is significant at the .10 level. This design yields 90% power to detect an 80% PD response rate, across patients, for either assay, with an overall 6% false positive for the two assays combined, under the null hypothesis that the agent has no biologic

Design 1: Defining a significant PD effect at the dose
level when the target PD response rate is
80% at the patient level

Treat three patients

⇓

Declare the PD effect statistically significant at the dose level
if at least two of the three patients demonstrate a PD response
at the .10 significance level

⇓

This yields 90% power, at the dose level,
to detect an 80% PD response rate at the patient level,
with an overall 6% false positive rate for both endpoints combined

FIGURE 2.18: Promising observed response rate for a dose level. The target PD response rate, across patients, is 80%. Power and false positive rate are derived from the binomial distribution.

effect. This is the design that was used in the NCI phase 0 trial of ABT-888, and it is illustrated in Figure 2.18.

To target a 60% PD response rate at each dose level, a two-stage design may be used. Three patients are accrued and the cohort is expanded to five patients if exactly one patient, for either PD assay, demonstrates a PD response which is significant at the .05 level. The dose level is declared effective with respect to either PD assay if at least two of the patients demonstrate a PD response which is significant at the .05 level. This design yields 89% power to detect a 60% PD response rate, across patients, for either assay, with an overall 4% false positive for the two assays combined, under the null hypothesis that the agent has no biologic effect. This design is illustrated in Figure 2.19.

2.4.3   Example of a Phase 0 Trial—the NCI PARP Inhibitor Trial—and Further Discussion of Phase 0 Statistical Issues

The NCI selected ABT-888, an inhibitor of the DNA repair enzyme poly (ADP-ribose) polymerase (PARP), for the first ever phase 0 trial for two reasons [47,48]. First, it was anticipated to have a wide margin of safety relative to target modulating doses in preclinical models. This is an essential characteristic for a phase 0 agent. Phase 0 trials cannot promise any benefit for the patients who participate, so there must be reasonable assurance that toxicity will be minimal. Second, it was anticipated to have wide therapeutic applicability if demonstrated effective. Elevated PARP levels are characteristic of tumors and can result in resistance to both chemotherapy (CT) and radiotherapy (RT). Therefore, PARP inhibitors hold promise of wide applicability as CT and RT sensitizers. The NCI trial demonstrated statistically significant reduction in PAR levels (a surrogate for PARP inhibition) in both tumor and PBMCs.

Design 2: Defining a significant PD effect at the dose
level when the target PD response rate is
60% at the patient level

Treat three patients

Treat an additional two patients if exactly one of the three patients
demonstrates a PD response at the .05 significance level

Declare the PD effect statistically significant at the dose level
if at least two of the three (or five) patients demonstrate a PD response
at the .05 significance level

⇓

This yields 89% power, at the dose level,
to detect a 60% PD response rate at the patient level,
with an overall 4% false positive rate for both endpoints combined

FIGURE 2.19:   Promising observed response rate for a dose level with a 2-stage design. The target PD response rate, across patients, is 60%. Power and false positive rate are derived from the binomial distribution.

There are a number of statistical issues relating to phase 0 trials that deserve further mention:

1. In the NCI phase 0 trial it was found that the variance of the pretreatment PD assay values was reduced if the logs of the values were used instead. It is often appropriate to log-transform PD assay values since geometric, rather than arithmetic, changes in value are thought to be qualitatively similar along the assay scale.

2. It will often be the case that assessing the PD treatment effect can be done with greater statistical power if the mean effect is measured across patients and then a test applied of the null hypothesis that the mean effect is equal to 0. Analogously, there have been proposals that phase II trials be assessed by testing whether the mean tumor shrinkage is statistically significant. The problem with this approach is that a statistically significant mean treatment effect does not necessarily imply a biologically relevant treatment effect for a meaningful proportion of the patients. For this reason, the NCI phase 0 trial investigators chose to impose the additional criterion of a biologically relevant level of PAR reduction for the individual patients. Likewise, it was felt appropriate to determine, for the individual patients, whether the PAR reduction observed was statistically significant. This follows the standard phase II model of determining what would constitute a response, for the individual patient, suggestive of benefit for that patient, and then assess the proportion of

patients demonstrating such a response. There may be phase 0 situations where this approach is too statistically demanding, and it is appropriate to resort to assessing the mean treatment PD effect.

3. For the tumor biopsy assay, multiple pretreatment assays per patient will generally not be available, for ethical reasons. Therefore, the interpatient SD of the pretreatment values must be used instead of the intrapatient SD, which cannot be determined. The interpatient variability will often be substantially greater than the intrapatient variability. This can seriously limit ability to declare statistically significant a treatment effect measured by the tumor assay. For example, in the NCI phase 0 trial, a 95% posttreatment reduction in the tumor assay value was required for statistical significance, while a 55% posttreatment reduction was sufficient for the PBMC assay.

References

[1] Rubinstein, LV (2000): Therapeutic studies. *Hematology/Oncology Clinics of North America* 14:849–876.

[2] Simon, R (2008): Design and analysis of clinical trials. In: DeVita, Hellman, and Rosenberg (eds): *Hellman and Rosenberg's Cancer Principles & Practice of Oncology*, 8th edn., pp. 571–589, Lippincot, Williams & Wilkins, Philadelphia, PA.

[3] Kummar, S, Kinders, R, Rubinstein, L, Parchment RE, Murgo, AJ, Collins, J, Pickeral, O, et al. (2007): Compressing drug development timelines in oncology using 'phase 0' trials. *Nature Reviews/Cancer* 7:131–139.

[4] Simon, R (1989): Optimal two-stage designs for phase II clinical trials. *Controlled Clinical Trials* 10:1–10.

[5] Therasse, P, Arbuck, SG, Eisenhauer, EA, Wanders, J, Kaplan, RS, Rubinstein, L, Verweij, J, et al. (2000): New guidelines to evaluate the response to treatment in solid tumors (RECIST guidelines). *Journal of the National Cancer Institute* 92:205–216.

[6] Brookmeyer, R and Crowley, JJ (1982): A confidence interval for the median survival time. *Biometrics* 38:29–41.

[7] Rubinstein, LV, Gail, MH, and Santner, TJ (1981): Planning the duration of a clinical trial with loss to follow-up and a period of continued observation. *Journal of Chronic Diseases* 34:469–479.

[8] Korn, EL and Freidlin, B (2006): Conditional power calculations for clinical trials with historical controls. *Statistics in Medicine* 25:2922–2931.

[9] Korn, EL, Liu, PY, Lee, SJ, Chapman, JW, Niedzwiecki, D, Suman, VJ, Moon, J, et al. (2008): Meta-analysis of phase II cooperative group trials in metastatic stage IV melanoma to determine progression-free and overall survival benchmarks for future phase II trials. *Journal of Clinical Oncology* 26:527–534.

[10] Zee, B, Melnychuk, D, Dancey, J, and Eisenhauer, E (1999): Multinomial phase II cancer trials incorporating response and early progression. *Journal of Biopharmaceutical Statistics* 9:351–363.

[11] Dent, S, Zee, B, Dancey, J, Hanauske, A, Wanders, J, and Eisenhauer E (2001): Application of a new multinomial phase II stopping rule using response and early progression. *Journal of Clinical Oncology* 19:785–791.

[12] Sill, MW and Yothers, G (2007): A method for utilizing bivariate efficacy outcome measures to screen agents for activity in 2-stage phase II clinical trials. Technical report 06-08, Department of Biostatistics, University at Buffalo. Accessed at: http://sphhp.buffalo.edu/biostat/research/techreports/index.php

[13] Herson, J and Carter, SK (1986): Calibrated phase II clinical trials in oncology. *Statistics in Medicine* 5:441–447.

[14] Ellenberg, SS and Eisenberger, MA (1985): An efficient design for phase III studies of combination chemotherapies. *Cancer Treatment Reports* 69:1147–1154.

[15] Simon, R, Wittes, RE, and Ellenberg, SS (1985): Randomized phase II clinical trials. *Cancer Treatment Reports* 69:1375–1381.

[16] Rubinstein, LV, Korn, EL, Freidlin, B, Hunsburger, S, Ivy, SP, and Smith, MA (2005): Design issues of randomized phase II trials and a proposal for phase II screening trials. *Journal of Clinical Oncology* 23:7199–7206.

[17] Simon, RM, Steinberg, SM, Hamilton, M, Hildesheim, A, Khleif, S, Kwak, LW, Mackall, CL, Schlom, J, Topalian, SL, and Berzofsky, JA (2001): Clinical trial designs for the early clinical development of therapeutic cancer vaccines. *Journal of Clinical Oncology* 19:1848–1854.

[18] Korn, EL, Arbuck, SG, Pluda, JM, Simon, R, Kaplan, RS, and Christian, MC (2001): Clinical trial designs for cytostatic agents: Are new designs needed? *Journal of Clinical Oncology* 19:265–272.

[19] Collett, D (1994): *Modeling Survival Data in Medical Research*, Chapman and Hall, Boca Raton, FL.

[20] Fleiss, JL, Tytun, A, and Ury, HK (1980): A simple approximation for calculating sample sizes for comparing independent proportions. *Biometrics* 36:343–346.

[21] Freidlin, B, Korn, EL, Hunsberger, S, Gray, R, Saxman, S, and Zujewski, JA (2007): Proposal for the use of progression-free survival in unblinded randomized trials. *Journal of Clinical Oncology* 25:2122–2126.

[22] Mantel, N and Haenszel, W (1959): Statistical aspects of the analysis of data from retrospective studies of disease. *JNCI* 22:719–748.

[23] DeGroot, MH (1986): Probability and Statistics, 2nd edn., Addison-Wesley Publishing Co., Reading, MA.

[24] Cox, DR (1972): Regression models and life tables. *Journal of Royal Statistical Society; B* 74:187–220.

[25] Pocock, SJ and Simon, R (1975): Sequential treatment assignment with balancing for prognostic factors in the controlled clinical trial. *Biometrics* 31:102–115.

[26] Lawless, JF (1982): *Statistical Models and Methods for Lifetime Data*, Wiley, New York.

[27] Bartle, RG and Sherbert, DR (1992): *Introduction to Real Analysis*, 2nd edn., Wiley, New York.

[28] Sellke, T and Siegmund, D (1983): Sequential analysis of the proportional hazards model. *Biometrika* 70:315–326.

[29] Schoenfeld, D (1981): The asymptotic properties of nonparametric tests for comparing survival distributions. *Biometrika* 68:316–319.

[30] Freedman, LS (1982): Tables of the number of patients required in clinical trials using the logrank test. *Statistics in Medicine* 1:121–129.

[31] Piantadosi, S. *Clinical Trials: A Methodologic Perspective*, Wiley, New York.

[32] Hsieh, FY and Lavori, PW (2000): Sample-size calculations for the cox-proportional hazards regression model with non-binary covariates. *Controlled Clinical Trials* 21:552–560.

[33] Peto R, et al. (1988): Randomized trial of prophylactic daily aspirin in British male doctors. *BMJ* 296:313–316.

[34] Steering Committee of the Physicians' Health Study Research Group (1989): Final report on the aspirin component of the ongoing Physicians' Health Study. *New England Journal of Medicine* 321:129–135.

[35] Hansson, L, et al. (1998): Effects of intensive blood-pressure lowering and low-dose aspirin in patients with hypertension: Principal results of the hypertension optimal treatment (HOT) randomised trial. *Lancet* 351:1755–1762.

[36] Schoenfeld, DA (1983): Sample-size formula for the proportional-hazards regression model. *Biometrics* 39(2):499–503.

[37] Wolfram S (2007): Wolfram Research Inc., Mathematica, Version 6.0, Champaign, IL.

[38] George, SL and Desu, MM (1974): Planning the size and duration of a clinical trial studying the time to some critical event. *Journal of Chronic Disease* 27:15–24.

[39] Pocock, SJ (1977): Group sequential methods in the design and analysis of clinical trials. *Biometrika* 64:191–199.

[40] O'Brien, PC and Fleming, TR (1979): A multiple testing procedure for clinical trials. *Biometrics* 35:549–556.

[41] Jennison, J and Turnbull, BW (2000): *Group Sequential Methods with Applications to Clinical Trials*, CRC Press, Boca Raton, FL.

[42] Lan, KKG and DeMets, DL (1983): Discrete sequential boundaries for clinical trials. *Biometrika* 70(3):659–663.

[43] Dmitrienko, A, Molenberghs, G, Chuang-Stein, C, and Offen, W. *Analysis of Clinical Trials Using SAS: A Practical Guide*, SAS Institute Inc., Cary, NC.

[44] Jennison, J and Turnbull, BW (1990): Statistical approaches to interim monitoring of medical trials: A review and commentary. *Statistical Science* 5(3):299–317.

[45] Lan, KKG, Simon, R, and Halperin, M (1982): Stochastically curtailed tests in long-term clinical trials. *Communications in Statistics: Sequential Analysis* 1(3):207–219.

[46] Wieand, S, Schroeder, G, and O'Fallon, JR (1994): Stopping when the experimental regimen does not appear to help. *Statistics in Medicine* 13:1453–1458.

[47] Murgo, AJ, Kummar, S, Rubinstein, L, Gutierrez, M, Collins, J, Kinders, R, Parchment, RE, et al. (2008): Designing phase 0 cancer clinical trials. *Clinical Cancer Research* 14:3675–3682.

[48] Kinders, R, Parchment, RE, Ji, J, Kummar, S, Murgo, AJ, Gutierrez, M, Collins, J, et al. (2007): Phase O clinical trials in cancer drug development: from FDA guidance to clinical practice. *Molecular Interventions* 7:325–334.

Chapter 3

Overview of Time-to-Event Parametric Methods

Karl E. Peace and Kao-Tai Tsai

Contents

3.1 Introduction

An overview of time-to-event parametric methods is presented in this chapter. The parameters *hazard function, death density function, survival function*, and *cumulative death distribution function* are first defined, and relationships between them are noted. Then five commonly used parametric models *exponential, Weibull, Rayleigh, Gompertz*, and *lognormal* are presented. These are followed by a discussion of how to incorporate concomitant, covariate, or regressor information into these models. Numerous applications from the literature, reflecting a broad range of time-to-event endpoints that are analyzed (estimation and hypothesis testing) by a variety of statistical methods, are then presented. Penultimately, examples illustrating applications of the parametric models is presented. The chapter ends with a discussion of the models, methods, and applications.

3.2 Parameters and Definitions

As indicated in Section 1.1, in many clinical trials, the primary endpoint is some critical event. In analgesic studies such as postdental extraction pain or postpartum pain, the event is relief of pain. In an anti-infective study of chronic urinary tract infection, the event is microbiological cure or the abatement of clinical signs and symptoms of the infection. In the study of bladder tumors, for example, important events in patient follow-up are remission or progression. In transplantation studies involving renal allografts, although death is *ultimately primary*, rejection may be the primary event reflecting the experimental objective. If the event is recurrence, then time-to-event is progression-free interval. If the event is death, then time-to-event is survival time.

Although parameters could be defined in terms of some general event, for ease of presentation in this chapter, we will assume that the event is death and that a population is undergoing some experience which may affect mortality or survival. Data on the times of the event and the times of censoring (as well as any information about the censoring mechanisms) from such a population provide meaningful information about survival parameters (see Section 1.1 for further discussion of censoring). Specifically what parameters, what data, and what method(s) of analysis will depend upon study objective(s), study design, study conduct, etc.

Parameters of widespread interest in depicting survival are *the hazard function* or *force of mortality, the death density function, the survival function*, and *the cumulative death distribution function*. These functions are symbolized in this chapter as $h(t)$, $f(t)$, $S(t)$, and $F(t)$, respectively, where t denotes survival time. These symbols are rather standard with the exception that $h(t)$ is often symbolized by $\lambda(t)$.

3.2.1 Hazard Function

The mathematical definition of the *hazard function* $h(t)$ is

$$h(t) = \lim_{\Delta t \to 0^+} \frac{\Pr[t \leq T \leq t + \Delta t | T \geq t]}{\Delta t},$$

where T denotes the random variable survival time. Ignoring limit considerations, $h(t)$ is the proportion of the population expiring in the interval $(t; t + \Delta t)$ among those at risk of expiring at the beginning of the interval, averaged over the length of the interval. So $h(t)$ may be thought of as the probability of dying at time $= t$, given that death did not occur prior to t; or $h(t)$ is the instantaneous risk of death at time t given that death did not occur prior to t.

A hazard function may remain constant with respect to time (corresponding to an exponential density); may increase as a function of time according to some power function (corresponding to a Weibull density); may increase linearly with time (corresponding to a Rayleigh density), or may increase exponentially with time (corresponding to a Gompertz density). In addition, there may be intervals of time where the hazard may alternatingly decrease or increase according to some power, linear, or exponential function of time.

The hazard function for a population of individuals whose only risks of death are accidents or rare illnesses would be expected to be constant. The hazard function for a population of retired persons would be expected to increase; e.g., Pr[dying prior to 66 | alive at 65] < Pr[dying prior to 71 | alive at 70]; i.e., from the U.S. Commerce life tables, these probabilities are respectively 0.0366 and 0.0580. The hazard function of a population of children who have undergone a complicated surgical procedure to correct a congenital defect would be expected to decrease. The hazard function of a population of individuals followed from birth to death would be expected to exhibit periods of increase and periods of decrease.

3.2.2 Death Density Function

The mathematical definition of the *death density function* $f(t)$ is

$$f(t) = \lim_{\Delta t \to 0^+} \frac{\Pr[t \leq T \leq t + \Delta t]}{\Delta t},$$

where T denotes the random variable survival time. Ignoring limit considerations, $f(t)$ is the proportion of all individuals in the population expiring in the interval $(t; t + \Delta t)$ divided by the length of the interval. So $f(t)$ may be thought of as the unconditional probability of dying at time $= t$; or $f(t)$ is the instantaneous unconditional risk of death at time t.

3.2.3   Survival Function

The mathematical definition of the *survival function* $S(t)$ is

$$S(t) = \Pr[T \geq t],$$

where T denotes the random variable survival time. The survival function $S(t)$ may be interpreted as the probability of surviving to at least time t, the t-year survival rate, the cumulative proportion surviving to at least time t, or the proportion of a population surviving to at least time t.

3.2.4   Cumulative Death Distribution Function

The *cumulative death distribution function* is the complement of the survival function, i.e., $F(t) = 1 - S(t)$.

3.2.5   Relationships between Parameters

The hazard, density, survival, and cumulative death distribution functions are interrelated. If one knows the survival function, its complement is the cumulative death distribution function, and the death density may be obtained by differentiating the negative of the survival function with respect to t; i.e., $f(t) = -d[S(t)]/dt$. The hazard function may then be obtained by dividing the death density by the survival function; i.e., $h(t) = f(t)/S(t)$. Alternatively, $h(t) = -d[\ln\{S(t)\}]/dt$. Also, if the hazard function is specified, the survival function may be obtained by exponentiating the negative integral of the hazard, i.e.,

$$S(t) = \exp\left[-\int_0^t h(u)du \right].$$

Thus knowledge of any one of the four enables one to determine the other three.

3.3   Five Commonly Used Parametric Models

Five commonly used parametric models are the exponential, Weibull, Rayleigh, Gompertz, and lognormal. Applications of these models in a variety of settings, in which interest is in modeling some critical, time-to-event endpoint, are summarized in Sections 3.5 and 3.6.

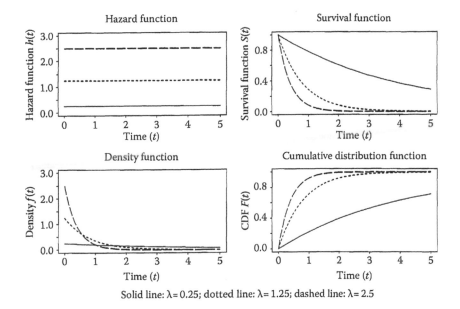

Solid line: $\lambda = 0.25$; dotted line: $\lambda = 1.25$; dashed line: $\lambda = 2.5$

FIGURE 3.1: Exponential model functions.

3.3.1 Exponential Model

The exponential model derives from a constant hazard function: $h(t) = \lambda_0$, where $\lambda_0 > 0$. The exponential death density function is $f(t) = \lambda_0 \exp(-\lambda_0 t)$. The exponential survival function is $S(t) = \exp(-\lambda_0 t)$. The cumulative death distribution function is $F(t) = 1 - \exp(-\lambda_0 t)$. Graphs of the hazard, density, survival, and cumulative event distribution functions for the exponential model appear in Figure 3.1.

3.3.2 Weibull Model

The Weibull model derives from a power-law hazard function: $h(t) = \lambda_0 \lambda_1 t^{(\lambda_1 - 1)}$, where $\lambda_0 > 0$ and $\lambda_1 > 0$. It may be noted that $\lambda_1 > 1$ guarantees that $h(t)$ is monotone increasing. The Weibull death density function is $f(t) = \lambda_0 \lambda_1 t^{(\lambda_1 - 1)} \exp[-\lambda_0 t^{\lambda_1}]$; the Weibull survival function is $S(t) = \exp[-\lambda_0 t^{\lambda_1}]$; and the Weibull cumulative death distribution function is $F(t) = 1 - \exp[-\lambda_0 t^{\lambda_1}]$. Graphs of the hazard, density, survival, and cumulative event distribution functions for the Weibull model appear in Figure 3.2.

3.3.3 Rayleigh Model

The Rayleigh model derives from a linear hazard function: $h(t) = \lambda_0 + 2\lambda_1 t$, where $\lambda_0 > 0$ and $\lambda_1 \geq 0$. It may be noted that if $\lambda_1 > 0$ then $h(t)$ is monotone increasing. The Rayleigh death density function is $f(t) = (\lambda_0 + 2\lambda_1 t) \exp[-(\lambda_0 t + \lambda_1 t^2)]$; the

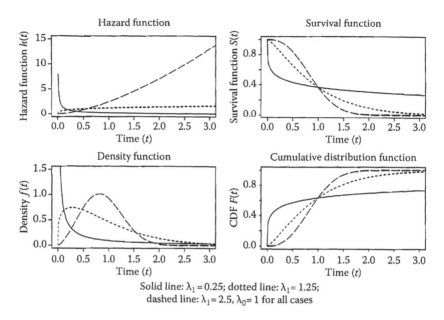

FIGURE 3.2:   Weibull model functions.

Rayleigh survival function is $S(t) = \exp[-(\lambda_0 t + \lambda_1 t^2)]$; and the Rayleigh cumulative death distribution function is $F(t) = 1 - \exp[-(\lambda_0 t + \lambda_1 t^2)]$. Graphs of the hazard, density, survival, and cumulative event distribution functions for the Rayleigh model appear in Figure 3.3.

3.3.4   Gompertz Model

The Gompertz model derives from an exponential hazard function; i.e., $h(t) = \exp(\lambda_0 + \lambda_1 t)$. Note that if $\lambda_1 > 0$ then $h(t)$ is monotone increasing. The Gompertz death density function is $f(t) = \exp(\lambda_0 + \lambda_1 t)\exp[(1/\lambda_1)\{\exp(\lambda_0) - \exp(\lambda_0 + \lambda_1 t)\}]$; the Gompertz survival function is $S(t) = \exp[(1/\lambda_1)\{\exp(\lambda_0) - \exp(\lambda_0 + \lambda_1 t)\}]$; and the cumulative death distribution function is $F(t) = 1 - \exp[(1/\lambda_1)\{\exp(\lambda_0) - \exp(\lambda_0 + \lambda_1 t)\}]$. Graphs of the hazard, density, survival, and cumulative event distribution functions for the Gompertz model appear in Figure 3.4.

3.3.5   Lognormal Model

The lognormal death density function is given by

$$f(t) = [1/(t\sigma(2\pi)^{1/2})] \exp[-(1/2\sigma^2)(\ln t - \mu)^2].$$

The lognormal survival function is $S(t) = 1 - \Phi\{(\ln t - \mu)/\sigma\}$, where Φ is the standard cumulative normal distribution. The hazard function is $h(t) = f(t)/S(t)$.

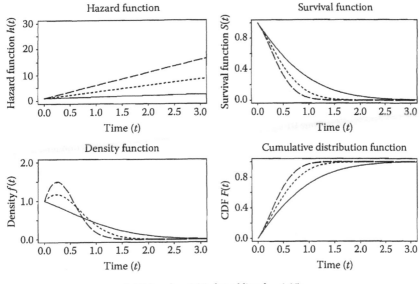

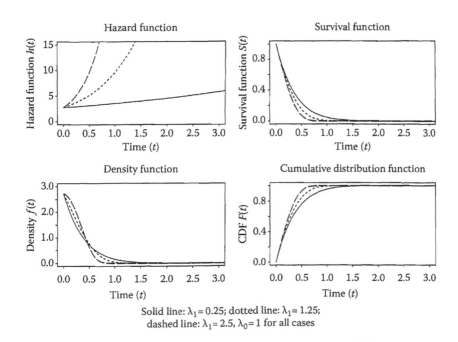

Solid line: $\lambda_1 = 0.25$; dotted line: $\lambda_1 = 1.25$;
dashed line: $\lambda_1 = 2.5$, $\lambda_0 = 1$ for all cases

FIGURE 3.3: Rayleigh model functions.

Solid line: $\lambda_1 = 0.25$; dotted line: $\lambda_1 = 1.25$;
dashed line: $\lambda_1 = 2.5$, $\lambda_0 = 1$ for all cases

FIGURE 3.4: Gompertz model functions.

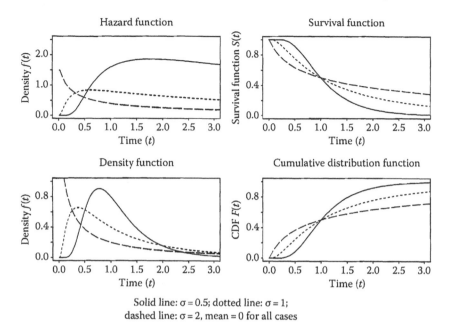

FIGURE 3.5:   Lognormal model functions.

The cumulative death distribution function is $F(t) = \Phi\{(\ln t - \mu)/\sigma\}$, where Φ is the standardized normal distribution. Graphs of the hazard, density, survival, and cumulative event distribution functions for the lognormal model appear in Figure 3.5.

3.4   Introduction of Concomitant or Regressor Information

The definitions presented in Sections 3.2 through 3.4 are explicitly functions of survival time t. Analysis of time-to-event data utilizing the models would consist of estimating their parameters and tests of hypotheses specified in terms of their parameters. In many experimental settings, particularly in the drug development or medical field, there exists concomitant, covariate, or regressor information on patients in addition to their times-to-event. In such settings, there is interest in assessing the significance of the concomitant information and how it may affect the distribution of times-to-event.

The parameters may be modified to allow the incorporation of concomitant, covariate, or regressor information and to assess the effect of such information on survival. Generally, this is accomplished using either the Cox proportional hazards model [1] or an accelerated failure time model [2–4].

3.4.1 Proportional Hazards Model

The hazard function reflecting the proportional hazards model [1] is specified as $\lambda(t \mid \mathbf{x}) = \exp(\mathbf{x}\boldsymbol{\beta})h(t)$, where $\mathbf{x}$ is a row vector of concomitant, covariate, or regressor information $(x_1, x_2, \ldots, x_p)$, $\boldsymbol{\beta}$ is a column vector of parameters $(\beta_1, \beta_2, \ldots, \beta_p)$ corresponding to $\mathbf{x}$, and $h(t)$ is the time-specific hazard function defined in Section 3.2.1 (which could assume any of the forms in Section 3.3), sometimes referred to as a homogeneous or baseline hazard function.

From the formulation, it is noticed that the concomitant information acts in a multiplicative fashion only on the time-dependent hazard function. Further, the term proportional hazards arises by observing that if an x_i is an indicator of treatment group membership ($x_i = 1$ if treatment group 1; $x_i = 0$ if treatment group 0), then the ratio of the hazard for treatment group 1 to the hazard of treatment group 0 is $\exp(\beta_i)$, or the hazard for treatment group 1 is proportional to the hazard of treatment group 0.

3.4.2 Accelerated Failure Time Model

The hazard function reflecting the accelerated hazards model [2–5] is specified as $\lambda(t \mid \mathbf{x}) = \exp(-\mathbf{x}\boldsymbol{\beta})h(t \exp(-\mathbf{x}\boldsymbol{\beta}))$, where again $\mathbf{x}$ is a row vector of concomitant, covariate, or regressor information $(x_1, x_2, \ldots, x_p)$, $\boldsymbol{\beta}$ is a column vector of parameters $(\beta_1, \beta_2, \ldots, \beta_p)$ corresponding to $\mathbf{x}$, and $h(\cdot)$ is the time-specific hazard function defined above. From the formulation, it is noticed that the concomitant information acts in a multiplicative fashion on time t; i.e., time is "accelerated" by multiplying it by $\exp(-\mathbf{x}\boldsymbol{\beta})$.

The accelerated failure time model may also be written in log-linear form as

$$\text{Log } T_i = \beta_0 + \beta_1 x_{i1} + \beta_2 x_{i2} + \cdots + \beta_p x_{ip} + \sigma \varepsilon_i,$$

where
T_i is the observed survival time of the ith subject $\{i = 1, 2, \ldots, n\}$,
σ is an unknown parameter to be estimated, and
the ε_i are independent and follow some common error distribution.

The $\sigma \varepsilon_i$ could be replaced by ε_i, but this would allow the variance of the ε_i to be different from 1.

The Weibull model and exponential model (since it is a special case of the Weibull) may be parameterized as either a proportional hazards model or an accelerated failure time model. These are the only two models that share this feature. The lognormal model may also be considered as an accelerated failure time model.

3.5 Statistical Methods and Applications

The parametric models presented here have been extensively studied and applied to time-to-event data: without censoring, without incorporating concomitant information, with censoring and incorporating concomitant information. Inferential methods based on maximum likelihood, least squares, resampling, and Bayesian approaches have been developed. Many excellent textbooks [3,5–15] and articles illustrating various analysis methods and applications of parametric models have been published. Some of the articles are summarized in Sections 3.5.1 through 3.5.5. Two are presented and discussed in detail in Sections 3.6.1 and 3.6.2.

3.5.1   Exponential Model

Feigl and Zelen [16] were among the first to incorporate concomitant information in an exponential model of survival time of patients with acute myelogonous leukemia. Concomitant information was white blood cell counts at diagnosis. Zippin and Armitage [17] extended Feigl and Zelen's work to allow for censored data. Zelen [18] presents other applications of the exponential model in biomedical sciences. Byar et al. [19] use an exponential model to relate censored survival data and concomitant information for patients with prostate cancer. Gage et al. [20] utilize an exponential model in validating a clinical classification scheme for predicting stroke.

Friedman [21] develops maximum likelihood-based procedures for providing inferences when fitting piecewise exponential models to censored survival data with covariates. Maller [22] considers an exponential model with covariates for censored survival times and develops sufficient conditions for the existence, consistency, and asymptotic normality of the regression coefficients.

3.5.2   Weibull Model

Menon [23] provides methods for estimating the parameters of the Weibull model. Cohen [24] derives maximum likelihood estimates for the parameters of the Weibull model based on complete and censored times-to-event. Harter and Moore [25] derive asymptotic variances and covariances of maximum likelihood estimators of the parameters of the Weibull model based on censored times-to-event. Dubey [26] also considers inferences on parameters of the Weibull model. And Crow [27] develops confidence interval procedures for the Weibull model with applications to reliability growth.

Anderson [28] considers the Weibull accelerated failure time regression model. Liao [29] used the Weibull model to elucidate the effect of pretreatment clinicopathologic variables on the prognosis of patients with hepatocellular carcinoma (HCCs) smaller than 5 cm in diameter treated by percutaneous ethanol injection (PEI) with or without transcatheter arterial chemoembolization. Carroll [30] examines the use and utility of the Weibull model in the analysis of times-to-event data from clinical trials.

3.5.3   Rayleigh Model

Bain [31] considers the Rayleigh model for complete and censored times-to-event and develops both least squares and maximum likelihood estimators for its parameters.

Bhattacharya and Tyagi [32] take a Bayesian approach to the analysis of times-to-event data following a Rayleigh model, from a clinical trial that is stopped after a predetermined number of events. Sen and Bhattacharya [33] develop maximum likelihood and least squares type estimation procedures for the parameters of the Rayleigh model based on censored times-to-event, and use the expectation-maximization (EM) algorithm for computing the maximum likelihood estimates. Indika and Hossain [34] also present estimation procedures for parameters of the Rayleigh model based on progressively censored data. Mahdi [35] investigates five methods: maximum likelihood, moments, probability weighted moments, least squares, and least absolute deviation, for estimating the parameters of the Rayleigh model.

3.5.4 Gompertz Model

Garg et al. [36] estimate the parameters of the Gompertz model by the method of maximum likelihood. Wu et al. [37] use the method of least squares to estimate the parameters of the Gompertz model. Wu and Li [38] obtain unweighted and weighted least squares estimates of the parameters of the Gompertz model for complete and censored data, and compare them to the maximum likelihood estimates.

Ananda et al. [39] utilize an adaptive Bayesian approach to estimate the parameters of the Gompertz model. Peter et al. [40] estimate cure rates from pediatric clinical trials using the Gompertz model with covariate information. Ricklefs and Scheuerlein [41] utilize the Gompertz model to describe the increase in age related mortality.

3.5.5 Lognormal Model

The lognormal model has been used extensively to model long-term survival and to estimate the proportion of patients cured following some intervention. Boag [42–44] is among the first to use this model to estimate the proportion of patients cured following radiation therapy and following gastric resection, using the method of maximum likelihood. Mould and Boag [45] utilized the lognormal model as well as other parametric models to estimate the success rate of treatment for carcinoma cervix uteri. Mould et al. [46] used the lognormal to model the distribution of survival of patients who died from head and neck cancer. Rutqvist [47] studied the utility of the lognormal model to describe the survival of breast cancer patients in Sweden.

Gamel et al. [48] provide a stable linear algorithm for fitting the lognormal model to survival data in estimating the proportion of patients cured. Gamel et al. [49] used the lognormal model to describe the long-term clinical course of patients with cutaneous melanoma.

Tai et al. [50] use the lognormal model in a 20-year follow-up study of long-term survival of patients with limited-stage small-cell lung cancer in which concomitant information was used. Tai et al. [51] use the lognormal model to study the long-term survival rates of patients with laryngeal cancer treated with radiation, surgery, or both. Tai et al. [52] use the lognormal model to assess cause-specific survival in patients with inflammatory breast cancer. Qazi et al. [53] use the lognormal model to calculate and compare survival statistics in the clinical treatment of patients with advanced metastatic pancreatic, breast, and colon cancer, and use meta-analysis techniques to identify effective treatment protocols.

3.6   Examples

3.6.1   Complete Data with Concomitant Information

Feigl and Zelen [16] provide data on patients diagnosed with Acute Myelogonous Leukemia who subsequently undergo chemotherapy. The data consist of survival times (t_i) following diagnosis and white blood cell count (WBC $= x_i$) at diagnosis. Patients are stratified into two groups: AG^+ or AG^-. Patients were AG^+ if Auer rods and/or significant granulature of leukemia cells in the bone marrow were present at diagnosis, and AG^-, otherwise. The data appear in Table 3.1. Survival times $(t_i^+$ and $t_i^-)$ are recorded as weeks from diagnosis and WBC $(x_i^+$ and $x_i^-)$ are recorded as thousands. Of interest is the assessment of whether WBC is related to survival. Feigl and Zelen fit a separate exponential model to the survival times in each group, with hazard function given by $h(t_i) = (a + bx_i)^{-1}$. They use a chi-square goodness-of-fit test to assess adequacy of the model, and find that WBC is correlated with survival (strongly so for the AG^+ group).

Alternatively, we fit [54] the exponential (Section 3.3.1), Weibull (Section 3.3.2), Rayleigh (Section 3.3.3), and Gompertz (Section 3.3.4) models to the data, incorporating WBC (log WBC for computational purposes) via the proportional hazards model (Section 3.4.1). Parameters are estimated by maximizing the log-likelihood using the Nelder–Mead simplex search procedure [55,56], and are summarized in Table 3.2. From this table it is noted that the estimate of λ_1 in the Weibull model is not different from 1, and is virtually 0 in the Rayleigh and Gompertz models. Therefore, these three models are reduced to the exponential model, and we may conclude that the exponential model describes the data well.

The likelihood ratio test is used to assess the significance of the correlation between survival and WBC (*Note*: This is equivalent to testing H_0: $\beta = 0$, where β is the parameter associated with WBC in the proportional hazards model.). The

TABLE 3.1: Survival times and WBC counts of myelogonous leukemia patients.

t_i^-	2	3	3	3	4	4	4	8	16	17	17	22	30	43	56	65
x_i^-	27	10	21	28	19	26	100	31	9	1.5	4	5.3	7.9	100	4.4	3
t_i^+	1	1	4	5	16	22	26	39	56	65	54	100	108	121	134	143	156
x_i^+	100	100	17	52	6	35	32	5.4	9.4	2.3	100	4.3	10.5	10	2.6	7	0.75

TABLE 3.2: Maximum likelihood estimates of model parameters.

Parameters	Group	Model Estimates			
		Exponential	**Weibull**	**Raleigh**	**Gompertz**
λ_0	AG^-	0.01031	0.01216	3.00986	0.26134
	AG^+	0.00021	0.00019	1.75090	−0.07376
λ_1	AG^-	NA	0.96701	-0.47×10^{-6}	0
	AG^+	NA	1.02121	-0.2×10^{-2}	0
B	AG^-	0.40564	0.39158	3.41591	1.42910
	AG^+	1.10730	1.10780	−1.22290	1.68040
Log likelihood	AG^-	62.16597	62.15592	62.16558	∞
	AG^+	83.87757	83.87258	98.47643	∞

TABLE 3.3: Hazard rates with and without WBC in exponential model.

AG^- **Group**	AG^+ **Group**
Without WBC in the model	Without WBC in the model
Mean survival time = 18.56 weeks,	Mean survival time = 62.47 weeks,
$\lambda_0 = 1/18.56 = 0.0539$	$\lambda_0 = 1/62.47 = 0.0160$
With WBC in the model	With WBC in the model
$\lambda_0 = 0.0103$	$\lambda_0 = 0.0002$
$\beta = 0.4056$	$\beta = 1.1073$
$\lambda = \lambda_0 \exp[\beta*\text{Median(WBC)}]$	$\lambda = \lambda_0 \exp[\beta*\text{Median(WBC)}]$
$= (0.0103)\exp(0.4056)(4.30)]$	$= (0.0002)\exp(1.1073)(4.00)]$
$= 0.0589$	$= 0.0166$
$H_0: \beta = 0$ vs. $H_a: \beta \neq 0$	$H_0: \beta = 0$ vs. $H_a: \beta \neq 0$
$-2 \ln LR = \chi^2 = 2.10$ ($P > 0.05$)	$-2 \ln LR = \chi^2 = 6.83$ ($P < 0.01$)

results are summarized in the bottom row of Table 3.3, which shows that survival and WBC are strongly correlated [$\chi^2 = 6.83$ ($P < 0.01$)] in the AG^+ group.

Table 3.3 also includes estimated hazard functions without and with the covariate WBC. It is interesting to note that the hazard function without WBC is virtually identical to the hazard function incorporating WBC, when evaluated at median WBC.

3.6.2 Censored Data with Concomitant Information

Kalbfleisch and Prentice [3, pp. 223–224], provide data on 137 patients with advanced, inoperable lung cancer who participated in the Veteran Administration's Lung Cancer Trial and were treated with either standard or test chemotherapy. The data consist of observed survival time in days (from the time of chemotherapy initiation to death or last follow-up), survival time status (0 if censored; 1 if death), and covariates: Karnofsky performance scale score (KPS: 100 is maximum), months since diagnosis (difference between the time of randomization and the time

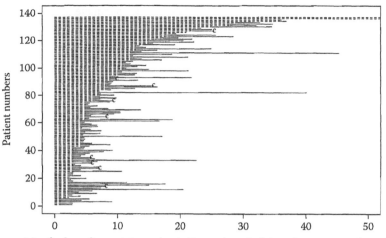

Months from diagnosis to randomization and survival time after treatment (months)
(dotted line: months from diagnosis; Solid line: survival time after treatment;
c: censored data)

FIGURE 3.6:   Patient enrollment and treatment profiles.

of diagnosis), age in years, prior therapy ($0 =$ no; $1 =$ yes), histological tumor type [squamous ($n = 35$), small cell ($n = 48$), adeno ($n = 28$), or large cell ($n = 27$)].

Patients were randomized to chemotherapy treatment groups. The objectives of the trial were to (A) compare the relative efficacy of the chemotherapy regimens in the treatment of male patients with advanced inoperable lung cancer in terms of survival; and (B) assess the correlation between survival and the covariates.

The data were analyzed to address the objectives as follows. First, months from diagnosis to randomization and survival times after treatment for all patients were plotted (Figure 3.6) as a continuum to get a feel for the total time from diagnosis to death (or censoring), to visually assess the possible predictive capacity of months from diagnosis on survival time, and to observe the pattern of censored observations across times to death. Second, the distribution of survival times was examined to determine a parametric model that fit the data well. Third, the covariates were examined to assess whether they satisfied the proportional hazards assumption of the Cox model. Fourth, the relationship between survival time and all covariates were examined. And finally, a regression analysis of survival time on the covariates was performed using S-PLUS. The results are summarized in the following sections.

3.6.2.1   Parametric Model Describing Survival Time

The monotonic transformation: $t^{0.12} - 0.75$ was applied to the original survival time data. A Weibull model with scale parameter (λ_0) $= 1$ and shape parameter (λ_1) $= 4.2$ described the transformed data well. The quantile–quantile plot is shown in Figure 3.7 and superimposed with a well-fitted 45° line. Minor deviations about

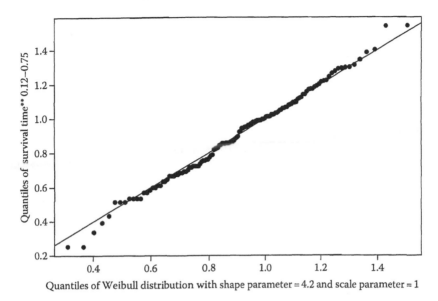

Quantiles of Weibull distribution with shape parameter = 4.2 and scale parameter = 1

FIGURE 3.7: Quantile plot of survival times.

the 45° line occur for a few data points at both two tails. However, these deviations do not present any major concern as real data hardly ever follow any theoretical distribution exactly.

3.6.2.2 Examining the Proportional Hazards Assumption

Figure 3.8 reflects the graphical diagnostic tests of the proportional hazards assumption (see Section 3.4.1 and Chapter 9) for each covariate. Even though there is some evidence that proportional hazards assumption holds for age, cell type, and months from diagnosis, it does not hold for the Karnofsky performance scores. Therefore, the Cox proportional hazards model (with the Weibull $h(t)$ to facilitate a parametric analysis) may provide misleading results if it is used to incorporate all covariate information simultaneously.

3.6.2.3 Relationship between Survival Time and Covariates

Survival times were plotted (Figure 3.9) against each covariate with a smooth curve superimposed to explore the possible relationship between the covariate and survival time. Age and month from diagnosis did not reveal any interesting relationship. The plot of survival times versus cell type appear to indicate that cell types 2 and 3 have shorter survival than the other two cell type categories. On the other hand, survival time and Karnofsky performance scores seem to be positively correlated (the higher the score, the longer the survival time).

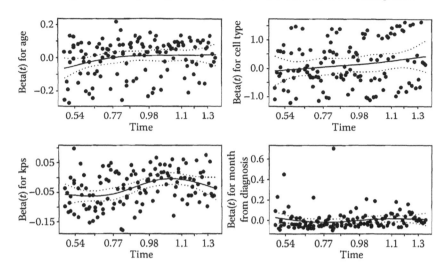

FIGURE 3.8: Assessing proportional hazards of regression model.

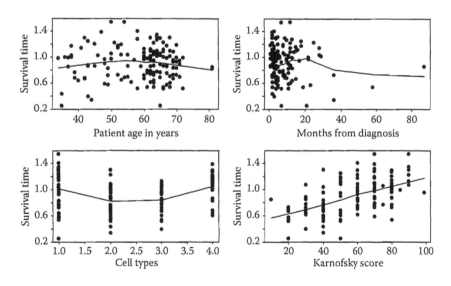

FIGURE 3.9: Relationship between survival time and key covariates.

3.6.2.4 Regression Analysis of Survival Time

Regression analysis of survival time (complete and censored data) on the covariates was performed using S-PLUS assuming the random error followed the Weibull model with parameters $\lambda_0 = 1$ and $\lambda_1 = 4.2$. Specifically, the nonrandom component of the regression model used is

TABLE 3.4: Summary of regression analysis of veterans administration (VA) lung cancer data.

Parameter	Estimate	Std. Err.	95% LCL	95% UCL	z-value	p-value
(Intercept)	−0.368478	0.15679	−0.67579	−0.06117	−2.3501	0.018
Treatment	−0.041538	0.03969	−0.11933	0.03626	−1.0465	0.295
Age	0.000528	0.00198	−0.00335	0.00440	0.2670	0.789
KPS	0.007720	0.00108	0.00561	0.00983	7.1813	<0.001
Cell_Type	−0.026021	0.01645	−0.05827	0.00623	−1.5815	0.114
Mo._Diag	−0.000100	0.00182	0.00367	0.00347	−0.0552	0.956

Note: −2 log-likelihood = −10.2 from the fitted model.

TABLE 3.5: Correlation coefficients for VA lung cancer covariates.

	(Intercept)	Treatment	AGE	KPS	Cell_Type
Treatment	−0.253				
AGE	−0.788	−0.157			
KPS	−0.545	−0.092	0.253		
Cell_Type	−0.265	0.114	0.000	−0.077	
Mo._Diag	−0.208	−0.037	0.085	0.131	0.016

$$\text{Survival time} = \text{Treatment} + \text{Age} + \text{KPS} + \text{Cell\_Type}$$
$$+ \text{Months\_from\_Diagnosis.}$$

The estimated coefficients, standard error, 95% confidence limits, z-values, and p-values appear in Table 3.4. Treatment groups did not differ statistically significantly, and Karnofsky performance score was the only covariate showing statistical significance.

Table 3.5 summarizes the correlation coefficients among all covariates.

3.7 Discussion

This chapter provides an overview of time-to-event parametric methods. The parameters: *hazard function, death density function, survival function*, and *cumulative death distribution function* were defined, and relationships between them noted. Five commonly used parametric models: *exponential, Weibull, Rayleigh, Gompertz*, and *lognormal* were then presented and discussed, and ways to incorporate concomitant, covariate, or regressor information into these models specified. Numerous applications from the literature, reflecting a variety of statistical methods for analyzing time-to-event endpoints were summarized. Two examples illustrating analysis and interpretation of the parametric models incorporating concomitant information were presented in detail.

References

[1] Cox DR (1972): Regression models and life tables. *Journal of Royal Statistical Society, Series B*, 34: 187–220.

[2] Prentice RL (1978): Linear rank tests with right censored data. *Biometrika*, 65: 167–179.

[3] Kalbfleisch JD and Prentice RL (1980): *The Statistical Analysis of Failure Time Data*. New York: Wiley.

[4] Wei LJ (1992): The accelerated failure time model: A useful alternative to the Cox regression model in survival analysis. *Statistics in Medicine*, 11(14–15): 1871–1879.

[5] Collett D (2003): *Modeling Survival Data in Medical Research*, 2nd edn. Chapman & Hall/CRC Boca Raton, FL.

[6] Gross AJ and Clark VA (1975): *Survival Distributions: Reliability Theory in the Biomedical Sciences*. New York: John Wiley & Sons.

[7] Elandt-Johnson RC and Johnson NL (1980): *Survival Models and Data Analysis*. New York: John Wiley & Sons.

[8] Miller RG Jr. (1981): *Survival Analysis*. New York: John Wiley & Sons.

[9] Lawless JF (1982): *Statistical Models and Methods for Lifetime Data*. New York: John Wiley & Sons.

[10] Cox DR and Oakes D (1984): *Analysis of Survival Data*. London: Chapman & Hall.

[11] Lee ET (1992): *Statistical Methods for Survival Data Analysis*, 2nd edn. New York: John Wiley & Sons.

[12] Allison PD (1995): *Survival Analysis using the SAS System: A Practical Guide*. Cary, NC: SAS Institute Press.

[13] Klein JP and Moeschberger ML (1997): *Survival Analysis: Techniques for Censored and Truncated Data*. New York: Springer Series in Statistics for Biology and Health.

[14] Harrell FE (2001): *Regression Modeling Strategies, with Applications to Linear Models, Survival Analysis and Logistic Regression*. New York: Springer Series in Statistics.

[15] Klein JP and Moeschberger ML (2003): *Survival Analysis: Techniques for Censored and Truncated Data*, 2nd edn. New York: Springer Series in Statistics for Biology and Health.

[16] Fiegl P and Zelen M (1965): Estimation of exponential probabilities with concomitant information. *Biometrics*, 21: 826–838.

[17] Zippin C and Armitage P (1966): Use of concomitant variables and incomplete survival information in the estimation of an exponential survival parameter. *Biometrics*, 22: 665–672.

[18] Zelen M (1966): Applications of exponential models to problems in cancer research. *Journal of the Royal Statistical Society, Series A*, 129: 368–398.

[19] Byar DP, Huse R, and Bailar JC (1974): An exponential model relating censored survival data and concomitant information for prostatic cancer patients. *Journal of the National Cancer Institute*, 52(2): 321–326.

[20] Gage BF, Waterman AD, Shannon W, Boechler M, Rich MW, and Radford MJ (2001): Validation of clinical classification schemes for predicting stroke: Results from the National Registry of Atrial Fibrillation. *Journal of the American Medical Association*, 285: 2864–2870.

[21] Friedman M (1982): Piecewise exponential models for survival data with covariates. *The Annals of Statistics*, 10(1): 101–113.

[22] Maller RA (1988): On the exponential model for survival. *Biometrika*, 75(3): 582–586.

[23] Menon M (1963): Estimation of the shape and scale parameters of the Weibull distributions. *Technometrics*, 5: 175–182.

[24] Cohen AC (1965): Maximum likelihood estimation in the Weibull distribution based on complete and censored samples. *Technometrics*, 5: 579–588.

[25] Harter HL and Moore AH (1967): Asymptotic variances and covariances of maximum likelihood estimators from censored samples of the parameters of Weibull and Gamma populations. *Annals of Mathematical Statistics*, 38: 557–570.

[26] Dubey SD (1967): Normal and Weibull distributions. *Naval Research Logistics Quarterly*, 14: 69–79.

[27] Crow LH (1982): Confidence interval procedures for the Weibull process with applications to reliability growth. *Technometrics*, 24: 67–72.

[28] Anderson KM (1991): A nonproportional hazards Weibull accelerated failure time regression model. *Biometrics*, 47: 281–288.

[29] Liao C (2003): Prognosis of small hepatocellular carcinoma treated by percutaneous ethanol injection and transcatheter arterial chemoembolization. *Journal of Clinical Epidemiology*, 55(11): 1095–1104.

[30] Carroll KJ (2003): On the use and utility of the Weibull model in the analysis of survival data. *Controlled Clinical Trials*, 24(6): 682–701.

[31] Bain L (1974): Analysis for the linear failure-rate life testing distribution. *Technometrics*, 15(4): 551–559.

[32] Bhattacharya SK and Tyagi RK (1990): Bayesian survival analysis based on the Rayleigh model. *Test*, 5(1): 81–92.

[33] Sen A and Bhattacharyya G (1995): Inference procedures for the linear failure rate model. *Journal of Statistical Planning and Inference*, 46: 59–76.

[34] Indika SHS and Hossain AM (2005): Rayleigh parameter estimation using progressive Type-II right censored data. *Journal of Statistical Studies*, 25: 43–53.

[35] Mahdi S (2006): Improved Parameter Estimation in Rayleigh Model. *Metodološki zvezki*, 3(1): 63–74.

[36] Garg ML, Rao BR, and Redmond CK (1970): Maximum-likelihood estimation of the parameters of the Gompertz survival function. *Applied Statistics*, 19(2): 152–159.

[37] Wu JW, Hung WL, and Tsai CH (2003): Estimation of parameters of the Gompertz distribution using the least squares method. *Journal of Applied Mathematics and Computation*, 158(1): 133–147.

[38] Wu JW and Li PL (2004): Optimal estimation of the parameters of the Gompertz distribution based on the doubly Type II censored sample. *Quality and Quantity*, 38: 753–769.

[39] Ananda MM, Dalpatadu RJ, and Singh AK (1996): Adaptive Bayes estimators for parameters of the Gompertz survival model. *Applied Mathematics and Computation*, 75(2–3): 167–177.

[40] Peter W, Gieser PW, Chang MN, Rao PV, Shuster JJ, and Pullen J (1998): Modeling cure rates using the Gompertz model with covariate information. *Statistics in Medicine*, 17(8): 831–839.

[41] Ricklefs RE and Scheuerlein A (2002): Biological implications of the Weibull and Gompertz models of aging. *The Journals of Gerontology Series A: Biological Sciences and Medical Sciences*, 57: B69–B76.

[42] Boag JW (1948): The presentation and analysis of the results of radiotherapy. Part I. Introduction. *British Journal of Radiology*, 21: 128–138.

[43] Boag JW (1948): The presentation and analysis of the results of radiotherapy. Part II. Mathematical theory. *British Journal of Radiology*, 21: 189–203.

[44] Boag JW (1949): Maximum likelihood estimates of the proportion of patients cured by cancer therapy. *Journal of the Royal Statistical Society (Series B)*, 11: 15–53.

[45] Mould RF and Boag JW (1975): A test of several parametric statistical models for estimating success rate in the treatment of carcinoma cervix uteri. *British Journal of Cancer*, 32: 529–550.

[46] Mould RF, Hearnden T, Palmer M, and White GC (1976): Distribution of survival times of 12,000 head and neck cancer patients who died with their disease. *British Journal of Cancer*, 34: 180–190.

[47] Rutqvist LE (1985): On the utility of the lognormal model for analysis of breast cancer survival in Sweden: 1961–1973. *British Journal of Cancer*, 52: 875–883.

[48] Gamel JW, Greenberg RA, and McLean IW (1988): A stable linear algorithm for fitting the lognormal model to survival data. *Computers and Biomedical Research*, 21: 38–47.

[49] Gamel JW, George SL, Edwards MJ, and Seigler HF (2002): The long-term clinical course of patients with cutaneous melanoma. *Cancer*, 95: 1286–1293.

[50] Tai P, Tonita J, Yu E, and Skarsgard D (2003): A 20-year follow-up study of the long-term survival of limited stage small cell lung cancer and an overview of prognostic and treatment factors. *International Journal of Radiation Oncology Biology Physics*, 56: 626–633.

[51] Tai P, Yu E, Shiels R, and Tonita J (2005): Long-term survival rates of laryngeal cancer patients treated by radiation and surgery, radiation alone, and surgery alone: Studied by lognormal and Kaplan–Meier survival methods. *BMC Cancer*, 5(13): doi: 10.1186/1471-2407-5-13.

[52] Tai P, Yu E, Shiels R, Pacella J, Jones K, Sadikov E, and Mahmood S (2005): Short- and long-term cause-specific survival of patients with inflammatory breast cancer. *BMC Cancer*, 5: 137: doi: 10.1186/1471-2407-5-137.

[53] Qazi S, DuMez D, and Uckun FM (2007): Meta analysis of advanced cancer survival data using lognormal parametric fitting: A statistical method to identify effective treatment protocols. *Current Pharmaceutical Design*, 13(15): 1533–1544.

[54] Peace KE (1976): Maximum likelihood estimation and efficiency assessments of tests of hypotheses on survival parameters. Doctoral Dissertation, Medical College of Virginia, Richmond.

[55] Olsson DM (1974): A sequential simplex program for solving minimization problems. *Journal of Quality Technology*, 6(1): 53–57.

[56] Olsson DM and Nelson LA (1974): The Nelder-Mead simplex procedure for function minimization. *Technometrics*, 17(1): 45–51.

Chapter 4

Overview of Semiparametric Inferential Methods for Time-to-Event Endpoints

Jianwen Cai and Donglin Zeng

Contents

4.1 Introduction

The parametric methods described in Chapter 3 can be useful in the analysis of survival data when the survival time can be assumed to follow a certain distribution. If the distribution is correctly assumed, the resulting estimates are most efficient. However, incorrect specification of the distribution can lead to misleading conclusions. Semiparametric models without having to specify the distribution of the survival time are desirable when it is unclear which distribution should be assumed.

In this chapter, we will discuss the inference associated with semiparametric Cox regression model. We will review the partial likelihood used for estimation of the regression parameters and discuss issues associated with tied data, time-dependent covariates, and model diagnostics. We will also review briefly on the extension of the Cox regression model to correlated events. Examples from biomedical studies will be used for illustration.

4.2   Methods

4.2.1   Cox Proportional Hazards Model and the Partial Likelihood

As mentioned in the previous chapters, what makes time-to-event endpoints data distinct from others is the issue of *censoring*, either intentional, for example, the termination of trials before the event of interest occurs, or unintentional, such as loss of follow-up. Another fundamental aspect with time-to-event endpoints data is the conditioning principle which corresponds to the concept of being at risk (of failure). For example, a subject is only at risk of death if the subject is alive currently. The conditioning principle naturally leads us to the discussion of the distribution of the failure time T via the hazard function $\lambda(t)$, which is defined as the instantaneous rate of failure probability, given that the subject has not failed at the beginning of the interval. Specifically, the hazard function $\lambda(t)$ is defined as

$$\lambda(t) = \lim_{h \downarrow 0} \frac{1}{h} \Pr(t \leq T < t + h | T \geq t).$$

The hazard rate function $\lambda(t)$ measures the instantaneous potential of failure at time t given survival up to time t. By definition, the hazard rate function uniquely determines the distribution of T. Particularly, the relationship between the survival function $S(t) = P(T \geq t)$ and the hazard rate function is $S(t) = \exp\{-\int_0^t \lambda(s)ds\}$.

Hazard ratio, defined as the ratio of the hazard rate functions for two groups, is commonly used as a summary statistic when comparing the survival distributions of two groups. When survival functions are compared across multiple groups or sub-populations, a commonly used model is to assume that hazard ratios are proportional across groups or subpopulations over time. This model is called the proportional hazards (PH) model. Cox PH model is a PH model without specifying the distribution of the time-to-event endpoint (Cox [6]).

Cox PH model specifies the hazard rate function $\lambda(t; \mathbf{Z})$ for an individual with covariate vector $\mathbf{Z}$ as

$$\lambda(t; \mathbf{Z}) = \lambda_0(t) \exp\{\boldsymbol{\beta}'\mathbf{Z}\}, \quad t \geq 0, \tag{4.1}$$

where
$\lambda_0(t)$ is an unknown and unspecified nonnegative function, and
$\boldsymbol{\beta}$ is a p-vector of unknown regression coefficients.

The function $\lambda_0(t)$ is referred to as the baseline hazard function and it corresponds to the hazard rate for an individual with covariate vector $\mathbf{Z} = 0$.

Since the functional form of $\lambda_0(t)$ is unspecified, this leaves the distribution of the failure times to be unspecified. On the other hand, the covariates are specified to influence the hazard rate function multiplicatively. Hence, model (Equation 4.1) is a semi parametric model, in that the effect of the covariates on the hazard is explicitly specified while the distribution of the failure time is unspecified. Each regression coefficient in model (Equation 4.1) represents the log hazard ratio for one unit increase in the corresponding covariate given that the other covariates in the model are held at the same value. For example, consider a clinical trial comparing a treatment group with a placebo group. Let $Z=1$ for the treatment group and $Z=0$ for the placebo group. Let Male be an indicator for male gender, i.e., Male $=1$ for male patients and Male $=0$ for female patients. The Cox PH model for studying the effect of treatment after adjusting for gender is $\lambda(t) = \lambda_0(t) \exp(\beta_{trt} Z + \beta_{Male} \text{Male})$. The coefficient β_{trt} is the log hazard ratio for comparing the treatment group to the placebo group for patients of the same gender, while β_{Male} is the log hazard ratio for comparing male patients to female patients within the same treatment group.

One important reason for specialized statistical methods for failure time data is the need to accommodate censoring in the data. Typical failure time data are subject to right-censoring, where some study subjects are only observed to survive beyond certain time points. Independent censoring mechanism is usually assumed; that is, the probability of failing in the interval $[t, t+dt)$ given all failure and censoring information as well as all information on the covariates up to time t is the same as the probability of failing in the interval $[t, t+dt)$ given that the subject survived up to time t and given all information on the covariates up to time t. Let C denote the potential censoring time. The observed time is $X = \min(T,C)$. Under independent censoring mechanism, i.e.,

$$P(t \leq T < t + dt | T \geq t, C \geq t, \mathbf{Z}) = P(t \leq T < t + dt | T \geq t, \mathbf{Z})$$

the estimation of the regression parameter β in Equation 4.1 can be carried out by applying standard asymptotic likelihood procedures to the "partial" likelihood function ([7])

$$\mathcal{L}(\beta) = \prod_{i=1}^{n} \left\{ \frac{e^{\beta' z_i}}{\sum_{j \in \mathcal{R}_i} e^{\beta' z_j}} \right\}^{\delta_i}, \tag{4.2}$$

where
$\mathbf{Z}_i$ is the covariate vector for subject i,
$\mathcal{R}_i = \{j : X_j \geq X_i\}$ where $X_1, \ldots, X_n$ are the observed times, and
δ_i is an indicator for failure.

In fact, the ith factor associated with $\delta_i = 1$ in Equation 4.2 is precisely the probability that the subject with covariate vector $\mathbf{Z}_i$ fails at X_i given the failure, censoring and covariate information prior to X_i on all subjects in the sample, and given that exactly one failure occurred at X_i. The estimator of β, denoted by $\hat{\beta}$, is obtained by maximizing the partial likelihood, which is equivalent to solving the score equation $\mathcal{U}(\boldsymbol{\beta}) = 0$, provided finite maximum exists, where the score is

$$\mathcal{U}(\boldsymbol{\beta}) = \nabla_{\boldsymbol{\beta}} \log \mathcal{L}(\boldsymbol{\beta}) = \sum_{i=1}^{n} \delta_i \{ \mathbf{Z}_i - \mathbf{E}_i(X_i; \boldsymbol{\beta}) \} \tag{4.3}$$

with

$$\mathbf{E}_i(X_i; \boldsymbol{\beta}) = \frac{\sum_{j \in \mathcal{R}_i} \mathbf{Z}_j e^{\boldsymbol{\beta}' z_j}}{\sum_{j \in \mathcal{R}_i} e^{\boldsymbol{\beta}' z_j}}.$$

Note that $\mathcal{U}(\boldsymbol{\beta})$ is the sum of random variables that have a conditional, and hence an unconditional, mean of zero so that $\mathcal{U}(\boldsymbol{\beta}) = 0$ provides an unbiased estimating equation for $\boldsymbol{\beta}$. It was pointed out that in the special case of the two sample problem $\mathcal{U}(0)$ reduces to the logrank test [16, 23]. Iterative procedures, such as Newton–Raphson method, is commonly used to solve the score equation.

The partial likelihood given in Equation 4.2, which differs from a marginal or conditional likelihood, was first introduced by Cox [7]. It was later justified (cf. [15]) that Equation 4.2 is also the profile likelihood function for $\boldsymbol{\beta}$. Hence, standard theory for parametric likelihood function is applicable under suitable regularity conditions. For example, the inverse of $-\nabla^2_{\boldsymbol{\beta}\boldsymbol{\beta}} \log \mathcal{L}(\hat{\boldsymbol{\beta}})$ is a consistent estimator of the asymptotic variance of $\hat{\boldsymbol{\beta}}$. The Wald's test, score test, or likelihood ratio test for comparing two nested models can also be carried out using the partial likelihood. The formal justification of the asymptotic properties for $\hat{\boldsymbol{\beta}}$ was given in Andersen and Gill [1] using the martingale theory.

After the Cox model fit, following Oakes [20] or Breslow [2], the estimator for the cumulative baseline hazard function, defined as $\Lambda_0(t) = \int_0^t \lambda_0(s) ds$, is given by

$$\hat{\Lambda}_0(t) = \sum_{X_i < t} \frac{\delta_i}{\sum_{j \in \mathcal{R}_i} e^{\hat{\boldsymbol{\beta}}' z_j}}. \tag{4.4}$$

Hence, for any given values of $\mathbf{Z}$, we can estimate the cumulative hazard function and survival function using $\hat{\Lambda}(t|\mathbf{Z}) = \hat{\Lambda}_0(t) e^{\hat{\boldsymbol{\beta}}' z}$ and $\hat{S}(t|\mathbf{Z}) = [\hat{S}_0(t)]^{e^{\hat{\boldsymbol{\beta}}' z}}$. In the special case of one homogenous population, i.e., there are no covariates, Equation 4.4 reduces to the Nelson–Aalen estimator for the cumulative hazard.

4.2.2   Counting Process Formulation

Counting process is commonly used in the statistical inference with censored event. By definition, a counting process is a stochastic process over time and the value at each time t is the count of the event occurrences by time t. We usually use $N_i(t)$ to denote the observed counting process for subject i. Thus, for survival data, $N_i(t)$ is equivalent to $\delta_i I(X_i \leq t)$, where X_i is the observed event time for subject i. Additionally, we use $Y_i(t)$ to denote the process on whether subject i is at risk at time t, i.e., $Y_i(t) = I(X_i \geq t)$. With the counting process notation, Equation 4.3 can be rewritten as

$$\sum_{i=1}^{n} \int \left\{ \mathbf{Z}_i - \frac{\sum_{j=1}^{n} Y_j(t)\mathbf{Z}_j e^{\boldsymbol{\beta}' \mathbf{z}_j}}{\sum_{j=1}^{n} Y_j(t) e^{\boldsymbol{\beta}' \mathbf{z}_j}} \right\} dN_i(t) = 0. \tag{4.5}$$

One key fact in the counting process theory is that under independent censorship, $N_i(t)$ can be decomposed into

$$N_i(t) = Y_i(t)\Lambda_i(t) + M_i(t),$$

or equivalently

$$dN_i(t) = Y_i(t)d\Lambda_i(t) + dM_i(t),$$

where
  $\Lambda_i(t)$ is the cumulative hazard function for subject i, and
  $M_i(t)$ is a martingale process with respect to some σ-field filter.

Such a decomposition is useful in deriving the asymptotic property for the estimators in the Cox model, owing to the fruitful results in the martingale theory. For example, since $\Lambda_i(t) = \Lambda_0(t)e^{\boldsymbol{\beta}' \mathbf{z}_i}$ under the Cox model, the left-hand side of Equation 4.5 is equivalent to

$$\sum_{i=1}^{n} \int \left\{ \mathbf{Z}_i - \frac{\sum_{j=1}^{n} Y_j(t)\mathbf{Z}_j e^{\boldsymbol{\beta}' \mathbf{z}_j}}{\sum_{j=1}^{n} Y_j(t) e^{\boldsymbol{\beta}' \mathbf{z}_j}} \right\} dM_i(t),$$

which has the form of $\sum_{i=1}^{n} \int H_i(t)dM_i(t)$ with $H_i(t)$ being some predictive process. Thus, from the martingale central limit theorem (cf. [9]), this type of process weakly converges to a Gaussian process. Similarly, using the martingale theory, we can show the derivative of the left-hand side of Equation 4.5 with respect to $\boldsymbol{\beta}$ divided by n converges to a nonsingular matrix. These two facts, along with some additional conditions, can be used to show that $\hat{\boldsymbol{\beta}}$ is consistent and has an asymptotical normal distribution.

In summary, the counting process theory has been extensively and successfully used in studying the asymptotic distribution of the estimators in the Cox model. Although the recent use of the empirical process theory has been demonstrated more powerful, the counting process formulation is still used by many users for its simplicity.

4.2.3   Modified Partial Likelihood for Stratified or Tied Data

The Cox partial likelihood function can be modified to include stratified or tied data. In the stratified data, study population may consist of more than one distinct subpopulations. The results without adjusting for the differences among strata can be biased and misleading. Thus, to account for systematic differences across different strata, a stratified Cox PH model assumes that for stratum $j, j = 1, \ldots, K$, the hazards rate function is given by

$$\lambda_j(t; \mathbf{Z}) = \lambda_{0j}(t)e^{\boldsymbol{\beta}' \mathbf{z}}. \tag{4.6}$$

In other words, the modified model allows for different baseline hazards rate function for different strata but assumes the common effect of $\mathbf{Z}$ across strata. The estimator for $\boldsymbol{\beta}$ under models (Equation 4.6) can be obtained by maximizing the following stratified partial likelihood function

$$\mathcal{L}_S(\hat{\boldsymbol{\beta}}) = \prod_{j=1}^{K} \prod_{i=1}^{n_j} \left\{ \frac{e^{\boldsymbol{\beta}'\mathbf{z}_{ij}}}{\sum_{l \in \mathcal{R}_{ij}} e^{\boldsymbol{\beta}'\mathbf{z}_{lj}}} \right\}^{\delta_{ij}},$$

where

n_j is the number of subjects in the jth stratum,

$\mathcal{R}_{ij}$ denote risk set of subject i in the jth stratum, and

$\mathbf{Z}_{ij}$ and δ_{ij} are the corresponding covariates and censoring indicators.

For fixed K, it can be shown that when $\min\{n_j, j = 1, \ldots, K\} \to \infty$, the estimator for $\boldsymbol{\beta}$ is consistent and asymptotically normal and that the asymptotic covariance can be consistently estimated by the inverse of $-\nabla^2_{\boldsymbol{\beta}\boldsymbol{\beta}} \log \mathcal{L}_S(\hat{\boldsymbol{\beta}})$. However, when the number of strata is large, for example, the stratum is determined by categorizing a continuous confounder, the above inference may be incorrect; instead, one can fit the usual Cox PH model by including the stratifying variable into the regression model.

Tied data are common in most of practice, due to imprecise measures of continuous times. In the tied data, the true time ordering of the ties is not observed. Thus, the partial likelihood function in Equation 4.2 should be modified to reflect this ordering. One approach is to consider all possible orderings for the tied events, for instance, if we see d tied observations, then the total number of the possible orderings among these d events is $d!$ Then the contribution of these d observations in the partial likelihood function should be the summation of the contributions from all these $d!$ possibilities. Mathematically, suppose we observe untied events $X_{(1)} < X_{(2)} < \cdots < X_{(m)}$ and there are d_i tied observations at $X_{(i)}$. Then the modified partial likelihood function should be

$$\prod_{i=1}^{m} \left[\sum_{X_{(i).1} < X_{(i).2} < \cdots < X_{(i).d_i}} \prod_{j=1}^{d_i} \frac{e^{\boldsymbol{\beta}'\mathbf{z}_{(i).j}}}{\sum_{k \in \mathcal{R}_{(i).j}} e^{\boldsymbol{\beta}'\mathbf{z}_k}} \right],$$

where

$X_{(i).1}, \ldots, X_{(i).d_i}$ are the potential times for the d_i tied events at $X_{(i)}$,

$\mathbf{Z}_{(i),j}$ is the corresponding covariates, and

$\mathcal{R}_{(i),j}$ is the corresponding risk set.

Since the above partial likelihood function reflects the actual probabilities of all the orderings, such a method of handling ties is exact. One drawback of the exact method is that computation can be very intensive if there are many tied observations. Instead, for most of the practical use, there are two approximation approaches which are relatively simple in computation to handle ties. Particularly, Breslow [2] suggests treating the ties actually occur sequentially as if they were distinct. Therefore, the partial likelihood function is

$$\prod_{i=1}^{m} \left[\frac{\prod_{j=1}^{d_i} e^{\beta' z_{(i)j}}}{\left(\sum_{k \in \mathcal{R}_{(i)}} e^{\beta' z_k} \right)^{d_i}} \right].$$

Alternatively, in the approach suggested by Efron [8], one replaces $\left(\sum_{k \in \mathcal{R}_{(i)}} e^{\beta' z_k} \right)^{d_i}$ in the above expression by

$$\prod_{j=1}^{d_i} \left\{ \frac{j}{d_i} \sum_{k \text{ is one of } d_i \text{ tied events}} e^{\beta' z_k} + \sum_{k \in \mathcal{R}_{(i)} \text{ excluding } d_i \text{ tied events}} e^{\beta' z_k} \right\}.$$

Empirically, Breslow approximation works well when the number of ties is relatively small; Efron's approximation yields results closer to the exact results than Breslow's approximation with only trivial increase in computer time. Most software uses Breslow approximation as default.

4.2.4 Cox Regression Model Incorporating Time-Dependent Covariates

So far, we have been discussing the Cox PH model with time-independent covariates. In practice, some covariates affecting the event may vary over time and they are termed time-dependent covariates. Time-dependent covariates can be further categorized into external and internal ([14], 6.3). The former refers to those which are not dependent on a subject's survival for their value at any time, for example, temperature and amount of pollution or radiation in an area; while the latter refers to those which can only be measured or only have meaning when the subject is alive. Examples of the internal time-dependent covariates include white blood cell (WBC) count over time, systolic blood pressure over time, and spread of cancer over time.

For time-dependent covariates $\mathbf{Z}(t)$, the Cox model can incorporate $\mathbf{Z}(t)$ into consideration by assuming

$$\lambda(t|\mathbf{Z}) = \lambda_0(t) e^{\beta' z(t)}.$$

Under this model, the hazard ratio for comparing subjects with $\mathbf{Z}(t)$ vs. subjects with $\tilde{\mathbf{Z}}(t)$ is equal to $e^{\beta'(z(t) - \tilde{z}(t))}$, which is no longer independent of t. In parallel, the partial likelihood function is modified to

$$\mathcal{L}(\beta) = \prod_{i=1}^{n} \left\{ \frac{e^{\beta' z_i(X_i)}}{\sum_{j \in \mathcal{R}_i} e^{\beta' z_j(X_i)}} \right\}^{\delta_i},$$

where $\mathbf{Z}_i(t)$ is the covariate process for subject i. Inference procedure for β can be carried out as before.

One caution of using internal time-dependent covariate in fitting Cox model is the interpretation of its effect, since such covariate often lies in the causal pathway about which one wants to make inferences. For example, in a clinical trial for the effect of immunotherapy in the treatment of metastatic colorectal carcinoma, adjusting for most recent depressed white blood cell count (WBC) would make treatment comparison among subjects with like prognosis at each time. However, immunotherapy might improve prognosis by improving WBC over time and adjustment for WBC over time might remove the apparent effect of treatment, since treated and control subjects with the same WBC might have similar prognosis.

4.2.5   PH Model Diagnostics

In the Cox PH model, one crucial assumption for the PH model is that the hazard ratio for different values of a time-independent covariate is constant over time. There are many ways to check such proportionality assumptions in practice. We review some diagnostic methods in the following.

The first way of checking proportionality is via parametric test. In this approach, we introduce an interaction term between the covariate being assessed and a specified function of time. Thus, to check the PH assumption, we can test the null hypothesis that the interaction is not significant. Obviously, this approach may not detect other forms of departure from the proportionality.

The second way of checking proportionality is to assess the time-varying effect of the covariates. In this approach, we fit a Cox PH model by assuming different effects of covariates in different time periods. By testing the equality of these effects, it can reveal the evidence of nonproportionality.

The third way is to assess the proportionality nonparametrically. Particularly, we use the fact that under the PH assumption,

$$\log\left(-\log S(t|\mathbf{Z})\right) = -\boldsymbol{\beta}'\mathbf{Z} + \log\left(-\log S_0(t)\right),$$

where

$S(t|\mathbf{Z})$ is the conditional survival function given $\mathbf{Z}$, and
$S_0(t) = \exp\{-\Lambda_0(t)\}$.

Therefore, the survival functions for all levels of $\mathbf{Z}$ should be parallel. We can then examine the plot of $\log(-\log \hat{S}(t|\mathbf{Z}))$ for assessing the PH assumption for a single discrete variable $\mathbf{Z}$, where $\hat{S}(t|\mathbf{Z})$ is estimated nonparametrically or using stratified Cox regression when other covariates need to be controlled for. When $\mathbf{Z}$ is continuous, we may stratify $\mathbf{Z}$ into some finite levels then carry out as a discrete covariate.

Residuals from fitting the Cox PH model can also be used for diagnostics. Particularly, the so-called Schoenfeld residuals, defined as $Z_{ij}(X_i) - \overline{Z}_j(X_i)$, where

$$\overline{Z}_j(t) = \frac{\sum_{l=1}^{n} I(X_l \geq t) Z_{lj}(t) e^{\hat{\boldsymbol{\beta}}' \mathbf{z}_l(t)}}{\sum_{l=1}^{n} I(X_l \geq t) e^{\hat{\boldsymbol{\beta}}' \mathbf{z}_l(t)}},$$

can be used. If the PH assumption holds, such residuals should be a random walk so they should be randomly scattered about zero if the PH assumption holds. Any clear trend in the Schoenfeld residuals reflects how the effect of the covariate is varying over time.

4.2.6 Extending Cox Model to Correlated Events

Correlated events are common in medical studies. In most of the cases, events are correlated due to either cluster events or multiple types of events. Clustered events refer to the events of the multiple subjects from the same cluster, for example, patients in the same clinic. Since these subjects are from the same cluster, their events tend to be correlated. Multiple types of events refer to the different types of events experienced by the same subject, for example, a patient with cardiovascular disease may experience stroke, and myocardial infarction. These events are of different types but are obviously dependent on each other.

The Cox PH model can be extended to correlated events. However, since correlated events may arise through different mechanism, the extension is different. Additionally, there are many different ways of modeling and inferences, we focus our attention to a marginal model where the marginal distribution of each event is modeled.

For clustered events, suppose that $\lambda_{ij}(t)$ denotes the hazards rate function for subject i in cluster j, $j = 1, \ldots, m$, $i = 1, \ldots, n_j$. We assume

$$\lambda_{ij}(t) = \lambda_0(t) e^{\beta' z_{ij}},$$

where $\mathbf{Z}_{ij}$ is the associated covariates. Again, β can be estimated by maximizing the following pseduopartial likelihood function

$$\prod_{j=1}^{m} \prod_{i=1}^{n_j} \left\{ \frac{e^{\beta' z_{ij}}}{\sum_{k \in \mathcal{R}_{ij}} e^{\beta' z_k}} \right\}^{\delta_{ij}},$$

where $\mathcal{R}_{ij}$ is the risk set for subject i in cluster j. Equivalently, the estimator solves equation

$$\mathcal{U}(\beta) = \sum_{j=1}^{m} \sum_{i=1}^{n_j} \delta_{ij} \left[\mathbf{Z}_{ij} - \frac{\sum_{k \in \mathcal{R}_{ij}} \mathbf{Z}_k e^{\beta' z_k}}{\sum_{k \in \mathcal{R}_{ij}} e^{\beta' z_k}} \right] = 0.$$

Since the events in the same cluster are correlated, the asymptotic variance for the estimator must be estimated using the sandwiched estimator as in the generalized estimating equation, that is, one consistent estimator for the asymptotic covariance is

$$m \left[\nabla_\beta \mathcal{U}(\hat{\beta}) \right]^{-1} \left[\sum_{j=1}^{m} \left\{ \sum_{i=1}^{n_j} \delta_{ij} \left[\mathbf{Z}_{ij} - \frac{\sum_{k \in \mathcal{R}_{ij}} \mathbf{Z}_k e^{\hat{\beta}' z_k}}{\sum_{k \in \mathcal{R}_{ij}} e^{\hat{\beta}' z_k}} \right] \right\}^{\otimes 2} \right] \left[\nabla_\beta \mathcal{U}(\hat{\beta}) \right]^{-1}.$$

When the correlated events are multiple types and suppose $\lambda_{ik}(t)$ denotes the hazards rate function of event type k for subject i, $i = 1, \ldots, n$, $k = 1, \ldots, K$, the Cox PH model can be extended by assuming

$$\lambda_{ik}(t) = \lambda_k(t)e^{\beta_k' z}.$$

That is, we use different baseline functions and different covariates effects for each event type. The estimator for β_k then maximizes the partial likelihood function

$$\prod_{i=1}^{n} \left\{ \frac{e^{\beta_k' z_i}}{\sum_{j \in \mathcal{R}_{ik}} e^{\beta_k' z_j}} \right\}^{\delta_{ik}},$$

where $\mathcal{R}_{ik}$ is the risk set for subject i associated with event k. The inference for estimating β_k can be obtained as the usual Cox model. However, the inference for the joint distribution of the estimators for $\beta_1, \ldots, \beta_K$ has to account for the correlations among the events and the sandwiched estimator must be used for estimating their asymptotic covariance.

4.3   Applications

4.3.1   Data Example Illustrating Model Building and Model Diagnostics for Cox PH Model

We illustrate how to fit the Cox PH model using a melanoma dataset from an Eastern Cooperative Oncology Group (ECOG) phase III clinical trial [24]. This trial was a two-arm clinical trial comparing high-dose interferon (IFN) to observation (OBS). The goal is to examine the effect of IFN on overall survival, as compared to OBS. IFN is approved by the U.S. Food and Drug Administration (FDA) as an adjuvant therapy for high-risk melanoma patients. Other risk factors included age at entry (in years), gender, performance status ($0 = $ excellent, $1 = $ ambulatory), number of positive nodes, breslow thickness of tumor, and stage of disease with four ordinal values. The data we use contain 234 subjects and the censoring rates for time-to-death is 42%.

Fitting the Cox model can be done either using "coxph" in R package or "PHREG" in SAS package. For this dataset, there are four tied death events so the Efron method is used to handle ties. Table 4.1 summarizes the results from such a model.

The results indicate that there exists no significant difference among different levels of disease stages or between two genders. Moreover, the effects of age and breslow thickness are not statistically significant. Thus, we refit another model by removing these covariates. The difference of the log-likelihood functions between

TABLE 4.1:   Analysis of melanoma data: Full model.

Covariates	Estimate	Standard Error	z-Stat	p-Value
IFN vs. OBS	−0.305	0.175	−1.745	0.081
Age	0.010	0.007	1.429	0.150
Sex	−0.123	0.183	−0.672	0.500
Perform	−0.581	0.322	−1.804	0.071
Nodes	0.396	0.112	3.552	0.0004
Breslow	−0.014	0.024	−0.570	0.570
Stage 2 vs. 1	0.0169	0.440	0.038	0.970
Stage 3 vs. 1	0.3447	0.448	0.769	0.440
Stage 4 vs. 1	0.0929	0.393	0.236	0.810

TABLE 4.2:   Analysis of melanoma data: Reduced model.

Covariates	Estimate	Standard Error	z-Stat	p-Value
IFN vs. OBS	−0.291	0.172	−1.68	0.092
Perform	−0.532	0.316	−1.68	0.093
Nodes	0.410	0.092	4.47	<0.0001

the reduced model and the previous model is −2.177 so the likelihood ratio test with six degrees of freedom yields the p-value 0.903, indicating that the reduced model is also a good fit for the data. The results from the reduced model are in Table 4.2. We conclude that the IFN treatment tends to reduce the risk of death by about 25% as compared to the OBS treatment but such evidence is only marginally significant; the patients with the ambulatory performance tend to have less risk of death than the patients with excellent performances; the patients with more nodes have significantly larger risk.

We may also concern that the patients with ambulatory performance and the patients with excellent performance are from very different populations. To address this issue, we can fit the Cox PH model by treating performance covariate as the stratified variable. It turns out that both the effects and significance levels of treatment and nodes covariates are very similar to before.

Finally, we assess the proportionality of three covariates in the last model. To check if the proportionality assumption holds between two treatment arms, we plot the log(−log) survival functions from these two groups where the survival functions are estimated using the Kaplan–Meier estimates. Figure 4.1 shows that the two curves are parallel. Thus, the proportionality assumption for the treatment arms is plausible. Moreover, the tests for the proportionality using the Schoenfeld residuals [10] reveal the p-values for each covariate as 0.197 (treatment), 0.917 (performance), and 0.193 (nodes), which again confirms the validity of using the Cox PH model.

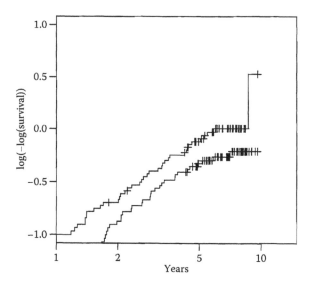

FIGURE 4.1:   Plot of log(−log) survival functions between two treatment arms.

4.3.2   Data Example with Time-Dependent Covariates

The data come from a burn management study [13] to evaluate a protocol change in disinfectant practices in a large midwestern university medical center. Infection can result in death so control of infection is important in burn management. The purpose of the study is to compare a routine bathing care method with a body-cleansing method. The study contains records from 154 patients, among which 70 patients received the routine bathing care and 81 patients were treated with the new bathing solution. The event of interest is time to infection in days and 48 patients had infections during the study.

Besides the different treatment methods, two time-dependent covariates are also important in affecting the infection occurrence: one is the time to excision and the other is time to prophylactic antibiotic treatment administered, namely, whether or not the patient's wound had been excised and whether or not the patient had been treated with an antibiotic sometime during the course of the study.

We fit a Cox regression model incorporating both treatment and two time-dependent covariates. The results are given in Table 4.3. There is no sufficient evidence to

TABLE 4.3:   Analysis of burn data.

Covariates	Estimate	Standard Error	z-Stat	p-Value
Body-cleansing method vs. routine care	−0.453	0.299	−1.519	0.129
Whether patient had excision	−0.952	0.481	−1.981	0.048
Whether patient had antibiotic	−0.019	0.376	−0.051	0.960

suggest that the body-cleansing method is different from the routine care method. However, the patients who had wound excision tend to have 60% less risk of infections than the patients who did not. Whether the patients had been treated with the antibiotic does not reduce the risk of infection.

4.3.3 Data Example Involving Marginal Model with Correlated Time-to-Event Data

The example comes from the well-known Diabetic Retinopathy Study [12], which was conducted to assess the effectiveness of laser photocoagulation in delaying visual loss among patients with diabetic retinopathy. One eye of each patient was randomly selected to receive the laser treatment while the other eye was used as a control. The failure time of interest is the time to visual loss as measured by visual acuity less than 5/200. We confine our attention to a subset of 197 high-risk patients, and consider three covariates: Z_{1ij} indicates, by the values 1 vs. 0, whether or not the jth eye ($j = 1$ for the left eye and $j = 2$ for the right eye) of the ith patient was treated with laser photocoagulation, $Z_{2i1} \equiv Z_{2i2}$ indicates, by the values 1 vs. 0, whether the ith patient had adult-onset or juvenile-onset diabetics, and $Z_{3ij} = Z_{1ij} * Z_{2ij}$.

We apply the Cox-type marginal hazards model to fit the data. Particularly, the time-to-visual loss from either eye follows the Cox PH model. The pseudo partial likelihood function as given in Section 4.2.6 is maximized for estimation and inference. Table 4.4 presents the fitted results. It shows that the effect of the treatment varies significantly between the two diabetic types. The treatment of laser photocoagulation significantly reduces the risk of visual loss by 35% for juvenile diabetes and by 72% for adult diabetes. Without the laser treatment, the patients with adult-type diabetics tend to have greater risk of visual loss than those with juvenile-type diabetics, however, with the laser treatment the patients with juvenile-type diabetics tend to have great risk.

4.4 Discussion

We have reviewed the Cox PH model in survival analysis. Especially, we have reviewed the model formulation, partial likelihood function, the counting process formulation, tied data, modeling of the time-dependent covariates, and marginal

TABLE 4.4: Analysis of diabetic retinopathy study.

Covariates	Estimate	Standard Error	z-Stat	p-Value
Treatment	−0.425	0.185	−2.30	0.022
Diabetic type (adult vs. juvenile)	0.341	0.196	1.74	0.081
Interaction	−0.846	0.304	−2.79	0.005

models for the correlated events. There have been much development in the extension of the Cox PH model during the past three decades. We list some directions which are not covered in this chapter in the following.

1. Apply the Cox PH model to event data with different censorship. Such work includes the Cox PH model to the current status data [11] and the Cox PH model to the interval censored data [25]. Other applications have been seen for event data with truncation, doubly censorship, or cure rate.

2. Generalize the Cox PH model to linear transformation models. The Cox PH can be also represented as

$$\log \Lambda_0(T) = -\boldsymbol{\beta}'Z + \varepsilon,$$

where ε follows the extreme-value distribution. If we further allow ε to be some different distribution from the extreme-value distribution, we then obtain a class of non-PH model, named linear transformation models. Particularly, the logistic distribution of ε yields the proportional odds model [5, 19]. The inference for linear transformation models is given [4]. More general class of linear transformation models with time-dependent covariates can be found in Refs. [26,27].

3. Use the frailty in the Cox PH model for correlated events. In this review, we focused on the marginal PH model for modeling correlated events. However, a completely different way of modeling correlated events is to introduce frailty into the Cox PH model to account for the dependence among the correlated events. The most popular model is the gamma-frailty model by assuming

$$\lambda_{ij}(t) = \lambda_0(t)\gamma_i e^{\boldsymbol{\beta}'\mathbf{z}_{ij}},$$

where $\lambda_{ij}(t)$ is the hazard rate function for subject i in cluster j and γ_i is an unobserved random variable following a gamma distribution with mean one. The inference for the gamma-frailty model is given in Refs. [17,18] and later by Ref. [21] for a more general correlation structure.

4. Generalize the concept of the Cox PH model to recurrent events. A recurrent event means that the same subject may experience one or more events over time, for example, multiple infections or cancer relapses. A recurrent event is one of the correlated events. However, it is very different from either clustered events or multiple type events due to the natural ordering of recurrent events. For recurrent event, the concept of the hazards rate is generalized to the so-called intensity function, the instantaneous probability of developing a new event given the past process. A model parallel to the Cox PH model is called the Andersen–Gill proportional intensity model. Additionally, the proportional rate model, which models the mean frequency of recurrent events, has also been developed and studied extensively [3, 22].

References

[1] Andersen, P.K. and Gill, R.D. (1982), Cox's regression model for counting processes: A large sample study. *The Annals of Statistics*, 10, 1100–1120.

[2] Breslow, N.E. (1972), Contribution to discussion of paper by D.R. Cox. *Journal of the Royal Statistical Society, B*, 34, 216–217.

[3] Cai, J. and Schaubel, D.E. (2004), Analysis of recurrent event data. *Handbook of Statistics*, vol. 23, pp. 603–623.

[4] Cheng, S.C., Wei, L.J., and Ying, Z. (1995), Analysis of transformation models with censored data. *Biometrika*, 82, 835–845.

[5] Clayton, D. and Cuzick, J. (1985), Multivariate generalizations of the proportional hazards model (with discussion). *Journal of the Royal Statistical Society, A*, 148, 82–117.

[6] Cox, D.R. (1972), Regression models and life-tables. *Journal of the Royal Statistical Society, B*, 34, 187–202.

[7] Cox, D.R. (1975), Partial likelihood. *Biometrika*, 62, 269–276.

[8] Efron, B. (1967), Efficiency of Cox's likelihood function for censored data. *Journal of the Americal Statistical Association*, 72, 557–565.

[9] Fleming, R.R. and Harrington, D.P. (1991), *Counting Processes and Survival Analysis*. Wiley, New York.

[10] Grambsch, P. and Therneau, T. (1994), Proportional hazards tests and diagnostics based on weighted residuals. *Biometrika*, 81, 515–526.

[11] Huang, J. (1996), Efficient estimation for the proportional hazard model with interval censoring. *Annals of Statistics*, 24, 540–568.

[12] Huster, W.J., Brookmeyer, R., and Self, S.G. (1989), Modelling paired survival data with covariates. *Biometrics*, 45, 145–156.

[13] Ichida, J.M., Wassell, J.T., Keller, M.D., and Ayers, L.W. (1993), Evaluation of protocol change in burn-care management using the Cox proportional hazards model with time-dependent covariates. *Statistics in Medicine*, 12, 301–310.

[14] Kalbfleisch, J.D. and Prentice, R.L. (2002), *The Statistical Analysis of Failure Time Data*. Wiley, New York.

[15] Johansen, S. (1983), An extension of Cox's regression model. *International Statistical Review*, 51, 258–262.

[16] Mantel, N. (1966), Evaluation of survival data and two new rank order statistics arising in its consideration. *Cancer Chemotherapy Reports* 50, 163–170.

[17] Murphy, S.A. (1994), Consistency in a proportional hazards model incorporating a random effect. *Annals of Statistics*, 22, 712–731.

[18] Murphy, S.A. (1995), Asymptotic theory for the frailty model. *Annals of Statistics*, 23, 182–198.

[19] Murphy, S.A., Rossini, A.J., and van der Vaart, A.W. (1997), Maximal likelihood estimate in the proportional odds model. *Journal of the American Statistical Association*, 92, 968–976.

[20] Oaks, D. (1972), Contribution to discussion of paper by D.R. Cox. *Journal of the Royal Statistical Society*, B, 34, 208.

[21] Parner, E. (1998), Asymptotic theory for the correlated gamma-frailty model. *Annals of Statistics*, 26, 183–214.

[22] Pepe, M. and Cai, J. (1993), Some graphical displays and marginal regression analysis for recurrent failure times and time dependent covariates. *Journal of the American Statistical Association*, 88, 811–820.

[23] Peto, R. and Peto, J. (1972), Asymptotically efficient rank invariant test procedures (with discussion). *Journal of the Royal Statistical Society*, A, 135, 185–206.

[24] Socinski, M.A., Schell, M.J., Peterman, A., Bakri, K., Yates, S., Gitten, R., Unger, P., Lee, J., Lee, J.H., Tynan, M., Moore, M., and Kies, M.S. (2002), Phase III trial comparing a defined duration of therapy versus continuous therapy followed by second-line therapy in advanced-stage IIIB/IV non-small-cell lung cancer. *Journal of Clinical Oncology*, 20, 1335–1343.

[25] Sun, J. (2006), *The Statistical Analysis of Interval-Censored Failure Time Data*. Springer, New York.

[26] Zeng, D. and Lin, D.Y. (2006), Maximum likelihood estimation in semiparametric transformation models for counting processes. *Biometrika*, 93, 627–640.

[27] Zeng, D. and Lin, D.Y. (2007), Maximum likelihood estimation in semiparametric models with censored data (with discussion). *Journal of the Royal Statistical Society*, B, 69, 507–564.

Chapter 5

Overview of Inferential Methods for Categorical Time-to-Event Data

Eric V. Slud

Contents

The setting for this chapter is time-to-event data in clinical studies, with discrete categorical responses and covariates observed for individual subjects at fixed or grouped discrete times. The topics covered in the chapter fall under the heading of *longitudinal data*, but that term covers a much broader array of data structures, including data observed irregularly at different times for different individuals, where responses may themselves be repeated quantitative measurements not restricted to occurrence times for clinical endpoints. For broader coverage of repeated measurements over time, we refer the reader elsewhere: for *categorical regression models* (both generalized-linear and loglinear) to Refs. [1,2]; for longitudinal-linear and generalized-linear models (GLMs) to Refs. [3,4]; for *repeated measures* and *panel data* models to Refs. [5]; for *ordinal and nominal data regression* topics to Ref. [6]; and for categorical-response models with specifically *time series* flavor to Ref. [7]. The literature on each of these topics is large, with extensive ramifications in the social sciences. The restrictions of scope in this chapter—to discrete times, categorical responses mostly from GLMs and possibly with random effects—are imposed in the interest of manageable length and a unified parametric theoretical framework in a biostatistical context. The focus on explanatory and likelihood-based models enables us also to treat goodness-of-fit topics and model criticism. Covariate measurements within this framework may be discrete or continuous, and the data structures are allowed to have possibly time-dependent covariates, multiple responses per subject, and general patterns of censoring.

Texts and monographs which can serve as general references for the topics covered here include Refs. [3,4,8]. There seems to be no text which has drawn together the longitudinal-data methods specifically applicable to time-to-event modeling, although perhaps Ref. [8] is closest to having done so.

5.1   Introduction

For definiteness, consider the basic notation and data structure:

$$(Y_{it}, x_{itk}, z_{itl}, r_{it}), \quad 1 \leq i \leq n, \quad 1 \leq t \leq M, \quad 1 \leq k \leq p, \quad 1 \leq l \leq d \qquad (5.1)$$

Here i and t are, respectively, subject and time indices; Y_{it} is a categorical response variable, usually a binary indicator or a count; X_{it} a covariate vector of dimension p (and components x_{itk}, $1 \leq k \leq p$) and Z_{it} another covariate vector within models with random effects, for each subject i and time t; and r_{it} an indicator of subject i being at risk and observable for the t time period. The responses Y_{it}, and sometimes also the covariates, are observable only for the (i, t) combinations for which $r_{it} = 1$.

Depending upon the application, the time index t may either be a fixed discrete time, such as a rounded occurrence time or the time of a periodic medical examination, or may refer to a fixed chronological time-interval $(a_{t-1}, a_t]$. A careful discussion in Ref. [4, Chapter 3] gives historical references for the different mechanisms that can lead to these discretized time indices t. When the responses Y_{it} are known only to have occurred within the time interval $(a_{t-1}, a_t]$, they are termed *interval censored* as in Ref. [9, Section 3.3].

While survival analysis in continuous time must necessarily also address continuous-time mechanisms of loss to follow-up or censoring, the discrete longitudinal setup considered here reports each individual i as either being followed up or not (respectively, $r_{it} = 1$, 0) in the t time period. This is an oversimplification, with the logical status of a notational convention. For each individual reported at risk and with observed response Y_{it} in $(a_{t-1}, a_t]$, the corresponding right-censored continuous-time data would have the time C_i of loss to follow-up occurring later than the response time T_i, with $a_{t-1} < T_i \leq \min(C_i, a_t)$. From the viewpoint of estimation of survival or endpoint-occurrence hazards, this means that the discrete longitudinal structure presents all such censoring times as having occurred just after the end of the interval, i.e., just after a_t. The use of an interval at-risk indicator r_{it} allows discrete longitudinal data with complicated drop-out and drop-in patterns. The standard requirement for avoiding bias in survival estimation is that the censoring mechanism must be *noninformative* or missing at random (MAR, as in Ref. [10]) with respect to the covariates of the problem, and such an assumption is required in this setting too. This assumption means essentially that the indicators r_{it} of being at risk and observed are conditionally independent of Y_{it} given $(X_{is}, s \leq t)$, and can be avoided only by modeling the otherwise nonindentifiable conditional distribution of r_{it} given Y_{it}, X_{it} directly. (This topic is discussed further in Section 5.3.4.)

The discrete longitudinal data structure (Equation 5.1) encompasses both the case of a single categorical endpoint for each clinical subject and the case of recurrent observations such as multiple times to tumor recurrences. The flexibility stems both from the indicators r_{it} of being at risk and observed, which can be nonzero either up to the occurrence of a single endpoint or beyond, and from inclusion within X_{it} of time-dependent covariates, such as numbers and times of previously observed endpoints.

5.2   Modeling Discrete Event-Times

Several authors (see Ref. [3]) distinguish between approaches which model only marginal means, those which locate within-subject random effects and those which explicitly model transitions among underlying states. This choice reflects modeling style and the preferred technique of analysis, and also the level of medical knowledge that can be plausibly incorporated into an explanatory model. For example, in some biostatistical problems one can directly model the transition intensities among intermediate states, such as indicators of platelet recovery or adverse graft-versus-host reactions in the extended bone marrow transplant model and data example in Ref. [9, Section 1.3*ff*]. Diseases that produce adverse outcomes after a period of latency can be described in terms of *illness–death models* [11, Section I.3.3*ff*]. However, as we see in the following sections, the boundary between the random-effects and transition-intensity descriptive models is blurred when time-dependent covariates are introduced as state variables and when longitudinal dependencies connect the within-subject random effects. Moreover, the voluminous literature on longitudinal-linear models of quantitative responses cited in Ref. [3] lends itself to a description of underlying states in terms of variables formed from linear combinations of measured covariates, subject-level random effects, and fixed or stochastic time effects which may also be subject specific.

5.2.1   From Accelerated Failure Times to Generalized Linear Models

We begin with a train of thought leading to regression models that can be adapted to discrete longitudinal data. The starting point is to consider continuous event times T_i which follow a parametric regression model:

$$\log T_i = -b'X_i^0 + e_i \tag{5.2}$$

with X_i^0 an observed baseline covariate p-vector and e_i random errors, independent and identically distributed (*iid*) across subject indices i, with specified distribution but possibly unknown scale parameter σ. Such *accelerated failure time* (AFT) or *accelerated life* regression models were originally introduced in reliability testing, and were used with covariates quantifying heightened stresses to extrapolate failure distributions to ordinary operating conditions. See Ref. [12] for many historical references and extensions. In a right-censored continuous-time biostatistical setting, these models have been intensively studied, parametrically [9, Chapter 2] and semiparametrically [11, Section VII.5.2]. Computational implementation of the models in **S** and **R** is documented in Ref. [13]. In a longitudinal setting, for a fixed set of time-interval endpoints a_t, the available data take the form of a sequence over t of binary indicator variables $Y_{it} = I[T_i \leq a_t]$ observed whenever $r_{it} = 1$. Here a right-censoring mechanism corresponds to $r_{it} = I[C_i \geq a_t]$.

There is a useful equivalent way to view the AFT model (Equation 5.2), in terms of the continuously distributed variate $A_i = e_i/\sigma$ with specified distribution function F_0, and of a set of time-dependent covariates X_{it} consisting of the baseline covariates X_i^0 augmented by the time-effect component $\log t$, where

$$T_i > t \quad \Leftrightarrow \quad A_i > \frac{1}{\sigma}(\log t + \beta'X_i^0) \equiv \beta'X_{it} \tag{5.3}$$

A useful class of regression models extending AFT allows a vector of time-dependent covariates X_{it} to affect an underlying but unobserved *cumulative damage* process $\eta_{it} = \beta'X_{it}$, resulting in a failure when this process exceeds the random and subject-specific threshold A_i. This is a well-known idea in a continuous time context and underlies the approach of Ref. [14] to hazard rate modeling and of Ref. [15] to survival regression. By encoding within components of X_{it} one or more cumulative times of exposure to various hazards or environments, the state-variable η_{it} can incorporate weighted sums of exposures, with weights to be estimated as regression coefficients.

What sorts of distributions will be specified for the random variates A_i in Equation 5.3? Viewed as a time-to-event model, Equation 5.3 is a censored lognormal regression when A_i is standard normal, and is a Weibull regression model when A_i has the complementary loglog (*cloglog*) distribution function $1 - \exp(-e^x)$ (see Ref. [11, p. 581], also for semiparametric extensions). For logistic distributed A_i, Equation 5.3 is equivalent to the *proportional odds* model [4, p. 76]. If the time to event is a threshold crossing by a Wiener process, then A_i is *inverse Gaussian* as in Ref. [15]. These distributions all make sense in Equation 5.3 whether t is continuous or discrete. The most commonly used distributions for A_i in discrete longitudinal models are the cloglog—because of its relation to the Cox proportional hazards model—and the logistic and normal. Along with "overdispersed" extensions in which responses exhibit variance indicative of heterogeneous parameter values, logistic and normal share primacy in the literature for a few different reasons. These two distributions are especially important partly for their early appearance, partly as instances of GLMs amenable to analysis methods based on generalized estimating equations (GEE), and partly because of their ease of use in connection with expectation-maximization (EM)-algorithm analyses of mixed-effects extensions of the model in Equation 5.3.

5.2.2 General Discrete Longitudinal Models

So far, we have considered only models of binary observations Y_{it} relating to single endpoints T_i, i.e., of response series $\{Y_{it}\}_t$ with a single change-point $T_i = \min\{t : Y_{it} = 1\}$ for each i. The other particularly important kinds of responses in clinical time-to-event studies are recurring binary endpoints or counts. These are respectively binary series $\{Y_{it}\}_t$ indicating multiple occurrences for each i, or nonnegative integer-valued tallies Y_{it} of adverse events (tumors, seizures, etc.) for subject i in successive intervals $(a_{t-1}, a_t]$ of time on study.

Motivated by the regression models of Section 5.2.1, we now introduce a unified and very broad family of models of the responses Y_{it} which cover almost all of the longitudinal models in frequent use. We restrict attention to models with linear state variables

$$\eta_{it} = X'_{it}\beta + Z'_{it}\varepsilon_{it}, \quad 1 \le i \le n, \quad 1 \le t \le M$$

where X_{it}, Z_{it} are one-step-ahead time-dependent covariates, i.e., covariates observable by time a_{t-1}, if the Y_{it} outcomes refer to the time period $(a_{t-1}, a_t]$, and the unobserved random-effect vectors ε_{it} are defined at the level of time or subject or both. Responses $\{Y_{it}\}_{i,t}$ are related to $\{\eta_{it}\}_{i,t}$ and an array $(A_{it}, 1 \le i \le n, 1 \le t \le M)$ of variables *of known distribution* and independent of all $(X_{js}, Z_{js}, \varepsilon_{js})_{j,s}$ variables, by an equation:

$$Y_{it} = h(A_{it}, \eta_{it}, \rho) \tag{5.4}$$

where h is assumed known except possibly for an identifiable finite-dimensional parameter vector ρ. The most important instances of this model, and the only ones to be discussed in detail in this chapter, are the binary-response models

$$Y_{it} = I[A_{it} \le \eta_{it}], \quad A_{it} \sim F \tag{5.5}$$

with F usually $\mathcal{N}(0, 1)$ or logistic, and the Poisson-count model

$$Y_{it} = \text{Poi}^{-1}(A_{it}; \eta_{it}), \quad A_{it} \sim \text{Uniform}[0, 1] \tag{5.6}$$

where
  Poi$(x; \lambda)$ denotes the Poisson(λ) distribution function
  Poi$^{-1}(u; \lambda) = \inf\{x : \text{Poi}(x; \lambda) \ge u\}$ the Poisson(λ) quantile function

An equivalent and more understandable form of the model in Equation 5.6 arises by defining $\zeta_{it}(\cdot)$ to be a unit-rate Poisson process and

$$Y_{it} = \zeta_{it}(\eta_{it}) \tag{5.7}$$

For ease of exposition, special cases of model (Equation 5.4) are described first for binary responses, within model (Equation 5.5). Corresponding Poisson models for counts, within Equation 5.7, are mentioned at the end of each subsection.

The models in Equation 5.5 or Equations 5.6 and 5.7 can take a great variety of forms, depending on the nature (time-dependent or not, stochastic or not) of predictor variables X_{it} and on the kind of dependence allowed among the variables A_{it} and random effects ε_{it} for different times t and the same subject i. The unifying idea in model of Equation 5.4 in all its forms, is that the binary or count responses Y_{it} are defined from crossings of latent thresholds A_{it} by state variables η_{it} constructed linearly from predictors X_{it} and time-by-subject random effects ε_{it}.

While X_{it}, Z_{it} can be time-dependent and stochastic in practical examples, they include information about responses only from the past (Y_{is}, $s < t$). For notational simplicity, in model assumptions made conditionally given all available past data on all subjects before time t, that conditioning is denoted by

$$\mathcal{F}_{t-1} = \sigma((X_{is}, Z_{is}, Y_{i,s-1}), s \le t, 1 \le i \le n) = \text{Data before } t \tag{5.8}$$

Throughout the rest of this section, all models conditionally specify the distribution of Y_{it} given $\mathcal{F}_{t-1}$. The unknown parameters for these models always consist (only) of the coefficient vectors β, the variance matrices D for the random effects ε_{it} and in cases with dependence among ε_{it}, parameters α specifying the associations among these random effects. Time-dependent effects on occurrence rates are handled through coefficients β_k of time-varying predictor components x_{itk}: useful complexity can be introduced through time-dependent, or stochastic, covariates X_{it}.

The latent variables A_{it} in Equation 5.4 are always assumed jointly independent of all random-effect variables ε_{it}, and whether they are modeled as independent or dependent, have distributions assumed to be completely known. Further assumptions and regularity conditions are listed in Section 5.2.6, but throughout this chapter,

$$\{(A_{it}, \varepsilon_{it})\}_{t=1}^{M} \text{ are } iid, \quad i = 1, 2, \ldots, n$$

REMARK 1

This assumption is imposed mostly for ease of exposition. The variables ε_{it} might not be independent across i: individuals may naturally group into higher level clusters (e.g., family or clinical center) for which a shared random effect is plausible.

5.2.3   Cumulative Models

The first major subclass of models is that of *cumulative models*, in the terminology of Ref. [4, Section 3.3]. In our setup, this class is characterized by the properties that within-subject responses Y_{it} are *ordinal* or increasing, and that there is only a single latent variable for each subject, i.e.,

$$Y_{it} \nearrow \text{ in } t, \quad \text{and} \quad A_{it} \equiv A_i \quad \text{for all } i, t \tag{5.9}$$

When responses are binary, the identical distribution of A_{it} means that with F denoting a distribution function, usually either the logistic or standard normal,

$$P(Y_{it} = 1 | X_{it}, Z_{it}, \varepsilon_{it}) = F(\eta_{it}) = F(X_{it}'\beta + Z_{it}'\varepsilon_{it}) \tag{5.10}$$

The combination of Equations 5.5, 5.9, and 5.10 sharply restricts the time-dependence of the covariates. Since subjects share the same A_i value in Equation 5.5 at all time points, nondecreasing Y_{it} implies nondecreasing state variables $\eta_{it} = X_{it}'\beta + Z_{it}'\varepsilon_{it}$. These models have most often been used without random effects (i.e., with $\varepsilon_{it} = 0$). In this case, let the X_{it} covariates and β coefficients be partitioned

$$X_{it} = \begin{pmatrix} X_i^0 \\ X_{it}^1 \end{pmatrix} \quad \text{and} \quad \beta = \begin{pmatrix} \gamma \\ \mu \end{pmatrix}$$

into respectively q_0 and q_1 dimensional sub-vectors, where the non-time-dependent baseline covariates X_i^0 have coefficients γ. Then $\mu'X_{it}^1$ must be increasing in t, and μ should take values in a known parameter set containing an open neighborhood. That implies, possibly after a linear transformation of X_{it}^1 in which a non-time-varying portion is subtracted and included within X_i^0 and the remaining portion of X_{it}^1 is rotated, that the time-varying components of X_{it} must be increasing and their coefficients restricted to be positive. For example, $\mu'X_{it}^1$ is monotone increasing if each component X_{itk}^1 is an operational-time variable increasing in t for subject i, and the corresponding coefficient μ_k is a positive weight. Random effects *can* be included in cumulative models, but reasoning similar to that above shows that inclusion of nontrivial mean-0 random effects ε_{it} in Equation 5.10 would ruin the within-subject monotonicity of η_{it}, unless $\varepsilon_{it} = \varepsilon_i$ and $Z_{it} = Z_i$ are constant within subject.

In summary, the restrictions on cumulative binary response models are

$$A_{it} = A_i, \quad \varepsilon_{it} = \varepsilon_i, \quad Z_{it} = Z_i, \quad \eta_{it} \nearrow \text{ in } t \quad \text{for all } i$$

resulting in the model form:

$$T_i = \inf\{t \geq 1 : Y_{it} = 1\} = \min\{t : \gamma'X_i^0 + Z_i'\varepsilon_i + \mu'X_{it}^1 \geq A_i\} \tag{5.11}$$

where
   X_i^0 are any baseline covariates and
   X_{it}^1 time-dependent covariates for which each component is nondecreasing in t

The unknown parameters consist of an arbitrary q_0-dimensional parameter vector γ, a q_1-dimensional vector μ with nonnegative entries, and any parameters α needed to specify the distribution of random effects ε_i.

Cumulative models of the type of Equation 5.11 with $\mu = 0$ and $\varepsilon_i = 0$ have already been discussed within Section 5.2.1, and can be rewritten in the form:

$$P(T_i = t|X_i^0) = F(\gamma'X_i^0 + \vartheta_t) - F(\gamma'X_i^0 + \vartheta_{t-1}) \qquad (5.12)$$

They include the proportional odds models (in the $F = $ logistic case) and grouped Cox model [4, p. 78] when F has the cloglog form. The terminology of *proportional odds* for the case of logistic F comes from the expression of the odds of failure by time t as

$$\frac{P(T_i \le t|X_i^0)}{1 - P(T_i \le t|X_i^0)} = \frac{F(\gamma'X_i^0 + \vartheta_t)}{1 - F(\gamma'X_i^0 + \vartheta_t)} = \exp(\gamma'X_i^0 + \vartheta_t) \qquad (5.13)$$

implying that the odds for two subjects, i and j with baseline covariate vectors X_i^0 and X_j^0, are proportional for all t, with proportionality factor $\exp\left(\gamma'(X_i^0 - X_j^0)\right)$. The *grouped Cox* terminology refers to the equivalence of the model of Equation 5.12 to a discrete multiplicative hazard model, shown in Section 5.2.4, when F has the cloglog form. Several other references where this cumulative model (Equation 5.12) has been used with different choices for F can be found in Ref. [4, p. 79]. Viewing T_i as an ordinal response, Ref. [2] calls Equation 5.13 a *cumulative link* model.

The model in Equation 5.11, with $\mu \ne 0$ and $\varepsilon_i = 0$ but with coordinates of X_{it}^1 taking a form equivalent to $w_i I_{[t \ge r]}$ for baseline non-time-dependent covariates w_i, has been proposed and applied by Fahrmeir and Tutz Ref. [4, pp. 79ff and Example 3.5] as an *extended cumulative model*. The model with coordinates of X_{it}^1 equal to cumulative times spent by subject i within specific exposure regimes has been known to writers on reliability for many years [16,17] and has been used recently by Lee et al. [18] in a continuous-time survival analysis. Such models could also find interesting applications in discrete-time longitudinal modeling in epidemiology.

Cumulative models (Equations 5.10 and 5.11) with random effects were proposed in Ref. [19] under the heading of mixed-effect ordinal regression. For later developments, including biostatistical time-to-event applications, see Ref. [6]. In particular, the proportional-odds frailty model of Zeng et al. [20] is a mixed-effect cumulative model.

When the responses Y_{it} are counts, a cumulative Poisson model would restrict Equation 5.7 to have a single latent subject-specific Poisson process $\zeta_i(\cdot)$ for each subject i, with state variables η_{it} increasing in t for fixed i. Such a model would equivalently describe independent Poisson counts in successive intervals (conditionally given X_{it}, Z_{it}, ε_{it}), a setting better handled by the *sequential* models treated in Section 5.2.4.

5.2.4   Discrete-Hazards or Sequential Models

Where the cumulative models in the form of Equation 5.12 define conditional probabilities of response given covariates through the probability masses for $T_i = t$, other models parameterize the discrete hazards

$$P(T_i = t | T_i \geq t, \mathcal{F}_{t-1}) = P(T_i = t | T_i \geq t, \eta_{it}) = F(\eta_{it}) \qquad (5.14)$$

Such a hazard formula arises in Equation 5.5 by taking the latent variables A_{it} to be *iid* over t within fixed subject i. The models (Equation 5.14) are termed *sequential* by Fahrmeir and Tutz [4], because they describe new responses conditionally at each time t given all previous response data and current covariates. In the binary-outcome case, when the A_{it} are *iid* with distribution function F, the model of Equation 5.5 says that the discrete first-occurrence time $T_i \equiv \inf\{t \geq 1: Y_{it} = 1\}$ has conditional probability mass function

$$P\big(T_i = t | \{X_{is}, Z_{is}, \varepsilon_{is}\}_{s=1}^t\big) = \left\{ \prod_{s=1}^{t-1} \big(1 - F(X_{is}'\beta + Z_{is}'\varepsilon_{is})\big) \right\} F\big(X_{it}'\beta + Z_{it}'\varepsilon_{it}\big) \quad (5.15)$$

Another way to view the distinction between binary-response cumulative and sequential models is that cumulative models describe data where the last observed response on a subject contains all of the information for that subject, while sequential models regard each binary response Y_{it} as the outcome of a separate binary trial. The sequential models allow recurrent-events data in which individual subjects exhibit multiple nonlethal responses, such as multiple times to tumor recurrence or other repeated adverse episodes like seizures or reinfections. Because sequential models allow analysis of multiple time period data, with possibly time-dependent covariates, most of the recent advances in longitudinal time-to-event modeling relate to these parameterizations.

REMARK 2

To handle recurrent events, a cumulative regression type model (say, a proportional odds model with logistic F) could be defined for the sequence of responses until the first time $T_i = t$ at which $Y_{it} = 1$, and the time-on-test clock then restarted at 0 with A_i replaced by an independent F-distributed variate after each positive response. In this approach, when there are no random effects ε_{it}, each portion of a subject's data between successive positive responses would be treated as though coming from a distinct independent "individual."

We now present several successively more complex models for binary responses of sequential type, that is, with A_{it} *iid* across all distinct pairs (i, t). Toward the end of the subsection, analogous models for Poisson count responses are described.

The first models considered have no random effects ε_{it}. They provide a sequential version of Equation 5.5, conditioned on the past defined by Equation 5.8:

$$P(Y_{it} = 1 | \mathcal{F}_{t-1}) = F\big(X_{it}'\beta\big) \qquad (5.16)$$

The model of Equation 5.16 is closely related to the grouped-data proportional hazards model [4, p. 318]. Suppose that the time indices t refer to endpoints falling in the fixed interval $(a_{t-1}, a_t]$, so that the possibly time-dependent covariates X_{it} are observable by chronological time a_{t-1}. A Cox proportional hazards model [21] for a continuous occurrence-time T_i with piecewise constant covariates $X_i(s) \equiv \xi_{it}$ on intervals $s \in (a_{t-1}, a_t]$ gives the continuous-time hazard intensity for T_i of the form

$$\lambda_{T_i}(s) = \lambda_0(s) \exp(X_i(s)'b) = \lambda_0(s) \exp(\xi_{it}'b) \quad \text{for } s \in (a_{t-1}, a_t]$$

for some nonrandom baseline hazard intensity function λ_0, which implies

$$P(T_i > a_t | T_i > a_{t-1}, \mathcal{F}_{t-1}) = \exp\left(-\int_{a_{t-1}}^{a_t} \exp(\xi_{it}'b)\lambda_0(s)ds\right)$$

or

$$P(a_{t-1} < T_i \leq a_t | T_i > a_{t-1}, \mathcal{F}_{t-1}) = 1 - \exp\left(-e^{\xi_{it}'b}\int_{a_{t-1}}^{a_t}\lambda_0(s)ds\right)$$

The last equation agrees precisely with the model of Equation 5.16 if $Y_{it} = I_{[a_{t-1} < T_i \leq a_t]}$, and X_{it} consists of the covariates ξ_{it} augmented by the dummy indicators ($I_{[t=s]}$, $1 \leq s \leq M$), where β consists of the coefficients b augmented by entries $\vartheta_s = \log\left(\int_{a_{s-1}}^{a_s} \lambda_0(u)du\right)$ and F has the cloglog form $F(x) = 1 - \exp(-e^x)$. Taking into account that the event $Y_{it} = 1$ in Section 5.2.3 is the same as the event which would be denoted $\sum_{s=1}^{t} Y_{is} = 1$ in this section, it is easy to check that the models of Equations 5.10 and 5.16 are the same when $F(x)$ in Equation 5.10 is cloglog.

Thus, the model in Equation 5.16 is compatible with one case of Equation 5.10, but the parameterizations are generally different. Equation 5.16 with logistic F, which is a common [22–25] discrete-time variant of the Cox proportional hazards model, is definitely *not* the same, even after accounting for the different Y_{it} notations, as the proportional-odds model (Equation 5.10) with logistic F. Similar comments can be made about the differences between probit models of Equations 5.16 and 5.10.

Even as a fixed-effect model, Equation 5.16 allows three types of time dependence: first, through the fixed time-period effects ϑ_s entering as coefficients of the components of X_{it} corresponding to dummy predictors $I_{[t=s]}$, $1 \leq s \leq M$, within the discrete Cox or logistic or probit hazards model; second, through the effects of exogenous time-dependent predictor columns of X_{it} (the "regressive logistic models" of Bonney [23], with many examples in Refs. [4,7]); and finally, the autoregressive effects arising when some columns of X_{it} are lagged (possibly recoded) values $Y_{i,t-l}$ for lags $l \geq 1$. Models of this last type were introduced by Zeger and Qaqish [26], and by many authors referenced by Kedem and Fokianos [7], as categorical time series models, but they are also natural as longitudinal models [27]. An example is studied in Section 5.5.3.

The models discussed in the previous paragraph are all still logistic or probit models with stochastic regressors, but much of the interest in longitudinal models derives from between-subject heterogeneity. Subject differences are generally modeled by shared random-effect (vector) parameters $\varepsilon_{it} \equiv \varepsilon_i$ across all responses by each subject. They reflect otherwise unmodeled *iid* differences between the subjects i, with distributions assumed known, usually specified as $\mathcal{N}(0, D)$ where the variance matrix is completely or partially unknown. The "general logistic-linear mixed model" of Stiratelli et al. [28] is an early instance of model (Equation 5.16) with logistic F and $\eta_{it} = X'_{it}\beta + Z'_{it}\varepsilon_i$ and *iid* normal subject-specific random effects ε_i. An analogous probit model is given by Chan and Kok [29], citing earlier references with more restrictive assumptions (diagonal D). Many papers in the late 1980s and early 1990s introduced such models, but often piecemeal reflecting incremental progress in the computational methods—EM algorithm, GEE methods, Bayesian Gibbs sampling—of estimating them. The models early combined fixed and stochastic time-dependent effects, and also autoregressive terms [28, p. 963], with random subject effects. Such models have naturally become more sophisticated over the years, modeling event occurrences jointly with underlying state processes and allowing random effects. Reference [30] provides an interesting current example within Equation 5.16: a random-effects Markov model of multiple sclerosis progression in terms of baseline covariates.

The literature on Cox's [21] regression model in continuous time introduced random subject effects under the terminology of *frailty* [11, Chapter IX]. The most-studied model is a random-intercept Cox model in continuous time, which in a discrete-time longitudinal setting and notation, takes the discrete-hazard form

$$P(T_i = t | T_i \geq t, \mathcal{F}_{t-1}) = \lambda_0(t) \exp(\xi'_{it} b + \varepsilon_i) \tag{5.17}$$

where b and $\lambda_0(t)$ are unknown, $1 \leq t \leq M$, and ε_i are *iid* random effects with distribution known except possibly for an unknown parameter ρ. Several distributions for $\exp(\varepsilon_i)$ have been used (see Ref. [31] for gamma, positive-stable, and Weibull; and Ref. [32] for normal). The model has often been introduced with cluster level of family (the *shared frailty model*, Ref. [31, Chapter 7]) rather than individual. The general discrete-hazard frailty model in Equation 5.14 is

$$P(T_i = t | T_i \geq t, \mathcal{F}_{t-1}) = F(X'_{it}\beta + \varepsilon_i) \tag{5.18}$$

which incorporates the discrete-Cox form (Equation 5.17) if $\vartheta_s \equiv \log \lambda_0(s)$ is the coefficient of the dummy predictor column $I_{[t=s]}$, $1 \leq s \leq M$, and X_{it} consists of these columns augmenting the predictors ξ_{it}. Usually, F will continue to be chosen as logistic or normal or cloglog distribution function. Equation 5.18 actually restricts the models of Equation 5.14 with subject random effects, to the case where $Z_{it} \equiv 1$ and ε_i is scalar. An analogous *proportional-odds frailty model* [20] has already been introduced above as a cumulative mixed-effects model.

The multilevel random-effect models mentioned in Remark 1 fall outside the scope of our discussion here because of the more subtle dependence they require among ε_{it} random effects. Multilevel analysis of longitudinal time-to-event data does not yet have a large literature, but borrows from the extensive work done by social scientists on multilevel modeling. See Ref. [33] for an introductory treatment, mostly of sequential-type models in the context of binary responses and logistic links. Cumulative-type multilevel models are treated in Refs. [6,19].

Mixed-effect regression models for counts, and especially Poisson and GLMs, are introduced in Ref. [2]. For fuller coverage of aspects related to stochastic regressors, including large-sample theory, see Ref. [7, Chapter 4], which also discusses variant models involving nonlinear transformation and truncation. For many authors, including these, Poisson regression is an example of GLM theory and quasilikelihood estimating equations, with particular reference to estimation in the presence of overdispersion [3,34]. For application of parametric models of the type (Equation 5.7) with $Z_{it} = 1$, subject-specific random effects ε_i, and baseline or exogenous covariates X_{it}, see Ref. [35]. Various authors [3,36] have proposed methods to handle random-effect heterogeneity within Poisson regression time series models. See Ref. [8] generally for Poisson regression models with random effects.

5.2.5   Partially Parameterized and Marginal Models

A dauntingly large literature has grown around models for GLM and longitudinal data parameterized only to the extent necessary for statistical estimation of regression parameters from estimating equations. The classic reference for the underlying GLM theory and estimating equations is Ref. [37], although Ref. [2] gives a good introduction. This is not a subject to which we can do justice here, beyond saying that the binary-response models (Equation 5.5) and Poisson models (Equation 5.7) are all GLM examples conditionally given the random effects ε_{it}. Much effort has gone into formulating longitudinal models in such a way that the response variables Y_{it} considered marginally, i.e., individually, are of GLM form. (Key references along this line are Refs. [3,38,39].) The value added by this formulation, in view of the seminal paper of Liang and Zeger [40] and its successors like Prentice and Zhao [41] further establishing the GEE method, is the ability to estimate regression parameters—with consistency and asymptotic normality to support inferential techniques—without having to specify more than the mean of the responses (with link) in terms of regression parameters. The covariance structure must also be specified in terms of auxiliary parameters, but of these specifications, only the mean need be correct.

There are both philosophical and practical reasons for formulating marginal models and estimating them, whether by GEE-related or likelihood methods. Many authors emphasize that the interpretation of marginal model parameters differs from that of corresponding parameters in random-effects "transition" models. See Refs. [3,8] for perspective on the differences between these models. When marginal GLMs are appropriate, the model assumptions required by GEE methods are very mild, far less than the complete specification of a parametric likelihood. Yet there are many "transition" model likelihoods within the general model of Equation 5.4 that are incompatible with marginal and GEE models. The GEE theory does not contain adequate tools to assess the validity of its mean specification. So GEE and marginal models should still be used in tandem with likelihood theory and testable models. Their best use may be in completing a likelihood-based exploratory analysis as in Section 5.5.2, after model criticism disqualifies standard models.

5.2.6 Large-Sample Regularity Conditions

The models of Equation 5.4 do require some conditions for the consistency and asymptotic normality of inferences to hold, particularly when covariates are time-varying and stochastic. We continue to assume $(A_{it}, \varepsilon_{it})$ *iid* across i, and r_{it} and $(A_{it}, \varepsilon_{it})$ conditionally independent given $\mathcal{F}_{it}$, a fairly strong form of MAR condition. In addition, it is important to assume large-sample stability of the joint empirical distribution of covariates $\{(X_{it}, Z_{it})\}_{i,t}$. If for convenience the covariates are restricted to lie in a bounded range of $\mathcal{R}^p \times \mathcal{R}^d$, then this stability restriction is essentially that there is a fixed positive constant $c \in (0, 1]$ and probability distribution ν on $\mathcal{R}^p \times \mathcal{R}^d$, such that for all bounded continuous real-valued functions $g(x, z)$ on $\mathcal{R}^p \times \mathcal{R}^d$, as n and perhaps M get large,

$$(nM)^{-1} \sum_{i=1}^{n} \sum_{t=1}^{M} r_{it} g(X_{it}, Z_{it}) \longrightarrow c \int g(x, z) d\nu(x, z) \tag{5.19}$$

For identifiability of parameters, the limiting distribution ν should not assign probability 1 to any linear subspace of $\mathcal{R}^p \times \mathcal{R}^d$ of dimension less than $p + d$. Further general assumptions are needed on the smoothness (and boundedness of derivatives) of h in Equation 5.4, and similarly of F in Equations 5.16 and 5.10, together with smoothness and identifiability assumptions on the distribution of ε_{it} as a function of its unknown parameters. (These last assumptions will always hold when F is logistic, normal, or cloglog and ε_{it} are normal with either general or diagonal covariance matrix.)

Assumptions of the type of Equation 5.19 were introduced in a right-censored survival context by Andersen and Gill [42] and adapted by the author of Refs. [24,27] (in settings without missing data or random effects, but the proofs would be essentially the same in the more general context) to prove large-sample consistency and asymptotic normality of maximum likelihood (ML) parameter estimators using martingale limit theorems. Kedem and Fokianos [7] deal primarily with long time series, where n is bounded and M gets large, but the case of interest for discrete longitudinal event-time data is where n gets large and M is bounded or grows slowly as n does. The restrictive condition is Equation 5.19, which indicates the kinds of large-sample behavior (requiring near-stationarity over time for long time series) needed on baseline and time-dependent covariates for large-sample inference.

5.3 Analysis Methods

5.3.1 Likelihood-Based Methods

For parametric likelihoods specified within Equation 5.4, regression coefficients are generally estimated by ML. In many cases, especially those with sophisticated dependence between random effects ε_{it} across t within subject (but also across subject in case of higher-level multisubject clusters), ML estimation is often accomplished via the EM algorithm [10] as well as its simulation-aided variants as in Ref. [43]. For many years, for ease of computer implementation, non-Bayesian estimation was often done by modified likelihood methods like the penalized quasilikelihood (PQL) of Breslow and Clayton [44], methods which are progressively being superseded by software enabling full-ML estimation. But see Ref. [45] for current work involving bias-corrected PQL in Poisson mixed models.

Hypothesis testing, particularly of treatment effects, within fully specified models can be based on score or Wald-type or likelihood ratio (LR) tests. Similarly, LR and Wald testing for significance of parameters is of great value in model building. However, since variance parameters with value 0 fall on the boundary of their parameter space, the large-sample distribution theory for LR tests for variance components must be modified, as in Ref. [46]. For testing fixed-effect terms and presence of nonzero off-diagonal random-effect variance components, the standard Wilks LR tests apply, with χ^2 distributions and degrees of freedom equal to the number of additional parameters in the alternative hypothesis model. For testing presence versus absence of single variance components, assumed independent of any previously entered variance components, the LR test statistic (twice the difference of maximized *logLik* with the extra variance term minus maximized *logLik* without it) is found in Ref. [46] to have asymptotic distribution equal to a mixture with weights $1/2$, $1/2$ of a point mass at 0 with a χ^2_1 distribution. Thus, the *p*-value for the LR statistic Λ is $(1 - F_{\chi^2_1}(\Lambda))/2$ in place of $1 - F_{\chi^2_1}(\Lambda)$.

Nonparametric weighted logrank-type tests of treatment effectiveness still have an important role to play in discrete-time longitudinal data [11]. Other modified score tests, designed for modified optimality criteria as in Ref. [47], can also be useful.

Bayesian methods in this subject generally fall under the heading of hierarchical GLMs [4, Section 2.3.2]. Such models were an important early arena for the application of Bayesian Gibbs sampling methodology [3]. An example falling squarely within the scope of this chapter is Ref. [48].

Among other likelihood-based methods, loglinear models [2] are still in common use for categorical data analysis in the social sciences, even in a specifically longitudinal-data context [1]. Nevertheless, these models seem to have fallen out of favor in biomedical statistics with the advent of GLM- and GEE-based methods.

5.3.2   Methods for Discrete Cox Models

The discrete hazard form of the Cox proportional hazards model [21] has already been seen to be equivalent to sequential model (Equation 5.16) with extreme-value distribution function F. However, standard Cox-model partial likelihood (PL) maximizing software (see Chapter 4), such as coxph in **R** [13,49], uses instead the discrete-hazard parameterization

$$P(T_i = t | T_i \geq t, \mathcal{F}_{t-1}) = \lambda_0(t) \exp(X'_{it}\beta) \tag{5.20}$$

An unavoidable issue in applying Cox model methods to discrete longitudinal data is the handling of tied observations. The cleanest form of large-sample theory for maximum PL Cox model estimators [42] relies on continuously distributed survival times without ties, but all of the large sample results have discrete-time counterparts [24,27]. In really large samples, the method used to account for tied survival times makes only a tiny difference to estimates. One can check computationally whether this is true in a moderately large dataset by rerunning Cox model software several times after adding small uniform random numbers to the individual survival times, which has the effect of breaking the ties and randomly ordering the observed survival times. In survival data of many hundred subjects, this kind of sensitivity checking will often show the method of handling ties to be unimportant. But most trials are not that large, so that some discussion of the handling of ties is useful, as in Ref. [9, Section 8.4]. There are two common methods of constructing the sum of at-risk hazard multipliers in the PL factor denominators. The first, due to Breslow, uses the whole sum of at-risk hazard factors for all observed failures at a particular time. The second method, due to Efron, constructs the at-risk sums for ordered individuals as when the failure times are not tied after replacing the risk multipliers $\exp(X_{it}'\beta)$ for all individuals failing at time t by their average. With Efron's replacement, the PL factor for time t would be precisely the same if the individuals with failure times tied at t were ordered in any way whatever. There is also a principled but computationally burdensome method of calculating PL for discrete-time models, suggested by Cox [21], but computational experience shows that the Efron method—which is the default in the survival package in **R**—gives a reasonably good approximation to it. In applications where the method of handling ties seems critical, Ref. [50] provides a theoretically supported EM-based approach.

One aspect of data analysis which is more difficult in the semiparametric Cox model framework than in parametric discrete-hazard variants is the checking of equality of nuisance hazards (i.e., of time-period effects) in subgroups or strata. There is no general partial likelihood ratio test for the equality of hazards, but there are methods based on supremum or other metrics of difference between estimated baseline hazards [51], which could be used in testing equality of baseline hazards within stratified models. By contrast, parametric likelihood ratio tests for time-effect differences among strata are simple and valid. Such a test is implemented in the example of Section 5.5.1.

5.3.3 Estimating Equations and GEE Methods

There is great benefit in being able to estimate regression parameters validly without having to specify precise distributions for observed response variables. Just as survival analysis methods received a tremendous boost from the semiparametric methodology initiated by Cox in Ref. [21], longitudinal methods based on estimating equations have flourished since the GEE approach of Liang and Zeger [40] extended GLM quasilikelihood scores to longitudinal data. In the setting of binary or count response models, the GEE estimators are defined in our notation as solutions $\hat{\beta}$ of the equation

$$\sum_{i=1}^{n}\sum_{s=1}^{M}\sum_{t=1}^{M}\nabla_{\beta}E(Y_{it}|X_{it})\mathbf{V}_{i,ts}^{-1}(\beta,\hat{\alpha})(Y_{is}-E(Y_{is}|X_{is}))=\mathbf{0} \qquad (5.21)$$

where the expectations $E(Y_{it}|X_{it})$ are ideally specified (the *marginal model* formulation) as functions of the unknown parameter-vector β alone. The variance matrix $\mathbf{V}_i$ of the vector $(Y_{it})_{t=1}^{M}$, with the (t, s) entry of its inverse denoted $\mathbf{V}_{i,ts}^{-1}$, is specified in terms of a diagonal depending on β, of an additional scale parameter ϕ which does not affect Equation 5.21, and of a correlation structure parameterized (not necessarily correctly) by other unknown parameters α which must be estimated with large-sample validity by estimators $\hat{\alpha}$.

The large-sample theory of consistency and asymptotic normality for $\hat{\beta}$, developed by Liang and Zeger [40] and later papers about GEE and marginal models, justifies significance tests for components of $\hat{\beta}$ and confirmatory tests of significance, e.g., for treatment effect in a randomized clinical trial. The same methods provide model-building tools, when only significant predictors are retained under a variable selection strategy. Although software outputs typically provide information only for Wald-type tests, score-type tests are also possible, as in Ref. [34]. It is known that GEE parameter estimates are (nearly) efficient when the variance specification is (nearly) correct. Effective strategies for specifying variance models are highly prized. In the overdispersed Poisson setting, Ref. [52] provides one such strategy.

GEE methods are susceptible to two known drawbacks. Despite developments [41] making variance estimation more systematic, this theory lacks machinery for model criticism or goodness-of-fit checking. A further criticism is that GEE provides no way to correct for missing-data mechanisms which are independent of responses only conditionally given covariates (MAR rather than MCAR, in the terminology of Ref. [10]), although the simulation evidence of Ref. [38] suggests that GEE still behaves well under MAR censoring mechanisms.

5.3.4   Approaches to Missing Data

Missing data within longitudinal models is another topic with a large literature, which cannot adequately be addressed here, even within the restricted scope of discrete time-to-event models. Various types of left, right, and interval censoring arise in the time-to-event setting and are introduced effectively in Ref. [9, Chapter 3] and Ref. [11, Chapter III]. The notation r_{it} appearing in Equation 5.1 and throughout this chapter does double duty, as an indicator that the study subject i is both *at risk* and is *accessible to observation* at time period t. This indicator signals that data for i is not missing at t, because subject i is both alive and not censored.

The distinctions of Ref. [10] among missing-data mechanisms has been highly influential in longitudinal statistics. Mechanisms operating completely at random (MCAR) have observability-indicators r_{it} which are independent of all of the random variables $(X_{it}, Z_{it}, \varepsilon_{it}, A_{it})$ affecting observations Y_{it} and are easiest to deal with; mechanisms which operate independently only within covariate-defined strata, i.e., for which r_{it} are conditionally independent of $(A_{it}, \varepsilon_{it})$ given (X_{it}, Z_{it}), are called MAR and can be handled theoretically by likelihood-based but not by estimating-equation methods; and finally, the *nonignorable* or non-MAR mechanisms for missing or censored data which must be modeled somehow to avoid biasing parameter estimates.

Two distinct problems in analyzing ignorable missing longitudinal time-to-event data are missing values of time-dependent covariates X_{it} needed in modeling, and missing responses Y_{it} (often for different subjects). References [53,54] address the first problem. Missing responses have often been handled in recent literature by methods involving weighting observed responses by their inverse probability of being observed, estimated according to a parametric model. Useful references with this flavor are Refs. [55,56]. For a current exposition of longitudinal analysis in clinical trials, taking account of both these strands of research, see Ref. [57]. The different approach in Ref. [58], which has also had impact, is to subset the data according to the pattern of missing observations by subject, and to model separately within the subsets.

5.3.5 Goodness-of-Fit Statistics

In discrete longitudinal analysis, as in many other areas of statistics, most testing of goodness of fit of models is done by comparison of nested models, via likelihood ratio or score tests, as part of model building. This can be done both in the likelihood and GEE frameworks, as regards fixed-effect predictors. Random-effect model components are not easily tested within GEE, and as mentioned in Section 5.3.1, likelihood ratio testing for the presence or absence of a variance component is nonstandard because the zero component lies on the boundary of its parameter range.

Goodness-of-fit tests in categorical and GLM data, usually in a setting of only fixed effects, can be found in Ref. [2]. Various other goodness-of-fit tests in Ref. [7, pp. 66–69, 110–115, and 159] are based on logistic-regression or other categorical time series residuals, with particular relevance to the longitudinal setting because of an explicit treatment of time-dependent and stochastic regressors. Within the Cox modeling framework, goodness-of-fit tests based on several types of model residuals are implemented in **R** [13,49]. One fundamental idea for Cox model residuals, due to Ref. [59], is to standardize observed and expected response counts within cells of a partition of covariate-by-time space, and to create an omnibus test of fit as a quadratic form in these standardized counts. This idea was adapted by Slud and Kedem [27] to a case including the binary-response sequential models with time-dependent covariates but without random effects. Because the idea is so natural for discrete time-to-event longitudinal data, we provide some details of the statistic here.

Define $U_{it} \equiv (X_{it}, t)$ as a set of state variables in the general model (Equation 5.4), and let the cells C_k, $k = 1, \ldots, K$, partition the state space. In the sequential binary response model (Equation 5.16) without random effects, let the respective vectors $\underline{M}$ and $\hat{E}(\beta)$ of observed and model-predicted cell-wise counts be defined, for $k = 1, \ldots, K$, by

$$M_k = \sum_{i,t} I_{[U_{it} \in C_k]} Y_{it}, \quad \hat{E}(\beta)_k = \sum_{i,t} I_{[U_{it} \in C_k]} F(X'_{it} \hat{\beta})$$

Then the goodness-of-fit statistic has the following ingredients:

$$\hat{G} = \sum_{i,t} X_{it}^{\otimes 2} \left(\frac{dF}{dx} (X'_{it} \hat{\beta}) \right)^2 \Big/ \left(F(X'_{it} \hat{\beta}) (1 - F(X'_{it} \hat{\beta})) \right)$$

estimates the information matrix (where $\mathbf{v}^{\otimes 2} = \mathbf{v}\mathbf{v}'$ for a column vector $\mathbf{v}$);

$$\hat{D} = \text{Diag}\left(\sum_{i,t} I_{[U_{it} \in C_k]} F(X'_{it}\hat{\beta})(1 - F(X'_{it}\hat{\beta})) \right)$$

estimates the diagonal variance–covariance matrix of the vector $\underline{M} - \underline{\hat{E}}(\beta)$ of cell-wise *observed minus expected* counts; and the $p \times K$ estimated cross-information matrix is

$$\hat{B} = \sum_{i,t} \frac{dF}{dx}(X'_{it}\hat{\beta})X_{it}(I_{[U_{it} \in C_1]}, \ldots, I_{[U_{it} \in C_K]})$$

Then the goodness-of-fit statistic becomes

$$\hat{\Gamma} = (\underline{M} - \underline{\hat{E}}(\hat{\beta}))'(\hat{D} - \hat{B}'\hat{G}^{-1}\hat{B})^{-1}(\underline{M} - \underline{\hat{E}}(\hat{\beta})) \qquad (5.22)$$

where the matrix inverse may be a generalized inverse, and under the regularity conditions described in Section 5.2.6, the statistic is chi-square distributed,

$$\hat{\Gamma} \sim \chi_q^2, \quad q \equiv \text{rank}(\hat{D} - \hat{B}'\hat{G}^{-1}\hat{B}) \qquad (5.23)$$

The justification of the χ^2 asymptotic distribution (Equation 5.23) under the large-sample regularity conditions of Section 5.2.6 is given by Slud and Kedem [27, Section 3]. A completely analogous χ^2 goodness-of-fit statistic can be given for the Poisson-regression case, also without random effects. To the author's knowledge, analogous statistics have not been developed for the sequential model (Equation 5.14) with random effects and for its Poisson-regression analog, but they could be.

5.4 Computational Methods

Discrete longitudinal data analysis is an applied field, and the hindrances and signposts to its development have had much more to do with computational technique than with statistical theory. Computational techniques are described here with particular reference to the **R** statistical package [49]. Algorithms for iterative maximization of fixed-effect GLM likelihoods and for their quasilikelihood estimating equations were developed early [37] and are well implemented in all major statistical packages: the **R** function is `glm`. Several GEE implementations exist in **R**: the one we use below is `geeglm`, based on Ref. [41]. EM algorithms and various simulation-based extensions [10] have been a staple of computation for mixed effect GLM models, but are very hard to unify and generally have to be coded *ad hoc*. Algorithms for mixed GLM estimation based on Ref. [44]'s PQL method are implemented in the function `glmmPQL` within the MASS library in **R**. As of the R 2.7.0 release, the function `glmer` within D. Bates' `lme4` package [60] provides effective and accurate iterative ML maximization for mixed GLM models of not too great complexity. The **R** package does not yet contain effective computational tools for true multilevel mixed GLM estimation, although reportedly the `STATA`, `MLwin`, and `SAS` packages do [8,33]. In longitudinal event data as in other areas of statistics, the models of greatest complexity are computed by Bayesians, using the Markov Chain Monte Carlo and Gibbs sampling algorithms embedded in the publicly available `BUGS` software. There is a `bugs` function in **R**, in package `R2WinBugs` [61].

5.5   Data Examples

In this section, we summarize three data analyses to illustrate various aspects of longitudinal time-to-event modeling and model fitting as described above. Section 5.5.1 compares the fits of Cox and other models to data on first recurrences of bladder cancer, and employs a time-dependent stratifying variable in checking whether a unified model can fit the data on later recurrences. Section 5.5.2 explores GEE model-fits for counts versus mixed GLM models for indicators of positive responses. Finally, modeling issues arising with time-dependent covariates for recurrent events are addressed in Section 5.5.3 using data from a clinical trial on basal cell carcinomas (BCCs).

All of the data analyses were done using `R 2.7.0` [49]. Many of the **R** functions used, from the `survival` package, are documented in Ref. [13]. Others, especially `glmer` for mixed effects GLM regression, are in the `lme4` package [60].

5.5.1   Bladder Cancer Recurrence Data

The data in this example are modified from the form published in Ref. [62], which is included in the files `bladder` and `bladder2` in the `survival` package in **R**. The data as published, and as analyzed previously by many authors, consist of TRT (indicator of treatment, thiotepa vs. placebo), baseline `number`, and `size` (in cm) of previous tumors, and follow-up and recurrence times measured in months for 86 bladder cancer patients. One patient with follow-up time 0 and no recurrences was dropped, after which follow-up times ranged from 1 to 59 months, and six patients followed up beyond the fourth recurrence were right-censored at their fourth recurrence time. The numbers of patients for whom 0, 1, 2, 3, and 4 recurrences were observed were, respectively, 38, 18, 7, 8, and 14.

Since our analyses concern the adequacy of parametric models with temporal effects and interactions with numbers of previous recurrences, we avoid overparameterization by redefining cumulative times so that between-recurrence intervals are recoded to 3-month intervals. (1–3 recoded to 1, 4–6 recoded to 2, etc. Thus patient 9, with cumulative recurrence times of 12, 16, and 18 months, had these times recoded to 4, 6, and 7.) In this modified form, the time-period index ranges from 1 to 20, but the time-period indices of observed first recurrences range only up to 13.

TABLE 5.1:   Summary of models fitted.

Term	CoxMod	GLM.clglg	GLM.logis	GLM.probit	Cum.logis
TRT	−0.5227	−0.5321	−0.5786	−0.5744	−0.6633
Number	0.2233	0.2313	0.2629	0.2621	0.2984
Size	0.0688	0.0723	0.0788	0.0655	0.0809
lghaz1	−1.4638	−1.3215	−1.1879	−1.2840	−1.1843
lghaz2	−1.9282	−1.7838	−1.7194	−1.8240	−0.6004
lghaz3	−2.8702	−2.7233	−2.7150	−2.7659	−0.4221
. . .	. . .	. . .	. . .	. . .	. . .
lghaz10	−2.4119	−2.2420	−2.2179	−2.3485	0.4950
lghaz12	−2.7329	−2.6078	−2.5932	−2.6984	0.6039
lghaz13	−2.4542	−2.2812	−2.2235	−2.2567	0.7342
logLik	−134.1	−133.7	−133.6	−133.5	−134.2
Chi-sq	*	0.708	0.863	0.900	*

Note: CoxMod fitted by max PL, others by ML, to first-recurrence bladder-cancer data. lghaz denotes discrete log-hazards for CoxMod, time-effects for other models. Coefficients and lghaz for GLM.probit multiplied by 1.8134.

Table 5.1 exhibits coefficients and summary statistics from several forms of model estimated for first recurrence times. First, the discrete hazard Cox model of Equation 5.20 was fitted, by maximum Partial Likelihood (maxPL) using coxph for the coefficients, and basehaz for the cumulative baseline hazards, in terms of the non-time-dependent covariates $X_i^0 = ($TRT, number, size$)$. The next three columns of Table 5.1 were fitted by maximum likelihood (ML) as binary response models (indicated as GLMs) of the sequential form (Equation 5.16), with F successively specified as complementary loglog, logistic, and standard-normal, using glm in **R** with the same three baseline covariates X_i^0 plus dummy time-period effects. However, since the normal approximates the logistic distribution only when scaled up by the logistic standard deviation $(\pi^2/3)^{1/2} = 1.8134$, for comparability between logistic and probit fits we have multiplied the fitted probit coefficients and time-period effects by the factor 1.8134. The final column of Table 5.1 is the ML fit to the cumulative logistic model (Equation 5.13), again with baselines covariates X_i^0 and time-period effects. If not for the right-censorship in these data, the cumulative ordinal regression model could be fitted using the **R** function polr in the MASS library. But there is no currently available **R** function to fit right-censored models of this type (where for some individuals, the final observation tells not the precise ordinal value T_i, but rather a value C_i for which $T_i > C_i$). So the cumulative regression model fit was separately coded in **R**, using the general nonlinear function minimizer nlm.

The log-likelihood values (*logLik*) in the table are calculated from right-censored binary-response likelihoods using the respective models for the probabilities $P(T_i = t | X_i^0)$. These values are automatic from the glm fits, and obtained from the ML calculation in the proportional odds model, but *logLik* had to be coded separately for the Cox model.

Note the similarity of the (TRT, size, number) coefficients from all models, and the very close *logLik* values. The closeness of the loghaz coefficients for the Cox

TABLE 5.2:   Cell counts, and aggregated estimated GLM means (*M*) and variances (*V*), for models of first recurrence times in bladder cancer data.

Size	Time	Recur	Obs	E.Clglg	E.Logis	E.Norm	V.Clglg	V.Logis	V.Norm
=1	1:4	15	161	16.43	16.39	16.36	14.14	14.08	14.03
>1	1:4	19	90	17.62	17.78	17.81	12.92	13.09	13.21
=1	6:13	7	116	7.04	6.90	6.75	6.50	6.37	6.23
>1	6:13	6	59	5.83	5.93	6.07	5.06	5.12	5.22

and GLM.cloglog models is no surprise in light of the equivalence of these models shown in Section 5.2.4: the differences are due to the fact that the fitted values are PL maximizers in the Cox case, but ML maximizers in the GLM. The similarity of loghaz values across the different GLMs show that these fits are not very sensitive to the choice of link, but the corresponding parameters in the proportional odds (cumulative logistic) model have a different meaning, except for the first one which is close to the loghaz1 parameter for the logistic GLM.

The last line of Table 5.1 consists of the calculated chi-square goodness-of-fit statistics described in Section 5.3.5, Equation 5.23. All had $q = 4$ degrees of freedom, based on 4 cells defined by whether the baseline tumor size code was $= 1$ or >1 and the (recoded) time was < 5 or ≥ 5. The Chi-square values suggest excellent fits for all of the models, with clglg performing best by a slight amount on this criterion. The numbers of recurrences (Recur) in these cells out of all observations (Obs), and the expected values and estimated variances of the cell counts in each of the sequential binary-response models, are given in Table 5.2.

Since previous authors have used these data from Ref. [62] to study analysis methods for recurrent events, we consider now Cox model fits on the full (time-recoded) dataset, using the number enum (equal to one plus the number of previous within-study recurrences) either as a predictive or a stratifying factor. In these analyses, the only fixed-effect baseline covariates included are TRT and number, since size never produced significant effects.

In the first-recurrence analyses above, the TRT effect was suggestive (*p*-value between 0.05 and 0.10). We now expand the analysis to the full recoded dataset up to time 13—since there are very few and isolated recurrences beyond that time—incorporating dummy variables for enum as predictors. A Cox model (with Efron method for ties) now shows TRT not at all significant ($p = 0.44$) but number and enum highly significant. However, closer analysis reveals the baseline hazards to be very different among the different enum groups. We compare three nested models, in which enum enters either as a four-level factor (effectively, a three-column time-dependent dummy predictor) or as a stratifying variable:

(1) The simplest has 2 baseline covariates (TRT, number), 3 time-dependent dummies (for enum), and implicitly 10 time-period effects (the discrete baseline hazards at the 10 distinct observed failure times).

(2) The second is stratified on four levels of enum for a total of 52 possible time-period effects, plus 2 common (TRT, number) terms.

(3) The third is four separate enum-stratified models with separate (TRT, num-ber) parameters. The total possible number of parameters was 58, but here and in (2) there are actually fewer parameters because all failure times do not all occur in all strata.

The full dataset has 85 subjects contributing 152 records to these analyses (respect-ively 85, 45, 27, 18 in the four enum strata), which is not large considering the large number of parameters contemplated in the stratified models. The Cox model fitting functions allow a PL calculation at each of these stages, and the corresponding glm fit with cloglog link allows parametric likelihood-based calculations. The results are as follows:

Model	ML.df	PL.df	logPL	logML
(1)	18	*	-428.78	-284.79
(2)	48	x	-320.91	-262.38
(3)	54	x+7	-317.39	-258.21

In this table, the PL degrees of freedom should include the nuisance hazards (which is why the PL.df column contains * and x), but in any case there is no theoretical basis for comparing them in the stratified cases (2) and (3) versus the unstratified (1). While a PL likelihood ratio test of (1) versus (2) does not make sense, the parametric ML likelihood ratio test statistic is $2(284.79 - 262.38) = 44.82$ with χ^2_{30} p-value .040, indicating that the time-period effects within the separate enum groups are different. The likelihood ratio test of (2) versus (3) could in principle be performed using either the log PL or the log ML calculation, but the ML degrees of freedom ML.df have been affected by the occurrences of failures at different times in the different enum groups. Nevertheless, twice the (3)–(2) log-likelihood difference is clearly not significantly large for a χ^2_7 deviate. Thus model (2) is preferable to (3).

In this example, the essential equivalence between the Cox and cloglog-link binary response GLM justifies likelihood ratio tests and establishes that the stratified Cox model describes the data as well as any model considered. For completeness, we also checked the proportional hazards assumption using the cox.zph function in **R**, and by refitting the enum-stratified Cox model on the recoded times without right-censoring at 13, and with the timescale changed to restart at successive recurrence times, and on the original timescale (without recoding) for the data of Ref. [62]. In all cases, number remains very significant (p-value ranging from 0.005 to 0.025) and TRT nonsignificant (p-value ranging from 0.10 to 0.20). To illustrate our finding that the underlying Cox nuisance hazards are different in the four enum strata, Figure 5.1 displays these stratumwise cumulative hazards for the data of Ref. [62]. If the curves were not normalized to be equal at $t = 30$, the baseline hazards would be seen to increase steadily with enum, but this scale difference was already incorporated into model (1). The different shapes of the curves, accounting for the *logLik* improvement of model (2) over (1), includes but is not limited to differences in convexity versus concavity.

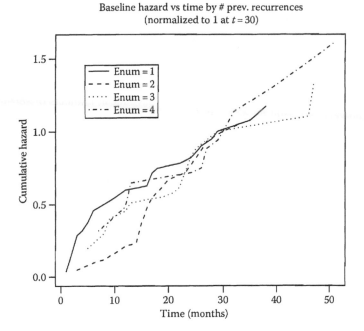

Baseline hazard vs time by # prev. recurrences
(normalized to 1 at $t = 30$)

FIGURE 5.1: Stratumwise cumulative baseline hazards for data of Ref. [62], within Cox model stratified by `enum` group, where `enum` is 1 plus the number of previous within-study recurrences. LR tests in text established differences between these curves.

5.5.2 Epileptic Seizure Count Data

The data for our second example, previously analyzed in Refs. [8,63], were downloaded from the supplementary data files `http://www.censtat.uhasselt.be/software/` of the Web site for Ref. [8]. The data are from a clinical trial [64] of the antiepileptic drug topiramate, and record weekly numbers of seizures for 89 patients, 44 of whom were randomized to the active treatment. The data consist of 1419 weekly records, incorporating demographic (`Age`, `Sex`, `Race`) variables and individual baseline covariates (`SeizRate`, `Height`, `Weight`). The interesting response variable is the weekly count Y_{it} = `NseizW` of seizures, especially in its relationship to treatment, and the time variable t is `StudyWk`.

The interesting aspect of these data for us is the ability of current tools—mixed effect models and GEE estimation methods—to compensate for the failure of simple fixed-effect Poisson regression models. The data are naturally longitudinal, in the sense that weekly seizure histories are available at the subject level. While `NseizW` turns out not to be directly correlated with `StudyWk`, there certainly is information—beyond the baseline seizure rate—about future numbers of seizures in the successive weekly patient seizure counts.

We begin with simple exploratory statistics related to the distribution of and correlations between the weekly counts Y_{it}. Let n_i denote the number of weekly observations available for patient i. Since the data contain considerable detail about individual subjects (eight having $n_i = 7$, while $n_i \geq 11$ for the rest), one sees immediately that there is considerable heterogeneity in individual seizure rates: the patients' mean numbers $\bar{Y}_{i\cdot}$ of weekly seizures have median 1.71, mean 3.42, and interquartile range (0.88, 4.00), and 13 patients have mean numbers of seizures > 8. Such heterogeneity would be compatible with the counts' having Poisson distribution, as long as the Poisson rates are sufficiently different. Nevertheless, the within-patient distributions of counts are found to have tails much heavier than the Poisson. The simplest way to see this is to calculate the Poisson patient-wise probabilities of seeing maximum counts at least as large as the observed maxima $\max_{1 \leq t \leq n_i} Y_{it}$, using the observed average counts $\bar{Y}_{i\cdot}$ (the patientwise ML estimates) as rates. Of the 89 probabilities calculated in this way, 12 are less than 5.e-4. This makes any Poisson regression model, with fixed effects or even with patient-specific random effects, untenable, although such models were fitted and interpreted in Ref. [8].

Next consider the correlations among weekly counts, within and across patients. The within-patient correlations between Y_{it} and t are very scattered, ranging from -0.80 to 0.52 (quartiles -0.28 and 0.13), with slightly negative bias apparently due to the patients with lower seizure rates tending to have longer follow-up. The overall correlation and partial correlation among NSEIZW and STUDYWK, correcting for ID, were slightly negative (both -0.066). Moreover, the within-patient correlation is negligible (-0.0056). So there seems to be no within-patient temporal structure in the data.

Although the Poisson distribution is excluded for counts, a few modeling strategies are possible. One is to look for an effect of the treatment in decreasing the incidence of weeks with at least one seizure. We give some results below for fixed and mixed effect binary-response models for I[NSEIZW>0]. Another strategy, followed by Molenberghs and Verbeke [8] and in a different way below, is to incorporate overdispersion and analyze the data by GEE methods. Still another approach, in Ref. [63], is to return to likelihood methods by allowing two different random effects within a Poisson model, one at patient level in the log of the Poisson mean, and another multiplicative effect on the Poisson mean at the level of single (i, t) observations. All of these analyses give similar results for the significance of effects of greatest interest, BSERATE and TRT, but while we find an adequate parametric model for binary responses, there seems to be no well-motivated one for the count data. That seems an excellent reason to rely on GEE methods for analyzing the count-response data.

To see why the reduction of detail in the response from the count NSEIZW to the indicator I[NSEIZW>0] is a promising method of analysis, consider Figure 5.2. Since within-patient temporal effects have been discounted, the plot exhibits the close and plausible relationship between seizure rates and fraction of weeks with seizures. A sequential-type logistic model for I[NSEIZW>0] in terms of all of the baseline predictors shows all but Race signficant. However, as often happens with large heterogeneous datasets, the significance is spurious and largely disappears when an appropriate random subject effect is introduced. Here, we used the **R**

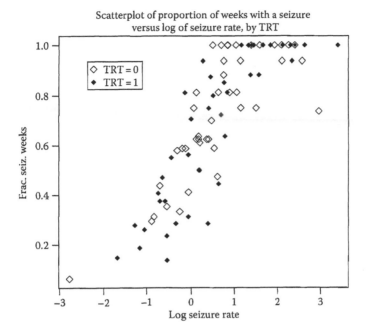

FIGURE 5.2: Log of patient mean seizure rate plotted by TRT symbol versus proportion of study weeks in which patient had at least one seizure.

function glmer in package lme4 to fit a model with random ID-level intercept: the comparison of *logLik* values is −806.95 (df = 8) for the fixed-effect model versus −712.74 (df = 9) for the mixed-effect model with a single normal ID random intercept. So the mixed model certainly fits better, and its only significant fixed coefficient is for BSERATE ($p=$ 6.e-7), with standardized TRT coefficient −1.56. When the insignificant baseline covariates are dropped in this random-ID intercept model, leaving only BSERATE and TRT, the *logLik* drops to −716.05 (now on df = 4), with standardized coefficient for TRT now nearly significant at −1.81. Adding a further random BSERATE effect improves *logLik* to −712.08 which is significantly better, but see Section 5.3.5 for why this likelihood ratio test for BSErate variance component has *p*-value $0.5(1 - F_{\chi_1^2}(2(716.05 - 712.08))) = 2.4\text{e-}3$ instead of $1 - F_{\chi_1^2}(2(716.05 - 712.08)) = 4.8\text{e-}3$. The model with independent random effects for Intercept (with fitted standard deviation 0.853) and BSErate (with fitted standard deviation 0.53) fits better than the one with only a random intercept; but the model with general correlated random Intercept and BSErate effects (*logLik* = −711.66) is not a sufficient improvement. Finally, STUDYWK is an additional highly significant fixed-effect predictor: entering it improves *logLik* to −704.09, and no additional or interaction terms give further significant improvements.

   The best model of this type (sequential binary-response mixed-effects logistic) appears to be one with fixed effects BSERATE, TRT, STUDYWK, and independent random effects for BSERATE and TRT (fitted standard deviations respectively 1.039 and 0.069). This model appears to fit adequately, and to be best by AIC-type criteria. It would be desirable to have a χ^2 goodness-of-fit test for such mixed models analogous to the tests described in Section 5.3.5, but the author is not aware of any. The fixed-effect coefficients, normalized coefficients, and two-sided Wald-test *p*-values for this best model are

Term	Coeff	Coeff.Stand	p-Value
Intercept	0.5436	1.667	0.0955
BSERATE	0.1150	4.942	1.e-06
TRT	−0.7880	−2.389	0.0169
STUDYWK	−0.0528	−4.029	5.6e-5

The TRT effect in this model is significant: the experimental drug has the effect of reducing the numbers of weeks containing seizures.

We checked also the GEE estimates and tests for TRT effect, based on the **R** function geeglm. With the binary response I[NSEIZW>0] (binary, logistic link), the GEE estimates closely confirm the likelihood-based findings above. However, the purpose of exploring GEE methods in this application is to be able to benefit from the more detailed form of the original count responses NSEIZW, and the GEE results with count response NSEIZW (Poisson log link) were interestingly different. STUDYWK is no longer significant, and surprisingly TRT is not either. However, the geeglm fit with terms TRT, BSERATE plus interaction TRT:BSERATE shows the interaction to be extremely highly significant (standardized coefficient −8.86), while the TRT coefficient is insignificantly positive. Thus the count data seem to show what the binary-responses could not: a signficant effect of treatment, operating differentially with much greater effect on patients with high baseline seizure rate. The results of this last analysis are confirmed when a GLM analysis allowing for overdispersion is performed using **R** function glm with the quasipoisson option, an analysis similar to others done by Molenberghs and Verbeke [8].

5.5.3   Basal Cell Carcinoma Study Data

Our final example is the analysis of data from a multiyear randomized clinical trial (the *ISOBCC* trial, Ref. [65]) of a drug treatment for BCCs, a form of nonmelanoma skin cancer which results in recurrent production of multiple skin tumors which are generally removed surgically. The trial consisted of 981 patients with previous BCCs, at eight clinical centers, with baseline covariates Age, Sex, Center, TRT, Nprior (= number of prior biopsy-proven BCCs, within 5 years before randomization), and measurements of skin Damage and SkinTyp. A few (9) patients had missing Damage and SkinTyp although they were followed up; so in this analysis, the missing covariates were imputed to typical moderate values. Patients were examined at staggered times measured in days from entry into the trial, when their new BCCs were counted and removed. Examinations were intended to occur after roughly 3 and 6 months, and every 6 months thereafter, so day-counts were recoded to exam numbers by

$$\texttt{Exam} = 1 + \texttt{trunc(round(Days/91.25)/2)}$$

and then, in the few cases where two separate examinations resulted in the same recoded Exam number, their NewBCC counts were aggregated to the single new Exam record. There were subjects who had 7 or fewer examinations, but 886 had 8 or more, and most had 11.

The objective of the trial was to study treatment effectiveness and adverse treatment-related events. A preliminary version of these data, with TRT omitted, was analyzed via logistic regression in Ref. [66] as an illustration of the calculation of relative efficiency of the logrank test for treatment effectiveness on Cox-model data. As it turned out, the drug treatment in ISOBCC was ineffective, and primary attention was devoted to side effects. The objective of this analysis, extending joint unpublished work done with Charles Brown of the National Cancer Institute in 1992, is to learn whether a unified explanatory model can give a clear picture of the dependence between earlier and later BCC counts: this is an exercise in the fitting and interpretation of time-dependent-covariate count-response longitudinal models. The interesting time-dependent predictors here are, for each Exam: CumBCC = the total of subject NewBCCs recorded at earlier Exams within the trial, and Nprev = number of previous Exams in the trial at which the subject had NewBCC ≥ 1.

A preliminary cross-tabulation of BCC rates per week, by Clinic and baseline number Nprior of BCCs, grouped by Nprior<3, Nprior=3:4, Nprior>4, shows that the occurrence rates per thousand person days increase sharply, from roughly 0.1 in the Nprior<3 group, to roughly 0.2 in the Nprior=3:4 group, to roughly 0.5 in the Nprior=5+ group, except that Clinic 8 shows a uniquely rapid increase across these groups, from 0.08 to 0.31 to 1.29. So all models must take into account not only a superlinear Nprior effect, but also a clear Clin8 interaction with Nprior.

The overall crude correlation between numbers of days between exams and NewBCC is −0.29, and a scatterplot confirms that while there is a positive relationship between Days and NewBCC within those exams which occurred within 400 days, for longer intervals the tendency was clearly negative. This may indicate that study subjects who tended to produce many BCCs maintained a regular exam schedule, while subjects who did not would wait until new BCCs appeared before having their exams. The following table shows the proportion of Exams with positive BCCs, in terms of Nprev and Days:

Nprev	= 0:2	3:4	5+
Days < 400	0.599	0.682	0.500
≥ 400	0.899	0.805	0.803

Thus, Days and Nprev have an interactive effect on BCC counts.

Poisson regression with baseline and time-dependent covariates and (pairwise) interactions leads rapidly by forward model-selection, with a final stage of pruning of nonsignificant terms, to a model in which SkinTyp and TRT play no role and Damage a very slight one, but with strikingly significant coefficients for Days (between successive exams), $Days^2$, $Nprior^k$, $k = 1, 2, \ldots, 5$, the Clin8 indicator, and interactions Nprior:CumBCC, Clin8:Nprev, CumBCC:Nprev, and Days:Nprior. This model, with 15 parameters, is very difficult to interpret in detail, although it shows clearly the variables that affect NewBCC production. The model is unavoidably complicated because of the subtle Days:Nprev and Clin8:Nprior interactions shown above.

Does the model fit adequately? There are several ways to check. One is to choose a partition of covariate-space into cells and see whether quadratic forms in the differences between aggregated observed and predicted NewBCCs for those cells are much larger than expected. For example, defining cells by Clinic and by Nprev up to a maximum of 5 yields the following table of standardized residuals (Obs BCC − Fitted count)/$\sqrt{\text{Fitted}}$:

	Clin=1	3	4	5	6	7	8	9
Nprev=0	2.96	1.45	0.21	1.23	−0.13	0.68	−1.14	1.17
1	0.04	−1.53	−1.35	−1.32	−0.22	−1.07	−0.04	−0.64
2	−0.54	0.35	0.32	−1.79	−0.26	−0.62	−1.31	−0.08
3	−1.01	−0.01	−0.80	−0.77	−0.53	−0.06	−0.35	0.82
4	2.34	−0.57	1.20	0.21	0.31	−0.37	0.12	0.63
5+	1.41	−0.33	−0.66	−0.12	0.10	1.05	−0.14	0.44

The sum of these squared residuals is 44.11, for 54 apparent degrees of freedom, and since 15 parameters were fitted and this quadratic form is larger than the minimum chi-square statistic (which does have asymptotic χ^2_{54-15} distribution), this display shows adequate fit despite the two large residuals in Clinic 1. Other such displays show similar behavior.

Models depending crucially on time-dependent covariates are difficult to interpret partly because some of the covariates are also responses. Note that while the correlation between observed and predicted counts in the model is a fairly noisy 0.52, the correlation between observed and predicted at the person level is 0.95, far better than the value 0.68 which was the correlation between observed and expected counts for the best person-level Poisson regression model it was possible to fit with baseline covariates alone. The improved correlation is partly due to the inclusion of running Nprev and CumBCC responses at the person level, but some thought shows the improvement is not automatic.

Further checks are possible. Fitting a random intercept to the Poisson regression model with the same fixed-effect predictors yields estimated variance essentially 0 for random effect at the patient level, which corresponds well with the finding that the dispersion scale-factor is close to 1 (actually 0.90) both by a glm quasilikelihood fit and with the geeglm fit. If the random intercept is introduced at the Observation level (i.e., the count at each Exam), a nonnegligible standard deviation of 0.6 is estimated, but almost exactly the same fixed-effect predictors are highly significant in all of these models, so it is not clear any of them is better than the purely fixed-effect model.

By searching, one can also find negative indications of fit. A likelihood ratio test of the same 15 fixed-effect coefficients appearing in the two subgroups of the data defined by `Nprev < 2` and `Nprev ≥ 2` gave the value 40.7, which is highly significant for a χ^2_{15} variate. The most reasonable conclusion is that the model is not quite statistically adequate in accounting for `Nprev` interactions in the Exam-level data.

5.6 Discussion

In this chapter, we have surveyed models and methods of analysis for discrete time-to-event data in a biostatistical setting. Regression models for longitudinal time-to-event data often have some or all of the following features:

- Time-dependent covariates including time-period dummy variables

- Subject-specific random effects, often treated as *iid* across subjects but which may also exhibit higher-level clustering (e.g., at a family or clinic or regional level)

- Recurrent endpoints, count data, or clinically meaningful state variables serving as covariates but calling for joint models with time-to-event responses

- Missing-data mechanisms involving drop-out or drop-in, seen as right or interval censorship, which may either be covariate mediated and ignorable (MAR) or nonignorable requiring explicit and usually parametric models

The rich variety of data structures and models of longitudinal time-to-event analysis has led to diverse methods of analysis: primarily likelihood methods whether estimation is done by scoring methods (in a GLM setting), by numerical maximization of (sometimes modified) likelihoods, or by EM algorithm; but also estimating equation and GEE methods based on marginal GLM likelihood formulations of longitudinal data models. We have touched on all of these, emphasizing in our discussion and examples the interplay between models of counts and point occurrences, the tools for checking goodness of fit, and the implementation of estimation and model checking in the **R** statistical computing platform [49].

Acknowledgment

The author is grateful to his colleagues Benjamin Kedem and Paul Smith for their careful reading of this chapter and very useful comments on it.

References

[1] N. Laird, Topics in likelihood-based methods for longitudinal data analysis, *Stat. Sinica*, 1, 33–50, 1991.

[2] A. Agresti, *Categorical Data Analysis*, 2nd ed. New York: Wiley, 2002.

[3] P. Diggle, P. Heagerty, K.-Y. Liang, and S. Zeger, S., *Longitudinal Data Analysis*, 2nd ed. Oxford: Oxford University, 2004.

[4] L. Fahrmeir and G. Tutz, *Multivariate Statistical Modeling Based on Generalized Linear Models*. New York: Springer-Verlag, 1994.

[5] J. Lindsey, *Models for Repeated Measurements*, 2nd ed. Oxford: Oxford University, 1999.

[6] D. Hedeker and R. Gibbons, *Longitudinal Data Analysis*. New York: Wiley, 2006.

[7] B. Kedem and K. Fokianos, *Regression Models for Time Series Analysis*. New York: Wiley, 2002.

[8] G. Molenberghs and G. Verbeke, *Discrete Longitudinal Models*. New York: Springer, 2005.

[9] J. Klein and M. Moeschberger, *Survival Analysis*, 2nd ed. New York: Springer, 2003.

[10] R. Little and D. Rubin, *Statistical Analysis of Missing Data*, 2nd ed. New York: Wiley, 2002.

[11] P. Andersen, Ø. Borgan, R. Gill, and N. Keiding, *Statistical Models Based on Counting Processes*. New York: Springer, 1993.

[12] V. Bagdonavicius and M. Nikulin, *Accelerated Life Models*. Boca Raton, FL: Chapman & Hall/CRC, 2002.

[13] T. Therneau, A package for survival analysis in S, Technical report, Rochester, MN: Mayo Clinic, 1999.

[14] O. Aalen and H. Gjessing, H., Understanding the shape of the hazard rate: A process point of view, *Stat. Sci.*, 8, 284–309, 2001.

[15] M.-L. Lee and G. Whitmore, Threshold regression for survival analysis: Modeling event times by a stochastic process reaching a boundary, *Stat. Sci.*, 21, 501–513, 2006.

[16] E. Çinlar and S. Özekici, Reliability of complex devices in random environments, *Prob. Eng. Informat. Sci.*, 1, 97–115, 1987.

[17] M. Hollander and E. Peña, Dynamic reliability models with conditional proportional hazards, *Lifetime Data Anal.*, 1, 377–402, 1995.

[18] M.-L. Lee, G. Whitmore, F. Laden, J. Hart, and E. Garshick, A case-control study relating railroad worker mortality to diesel exhaust exposure using a threshold regression model, *J. Stat. Planning Inference*, in press.

[19] D. Hedeker and R. Gibbons, A random-effects ordinal regression model for multilevel analysis, *Biometrics*, 50, 933–944, 1994.

[20] D. Zeng, D. Lin, and G. Yin, Maximum likelihood estimation for the proportional odds model with random effects, *J. Am. Stat. Assoc.*, 100, 470–483, 2005.

[21] D.R. Cox, Regression models and life tables (with discussion), *J. Roy. Stat. Soc. Ser. B*, 74, 187–220, 1972.

[22] W. Thompson, On the treatment of multiple observations in life studies, *Biometrics*, 33, 463–470, 1977.

[23] E. Bonney, Logistic regression for dependent binary observations, *Biometrics*, 43, 951–973, 1987.

[24] E. Arjas and P. Haara, A logistic regression model for hazard: Asymptotic results, *Scand. J. Stat.*, 14, 1–18, 1987.

[25] D. Stablein, K. Nolph, and A. Lindblad, Timing and characteristics of multiple peritonitis episodes: A report of the National CAPD Registry, *Am. J. Kidney Dis.*, 14, 44–49, 1989.

[26] S. Zeger and B. Qaqish, Markov regression models for time series: A quasi-likelihood approach, *Biometrics*, 44, 1019–1031, 1988.

[27] E. Slud and B. Kedem, Partial likelihood analysis of logistic regression and autoregression, *Stat. Sinica*, 4, 89–106, 1994.

[28] R. Stiratelli, N. Laird, and J. Ware, Random-effects models for serial observations with binary response, *Biometrics*, 40, 961–971, 1984.

[29] J. Chan and A. Kuk, Maximum likelihood estimation for probit-linear mixed models with correlated random effects, *Biometrics*, 53, 86–97, 1997.

[30] M. Mandel and R. Betensky, Estimating time-to-event from longitudinal ordinal data using random-effects Markov models: Application to multiple sclerosis progression, *Biostatistics*, 9, 750–764, 2008.

[31] P. Hougaard, *Analysis of Multivariate Survival Data.* New York: Springer, 2000.

[32] D. Zeng, D. Lin, and X. Lin, Semiparametric transformation models with random effects for clustered failure time data, *Stat. Sinica*, 18, 355–377, 2008.

[33] H. Goldstein, H. Pan, and J. Bynner, A flexible procedure for analyzing longitudinal event histories using a multilevel model, *Underst. Stat.*, 3, 85–99, 2004.

[34] N. Breslow, Tests of hypotheses in overdispersed Poisson regression models and other quasi-likelihood models, *J. Am. Stat. Assoc.*, 85, 565–571, 1990.

[35] P. Thall, Mixed Poisson likelihood regression models for longitudinal interval count data, *Biometrics*, 44, 197–209, 1988.

[36] R. Davis, W. Dunsmuir, and Y. Wang, On autocorrelation in a Poisson regression model, *Biometrika*, 87, 491–505, 2000.

[37] P. McCullagh and J. Nelder, *Generalized Linear Models*, 2nd ed. London: Chapman & Hall, 1989.

[38] G. Fitzmaurice, N. Laird, and A. Rotnitzky, Regression models for discrete longitudinal responses, *Stat. Sci.*, 8, 284–309, 1993.

[39] P. Heagerty, Marginalized transition models and likelihood inference for longitudinal categorical data, *Biometrics*, 58, 342–351, 2002.

[40] K.-Y. Liang and S. Zeger, Longitudinal data analysis using generalized linear models, *Biometrika*, 73, 13–22, 1986.

[41] R. Prentice and L.-P. Zhao, Estimating equations for parameters in means and covariances of multivariate datasets and continuous responses, *Biometrics*, 47, 825–839, 1991.

[42] P. Andersen and R. Gill, Cox's regression model for counting processes: A large sample study, *Ann. Statist*, 10, 1100–1120, 1982.

[43] R. Guieorguieva and A. Agresti, A correlated probit model for joint modeling of clustered binary and continuous responses, *J. Am. Stat. Assoc.*, 96, 1102–1112, 2001.

[44] N. Breslow and D. Clayton, Approximate inference in generalized linear mixed models, *J. Am. Stat. Assoc.*, 88, 9–25, 1993.

[45] X. Lin, Estimation using penalized quasilikelihood and quasi-pseudo-likelihood in Poisson mixed models, *Lifetime Data Anal.*, 13, 533–544, 2007.

[46] S. Self and K.-Y. Liang, Asymptotic properties of maximum likelihood estimators and likelihood ratio tests under nonstandard conditions, *J. Am. Stat. Assoc.*, 82, 605–610, 1987.

[47] B. Freidlin, M. Podgor, and J. Gastwirth, Efficiency robust tests for survival or order categorical data, *Biometrics*, 55, 883–886, 1999.

[48] N. Lange, B. Carlin, and A. Gelfand, Hierarchical Bayes models for the progression of HIV infection using longitudinal CD4 T-Cell numbers, *J. Am. Stat. Assoc.*, 87, 615–626, 1992.

[49] R Development Core Team, *R: A Language and Environment for Statistical Computing.* Vienna: R Foundation for Stat. Comp., http://www.R-project.org, 2008.

[50] T. Scheike and Y. Sun, Maximum likelihood estimation for tied survival data under Cox regression model via EM algorithm, *Lifetime Data Anal.*, 13, 399–420, 2007.

[51] N. Hjort, Goodness of fit tests in models for life history data based on cumulative hazard rates, *Ann. Stat.*, 18, 1221–1258, 1990.

[52] P. Thall and S. Vail, Some covariance models for longitudinal count data with overdispersion, *Biometrics*, 46, 657–671, 1990.

[53] J. Robins, A. Rotnitzky, and L. Zhao, Estimation of regression coefficients when some regressors are not always observed, *J. Am. Stat. Assoc.*, 89, 846–866, 1994.

[54] S. Lipsitz, J. Ibrahim, and G. Fitzmaurice, Likelihood methods for incomplete longitudinal binary responses with incomplete categorical covariates, *Biometrics*, 55, 214–223, 1999.

[55] D. Scharfstein, A. Rotnitzky, and J. Robins, Adjusting for nonignorable dropout using semiparametric nonresponse models, *J. Am. Stat. Assoc.*, 94, 1096–1120, 1999.

[56] G. Fitzmaurice, G. Molenberghs, and S. Lipsitz, Regression models for longitudinal binary responses with informative drop-outs, *J. Roy. Stat. Soc. Ser. B*, 57, 691–704, 1995.

[57] I. Jansen, C. Beunckens, G. Molenberghs, G. Verbeke, and C. Mallinckrodt, Analyzing incomplete discrete clinical trial data, *Stat. Sci.*, 21, 52–69, 2006.

[58] R. Little, Pattern-mixture models for multivariate incomplete data, *J. Am. Stat. Assoc.*, 88, 125–134, 1993.

[59] D. Schoenfeld, Chi-squared goodness of fit tests for the proportional hazards regression model, *Biometrika*, 67, 145–153, 1980.

[60] D. Bates, Documentation for lme4 package http://rweb.stat.umn.edu/R/library/lme4/doc/, 2008.

[61] A. Gelman, Running BUGS and WinBugs from **R** http://www.stat.columbia.edu/ gelman/bugsR/, 2008.

[62] L.-J. Wei, D.-Y. Lin, and L. Weissfeld, Regression analysis of multivariate incomplete failure time data by modeling marginal distributions, *J. Am. Stat. Assoc.*, 84, 1065–1073, 1989.

[63] G. Molenberghs, G. Verbeke, and C. Demetrio, An extended random-effects approach to modeling repeated, overdispersed count data, *Lifetime Data Anal.*, 13, 513–531, 2007.

[64] E. Faught, B. Wilder, R. Ramsay, R. Reife, L. Kramer, G. Pledger, and R. Karim, Topiramate placebo-controlled dose-ranging trial in refractory partial epilepsy using 200-, 400- and 600-mg daily dosages, *Neurology*, 46, 1684–1690, 1996.

[65] J. Tangrea, B. Edwards, P. Taylor, and A. Hartman, and other members of the Isotretinoin-Basal Cell Carcinoma Study Group, Long-term therapy with low-dose isotretinoin for prevention of basal cell carcinoma: A multicenter clinical trial, *J. Nat. Cancer Inst.*, 84(5), 328–332, 1992.

[66] E. Slud, Relative efficiency of the log rank test within a multiplicative intensity model, *Bimetrika*, 78, 621–630, 1991.

Chapter 6

Overview of Bayesian Inferential Methods Including Time-to-Event Endpoints

Laura H. Gunn

Contents

This chapter provides an overview of the Bayesian framework to analytic methods for public health data and time-to-event data in clinical trials, including parametric survival models. Section 6.1 presents an overview of Bayesian methods of analysis, with an application of these methods to public health data provided in Section 6.2. Section 6.3 provides a brief overview of the commonly used Weibull and Exponential parametric survival models for time-to-event data. Section 6.4 shows an example of Bayesian methods for time-to-event data in a clinical trial, while Section 6.5 concludes the chapter with a discussion.

6.1   Brief Overview of Bayesian Analysis

Although much of the literature in clinical trial, public health, and biomedical research is saturated with classical, or frequentist, approaches to statistical analyses, the Bayesian paradigm of analysis continues to gain greater attention and support. It was 10 years ago in the February 1998 International Medical Device Regulatory Monitor that Food and Drug Administration (FDA) officials endorsed Bayesian methods for incorporating "historical information into medical device clinical trial data" [1]. Berry [2] and Irony and Simon [3] offer a more detailed discussion of Bayesian methods in medical device development and trials. Today, 10 years later, Bayesian analyses are accepted as a standard approach for medical device development by the Center for Devices and Radiological Health (CDRH) of the FDA, with approximately 10% of FDA approvals for medical and radiological devices based on Bayesian approaches [4].

In the clinical trial setting, investigators are often concerned with the information that can be gained from the trial. For example, what prior evidence exists on the benefits of the treatment under study [5]? This prior information, or evidence, by which a prior distribution is constructed is updated with current evidence from the trial, which is described through the likelihood function. The updating of the prior evidence (in the form of a prior probability distribution) with the current evidence (in the form of a likelihood function) results in a posterior distribution on which Bayesian inferences are made, including the computation of predictive characteristics. The core of Bayesian analysis rests on the theory of updating evidence or beliefs.

Under the classical paradigm of statistical analysis, probability is objective. Inferences based on a classical approach, in which parameters are fixed, begin by specifying a model and null hypothesis (H_0) and continues with collecting data, calculating a p-value (i.e., the probability of obtaining results that are as extreme or more extreme than the observed data given H_0 is true), and making inferences based on significance levels to determine the size and direction of model effects.

In contrast, the Bayesian approach to statistical analysis is based on the notion of subjective probability. Bayesian inference considers parameters as random by which each model in a set of plausible models is assigned a prior probability. Data is collected, and Bayes' theorem is used to compute the posterior probability of each model given the observed data: it is important to note the absence of p-values in Bayesian analysis. Inferences are then drawn from posterior probabilities to guide decision making. In particular under the Bayesian framework, credible intervals are used to make direct inferences from the posterior distribution, compared to the frequentist confidence intervals which are based on hypothetical repetitions of the study and do not allow for direct probability statements. In other words, Bayesians are able to make a direct statement with a credible interval (i.e., there is a 95% chance that the parameter lies in the credible interval), whereas frequentists indirectly imply something similar (i.e., if the sampling were repeated in the same manner 100 times, then 95 of the 100 intervals would contain the true parameter value). Since the prior distribution contributes an additional component of variability to the Bayesian model, credible intervals can be wider than their classical confidence interval counterparts.

The posterior distribution is calculated using Bayes' theorem and is proportional to the prior multiplied by the likelihood:

$$p(\theta|\text{data}) \propto p(\theta)p(\text{data}|\theta), \tag{6.1}$$

where
  $p(\theta)$ is the prior belief on the parameter θ,
  $p(\text{data}|\theta)$ is the likelihood function, and
  $p(\theta|\text{data})$ represents the updated belief (i.e., the posterior distribution) combining the prior belief with the current evidence.

The constant of proportionality can be found by simply integrating (in the continuous case) or summing (in the discrete case) the right side of the proportionality statement with respect to θ.

The shape of the posterior distribution depends on the distributions of the prior and likelihood function. Choosing a conjugate prior will result in the posterior distribution following a closed-form expression in the same parametric form as the prior distribution. For example, if data are represented by y, then the likelihood function can be expressed in terms of a binomial distribution:

$$p(y|\theta) = \text{Bin}(y|n, \theta) \propto \theta^y(1 - \theta)^{n-y}, \tag{6.2}$$

with a beta conjugate prior on the parameter, θ:

$$p(\theta) = \text{Be}(\theta|\alpha, \beta) \propto \theta^{\alpha-1}(1 - \theta)^{\beta-1}, \tag{6.3}$$

where α and β are considered hyperparameters. Hyperparameters can be fixed or assigned a prior distribution; assume the hyperparameters are fixed in this example. Since the beta prior distribution is a conjugate family for the binomial likelihood function, then the posterior distribution, $p(\theta|y)$, follows a beta parametric form:

$$p(\theta|y) = \text{Be}(\theta|\alpha + y, \beta + n - y) \propto \theta^{\alpha+y-1}(1 - \theta)^{\beta+n-y-1}. \tag{6.4}$$

Another example of a conjugate family is an exponential distribution as the likelihood, which is commonly seen with time-to-event data, combined with a Gamma prior yielding a Gamma posterior distribution. Bernado and Smith [6] and Gelman et al. [7] provide more details regarding conjugate prior specification. The influence of a conjugate prior can be measured when multiplying the likelihood by the prior produces the same effect as increasing the sample size [8]. While conjugate priors simplify computation, provide good approximations, and produce results that are easy to comprehend, nonconjugate priors are often necessary for analyzing more complex models [7]. Updating a nonconjugate prior with the likelihood results in a posterior distribution with no closed-form expression. The methods for updating are similar when using a nonconjugate prior; however, the computation often becomes more involved in such cases.

Prior elicitation receives great attention in the model specification phase. In the clinical trial setting, agreement upon a prior specification can sometimes be difficult among members of a Data and Safety Monitoring Board (DSMB). Investigators assign informative or noninformative priors to model parameters. A noninformative diffuse, or flat, prior is assigned to a parameter when the researcher does not have strong evidence for particular parameter values and a large range of possible values exists in which all potential values are approximately equally probable. However, when a prior is so diffuse that it does not integrate to one, this is known as an improper prior. A uniform distribution is a good example of a noninformative prior in which the prior has little effect on the posterior, hence the posterior is proportional to the likelihood in this case (see [6, 7, 9–11] for more details about noninformative prior elicitation). In contrast, with a highly informative prior consisting of a point mass at a particular value, the posterior reflects the prior distribution. There are numerous priors in between these extreme cases, and the process of choosing the most appropriate prior involves a mixture of art and science. Essentially, when strong prior evidence exists, an informative prior elicitation is key to most appropriately specifying the model. More details regarding prior specification can be found in Gelman et al. [7], Chaloner [12], Kadane and Wolfson [13], Kass and Wasserman [14], O'Hagan [15], and Varshavsky and David [16].

Once a Bayesian model is specified, computational methods are needed to obtain posterior estimates for making inferences and guiding decision making. Markov chain Monte Carlo (MCMC) methods are a simulation-based procedure used to draw random samples from the posterior in order to approximate the posterior distribution. For example, the estimated posterior mean is found by computing the average of the random samples. MCMC derives its name from "Monte Carlo" referring to drawing random numbers from a certain distribution, and "Markov chain" representing the dependence of each sample on the previous sample. One advantage of MCMC methods is that they provide a relatively simple approach to solving analytically complex problems. Biostatisticians rely on computational power to generate random samples from the posterior, which is one reason MCMC methods have become more and more prominent over the last decade or so with advances in computer technology.

Gibbs sampling is one of the most commonly used MCMC techniques. It is an iterative updating scheme that generates new parameter values based on full conditional distributions. If θ is a parameter vector composed of k components, then at each iteration, m, of the sampler, there are k steps to the iteration. At every iteration m, each θ_j^m is sampled from the full conditional distribution, $p(\theta_j|\theta_{-j}^{m-1}, y)$, where θ_{-j}^{m-1} represents all the remaining components of θ, except for θ_j, at their current values (i.e., $\theta_1^m, \ldots, \theta_{j-1}^m$ for those up to θ_j and $\theta_{j+1}^{m-1}, \ldots, \theta_k^{m-1}$ after θ_j) [7]. The Gibbs sampler is widely used in Bayesian analysis, as are other computational methods such as the Metropolis-Hastings algorithm and importance sampling, to name two additional techniques. Gelman et al. [7], Gelfand and Smith [17], Casella and George [18], and Gamerman [19] provide much more depth into the theory and explanation of MCMC methods, including the Gibbs sampler and MCMC convergence diagnostics, with numerous applications provided by Gilks et al. [20].

While this is only a brief overview of Bayesian analysis, this section is hopefully helpful in providing a general framework for Bayesian methods of analysis. The further readings suggested within this section allow the reader to gain a greater understanding of Bayesian analysis than what is presented here. Prior to presenting Bayesian methods and an application for time-to-event data, specifically in the clinical trial setting, in Sections 6.3 and 6.4, Section 6.2 provides an application of Bayesian methods to public health data.

6.2 Application of a Bayesian Approach to Modeling the Proportion of HIV/AIDS Patients Prescribed Aggressive Care

6.2.1 Public Health Application Background

The advent of potent combination antiretroviral therapy has transformed HIV infection from a debilitating, universally fatal disease to a chronic, manageable disease. Morbidity and mortality from HIV infection has decreased significantly because of these "aggressive" treatments [21]. Aggressive treatment regimes continue to be defined and modified: in the late 1990s to early 2000s aggressive treatment was defined by combination antiretroviral drug therapy. Combination therapy consisted of at least three antiretroviral drugs, including protease inhibitors and nonnucleoside analogs, and was endorsed and implemented as practice guidelines by the Department of Health and Human Services in 1997 [22, 23].

Despite these recommendations, not all HIV-infected patients receive combination antiretroviral therapy. In a nationally representative survey of HIV-infected persons receiving care in the United States, only 55% of patients surveyed received a protease inhibitor or nonnucleoside analog, key elements of potent combination antiretroviral therapy, at some time prior to the end of 1996 [24]. Furthermore, as part of the HIV Practice Cooperative, reviews of 600 randomly selected charts at six HIV clinics across the United States showed that only 34% of patients received the preferred combination therapy recommended by the Department of Health and Human Services at the end of 1997 [25].

Prescription of combination antiretroviral therapy varies by patient characteristics. In a nationally representative survey of HIV-infected patients in the United States, 85% of patients with reported CD4 + lymphocyte counts less than 500 cells/mm^3 received a protease inhibitor or nonnucleoside analog by January 1998 [26]. Women, minorities, and the under-insured were less likely to have received these potent drugs. In a survey of 1034 patients enrolled in an AIDS Service Organization in Los Angeles, 66% reported treatment with a protease inhibitor. Multivariate logistic regression showed that patients who did not speak English or who had a lower income were less likely to receive a protease inhibitor [27].

Similar findings have been made in other industrialized countries. In a survey of physicians of patients seen as part of the Swiss HIV Cohort Study, 69% of patients received highly active antiretroviral therapy (HAART), defined as 1 to 2 nucleoside analogs plus 1 to 2 protease inhibitors, in the fall of 1997 [28]. Sixteen percent of patients did not receive HAART although their clinical condition warranted it according to official Swiss guidelines. Multivariate logistic regression showed that patients with lower educational level, active injection drug use and injection drug use as the mode of acquisition of HIV were less likely to receive HAART when indicated [28].

Less information has been available about patient characteristics that influence aggressive care prescription practices in the southeastern region of the United States. The North Carolina Special Project of National Significance (SPNS) Integration Project, funded by Health Resources and Services Administration (HRSA), began in the fall of 1996. The project's goal was to study the effects of an integrated service delivery model on HIV-infected persons living in the southeastern United States. This project has provided a unique opportunity to determine antiretroviral prescription practices in a region where the HIV infection rate has been growing most rapidly and where there exists a heterogeneous population from both urban and rural communities [29]. A cohort of patients was recruited in this project to determine the patient characteristics associated with the prescription of combination antiretroviral therapy. For regulation and monitoring purposes, it is important to understand which patients living with HIV and AIDS are prescribed aggressive treatment.

6.2.2   Study Design and Data

During the summer of 1997, 802 consecutive patients receiving Medicaid, or who were Medicaid-eligible, and attending one of six HIV clinics in the Southeast were asked if they would be willing to have their medical records reviewed and participate in a periodic telephone survey. The project was approved by the Institutional Review Board for each of the six participating sites and received a federal certificate of confidentiality from the Department of Health and Human Resources.

The study was conducted as an observational case-reference study. The primary outcome measure was the most recent antiretroviral regimen recorded at the time of the chart review in the fall of 1997. Combination antiretroviral therapy, represented here as aggressive care, was defined as (1) prescription of at least three antiretrovirals including a protease inhibitor or nonnucleoside analog, or (2) enrollment in an antiretroviral study protocol, regardless of the number of antiretrovirals prescribed. This definition is in accordance with 1997 treatment guidelines [22,23], in which the preferred initial regimen consisted of two nucleosides in addition to a protease or nonnucleoside analog. Enrollment in an antiretroviral study protocol was included in the definition because it was assumed that both the patient and health care provider wanted the patient to take a state-of-the-art regimen, even if the patient was receiving only two active antiretrovirals.

This study was performed on patient medical record abstractions as well as phone interviews from the fall of 1997. The consent rate for record review was 94%, while the response rate for the surveys was approximately 70% [30]. Twenty-six patient characteristics were collected via medical records and phone surveys. Variables collected describe demographics, housing and transportation characteristics, social support, adherence, drug use, other HIV risk factors, and disease stage. The demographics of this population were representative of previously published surveys of HIV-infected persons in the southern United States [29]. Data abstracted by hired clinicians include gender, race, date of birth, place of residence, risk factors for HIV, substance abuse history, general medical problems, and HIV-specific diagnoses. Antiretrovirals prescribed, CD4 + lymphocyte counts and plasma HIV-1 RNA measurements were recorded for the 12 month period prior to the date of chart abstraction. Baseline CD4 + lymphocyte counts and plasma HIV-1 RNA levels were defined as the first value recorded during the 12 month time period. Furthermore, the chart abstractor determined the primary HIV health care provider to be the physician who saw the patient most frequently.

All variables were collected dichotomously—which, as biostatisticians, we know is not always the most appropriate study design—and the coding scheme (1/0) is presented with each variable. The patient demographic characteristics include race (black/other), other race (not black or white/black or white), sex (male/female), age-old (50 or older/under 50), and age-young (under 34/34 or older). Housing and transportation variables include living distance from clinic (50 miles or more/under 50), unstable housing (yes/no), living in rural surroundings (yes/no), and available transportation to clinic (yes/no). A social support variable codes whether someone reminds the patient to take medications (yes/no). An adherence variable codes for adherence to treatment (yes/no). Drug use variables collected from medical records include: current drug abuse (yes/no), and history of drug use (yes/no). Drug use variables collected from the phone survey include ever used drugs (yes/no), drug use in the past 6 months (yes/no), drug use in the past 3 months (yes/no), IV drug use (yes/no), and IV drug use and heterosexual (yes/no). Nondrug-related HIV risk factors collected include male sex with male (yes/no), other risk factor (yes/no), and unknown risk factor (yes/no). Finally, disease state variables include low CD4 + cell count (<200 cells/mm^3/≥ 200 cells/mm^3), medium CD4 + cell count (200–499 cells/mm^3/<200 or ≥ 500 cells/mm^3), CDC clinical stage B—symptomatic, but no AIDS diagnosis—(yes/no), CDC clinical stage C—AIDS diagnosis—(yes/no), and plasma HIV-1 RNA viral load medium to high (>400 copies/mL/≤ 400 copies/mL).

Table 6.1 describes the sample from each clinic by these variables. The proportion of patients receiving aggressive care is quite variable across clinics, ranging from 47% to 82%, with 64% of patients prescribed aggressive treatment across all clinics. There is also considerable variability in patient characteristics across the clinics. For example, the proportion of patients who are male ranges from about 44% to about 76%. Many variables show ranges of 20% or more across clinics.

Prior to specifying a Bayesian model, missing data was imputed to complete the dataset. Five covariates contained missing observations, including low CD4 + counts, medium CD4 + counts, medium-to-high viral load, current drug use, and adherence to treatment. The percentages of missing data for these covariates range from 0.25% for medium CD4 + counts to 31.1% for adherence. The decision not to delete observations corresponding to missing values stems from the fact that some of the missing values correspond to a patient who is a physician's only patient, so

TABLE 6.1:   Observed patient characteristics by clinic.

	Clinic 1	Clinic 2	Clinic 3	Clinic 4	Clinic 5	Clinic 6
# Physicians	15	4	3	6	14	13
# Patients	227	130	91	59	71	224
% Aggressive care prescription	60.48	60.16	82.13	70.16	74.96	46.86
% Treatment adherence	62.76	61.30	67.18	67.48	49.40	59.86
% Reminded to take medication	21.15	20.77	17.58	25.42	28.17	23.66
% CD4 + count low	46.39	51.27	61.49	51.67	49.74	34.70
% CD4 + count medium	33.08	33.76	22.74	40.92	32.89	47.17
% Viral load medium to high	65.77	60.33	79.61	58.20	47.67	49.93
% Stage B disease	23.35	18.46	16.48	27.12	26.76	36.16
% Stage C disease	38.77	44.62	48.35	40.68	39.44	40.63
% Male	73.58	43.96	56.88	68.11	75.86	57.75
% Black	68.91	83.96	62.56	54.33	54.70	59.20
% Other race	4.41	0.77	2.20	1.69	1.41	4.91
% Age ≥ 50	11.01	3.85	6.60	15.25	8.45	4.91
% Age < 34	24.67	39.23	43.96	22.03	38.03	36.61
% Unstable housing	22.47	23.85	29.67	33.90	32.39	30.36
% Rural living	48.46	62.31	31.87	45.76	36.62	47.32
% Transportation available	11.45	10.00	10.99	18.64	18.31	11.16
% Current drug use (chart)	15.51	9.63	34.76	19.35	28.06	28.87
% History of drug use (chart)	59.91	44.62	45.05	57.63	52.11	50.45
% Ever used drugs (survey)	43.17	37.69	41.76	52.54	46.48	42.86
% Drug use in past 6 months (survey)	15.86	13.08	23.08	18.64	18.31	20.09
% Drug use in past 3 months (survey)	11.01	11.54	19.78	13.56	16.90	16.96
% Heterosexual and IV drug use	1.32	4.62	13.19	11.86	4.23	8.93
% IV drug use	18.94	10.00	3.30	6.78	1.41	7.14
% Homosexual	24.23	13.08	21.98	27.12	45.07	25.45
% Other risk	11.89	10.00	17.58	16.95	11.27	14.29
% Unknown risk	19.40	27.12	6.58	17.47	13.13	29.59

eliminating the patient would also discount the physician from the analysis. Therefore, missing data was imputed using

$$x_{ijk} \sim \text{Bernoulli}(\%\text{success}), \tag{6.5}$$

where

x_{ijk} is the jth covariate value for the ith patient under physician k and
%success represents the proportion of positive responses to each covariate containing missing values.

6.2.3 Bayesian Model Specification

The structure of the data requires Bayesian hierarchical modeling strategies. Patients are nested within 55 physicians and 6 southeastern academic clinics. To account for unmeasured factors that are correlated within physician, a physician random effect is included in the model. By including this random effect, one can account for a provider's inclination toward prescribing aggressive treatment over that specified by the fixed patient characteristic effects.

The basic model structure is a logistic regression function

$$\log\left(\frac{p_{ik}}{1 - p_{ik}}\right) = X_{ijk}\beta_j + r_k, \tag{6.6}$$

where

p_{ik} is the probability that patient i under physician k is prescribed aggressive care,
X_{ijk} is covariate j for patient i under physician k,
β_j is the regression coefficient corresponding to covariate j, and
r_k is the random effect for physician k.

Six indicator variables are included as part of the covariates in the model to represent the six clinics. The following priors are specified for β_j and r_k:

$$\beta_j \sim N(\text{MLE}, 10.0) \tag{6.7}$$

$$r_k \sim N(0, \sigma^2). \tag{6.8}$$

The prior variance of β_j is large at a value of 10.0, since it is centered at the maximum likelihood (MLE) estimate. The random physician effect is centered at zero with physician variability represented by σ^2.

The hierarchical structure of the model requires that a prior also be assigned to σ^2, the between-physician variability. Although the inverse-gamma distribution is a common and convenient prior to assign to σ^2, it places much of its probability on large values of σ^2 [31]. Therefore, a more appropriate log-logistic prior is assigned to σ [32]

$$\pi(\sigma) = \frac{s_0}{(s_0 + \sigma)^2} \quad \text{for } \sigma \geq 0, \tag{6.9}$$

where $s_0^2 = K/\sum_{k=1}^{K} s_k^{-2}$ is the harmonic mean of the $K = 55$ physician variances, s_k^2. This prior has several advantages. First, $\pi(\sigma)$ is a proper prior. Second, the prior is a decreasing function of σ and has a maximum at zero implying that values of σ near zero are possible [32]. Another advantage is that this choice of prior prevents results from being affected by the inclusion of physicians with a lot of variability. DuMouchel and Normand [32] discuss how this aforementioned advantage is due to s_0 being weighted toward smaller s_k values whose corresponding y_{ik} values (i.e., the outcome of whether a patient receives aggressive treatment) are more informative about σ.

Once the model is specified, a variable selection procedure is conducted in order to determine factors affecting prescription of aggressive care. With 26 patient characteristics, it is highly unlikely that the full model containing all covariates is the most efficient or significant model to implement. The Bayesian information criterion (BIC) was used to select covariates for the model

$$BIC(M_z) = \text{Deviance}(M_z) + p_z \log (802), \qquad (6.10)$$

where

M_z is the zth model under consideration,

p_z is the number of parameters in the zth model, and

802 is the number of observations in the study.

A standard backward elimination variable selection procedure based on a drop in deviance was also used to compare model selections. Although the order of covariate elimination was slightly different between the two approaches, the resulting model using backward elimination was identical to the model yielding the smallest BIC value.

MCMC methods are used to obtain posterior estimates for the model parameters. In particular, a Metropolis-Hastings algorithm is used to sample σ, r_k (for $k = 1, \ldots, 55$), and β_j (for $j = 1, \ldots, 14$: the choice of $J = 14$ is explained in Section 6.2.4) from their full conditional distributions.

6.2.4   Results

Variable selection results using BIC suggest that six patient covariates be included in the model: black, male, low CD4 + counts, medium CD4 + counts, medium-to-high viral load, and available transportation to the clinic. Although BIC results suggest the aforementioned variables to be significant for model inclusion, additional variables, such as those recommended by Shapiro et al. [26], Bing et al. [27], and Bassetti et al. [28], could be significant based on a more practical than statistical level. Therefore, unknown risk, adherence, and each of the drug variables were considered for model inclusion in addition to IV drug use, stage C, and distance from clinic. Hence, the model was first run with the initial six variables selected using BIC in addition to IV drug use, stage C, distance from clinic, and unknown risk of contracting HIV. This model was run five times, once with each of the five drug variables: ever used drugs, used drugs in the past 6 months, used drugs in the past

3 months, current drug use, and history of drug use. Inclusion of current drug use produced the smallest BIC value, which is not surprising given that the physician's impression as to whether the patient is a current drug user would likely have the greatest effect as to whether that physician prescribes the patient aggressive care. Collinearity was also considered and evaluated during the variable selection process. Therefore, the resulting model includes: male, black, unknown risk of HIV contraction, low and medium CD4 + counts, medium-to-high viral load, current drug use, adherence to prescribed treatment, and each of the six clinics.

The MCMC algorithm was run using C programming language, and history plots of the simulated iterations were evaluated using S-PLUS. By reviewing all the plots for each sampled parameter, it was clear that a burn-in of 2500 iterations was sufficient for this MCMC. The burn-in allows the effect of initial values to wear off so that the simulated values are distributed from the posterior distribution. Initial values were set at the MLEs for the first simulation, then they were altered to a generic value of 2.0 to ascertain chain convergence. However in order to obtain convergence and smoother posterior densities, a total of 50,000 iterations were simulated.

Visual and numerical convergence diagnostics were implemented, and various diagnostic tests were evaluated for convergence. For example, history plots of the parameters revealed no apparent trends in the behavior of the chain: this implies chain convergence. Another visual test deals with autocorrelation plots. Since autocorrelation measures the degree of dependence between successive iterates of the chain, then it is necessary to have autocorrelations as close to zero as possible. Most of the first-order correlations were near zero, with few exceptions. Two numerical convergence tests using Bayesian output analysis (BOA) software were then considered. Results of the Geweke diagnostic consist of all but four physician effects yielding z-scores between approximately ± 2, and Raftery and Lewis diagnostic results show that most of the dependence factors were close to one (see [20] and [33] for more details on these and other MCMC convergence diagnostics). Therefore based on the results of the visual and numerical diagnostic tests, one can conclude apparent chain convergence.

Table 6.2 incorporates a classification of covariates by the direction of effect, based on exclusion of zero from the 95% posterior intervals. The table shows negative effects, or lower probabilities of being prescribed aggressive treatment, for blacks and patients at clinics 1 and 6. The table shows positive effects, or higher probabilities of aggressive treatment prescription, for males and patients with (1) low- and (2) medium-CD4 + counts as well as (3) medium-to-high plasma HIV-1 RNA viral loads. Table 6.2 also provides model coefficients with standard deviations as well as 95% credible intervals and odds ratios. Table 6.2 shows the odds that a patient receives aggressive treatment is 5.64 times higher if the patient has a low CD4 + count, and 3.67 times higher if the patient has a medium CD4 + count. The odds of receiving aggressive care are about 2:1 for patients with medium to high plasma HIV-1 RNA viral load versus those with low viral load, while the odds are about 1.5:1 for males to females and approximately 0.6:1 for blacks to nonblacks. After controlling for all other variables, patients at clinic 3 had higher odds of receiving aggressive care, though not statistically significant based on

TABLE 6.2:   Summary statistics of model patient predictors of aggressive care prescription, including clinics.

Parameter	Coefficient	Standard Deviation	95% Credible Interval	Odds Ratio	Significant Effect
Low CD4 + count	1.73	0.26	(1.23, 2.26)	5.64	Positive
Medium CD4 + count	1.30	0.26	(0.82, 1.82)	3.67	Positive
Medium-to- high viral load	0.73	0.19	(0.37, 1.09)	2.07	Positive
Treatment adherence	0.34	0.17	(−0.0065, 0.68)	1.40	None
Sex (male)	0.45	0.18	(0.096, 0.78)	1.56	Positive
Race (black)	−0.53	0.19	(−0.91, −0.14)	0.59	Negative
Current drug use (chart)	−0.43	0.22	(−0.86, 0.0072)	0.65	None
Unknown risk	−0.36	0.22	(−0.80, 0.079)	0.70	None
Clinic 1	−0.86	0.34	(−1.53, −0.16)	0.42	Negative
Clinic 2	−0.77	0.39	(−1.50, 0.058)	0.46	None
Clinic 3	0.26	0.53	(−0.76, 1.31)	1.30	None
Clinic 4	−0.78	0.46	(−1.71, 0.17)	0.46	None
Clinic 5	−0.26	0.43	(−1.07, 0.62)	0.77	None
Clinic 6	−1.26	0.35	(−2.00, −0.63)	0.28	Negative

its 95% credible interval, while patients at clinics 1 and 6 had significantly lower odds. Figure 6.1 portrays a visual representation of the 95% credible intervals for the covariates and the between-provider variability, σ.

The physician random effects convey which physicians are most to least likely to prescribe aggressive care after controlling for patient characteristics. Table 6.3 presents summary statistics for all 55 physicians, while Figure 6.2 provides 95% credible intervals for these physicians, with the mean posterior proportion at 0.493. Figure 6.2 indicates that provider 6 is the only physician who clearly stands out from the others on aggressive care prescription. In particular, this doctor has a positive effect, indicating that provider 6 has a positive inclination toward prescribing aggressive therapy after controlling for patient characteristics. Similarly to interpreting the exclusion of zero in a frequentist confidence interval, this conclusion is based on the exclusion of zero in the 95% posterior interval for the effect corresponding to provider 6. Table 6.3 indicates that provider 6 practiced at clinic 1 with 46 patients: he/she prescribed aggressive care to 84.8% of his/her patients, while his/her estimated posterior proportion was shrunk to 71.3%. The remaining 95% credible intervals for all other physicians cover zero, indicating no inclination to prescribe or underprescribe aggressive treatment.

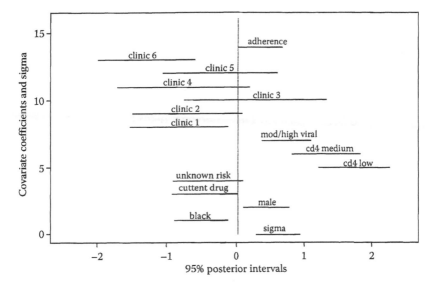

FIGURE 6.1: The above plot portrays 95% posterior credible intervals for the coefficients corresponding to patient characteristics, clinics, and σ (the between—physician standard deviation).

TABLE 6.3: Observed and posterior proportions (with 95% credible intervals) of aggressive care prescription for physician effects, including clinic affiliation and number of patients per physician.

Physician	Observed Proportion	Posterior Proportion	95% Credible Interval	Clinic	# Patients
1	0.694	0.506	(0.342, 0.672)	2	36
2	0.550	0.464	(0.266, 0.636)	1	20
3	0.000	0.453	(0.178, 0.679)	6	1
4	1.000	0.555	(0.288, 0.804)	5	4
5	0.714	0.602	(0.419, 0.781)	6	21
6	0.848	0.713	(0.556, 0.850)	1	46
7	0.636	0.485	(0.291, 0.701)	1	11
8	0.875	0.539	(0.322,0.758)	4	8
9	0.500	0.463	(0.229, 0.694)	5	2
10	0.583	0.424	(0.197, 0.650)	4	12
11	0.488	0.464	(0.286, 0.646)	6	43
12	0.333	0.451	(0.179, 0.712)	4	3
13	0.250	0.442	(0.190, 0.699)	6	4
14	0.667	0.551	(0.364, 0.741)	6	24
15	0.511	0.449	(0.280, 0.622)	6	47

(continued)

TABLE 6.3 (continued):   Observed and posterior proportions (with 95% credible intervals) of aggressive care prescription for physician effects, including clinic affiliation and number of patients per physician.

Physician	Observed Proportion	Posterior Proportion	95% Credible Interval	Clinic	# Patients
16	1.000	0.527	(0.275, 0.790)	5	1
17	0.541	0.430	(0.233, 0.601)	2	37
18	0.677	0.499	(0.324, 0.666)	1	31
19	1.000	0.510	(0.269, 0.779)	6	1
20	0.700	0.506	(0.275, 0.718)	5	10
21	0.800	0.498	(0.233, 0.739)	5	5
22	0.500	0.463	(0.240, 0.685)	6	8
23	0.622	0.477	(0.288, 0.647)	2	37
24	0.393	0.349	(0.187, 0.528)	6	28
25	0.619	0.505	(0.317, 0.715)	6	21
26	1.000	0.608	(0.373, 0.869)	3	16
27	0.667	0.465	(0.234, 0.692)	5	6
28	0.000	0.487	(0.243, 0.729)	6	1
29	0.500	0.454	(0.222, 0.681)	1	6
30	0.750	0.681	(0.485, 0.866)	6	20
31	1.000	0.515	(0.251, 0.792)	5	1
32	0.550	0.441	(0.232, 0.635)	2	20
33	0.500	0.451	(0.217, 0.706)	5	4
34	0.667	0.410	(0.132, 0.649)	3	6
35	0.797	0.417	(0.189, 0.618)	3	69
36	0.143	0.321	(0.105, 0.545)	1	7
37	0.500	0.469	(0.251, 0.690)	1	6
38	0.909	0.549	(0.330, 0.767)	5	11
39	0.857	0.562	(0.316, 0.812)	4	7
40	0.667	0.502	(0.219, 0.774)	5	3
41	0.818	0.522	(0.314, 0.737)	5	11
42	0.833	0.497	(0.247, 0.736)	5	6
43	1.000	0.574	(0.361, 0.826)	1	4
44	0.600	0.420	(0.192, 0.644)	5	5
45	0.583	0.468	(0.280, 0.664)	1	12
46	0.500	0.481	(0.204, 0.786)	5	2
47	0.200	0.367	(0.134, 0.601)	6	5
48	0.786	0.603	(0.390, 0.790)	1	14
49	0.833	0.563	(0.355, 0.777)	4	18
50	0.800	0.496	(0.264, 0.739)	1	5
51	0.720	0.560	(0.379, 0.739)	1	25
52	0.727	0.498	(0.287, 0.711)	4	11
53	0.682	0.509	(0.326, 0.683)	1	22
54	0.647	0.407	(0.206, 0.607)	1	17
55	0.000	0.465	(0.212, 0.714)	1	1

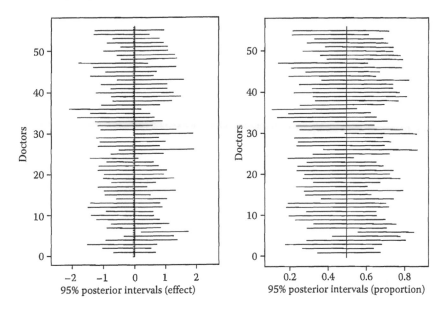

FIGURE 6.2: The left plot portrays 95% posterior credible intervals for the random physician effects, with the dashed vertical line representing the mean physician effect at 0.0319. The right plot shows 95% posterior credible intervals for the proportion of patients receiving aggressive care, with the vertical line drawn at 0.493 representing the posterior mean proportion estimated from the model.

Figure 6.3 portrays a shrinkage plot with the providers' observed proportion of aggressive care prescription across the top of the figure and the providers' corresponding estimated posterior proportion along the bottom of the plot. Since posterior estimates are a compromise between the prior and the data, it is natural for some degree of shrinkage to occur. If a completely noninformative, diffuse prior were used, then the posterior estimates would reflect the data, with very little shrinkage occurring. For larger sample sizes, the data has greater control over the compromise between the prior and the likelihood, resulting in a smaller degree of shrinkage [7].

Bayesian hierarchical modeling using a BIC variable selection process was used to determine the best predictors of prescription of combination antiretroviral therapy. By incorporating a random physician effect, a more comprehensive model than has been previously studied in this particular type of public health application is specified and one that controls for an important variance component, variability among physicians. Using this method, disease factors such as low and medium CD4 + lymphocyte counts and medium-to-high plasma HIV-1 RNA levels were positively associated with prescription of combination antiretroviral therapy. These factors have been described in previous studies [24,26,28] and are logical parameters upon which to base treatment decisions.

Unfortunately, not all treatment decisions appear to be made based on disease status. In this analysis, blacks and women were less likely to receive combination antiretroviral therapy. AIDS is currently one of the leading causes of death for blacks, perhaps because several types of medications and diagnostic procedures

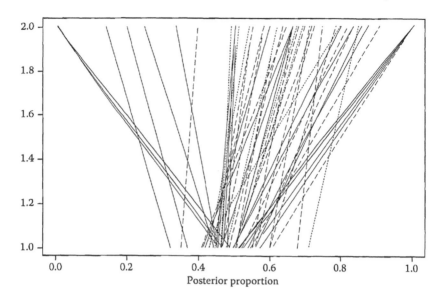

FIGURE 6.3:   The above is shrinkage plot where physician's observed proportion of aggressive treatment prescription is shown across the top, and the posterior proportion of prescribing aggressive care estimated from the model is indicated across the bottom.

are not given to blacks as often as to whites [34]. In one study, blacks were not as likely as whites to receive azidothymidine (AZT) medication and prophylactic drugs at an initial appearing for treatment as well as during a follow-up time [35]. Among patients at a teaching hospital appearing for treatment, blacks were 40% less likely than whites to have already received antiretroviral medication or prophylaxis against opportunistic infection, regardless of income and insurance coverage [36]. In a study of the use of recently developed antiretroviral drugs among a large sample of Medicaid-insured patients with HIV and AIDS, blacks were significantly less likely than whites to be prescribed protease inhibitors and nucleoside antagonists [37].

The analysis also found gender to have a negative effect on the prescription of aggressive treatment. Undertreatment of women was also found in another recent survey [26]. Several studies have shown that women were less likely than men to receive established treatment for myocardial infarction [38], and to undergo invasive procedures such as cardiac catheterization, angioplasty, and coronary bypass grafting [39,40]. Women have also been found to be less likely than men to undergo other procedures such as kidney transplantation [41], heart transplantation, defibrillator implants, pacemaker placement, and hip replacement [42]. There is growing evidence in the literature that the natural history of cardiac disease is different between men and women, which may account for some of the differences in treatment and outcome [43,44].

This study provides important insights into patient characteristics that influence the prescription of combination antiretroviral therapy, but is limited in several regards. First, the patient population is somewhat homogeneous because only Medicaid or Medicaid-eligible subjects were recruited into the study. Second, the differences found between men and women in this study may have been skewed by the manner in which patients qualify for Medicaid in North Carolina. Men can only qualify for Medicaid if they are found to be disabled. Women can qualify for Medicaid based on disability, or by being a mother of young children. This requirement means that, in general, women on Medicaid in North Carolina have less advanced HIV infection than men. Although the analysis controlled for CD4+ lymphocyte count and plasma HIV-1 RNA level, this bias may have overestimated the difference between treatment of men and women in this study. Third, there is a clear bias toward patients who seek medical care at major medical institutions, as that is where patients were recruited. This bias is further accentuated because the patients who attended clinic more regularly were more likely to be recruited during the enrollment period. Future studies should focus on a more appropriate study design, including: (1) more representative samples of patients and providers, with data on provider characteristics also collected; (2) collection of data in the appropriate format rather than collecting all the data as binary responses; (3) investigate differences among clinic sites more thoroughly; and (4) conduct a sensitivity analysis for evaluating the robustness of the prior choice.

Persons infected with HIV should receive the best available care for their disease. Treatment should be based on disease parameters, which are then tailored to the individual patient. Care needs to be taken to overcome systemic bias against effectively treating certain groups, such as women and blacks. Health care providers should compare their treatment patterns with current recommendations and be vigilant for their personal bias influencing treatment decisions.

6.3 Continuous Distributions for Modeling Time-to-Event Data

Now that the reader has been introduced to Bayesian methods and provided an example of a Bayesian analysis applied to public health data, it is time to switch gears a bit and move toward a Bayesian analysis of time-to-event data, particularly in the clinical trial setting. This section offers a review of basic survival analysis with focus on the Weibull and exponential distributions for time-to-event data, while Section 6.4 offers a Bayesian perspective to analyzing time-to-event data through a clinical trial application.

6.3.1 Brief Overview of Survival Analysis

In modeling continuous time-to-event data, begin by defining a continuous random variable T, for $T \geq 0$, to represent an event time, such as a failure or survival time of subjects. I will follow closely the overview of survival analysis provided by Ibrahim et al. [45]. The cumulative distribution function of T is

$$F(t) = P(T \leq t) = \int_0^t f(x)dx, \tag{6.11}$$

where $f(t)$ denotes the probability density function (pdf) of T. The survival function, $S(t)$, represents the probability that a subject survives to time T and is expressed as

$$S(t) = P(T > t) = 1 - F(t), \tag{6.12}$$

where $S(0) = 1$ and $S(t)$ decreases monotonically until $S(\infty) = \lim_{t \to \infty} S(t) = 0$.

The hazard function, $\lambda(t)$, which represents the instantaneous failure rate at time t, can be expressed in terms of the survival function:

$$\lambda(t) = \lim_{\Delta t \to 0} \frac{P(t < T \leq t + \Delta t | T > t)}{\Delta t} = \frac{f(t)}{S(t)}. \tag{6.13}$$

Furthermore, $\lambda(t)$ can also be expressed as

$$\lambda(t) = -\frac{d}{dt} \log(S(t)), \tag{6.14}$$

where $\lambda(t) \geq 0$ and $\int_0^\infty \lambda(t)dt = \infty$. Then, solving Equation 6.14 for $S(t)$ yields

$$S(t) = \exp\left(-\int_0^t \lambda(x)dx\right). \tag{6.15}$$

By revisiting Equation 6.13 and solving for $f(t)$, $f(t) = \lambda(t)S(t)$. Therefore, $f(t)$ can be expressed in terms of Equations 6.14 and 6.15:

$$f(t) = \lambda(t) \exp\left(-\int_0^t \lambda(x)dx\right). \tag{6.16}$$

6.3.2   Weibull and Exponential Survival Models

The Weibull distribution is one of the most commonly used parametric survival models for describing time-to-event data. If T follows a Weibull distribution, then we say that

$$t \sim \text{Weibull}(\theta, \alpha), \tag{6.17}$$

where T has probability density function:

$$f(t; \theta, \alpha) = \theta \alpha t^{\alpha-1} \exp(-\theta t^\alpha), \quad \text{for } t > 0, \theta > 0, \alpha > 0, \tag{6.18}$$

with θ and α the scale and shape parameters, respectively. The survival function of T is

$$S(t; \theta, \alpha) = \exp(-\theta t^{\alpha}), \tag{6.19}$$

and its hazard function is

$$\lambda(t; \theta, \alpha) = \theta \alpha t^{\alpha-1}, \tag{6.20}$$

where $\lambda(t)$ increases monotonically with time when $\alpha > 1$ and monotonically decreases with time when $0 < \alpha < 1$. The hazard is constant for $\alpha = 1$, and the Weibull distribution simplifies to the fundamental exponential distribution, $Exp(\theta)$. Furthermore, the cumulative hazard function of T is

$$\Lambda(t; \theta, \alpha) = \theta t^{\alpha}. \tag{6.21}$$

Since the exponential distribution, which is also a commonly used parametric survival model for time-to-event data, is a special case of the Weibull distribution, then focus is contained on the Weibull survival model with its more general form and appeal. Details focused on Bayesian survival analysis are found in Ibrahim et al. [45] and Congdon [46], while more primarily classical approaches to survival analysis include Hosmer and Lemeshow [47], Kleinbaum and Klein [48], Klein and Moeschberger [49], and Therneau and Grambsch [50].

Section 6.4 provides an application of a Bayesian Weibull survival model relevant to clinical trials. In particular, the application was conducted by Qian et al. [51]. They show how monitoring issues in clinical trials can be handled with inferences from posterior and predictive distributions, providing a Bayesian approach to typical classical assessments of stopping times in clinical trials.

6.4 Application of a Bayesian Weibull Survival Model in a Clinical Trial

6.4.1 Background of Clinical Trial Application

Qian et al. [51] performed an analysis of a phase III clinical trial conducted by the Cancer and Leukemia Group B (CALGB) for patients diagnosed with stage III nonsmall cell lung cancer (NSCLC). Lung cancer can be divided into two categories based on cell type at diagnosis, with the NSCLC as the larger group—accounting for approximately 87% of lung cancer cases [52]. In order for appropriate treatment regimes to be assigned to patients diagnosed with NSCLC, the disease stage must be identified. Patients in disease stage III NSCLC were used in this clinical trial. Those with stage III NSCLC "have no demonstrable distant metastases but do have locally extensive or invasive disease or involvement of mediastinal lymph nodes" [51].

A randomized phase III clinical trial performed by the CALGB was conducted on stage III NSCLC patients. The aim of this trial was to compare survival rates of the standard treatment (radiation therapy only) to that of those on the experimental treatment (two courses of combination chemotherapy prior to radiation therapy) [51]. The dose, volume, and schedule of the radiation therapy were the same between the standard and experimental arms.

The trial was initially designed to have a fixed sample size of 240 patients, with 120 patients randomly assigned to each treatment arm [51]. However, group sequential methods utilizing a truncated (at three standard deviations) O'Brien-Fleming [53] stopping rule implemented using a Lan-Demets [54] α-spending function were applied early in the study. Qian et al. [51] provide further details of patient eligibility criteria for inclusion into the trial.

Five interim analyses between May 1984 and May 1987 were presented to a data monitoring committee (DMC). Results of a Cox [55] proportional hazards model at the fifth interim analysis yielded a p-value of $p = 0.0008$ for the treatment comparison, hence crossing the truncated O'Brien-Fleming stopping boundary significance level of 0.0013 and indicating a treatment effect [51]. This result led to a unanimous vote by the DMC to stop the trial in April 1987 after only 155 of the 180 accrued patients (77 patients in the standard radiation only treatment and 78 patients in the experimental chemotherapy and radiation combined treatment) were eligible, with 56 patients dead of the 105 patients with follow-up data. Table 6.4 presents summary statistics and boundary significance levels used by the DMC, including the decision to keep open or close the trial [51]. Qian et al. [51] constructed Kaplan–Meier curves at each interim analysis. These curves are shown in Figure 6.4 and further portray a treatment effect with: (1) differences between treatment arms, particularly in the earlier interim analyses, and (2) longer survival times for patients on the experimental arm receiving combined chemotherapy and radiation therapy.

6.4.2   Model Specification

Following Qian et al. [51], let t_{ij} be the survival time of the jth patient in the ith treatment, for $i = 1, 2$ (where 1 denotes the standard radiation only therapy and 2 denotes the experimental radiation plus chemotherapy treatment); and, $j = 1, 2, \ldots, n_i$, for n_i representing the number of patients receiving treatment i. Let d_i represent the number of deaths, at any given time, on treatment i. Qian et al. [51] redefine j (i.e., $j = d_i + 1, \ldots, n_i$) to be the number of patients who died and survived, respectively, on treatment i. Patient indices must be reordered at each interim analysis.

A Bayesian hierarchical model is constructed such that a parametric survival model for lifetime t_{ij} is specified. In particular, Qian et al. [51] show that t_{ij} are independent and identically distributed such that

$$t_{ij} \sim \text{Weibull}(\theta_i, \alpha_i). \tag{6.22}$$

Prior distributions must now be chosen for the unknown model parameters, θ_i and α_i. Stangl [56] and Li [57] provide a parameterization such that:

TABLE 6.4: Summary statistics and boundary significance levels used by the DMC.

Analysis	d_1	n_1	$\sum_1^{n_1} t_{1j}$	d_2	n_2	$\sum_1^{n_2} t_{2j}$	Logrank p-Value	Truncated O'Brien-Fleming Boundary Significance Level	Pocock Boundary Significance Level	Decision
Sept. 1985	7	25	135.9	3	25	174.7	—[a]	0.0013	0.0041	Keep open
Mar. 1986	12	41	279.5	4	38	340.6	0.0210	0.0013	0.0034	Keep open
Aug. 1986	20	41	279.5	14	47	407.3	0.0071	0.0013	0.0078	Keep open
Oct. 1986	24	46	356.0	18	49	431.9	0.0015	0.0013	0.0061	Keep open
Mar. 1987	32	51	406.1	24	54	517.4	0.0015	0.0013	0.0081	Close

Source: From Qian, J., Stangl, D.K., and George, S., in *Bayesian Biostatistics*, Marcel Dekker, Inc., New York, 1996, 187–205. With permission.

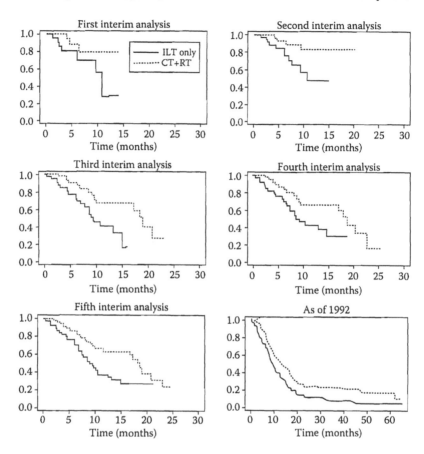

FIGURE 6.4: Kaplan–Meier plots at each interim analysis and as of 1992. (From Qian, J., Stangl, D.K., and George, S., in *Bayesian Biostatistics*, Marcel Dekker, Inc., New York, 1996, 187–205. With permission.)

$$\eta = \log\left(\frac{\theta_2}{\theta_1}\right), \tag{6.23}$$

where solving for θ_2 yields

$$\theta_2 = \theta_1 e^{\eta}. \tag{6.24}$$

This parameterization defines η as the log-hazard ratio of the experimental treatment to the standard therapy and allows the survival distributions for both treatments to be simplified to the exponential case when $\alpha_1 = \alpha_2 = 1$ [51]. Thus, Qian et al. [51] specify the following priors:

$$\alpha_i | u_\alpha, v_\alpha \sim Ga(u_\alpha, v_\alpha) \tag{6.25}$$

$$\theta_1 | u_\theta, v_\theta \sim Ga(u_\theta, v_\theta) \tag{6.26}$$

$$\eta | \mu_\eta, \sigma_\eta^2 \sim N\left(\mu_\eta, \sigma_\eta^2\right). \tag{6.27}$$

Qian et al. [51] chose independent gamma priors for α_i with a mode (i.e., $(u_\alpha - 1)/v_\alpha$) equal to one, $u_\alpha = 10,001$, and $v_\alpha = 10,000$. The prior standard deviation (i.e., $\sqrt{u_\alpha}/v_\alpha$) is small at approximately 0.01. Qian et al. [51] provide a sensitivity analysis where they vary the magnitude of the standard deviation of prior (Equation 6.25). Specification of prior (Equation 6.25) on the Weibull model parameters corresponds to the simplified exponential survival model, as seen, for example, in George et al. [58].

An independent gamma prior was also chosen for θ_1 whose median survival was 8.3 months, $u_\alpha = 2$, and $v_\alpha = 20$ [51]. Prior (Equation 6.26) was specified based on historical information that showed the median survival time for NSCLC patients to be approximately 9 months, with a 2- and 3-year survival of approximately 15% and 5%, respectively [51]. Finally, prior (Equation 6.27) was chosen with mean zero (i.e., $\mu_\eta = 0$) and variance one (i.e., $\sigma_\eta^2 = 1$) to represent the belief that both treatments are equally likely to be more effective, since η is the log-hazard ratio of the experimental treatment to the standard treatment [51].

The likelihood function, $L(\theta_1, \eta, \alpha_1, \alpha_2)$, as presented by Qian et al. [51] is

$$
\begin{aligned}
L(\theta_1, \eta, \alpha_1, \alpha_2) &= \prod_{i=1}^{2} \left\{ \prod_{j=1}^{d_i} f(t_{ij}; \theta_i, \alpha_i) \prod_{j=d_i+1}^{n_i} S(t_{ij}; \theta_i, \alpha_i) \right\} \\
&= \prod_{i=1}^{2} \left\{ (\theta_i \alpha_i)^{d_i} \left(\prod_{j=1}^{d_i} t_{ij} \right)^{\alpha_i - 1} \exp\left(-\theta_i \sum_{j=1}^{n_i} t_{ij}^{\alpha_i} \right) \right\}
\end{aligned}
\tag{6.28}
$$

$$
\begin{aligned}
L(\theta_1, \eta, \alpha_1, \alpha_2) &= (\theta_1 \alpha_1)^{d_1} \left(\prod_{j=1}^{d_1} t_{1j} \right)^{\alpha_1 - 1} \exp\left(-\theta_1 \sum_{j=1}^{n_1} t_{1j}^{\alpha_1} \right) \\
&\quad (\theta_1 e^\eta \alpha_2)^{d_2} \left(\prod_{j=1}^{d_2} t_{2j} \right)^{\alpha_2 - 1} \exp\left(-\theta_1 e^\eta \sum_{j=1}^{n_2} t_{2j}^{\alpha_2} \right)
\end{aligned}
$$

Following posterior computational methods introduced in Section 6.1, Qian et al. [51] use Gibbs sampling techniques to calculate the posterior, $p(\theta_1, \eta, \alpha_1, \alpha_2)$, by multiplying the likelihood, $L(\theta_1, \eta, \alpha_1, \alpha_2)$, by the prior, $\pi(\theta_1, \eta, \alpha_1, \alpha_2)$:

$$
\begin{aligned}
p(\theta_1, \eta, \alpha_1, \alpha_2) &= L(\theta_1, \eta, \alpha_1, \alpha_2) \pi(\theta_1, \eta, \alpha_1, \alpha_2) \\
&= (\theta_1 \alpha_1)^{d_1} \left(\prod_{j=1}^{d_1} t_{1j} \right)^{\alpha_1 - 1} \exp\left(-\theta_1 \sum_{j=1}^{n_1} t_{1j}^{\alpha_1} \right) \\
&\quad (\theta_1 e^\eta \alpha_2)^{d_2} \left(\prod_{j=1}^{d_2} t_{2j} \right)^{\alpha_2 - 1} \exp\left(-\theta_1 e^\eta \sum_{j=1}^{n_2} t_{2j}^{\alpha_2} \right) \\
&\quad \theta_1^{u_\theta - 1} e^{-v_\theta \theta_1} e^{-\frac{1}{2\sigma_\eta^2}(\eta - \mu_\eta)^2} \alpha_1^{u_\alpha - 1} e^{-v_\alpha \alpha_1} \alpha_2^{u_\alpha - 1} e^{-v_\alpha \alpha_2}
\end{aligned}
\tag{6.29}
$$

As seen in the example in Section 6.2, posterior distributions of parameters often directly summarize model effects such as treatment effects. Under the simple exponential case for survival times of both treatments, treatment effects can be directly identified from the posterior distribution of η [51]. In the case of survival times following a Weibull model, treatment comparisons are not as straightforward. Qian et al. [51] calculate the predictive probability of a longer survival on the experimental treatment (involving combined chemotherapy and radiation) than on the standard therapy (involving only radiation treatment) at time t:

$$D(t) = P(S_1(t) < S_2(t)|\text{data}), \qquad (6.30)$$

where $S_i(t)$ is the survival function for treatment $i = 1, 2$. The authors also use the measure

$$d(t) = E(S_1(t) - S_2(t)|\text{data}) \qquad (6.31)$$

to compute the predictive mean difference between survival probabilities, at time t, on the standard and experimental therapies.

6.4.3   Results and Discussion

Figure 6.5 presents the prior and posterior distributions that Qian et al. [51] construct for the Weibull model parameters $(\theta_1, \eta, \alpha_1, \alpha_2)$ as well as the predictive measures $D(t)$ and $d(t)$. The posterior modes at the different interim analyses of θ_1, the scale parameter of the Weibull survival model, range from 0.04 at the second interim analysis to 0.075 at the fifth interim analysis, corresponding to survival times ranging from 16 to 25 months [51]. Posterior modes for η, the log-hazard ratio of the experimental to standard treatments, range from -1.2 (occurring at the second interim analysis where the difference in treatments is largest) to -0.6, which when exponentiated represent hazard ratios ranging from 0.3 to 0.55 [51]. This result shows longer survival for those on the experimental treatment (i.e., radiation and chemotherapy combined) compared to patients on the standard radiation only therapy. It is not surprising that the posteriors for the shape parameters of the Weibull model, α_1 and α_2, are centered approximately around one, with posterior modes also at one.

Recall that prior (Equation 6.25) assigned to α_i, for $i = 1, 2$, is centered at approximately one with small standard deviation, 0.01. Since α_1 and α_2 are both approximately one hence simplifying to an exponential model, then $D(t)$ (i.e., the predictive probability that the survival is longer for those on the experimental treatment over those on the standard therapy) is roughly constant across time [51]. Figure 6.5 shows values for $D(t)$ above 0.98, with the exception of the first interim analysis, indicating strong evidence for the support of the experimental treatment over the standard therapy. Finally, the predictive mean differences in survival between the two treatments, at 20 months after treatment, range from approximately -0.35 at the second interim analysis, where the difference in treatments is largest, to approximately -0.18 as of 1992, further supporting the experimental treatment [51].

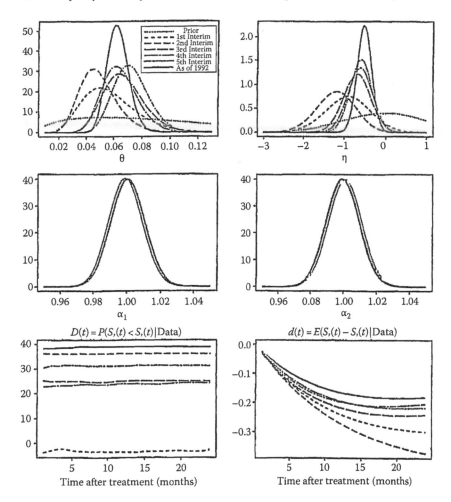

FIGURE 6.5: Posterior distributions of θ_1, η, α_1, α_2 and predictive characteristics under the following priors: $\alpha_1 \sim Ga(10{,}001,10{,}000)$, $\theta_1 \sim Ga(2,20)$, $\eta \sim N(0,1)$. (From Qian, J., Stangl, D.K., and George, S., in *Bayesian Biostatistics*, Marcel Dekker, Inc., New York, 1996, 187–205. With permission.)

Qian et al. [51] conducted a sensitivity analysis to examine the robustness of the model based on the prior specifications. Figure 6.6 shows results using a different prior specification on the shape parameters, α_1 and α_2, of the Weibull survival model. Prior (Equation 6.25) is still assigned to α_1 and α_2 having mean one, however the standard deviation is larger at 0.1: in particular, $u_\alpha = 101$ and $v_\alpha = 100$ [51]. Since interest focuses on differences in survival between treatments, the plots of $D(t)$ and $d(t)$ are of particular significance. Notice that $D(t)$, the difference in predictive survival probabilities at time t between treatments, is no longer constant with time—a result based on the posteriors of α_1 and α_2 which show that the posterior modes are not one and hence the Weibull model no longer follows a simplified exponential

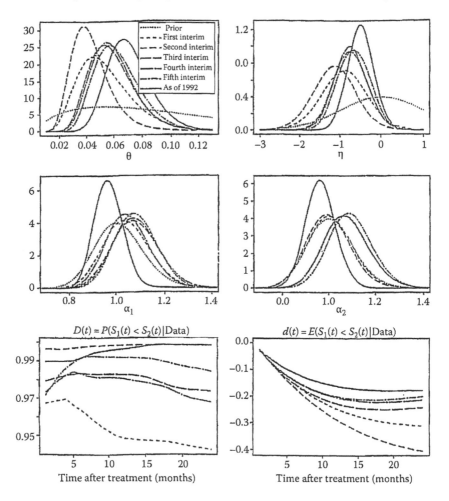

FIGURE 6.6: Posterior distributions of θ_1, η, α_1, α_2 and predictive characteristics under the following priors: $\alpha_1 \sim Ga(101,100)$, $\theta_1 \sim Ga(2,20)$, $\eta \sim N(0,1)$. (From Qian, J., Stangl, D.K., and George, S., in *Bayesian Biostatistics*, Marcel Dekker, Inc., New York, 1996, 187–205. With permission.)

form. Furthermore, Figure 6.6 shows little change in the plot of $d(t)$, the predictive mean differences in survival across time between the two treatments.

The sensitivity analysis that Qian et al. [51] conducted also consisted of 10 additional values of the standard deviation of η, the log-hazard ratio of the experimental to standard treatments, including 0.01 and increments of 0.1 from 0.1 to 0.9. Since prior (Equation 6.27) is centered at zero, then larger standard deviation values yield a higher probability of a treatment effect toward either treatment. Results of the sensitivity analysis show evidence in support of a treatment effect for the experimental treatment involving the radiation plus chemotherapy combined over the standard radiation only therapy [51].

In this study, the trial had already ceased, and interest focused on whether that was the correct decision [51]. However, these methods can be used for decision making regarding stopping times of clinical trials. For example, predictive distributions could be compared based on accruing additional patients [51]. Qian et al. [51] conducted a simulation study for the CALGB trial in which accrual of patients after the trial stopped in April 1987 were simulated at the same patient accrual rate throughout the trial, which in this example was six patients per month. Lifetimes were simulated from Weibull distributions whose parameters were sampled from the parameters' posterior distribution given all the data up to the trial's stopping time of April 1987. Results of the simulation study for 500 samples show that the accrual of 85 additional patients to reach the original accrual goal of 240 patients would not have altered the direction or size of the treatment effect [51]. More generally, DMCs could compare posterior distributions, which incorporate observed data, to predictive distributions, which combine observed data with additional simulated observations, to address the question of whether further patient accrual is necessary [51]. Such decisions can guide practitioners toward improved patient care.

6.5 Discussion

Bayesian methods of analysis are seen throughout the literature across a wide range of biostatistical applications. Section 6.1 provided an overview of Bayesian analysis in order that the reader may gain a general understanding of the methods. Further readings were suggested throughout the section to expand upon this intro-duction and provide resources through which the reader may learn to apply Bayesian methods to his/her own applications in clinical trials, public health, or biomedicine. The application in public health presented in Section 6.2 provided an example of how Bayesian methods are used in practice, in particular via Bayesian hierarchical modeling of aggressive care prescription of HIV/AIDS patients in the southeast.

The second half of this chapter focused on time-to-event data and methods of analysis of such data under the Bayesian paradigm. Section 6.3 provided an over-view of survival analytic methods, with emphasis on the most commonly used parametric models, the Weibull and exponential, for modeling time-to-event data. Section 6.4 provided an example of Bayesian inferential methods using a Weibull survival model in the clinical trial setting. In particular, an analysis conducted by Qian et al. [51] was presented of a phase III clinical trial administered by the CALGB for patients diagnosed with stage III nonsmall cell lung cancer.

This is merely a sample of the types of models that exist for describing time-to-event data. Other parametric models include the Log-normal and gamma models for modeling survival data (see [45]). Frailty models—both fully parametric, as found in Sahu et al. [59], and semiparametric, as presented by Clayton [60], Sinha [61], and Pennell and Dunson [62]—have also been widely used to model time-to-event data. Bayesian inference in cure rate models has been used to model survival data (see [63, 64]). Time-to-event data can also be modeled using Bayesian order-restricted inferential methods (see [65]).

In addition to Bayesian inferential methods for modeling time-to-event data, Bayesian analysis is used in other contexts throughout the study of clinical trials. For example, Bayesian meta-analysis is used to combine results of multiple trials, potentially in combination with additional evidence (see [63–71] for further readings on concepts and applications of Bayesian meta-analysis). Bayesian adaptive designs are also gaining greater attention (see [72–76]). Finally, for additional references in Bayesian clinical trials see Berry [77,78], Spiegelhalter et al. [79], and Racine et al. [80].

Acknowledgments

The author would like to thank Jiang Qian, Dalene Stangl, and Stephen George for use of their analysis presented in Section 6.4: their research was supported in part by grant CA 33601 from the National Cancer Institute. The author would also like to thank Kathryn Whetten and Dalene Stangl for their contributions to Section 6.2. The data provided in Section 6.2 was made possible in part through the support of the HIV/AIDS Bureau's Special Projects of National Significance, Domestic Assistance number 39–928, from the Health Resources and Services Administration, Department of Health and Human Services.

References

[1] FDA officials endorse statistical model that uses historical data in clinical trials (1998). In: *International Medical Device Regulatory Monitor*. Lanham, MD: Newsletter Services, Inc., 6(2), 2.

[2] Berry, D.A. (1997): Using a Bayesian approach in medical device development. Technical report available from Division of Biostatistics, Center for Devices and Radiological Health, FDA.

[3] Irony, T.Z. and Simon, R. (2005): Applications of Bayesian methods to medical device trials. In: Becker, K.M. and Whyte, J.J., eds. *Clinical Evaluation of Medical Devices: Principles and Case Studies, Second Edition*. Totowa, NJ: Humana Press Inc., pp. 99–116.

[4] Moyé, L.A. (2008): *Elementary Bayesian Biostatistics*. Boca Raton, FL: Chapman & Hall/CRC.

[5] Ashby, D. (2001): Bayesian methods. In: Redmond, C. and Colton, T., eds. *Biostatistics in Clinical Trials*. New York: John Wiley & Sons, pp. 13–18.

[6] Bernado, J.M. and Smith, A.F.M. (1994): *Bayesian Theory*. New York: John Wiley & Sons.

[7] Gelman, A., Carlin, J.B., Stern, H.S., and Rubin, D.B. (2003): *Bayesian Data Analysis, Second Edition*. Boca Raton, FL: Chapman & Hall/CRC.

[8] Berry, D.A. and Stangl, D.K. (1996): Bayesian methods in health-related research. In: Berry, D.A. and Stangl, D.K., eds. *Bayesian Biostatistics*. New York: Marcel Dekker, Inc., pp. 3–66.

[9] Box, G.E.P. and Tiao, G. (1973): *Bayesian Inference in Statistical Analysis*. New York: John Wiley & Sons.

[10] Berger, J.O. (1985): *Statistical Decision Theory and Bayesian Analysis, Second Edition*. New York: Springer.

[11] Carlin, B.P. and Louis, T.A. (2000): *Bayes and Empirical Bayes Methods for Data Analysis, Second Edition*. Boca Raton, FL: Chapman & Hall/CRC.

[12] Chaloner, K. (1996): Elicitation of prior distributions. In: Berry, D.A. and Stangl, D.K., eds. *Bayesian Biostatistics*. New York: Marcel Dekker, Inc., pp. 141–156.

[13] Kadane, J.B. and Wolfson, L.J. (1996): Priors for the design and analysis of clinical trials. In: Berry, D.A. and Stangl, D.K., eds. *Bayesian Biostatistics*. New York: Marcel Dekker, Inc., pp. 157–184.

[14] Kass, R.E. and Wasserman, L.A. (1995): Formal rules for selecting prior distributions: a review and annotated bibliography. Technical report 583, Carnegie-Mellon University, Pittsburgh, PA.

[15] O'Hagan, A. (1998): Eliciting expert beliefs in substantial practical applications. *The Statistician*. 47: 21–35 (with discussion, 55–68).

[16] Varshavsky, J.A. and David, S.R. (2000): Bayesian statistics. In: Chow, S.-C., ed. *Encyclopedia of Biopharmaceutical Statistics*. New York: Marcel Dekker, Inc., pp. 31–39.

[17] Gelfand, A.E. and Smith, A.F.M. (1990): Sampling based approaches to calculating marginal densities. *Journal of the American Statistical Association*. 85: 398–409.

[18] Casella, G. and George, E.I. (1992): Explaining the Gibbs sampler. *The American Statistician*. 46(3): 167–174.

[19] Gamerman, D. (1997): *Markov Chain Monte Carlo: Stochastic Simulation for Bayesian Inference*. London: Chapman & Hall.

[20] Gilks, W.R., Richardson, S., and Spiegelhalter, D.J. (1996): *Markov Chain Monte Carlo in Practice*. Boca Raton, FL: Chapman & Hall/CRC.

[21] Palella Jr., F.J., Delaney, K.M., Moorman, A.C., Loveless, M.O., Fuhrer, J., et al. (1998): Declining morbidity and mortality among patients with advanced human immunodeficiency virus infection. *New England Journal of Medicine.* 338(13): 853–860.

[22] Carpenter, C.C.J., Fischl, M.A., Hammer, S.M., Hirsch, M.S., Jacobson, D.M., et al. (1997): Antiretroviral therapy for HIV infection in 1997: updated recommendations of the International AIDS Society-USA panel. *Journal of the American Medical Association.* 277(24): 1962–1969.

[23] Centers for Disease Control and Prevention [CDC]. (1998): Guidelines for the use of antiretroviral agents in HIV-infected adults and adolescents: Department of Health and Human Services and the Henry J. Kaiser Family Foundation. *MMWR: Morbidity & Mortality Weekly Report.* 47(5): 42–82.

[24] Bozzette, S.A., Berry, S.H., Duan, N., Frankel, M.R., Leibowitz, A.A., et al. (1998): The care of HIV-infected adults in the United States. *New England Journal of Medicine.* 339(26): 1897–1904.

[25] Wolde-Rafael, D., Campo, R., and De Caprariis, P.J. (1999): How well are we doing in adopting HIV treatment guidelines? *Sixth Conference on Retroviruses and Opportunistic Infections.* Chicago, IL: Foundation for Retrovirology and Human Health.

[26] Shapiro, M.F., Morton, S.C., McCaffrey, D.F., Senterfitt, J.W., Fleishman, J.A., et al. (1999): Variations in the care of HIV-infected adults in the United States: results from the HIV cost and services utilization study. *Journal of the American Medical Association.* 281: 2305–2315.

[27] Bing, E.G., Kilbourne, A.M., Brooks, R.A., Lazarus, E.F., and Senak, M. (1999): Protease inhibitor use among a community sample of people with HIV disease. *Journal of Acquired Immune Deficiency Syndromes.* 20: 474–480.

[28] Bassetti, S., Battegay, M., Furrer, H., Rickenbach, M., Flepp, M., et al. (1999): Why is highly active antiretroviral therapy (HAART) not prescribed or discontinued? *Journal of Acquired Immune Deficiency Syndromes.* 21(2): 114–119.

[29] CDC. (1998): Risks for HIV infection among persons residing in rural areas and small cities—selected sites, southern United States, 1995–1996. *MMWR.* 47(45): 974–978.

[30] Whetten-Goldstein, K., Nguyen, T.Q., and Heald, A.E. (2001): Characteristics of individuals infected with the human immunodeficiency virus and provider interaction in the predominantly rural southeast. *Southern Medical Journal.* 94(2): 212–222.

[31] Pauler, D.K. and Wakefield, J. (2000): Modeling and implementation issues in Bayesian meta-analysis. In: Stangl, D.K. and Berry, D.A., eds. *Meta-Analysis in Medicine and Health Policy*. New York: Marcel Dekker, Inc., 205–230.

[32] DuMouchel, W. and Normand, S.L. (2000): Computer-modeling and graphical strategies for meta-analysis. In: Stangl, D.K. and Berry, D.A., eds. *Meta-Analysis in Medicine and Health Policy*. New York: Marcel Dekker, Inc., 127–178.

[33] Cowles, M.K. and Carlin, B.P. (1996): MCMC convergence diagnostics: a comparative review. *Journal of the American Statistical Association*. 91(434): 883–904.

[34] Geiger, H.J. (2002): Racial and ethnic disparities in diagnosis and treatment: a review of the evidence and a consideration of causes. In: Smedley, B.D., Smith, A.Y., and Nelson, A.R., eds. *Unequal Treatment: Confronting Racial and Ethnic Disparities in Health Care*. Washington, DC: National Academy Press, 192–223.

[35] Easterbrook, P., Keruly, J.C., Creagh-Kirk, T., Richman, D., Chaisson, R.E., et al. (1991): Racial and ethnic differences in outcome in Zivoduvine-treated patients with advanced HIV disease. *Journal of the American Medical Association*. 266: 2713–2718.

[36] Moore, R.D., Stanton, D., Gopalan, R., and Chaisson, R.E. (1994): Racial differences in the use of drug therapy for HIV disease in an urban community. *New England Journal of Medicine*. 330: 763–768.

[37] Anderson, K.H. and Mitchell, J.M. (2000): Differential access in the receipt of antiretroviral drugs for the treatment of AIDS and its implications for survival. *Archives of Internal Medicine*. 160: 3114–3120.

[38] Norhia, A., Vaccarino, V., and Krumholz, H.M. (1998): Gender differences in mortality after myocardial infarction: Why women fare worse than men. *Cardiology Clinics*. 16: 45–57.

[39] Tobin, J.N., Wassertheil-Smoller, S., Wexler, J.P., Steingart, R.M., Budner, N., et al. (1987): Sex bias in considering coronary bypass surgery. *Annals of Internal Medicine*. 107: 19–25.

[40] Ayainian, J.Z. and Epstein, A.M. (1991): Differences in the use of procedures between women and men hospitalized for coronary heart disease. *New England Journal of Medicine*. 325: 221–225.

[41] Bloembergen, W.E., Port, K.F., Mauger, E.A., Briggs, J.P., and Leichtman, A.B. (1996): Gender discrepancies in living related renal transplant donors and recipients. *Journal of the American Society of Nephrology*. 7: 1139–1144.

[42] Giacomini, M.K. (1996): Gender and ethnic differences in hospital-based procedure utilization in California. *Archives of Internal Medicine*. 156: 1217–1224.

[43] Hochman, J.S., Tamis, J.E., Thompson, T.D., Weaver, W.D., White, H.D., et al. (1999): Sex, clinical presentation, and outcome in patients with acute coronary syndromes. *New England Journal of Medicine.* 341(6): 226–232.

[44] Vaccarino, V., Parsons, L., Every, N.R., Barron, H.V., and Krumholz, H.M. (1999): Sex-based differences in early mortality after myocardial infarction. *New England Journal of Medicine.* 341: 217–225.

[45] Ibrahim, J.G., Chen, M.-H., and Sinha, D. (2001): *Bayesian Survival Analysis.* New York: Springer.

[46] Congdon, P. (2003): *Applied Bayesian Modeling.* New York: John Wiley & Sons.

[47] Hosmer, D.W., Jr. and Lemeshow, S. (1999): *Applied Survival Analysis: Regression Modeling of Time to Event Data.* New York: John Wiley & Sons.

[48] Kleinbaum, D. and Klein, M. (2005): *Survival Analysis: A Self-Learning Text, Second Edition.* New York: Springer.

[49] Klein, M. and Moeschberger, M.L. (2005): *Survival Analysis, Second Edition.* New York: Springer.

[50] Therneau, T.M. and Grambsch, P.M. (2000): *Modeling Survival Data: Extending the Cox Model.* New York: Springer.

[51] Qian, J., Stangl, D.K., and George, S.A. (1996): Weibull model for survival data: using prediction to decide when to stop a clinical trial. In: Berry, D.A. and Stangl, D.K., eds. *Bayesian Biostatistics.* New York: Marcel Dekker, Inc., pp. 187–205.

[52] American Cancer Society. (2008): *Cancer facts & figures 2008.* Atlanta, GA: American Cancer Society.

[53] O'Brien, P.C. and Fleming, T.R. (1979): A multiple testing procedure for clinical trials. *Biometrics.* 35: 549–556.

[54] Lan, K.K.G. and Demets, D.L. (1983): Discrete sequential boundaries for clinical trials. *Biometrika.* 70: 659–663.

[55] Cox, D.R. (1972): Regression models and life-tables (with discussion). *Journal of the Royal Statistical Society Series B.* 34: 187–220.

[56] Stangl, D.K. (1996): Hierarchical analysis of continuous-time survival models. In: Berry, D.A. and Stangl, D.K., eds. *Bayesian Biostatistics.* New York: Marcel Dekker, Inc., pp. 429–450.

[57] Li, C. (1994): Comparing survival data for two therapies: Nonhierarchical and hierarchical Bayesian approaches. PhD dissertation. Durham, NC: ISDS, Duke University.

[58] George, S.L., Li, C., Berry, D.A., and Green, M.R. (1994): Stopping a clinical trial early: frequentist and Bayesian approaches applied to a CALGB trial in non-small-cell lung cancer. *Statistics in Medicine.* 13: 1313–1327.

[59] Sahu, S.K., Dey, D.K., Aslanidou, H., and Sinha, D. (1997): A Weibull regression model with gamma frailties for multivariate survival data. *Lifetime Data Analysis*. 3: 123–137.

[60] Clayton, D.G. (1991): A Monte Carlo method for Bayesian inference in frailty models. *Biometrics*. 47: 467–485.

[61] Sinha, D. (1997): Semiparametric Bayesian analysis of multiple event time data. *Canadian Journal of Statistics*. 25: 445–456.

[62] Pennell, M.L. and Dunson, D.B. (2006): Bayesian semiparametric dynamic frailty models for multiple event time data. *Biometrics*. 62: 1044–1052.

[63] Stangl, D.K. and Greenhouse, J.B. (1998): Assessing placebo response using Bayesian hierarchical survival models. *Lifetime Data Analysis*. 4: 5–28.

[64] Chen, M.-H., Ibrahim, J.G., and Sinha, D. (2002): Bayesian inference for multivariate survival data with a cure fraction. *Journal of Multivariate Analysis*. 80(1): 101–126.

[65] Gunn, L.H. and Dunson, D.B. (2005): Bayesian methods for assessing ordering in hazard functions. *Discussion paper 2005–19*. Department of Statistical Science, Duke University, Hillsborough, NC.

[66] Stangl, D.K. and Berry, D.A. (2000): *Meta-Analysis in Medicine and Health Policy*. New York: Marcel Dekker, Inc.

[67] Carlin, J.B. (1992): Meta-analysis for 2×2 tables: A Bayesian approach. *Statistics in Medicine*. 11: 141–158.

[68] Sutton, A.J., Abrams, K.R., Jones, D.R., Sheldon, T.A., and Song, F. (2000): *Methods for Meta-Analysis in Medical Research*. New York: John Wiley & Sons.

[69] Higgins, J.P.T. and Spiegelhalter, D.J. (2002): Being skeptical about meta-analyses: A Bayesian perspective on magnesium trials in myocardial infarction. *International Journal of Epidemiology*. 31: 96–104.

[70] Dukic, V. and Gatsonis, C. (2003): Meta-analysis of diagnostic test accuracy assessment studies with varying number of thresholds. *Biometrics*. 59(4): 936–946.

[71] Sutton, A.J. and Higgins, J.P. (2008): Recent developments in meta-analysis. *Statistics in Medicine*. 27(5): 625–650.

[72] Berry, D.A., Müller, P., Grieve, A.P., Smith, M.K., Parke, T., Blazek, R., Mitchard, N., and Krams, M. (2001): Adaptive Bayesian designs for dose-ranging trials. In: Gatsonis, C., Kass, R.E., Carlin, B., Carriquiry, A., Gelman, A., Verdinelli, I., and West, M., eds. *Case Studies in Bayesian Statistics V*. New York: Springer, pp. 99–181.

[73] Cheng, Y. and Shen, Y. (2005): Bayesian adaptive designs for clinical trials. *Biometrika*. 92(3): 633–646.

[74] Chang, M. and Chow, S.C. (2005): A hybrid Bayesian adaptive design for dose response trials. *Journal of Biopharmaceutical Statistics*. 15(4): 677–691.

[75] Lewis, R.J., Lipsky, A.M., and Berry, D.A. (2007): Bayesian decision-theoretic group sequential clinical trial design based on a quadratic loss function: A frequentist evaluation. *Clinical Trials*. 4(1): 5–14.

[76] Zhou, X., Liu, S., Kim, E.S., Herbst, R.S., and Lee, J.J. (2008): Bayesian adaptive design for targeted therapy development in lung cancer—a step toward personalized medicine. *Clinical Trials*. 5(3): 181–193.

[77] Berry, D.A. (2005): Introduction to Bayesian methods III: Use and interpretation of Bayesian tools in design and analysis. *Clinical Trials*. 2(4): 295–300.

[78] Berry, D.A. (2006): A guide to drug discovery: Bayesian clinical trials. *Nature Reviews Drug Discovery*. 5: 27–36.

[79] Spiegelhalter, D.J., Abrams, K.R., and Myles, J.P. (2004): *Bayesian Approaches to Clinical Trials and Health-Care Evaluation*. New York, John Wiley & Sons, Ltd..

[80] Racine, A., Grieve, A.P., Fluhler, H., and Smith, A.F.M. (1986): Bayesian methods in practice: experiences in the pharmaceutical industry. *Applied Statistics*. 35(2): 93–150.

Chapter 7

An Efficient Alternative to the Cox Model for Small Time-to-Event Trials

Devan V. Mehrotra and Arthur J. Roth

Contents

7.1 Introduction

The standard tool for analyzing time-to-event data from a randomized two-group trial is the Cox proportional hazards model [1]. The Cox model is an attractive semiparametric option when the trial size is reasonably large. However, for small trials, such as many cancer clinical trials or pilot/early phase trials in other areas, point and interval estimates of the relative risk (hazard ratio) based on the Cox model can be inefficient, thereby adversely impacting the design of potential follow-up trials. Mehrotra and Roth [2] provided a heuristic explanation for the small sample inefficiency of the Cox model and developed a more efficient method for relative risk estimation and inference based on a generalized logrank (GLR) statistic. They showed that the GLR method and the Cox model yield similar results for large trials (>100 subjects per treatment group), but the GLR-based estimates of the relative risk have notably smaller mean squared errors (MSEs) for small trials.

In this chapter, we elaborate on the construction of the original GLR statistic for the case of no ties and provide two natural extensions of GLR for use in settings with tied event times; we refer to the extensions as GLR^{KP} and GLR^E, which are identical to GLR when there are no ties. In Section 7.2, we present score statistics for relative risk estimation and inference based on partial likelihoods proposed by Cox [1], Kalbfleisch and Prentice [3], and Efron [4] for the proportional hazards model, including Mantel's [5] logrank statistic based on Cox's partial likelihood. In Section 7.3, we describe the GLR, GLR^{KP}, and GLR^E methods. In Section 7.4, we show the link between the different score statistics based on the Cox model and their corresponding GLR counterparts. Two illustrative examples are provided in Section 7.5 to reinforce the key points. In Section 7.6, we report simulation results to quantify the efficiency gains of GLR, GLR^{KP}, and GLR^E relative to the corresponding approaches based on the Cox model, followed by concluding remarks in Section 7.7.

Throughout, we assume that subjects are randomized to either treatment A or treatment B, and that the event time distributions have proportional hazard functions, i.e., $\theta = \lambda_A(t)/\lambda_B(t)$ is constant over time, where $\lambda_A(t)$ and $\lambda_B(t)$ denote the hazard rates at time t for treatments A and B, respectively. The constant (time-invariant) hazard ratio, θ, is interchangeably referred to as the relative risk.

7.2   Estimation and Inference Using the Cox Proportional Hazards Model

Suppose N_A and N_B subjects are randomized to treatment groups A and B, respectively. With the time origin for each subject corresponding to his/her time of randomization, let $t_1 < t_2 < \cdots < t_k$ denote the ordered event (failure) times for the combined data. We assume throughout that censoring, if any, is noninformative.

If at t_i there are d_i events (failures) among n_i subjects at risk just before t_i, then the data at t_i can be summarized in a 2×2 table as follows:

	Failed	**Survived**	**Total**
Group A	d_{iA}	$n_{iA} - d_{iA}$	n_{iA}
Group B	d_{iB}	$n_{iB} - d_{iB}$	n_{iB}
Total	d_i	$n_i - d_i$	n_i

7.2.1   No Tied Event Times

For now, assume that there are no tied event times (i.e., $d_i = 1 \ \forall i$), and let the treatment indicator Z_i be 1 or 0 according to whether the event at t_i is in group A or group B, respectively. The Cox [1] partial likelihood function, typically expressed in terms of $\beta = \ln(\theta)$, can be written as

$$L(\beta) = \prod_{i=1}^{k} \frac{e^{Z_i\beta}}{\sum\limits_{j \in R(t_i)} e^{Z_j\beta}} = \prod_{i=1}^{k} \frac{e^{d_{iA}\beta}}{n_{iA}e^{\beta} + n_{iB}}, \tag{7.1}$$

where $R(t_i)$ is the indicator set for subjects at risk just prior to t_i. The score function arising from Equation 7.1, defined by $S(\beta) = \partial \ln L(\beta) / \partial \beta$, is given by

$$S(\beta) = \sum_{i=1}^{k} \left(d_{iA} - \frac{n_{iA} e^{\beta}}{n_{iA} e^{\beta} + n_{iB}} \right) = \sum_{i=1}^{k} \left(d_{iA} - \frac{n_{iA} \theta}{n_{iA} \theta + n_{iB}} \right). \tag{7.2}$$

The maximum partial likelihood estimator of β, say $\tilde{\beta}_C$, is obtained as the iterative solution of $S(\beta) = 0$. Under mild regularity conditions [6, 7], $\tilde{\beta}_C$ has an asymptotic normal distribution with mean β and approximate variance given by $V(\tilde{\beta}_C) = I(\tilde{\beta}_C)^{-1}$, where

$$I(\beta) = -\frac{\partial^2 \ln L(\beta)}{\partial \beta^2} = \sum_{i=1}^{k} \frac{n_{iA} n_{iB} e^{\beta}}{(n_{iA} e^{\beta} + n_{iB})^2} = \sum_{i=1}^{k} \frac{n_{iA} n_{iB} \theta}{(n_{iA} \theta + n_{iB})^2}. \tag{7.3}$$

Typically, in addition to obtaining a point estimate of β (or equivalently, θ), interest lies in testing $H_0: \beta = \beta_0$ and providing a confidence interval for β. This is commonly done using either the Wald or score approach based on the Cox model; the former is more popular presumably because of its availability in commercial software. For the Wald approach, the test statistic is $Z(\beta_0) = (\tilde{\beta}_C - \beta_0) / \sqrt{\hat{V}(\tilde{\beta}_C)}$, and an approximate $100(1 - \alpha)\%$ confidence interval for β is $\tilde{\beta}_C \pm Z_{\alpha/2} \sqrt{\hat{V}(\tilde{\beta}_C)}$, where $\hat{V}(\tilde{\beta}_C)$ is obtained by replacing β with $\tilde{\beta}_C$ in Equation 7.3 taking the reciprocal. The test statistic based on the score approach is given by

$$U(\beta_0) = \frac{\{S(\beta_0)\}^2}{I(\beta_0)}. \tag{7.4}$$

Note that the Cox maximum partial likelihood estimator, $\tilde{\beta}_C$, can be viewed as the value of β which satisfies

$$U(\tilde{\beta}_C) = \inf_{\beta} U(\beta). \tag{7.5}$$

Provided the number of events is sufficiently large, $U(\beta_0)$ is approximately distributed as a $\chi^2_{(1)}$ variate under the null hypothesis. Accordingly, a $100(1 - \alpha)\%$ confidence interval for β based on the score test, with endpoints defined by (β^L, β^U), can be constructed using

$$\beta^L = \inf_{\beta} \left\{ \beta : U(\beta) \le \chi^2_{(1),\alpha} \right\} \tag{7.6}$$

and

$$\beta^U = \sup_{\beta} \left\{ \beta : U(\beta) \le \chi^2_{(1),\alpha} \right\}. \tag{7.7}$$

For the special case of testing $H_0: \beta = 0$ (i.e., $H_0: \theta = 1$), setting $\beta_0 = 0$ in Equation 7.4 yields, upon simplification, Mantel's [5] logrank statistic for the case of no ties:

$$U(\beta_0 = 0) = \frac{\left\{\sum_{i=1}^{k} (d_{iA} - (n_{iA}/(n_{iA} + n_{iB})))\right\}^2}{\sum_{i=1}^{k} n_{iA} n_{iB}/(n_{iA} + n_{iB})^2}. \quad (7.8)$$

It is helpful to note that when $\beta_0 = 0$, conditional upon n_{iA}, n_{iB} and d_i, d_{iA} has a central hypergeometric distribution with mean given by

$$E(d_{iA}|n_{iA}, n_{iB}, d_i = 1, \beta_0 = 0) \equiv E_{iA}(\beta_0 = 0) = \frac{n_{iA}}{n_{iA} + n_{iB}} \quad (7.9)$$

and variance given by

$$V(d_{iA}|n_{iA}, n_{iB}, d_i = 1, \beta_0 = 0) \equiv V_{iA}(\beta_0 = 0) = \frac{n_{iA} n_{iB}}{(n_{iA} + n_{iB})^2}. \quad (7.10)$$

Accordingly, Mantel's logrank statistic can be conveniently expressed as

$$U(\beta_0 = 0) = \frac{\left[\sum_{i=1}^{k} \{d_{iA} - E_{iA}(\beta_0 = 0)\}\right]^2}{\sum_{i=1}^{k} V_{iA}(\beta_0 = 0)}. \quad (7.11)$$

7.2.2   Tied Event Times

So far we have assumed that there are no tied event times. However, in practice, ties will occur if the data are "grouped" by virtue of rounding to the nearest day, week, etc., in which case Equation 7.1 is no longer directly applicable. Several approaches have been proposed for dealing with ties. For example, Cox [1], Kalbfleisch and Prentice [3], Breslow [8], and Efron [4] proposed approximate tie-handling extensions of the partial likelihood in Equation 7.1, all of which are implemented in the PHREG procedure of SAS; even though the Breslow option is the PHREG default, we do not discuss it further because it performs poorly when there are many ties [9].

To allow for ties, additional notation is necessary. Let $Z_{i1}, Z_{i2}, \ldots, Z_{in_i}$ denote treatment indicators for the n_i subjects at risk just before t_i, where Z_{ij} equals 1 or 0 depending on whether subject j is from group A or group B, respectively. We work with the usual convention that all events reported at time t_i precede any censorings reported at t_i so that all censored subjects contribute fully to the corresponding risk set(s).

The partial likelihood extension of Equation 7.1 based on the Cox [1] tie-handling approximation (implemented using TIES = DISCRETE in PROC PHREG) is given by

$$L^C(\beta) = \prod_{i=1}^{k} \frac{\prod_{j=1}^{d_i} e^{Z_{ij}\beta}}{\sum_{l \in R(t_i,d_i)} e^{S_l\beta}} = \prod_{i=1}^{k} \frac{e^{d_{iA}\beta}}{\sum_{j=1}^{d_i} \binom{n_{iA}}{j}\binom{n_{iB}}{d_i-j} e^{j\beta}}, \quad (7.12)$$

where $S_l = \sum_j Z_{lj}$, and the sum in the first denominator is taken over all the distinct selections of d_i subjects drawn without replacement from the n_i at risk just before t_i.

The score statistic for testing $H_0 : \beta = \beta_0$ based on Equation 7.12, denoted by $U^C(\beta_0)$, is analogous to Equation 7.4, with

$$S^C(\beta_0) = \sum_{i=1}^{k} \left(d_{iA} - \frac{\sum_{j=1}^{d_i} j \binom{n_{iA}}{j}\binom{n_{iB}}{d_i-j} e^{j\beta_0}}{\sum_{j=1}^{d_i} \binom{n_{iA}}{j}\binom{n_{iB}}{d_i-j} e^{j\beta_0}} \right) \quad (7.13)$$

and

$$I^C(\beta_0) = \sum_{i=1}^{k} \frac{\left[\sum_{j=1}^{d_i} j^2 \binom{n_{iA}}{j}\binom{n_{iB}}{d_i-j} e^{j\beta_0}\right]\left[\sum_{j=1}^{d_i} \binom{n_{iA}}{j}\binom{n_{iB}}{d_i-j} e^{j\beta_0}\right] - \left[\sum_{j=1}^{d_i} j \binom{n_{iA}}{j}\binom{n_{iB}}{d_i-j} e^{j\beta_0}\right]^2}{\left[\sum_{j=1}^{d_i} \binom{n_{iA}}{j}\binom{n_{iB}}{d_i-j} e^{j\beta_0}\right]^2}.$$

$$(7.14)$$

For the special case of testing $H_0 : \beta = 0$, setting $\beta_0 = 0$ in Equations 7.13 and 7.14 leads to Mantel's logrank statistic in the presence of ties, which can still be expressed in the form given by Equation 7.11 with

$$E_{iA}(\beta_0 = 0) = \frac{d_i n_{iA}}{n_{iA} + n_{iB}} \quad (7.15)$$

and

$$V_{iA}(\beta_0 = 0) = \frac{n_{iA} n_{iB} d_i (n_{iA} + n_{iB} - d_i)}{(n_{iA} + n_{iB})^2 (n_{iA} + n_{iB} - 1)}. \quad (7.16)$$

Given the popularity of the logrank test for inference, it is natural to want to estimate β in the presence of ties by using $U^C(\beta)$ in lieu of $U(\beta)$ in Equation 7.5, but that is not recommended because the resulting estimator is generally biased, with the degree of bias increasing as the number of ties increases and as β deviates further from zero. More desirable estimators of β in the presence of ties are obtained using the partial likelihoods proposed by Kalbfleisch and Prentice [3] and Efron [4].

The Kalbfleisch and Prentice [3] extension of Equation 7.1 to accommodate ties for the Cox proportional hazards model can be implemented using the TIES = EXACT option in PROC PHREG; it uses the following expression of the partial likelihood function for efficient computation [10]:

$$L^{\text{KP}}(\beta) = \prod_{i=1}^{k} \int_{0}^{\infty} \prod_{j=1}^{d_i} \left\{ 1 - \exp\left[-\frac{e^{(Z_j\beta)t}}{\sum\limits_{l \in C(t_i)} e^{(Z_l\beta)t}} \right] \right\} e^{-t} dt. \tag{7.17}$$

Letting

$$\alpha_i = \frac{e^{\beta}}{(n_{iA} - d_{iA})e^{\beta} + (n_{iB} - d_{iB})}$$

and

$$\lambda_i = \frac{1}{(n_{iA} - d_{iA})e^{\beta} + (n_{iB} - d_{iB})},$$

it follows that

$$L^{\text{KP}}(\beta) = \prod_{I=1}^{K} \int_{0}^{\infty} (1 - e^{-\alpha_i t})^{d_{iA}} (1 - e^{-\lambda_i t})^{d_{iB}} e^{-t} dt.$$

Since a straightforward application of the Binomial theorem yields

$$(1 - e^{-\alpha_i t})^{d_{iA}} = \sum_{x=0}^{d_{iA}} \binom{d_{iA}}{x} (-1)^x e^{-\alpha_i t x},$$

we can reexpress $L^{\text{KP}}(\beta)$ as

$$L^{\text{KP}}(\beta) = \prod_{i=1}^{k} \sum_{x=0}^{d_{iA}} \sum_{y=0}^{d_{iB}} (-1)^{x+y} \binom{d_{iA}}{x} \binom{d_{iB}}{y} \frac{e^{\beta}(n_{iA} - d_{iA}) + (n_{iB} - d_{iB})}{e^{\beta}(n_{iA} - d_{iA} + x) + (n_{iB} - d_{iB} + y)}. \tag{7.18}$$

Straightforward but tedious algebra reveals that the score statistic for testing $H_0 : \beta = \beta_0$ using the Kalbfleisch and Prentice [3] partial likelihood in Equation 7.18, denoted by $U^{\text{KP}}(\beta_0)$, is analogous to Equation 7.4, with

$$S^{\text{KP}}(\beta_0) = \sum_{i=1}^{k} \frac{\sum\limits_{x=0}^{d_{iA}} \sum\limits_{y=0}^{d_{iB}} D_{ixy} E'_{ixy}(\beta_0)}{\sum\limits_{x=0}^{d_{iA}} \sum\limits_{y=0}^{d_{iB}} D_{ixy} E_{ixy}(\beta_0)} \tag{7.19}$$

and

$$I^{\text{KP}}(\beta_0) = \sum_{i=1}^{k} \frac{\left(\sum_{x=0}^{d_{iA}} \sum_{y=0}^{d_{iB}} D_{ixy} E'_{ixy}(\beta_0)\right)^2 - \left(\sum_{x=0}^{d_{iA}} \sum_{y=0}^{d_{iB}} D_{ixy} E''_{ixy}(\beta_0)\right)\left(\sum_{x=0}^{d_{iA}} \sum_{y=0}^{d_{iB}} D_{ixy} E_{ixy}(\beta_0)\right)}{\left(\sum_{x=0}^{d_{iA}} \sum_{y=0}^{d_{iB}} D_{ixy} E_{ixy}(\beta_0)\right)^2},$$

$$(7.20)$$

where

$$D_{ixy} = (-1)^{x+y}\binom{d_{iA}}{x}\binom{d_{iB}}{y}, \quad E_{ixy}(\beta_0) = \frac{e^{\beta_0}(n_{iA} - d_{iA}) + (n_{iB} - d_{iB})}{e^{\beta_0}(n_{iA} - d_{iA} + x) + (n_{iB} - d_{iB} + y)},$$

$$E'_{ixy}(\beta_0) = \frac{e^{\beta_0}[(n_{iA} - d_{iA})y - (n_{iB} - d_{iB})x]}{[e^{\beta_0}(n_{iA} - d_{iA} + x) + (n_{iB} - d_{iB} + y)]^2},$$

and

$$E''_{ixy}(\beta_0) = \frac{e^{\beta_0}[(n_{iA} - d_{iA})y - (n_{iB} - d_{iB})x][(n_{iB} - d_{iB} + y) - e^{\beta_0}(n_{iA} - d_{iA} + x)]}{[e^{\beta_0}(n_{iA} - d_{iA} + x) + (n_{iB} - d_{iB} + y)]^3}.$$

The Efron [4] version of Equation 7.1 to accommodate ties for the Cox model can be implemented using the TIES = EFRON option in PROC PHREG; it uses the following partial likelihood function:

$$L^{\text{E}}(\beta) = \prod_{i=1}^{k} \frac{e^{d_{iA}\beta}}{\prod_{j=1}^{d_i}[(n_{iA}e^{\beta} + n_{iB}) - ((j-1)/d_i)(d_{iA}e^{\beta} + d_{iB})]}.$$

$$(7.21)$$

The score statistic for testing $H_0: \beta = \beta_0$ using Efron's partial likelihood in Equation 7.21, denoted by $U^{\text{E}}(\beta_0)$, is analogous to Equation 7.4, with

$$S^{\text{E}}(\beta_0) = \sum_{i=1}^{k}\left(d_{iA} - \sum_{j=1}^{d_i} \frac{n_{iA}e^{\beta_0} - (j-1)(d_{iA}e^{\beta_0}/d_i)}{(n_{iA}e^{\beta_0} + n_{iB}) - (j-1)(d_{iA}e^{\beta_0} + d_{iB})/d_i}\right)$$

$$(7.22)$$

and

$$I^{\text{E}}(\beta_0) = \sum_{i=1}^{k} \sum_{j=1}^{d_i} \frac{[n_{iA}e^{\beta_0} - (j-1)(d_{iA}e^{\beta_0}/d_i)][n_{iB} - (j-1)(d_{iB}/d_i)]}{[(n_{iA}e^{\beta_0} + n_{iB}) - (j-1)(d_{iA}e^{\beta_0} + d_{iB})/d_i]^2}.$$

$$(7.23)$$

Point and interval estimates of β based on the Kalbfleisch and Prentice [3] and Efron [4] methods can be obtained by replacing $U(\beta)$ with $U^{\text{KP}}(\beta)$ and $U^{\text{E}}(\beta)$, respectively, in Equations 7.5 through 7.7. Of note, with no ties (i.e., when $d_i = 1 \ \forall i$), $L(\beta) = L^{\text{C}}(\beta) = L^{\text{KP}}(\beta) = L^{\text{E}}(\beta)$, and hence $U(\beta) = U^{\text{C}}(\beta) = U^{\text{KP}}(\beta) = U^{\text{E}}(\beta)$, so the Cox, Kalbfleisch and Prentice, and Efron methods lead to identical results.

The preceding material on partial likelihoods and associated score statistics for the Cox proportional hazards model provides the necessary background for a discussion of the material in Section 7.3. Specifically, we will now elaborate on the construction of Mehrotra and Roth's [2] GLR method for the case of no tied event times and extend GLR to accommodate ties, leading to GLR^{KP} and GLR^E.

7.3   Estimation and Inference Using Generalized Logrank Methods

7.3.1   No Tied Event Times (GLR)

To motivate the development of the GLR method, note that if T is a time-to-event variable with survival function $S(t) = P\{T > t\}$, the hazard function can be written as $h(t) = -(d/dt)(\ln[S(t)])$. Hence, $S(t) = e^{-\int_0^t h(x)dx}$ and

$$P\{t_{i-1} < T \le t_i | T > t_{i-1}\} = 1 - P\{T > t_i | T > t_{i-1}\} = 1 - e^{-p_i}, \quad (7.24)$$

where $p_i = \int_{t_{i-1}}^{t_i} h(x)dx$. Note that $1 - e^{-p_i} \approx p_i$ if p_i is small. Accordingly, at each t_i, given n_{iA} and n_{iB}, if we think of the number of events for group B as having arisen from a binomial distribution with failure probability p_i, under proportional hazards the corresponding failure probability for group A will be approximately $\theta p_i (= e^\beta p_i)$, where $0 \le p_i \le \min(1, \theta^{-1})$. It is clear from Equation 7.24 that this approximation will become increasingly more reasonable as the width of the time interval represented by the 2×2 table at each t_i decreases, so that the cumulative hazard between t_{i-1} and t_i becomes small. Hence, the GLR method described below is not recommended for situations in which tied event times arise from a coarse grouping of continuous event times; for reasons explained below, GLR^{KP} and GLR^E are better options.

If the random variable D_{iA} denotes the number of events in group A at t_i, then the conditional distribution of D_{iA} given $(n_{iA}, n_{iB}, d_i, \theta, p_i)$ can be approximated by the following noncentral hypergeometric distribution:

$$P(D_{iA} = d_{iA}|n_{iA}, n_{iB}, d_i, p_i, \theta) = \pi_{iA} = \frac{\binom{n_{iA}}{d_{iA}}\binom{n_{iB}}{d_{iB}}\theta^{d_{iA}}(1 - \theta p_i)^{n_{iA}-d_{iA}}(1 - p_i)^{n_{iB}-d_{iB}}}{\sum_{j \in G_i}\binom{n_{iA}}{j}\binom{n_{iB}}{d_i - j}\theta^j(1 - \theta p_i)^{n_{iA}-j}(1 - p_i)^{n_{iB}-d_i+j}}. \quad (7.25)$$

In Equation 7.25, $G_i = \{j : \max(0, d_i - n_{iB}) \le j \le \min(d_i, n_{iA})\}$. Let $E_{iA}(\theta, p_i) = \sum_{G_i} d_{iA}\pi_{iA}$ and $V_{iA}(\theta, p_i) = \sum_{G_i} d_{iA}^2 \pi_{iA} - (\sum_{G_i} d_{iA}\pi_{iA})^2$ denote, respectively, the mean and variance of D_{iA} based on the conditional distribution in Equation 7.25. With no ties (i.e., $d_i = 1 \; \forall i$), the following closed form expressions are available:

$$E_{iA}(\theta, p_i) = \frac{n_{iA}\theta(1 - p_i)}{n_{iA}\theta(1 - p_i) + n_{iB}(1 - \theta p_i)} \tag{7.26}$$

and

$$V_{iA}(\theta, p_i) = \frac{n_{iA}n_{iB}\theta(1 - p_i)(1 - \theta p_i)}{[n_{iA}\theta(1 - p_i) + n_{iB}(1 - \theta p_i)]^2}. \tag{7.27}$$

Assume for now that the vector of nuisance parameters $\underline{p} = (p_1, p_2, \ldots, p_k)$ is known. The GLR statistic to test $H_0 : \theta = \theta_0$ takes the same form as Equation 7.11 and is given by

$$\text{GLR}(\theta_0, \underline{p}) = \frac{\left[\sum_{i=1}^{k}\{d_{iA} - E_{iA}(\theta_0, p_i)\}\right]^2}{\sum_{i=1}^{k} V_{iA}(\theta_0, p_i)}. \tag{7.28}$$

To implement the GLR test when $\theta_0 \neq 1$, we need to (1) estimate the nuisance parameters $\{p_i\}$ and (2) determine a reference distribution for the resulting test statistic. Note that when $\theta = 1$, the conditional distribution given by Equation 7.25 does not depend on p_i, so that $\text{GLR}(\theta_0 = 1, \underline{p})$ does not depend on $\underline{p}$. Moreover, this special case of Equation 7.28 is Mantel's logrank statistic, for which the usual reference distribution is $\chi^2_{(1)}$. Hence neither (1) nor (2) above is necessary, and the term generalized logrank test is justified.

There are various ways to estimate p_i; Mehrotra and Roth [2] recommend that $\tilde{p}_{i,\theta}$ be the estimate of p_i that maximizes

$$L(p_i | \theta) = (\theta p_i)^{d_{iA}}(1 - \theta p_i)^{n_{iA} - d_{iA}}(p_i)^{d_{iB}}(1 - p_i)^{n_{iB} - d_{iB}}, \tag{7.29}$$

an objective function that is proportional to the product of the two unconditional binomial likelihoods $B(n_{iA}, \theta p_i)$ and $B(n_{iB}, p_i)$. It can be easily shown that Equation 7.29 is maximized in the domain $0 \leq p_i \leq \min(1, \theta^{-1})$ at

$$\tilde{p}_{i,\theta} = \frac{x_i - \left(x_i^2 - 4n_i d_i \theta\right)^{1/2}}{2n_i\theta}, \tag{7.30}$$

where $x_i = \theta(n_{iA} + d_{iB}) + (n_{iB} + d_{iA})$. Let $\underline{\tilde{p}}(\theta)$ denote the vector $(\tilde{p}_{1,\theta}, \tilde{p}_{2,\theta}, \ldots, \tilde{p}_{k,\theta})$. Replacing p_i in Equation 7.28 with $\tilde{p}_{i,\theta_0}$ from Equation 7.30 leads to the GLR statistic for testing $H_0 : \theta = \theta_0$:

$$\text{GLR}[\theta_0, \underline{\tilde{p}}(\theta_0)] = \frac{\left\{\sum_{i=1}^{k}[d_{iA} - E_{iA}(\theta_0, \tilde{p}_{i,\theta_0})]\right\}^2}{\sum_{i=1}^{k} V_{iA}(\theta_0, \tilde{p}_{i,\theta_0})}. \tag{7.31}$$

Next, we need a reference distribution for the statistic in Equation 7.31. For the special case of $\theta_0 = 1$, i.e., when the GLR test is Mantel's logrank test, $H_0 : \theta = \theta_0$ can be tested, as mentioned earlier, by treating Equation 7.31 as a $\chi^2_{(1)}$ variate under the null hypothesis as long as the number of events is sufficiently large. However, when $\theta_0 \neq 1$, the presence of the estimated nuisance parameters $\tilde{p}_{i,\theta_0}$ makes it difficult, if not impossible, to determine the true null distribution of $GLR[\theta_0, \tilde{p}(\theta_0)]$. Fortunately, when the group sample sizes (or more accurately, the risk sets) are very large, $\tilde{p}_{i,\theta_0} \approx 0$ for most i. In that case, for reasons that will become clear later, it is reasonable to expect that using $\chi^2_{(1)}$ to approximate the true null distribution will remain accurate enough to produce a test with acceptable Type I error rates. However, to ensure inferential validity with small to moderate sample sizes, an alternative reference distribution is required, one that converges to $\chi^2_{(1)}$ as the sample sizes increase. Based on an extensive numerical investigation, Mehrotra and Roth [2] recommended using $F(1, k^*)$ as an approximate reference distribution for $GLR[\theta_0, \tilde{p}(\theta_0)]$, where $k^* = \sum_i \min(d_i, n_i - d_i, n_{iA}, n_{iB})$ and $F(f_n, f_d)$ denotes a central F-distribution with (f_n, f_d) degrees of freedom. Note that the data-dependent reference distribution $F(1, k^*)$ converges to $\chi^2_{(1)} = F(1, \infty)$ as $k^* \to \infty$, and, with no ties, k^* is the number of 2×2 tables that contribute information toward θ. In summary, the GLR test rejects $H_0 : \theta = \theta_0$ at level approximately α if Equation 7.31 is greater than $F_\alpha(1, k^*)$; simulation-based support for the inferential validity of this testing procedure is provided in Mehrotra and Roth [2].

To obtain point and interval estimates of θ, note that $GLR[\theta, \tilde{p}(\theta)]$ is strictly decreasing in θ until it reaches a unique minimum (approximately zero), after which it is strictly increasing. Since small values of $GLR[\theta_0, \tilde{p}(\theta_0)]$ support the null hypothesis $H_0 : \theta = \theta_0$, a natural estimate of the relative risk is the θ that minimizes $GLR[\theta, \tilde{p}(\theta)]$. Accordingly, by analogy to Equation 7.5, the obvious estimator of θ based on the GLR test, which we denote by $\tilde{\theta}_{GLR}$, is defined to be the θ which satisfies

$$GLR[\tilde{\theta}_{GLR}, \tilde{p}(\tilde{\theta}_{GLR})] = \inf_\theta GLR[\theta, \tilde{p}(\theta)], \qquad (7.32)$$

and the endpoints of a $100(1 - \alpha)\%$ confidence interval for θ based on the GLR test, $(\theta^L_{GLR}, \theta^U_{GLR})$, are defined by

$$\theta^L_{GLR} = \inf_\theta \{\theta : GLR[\theta, \tilde{p}(\theta)] \leq F_\alpha(1, k^*)\} \qquad (7.33)$$

and

$$\theta^U_{GLR} = \sup_\theta \{\theta : GLR[\theta, \tilde{p}(\theta)] \leq F_\alpha(1, k^*)\}. \qquad (7.34)$$

7.3.2   Tied Event Times (GLR^{KP} and GLR^E)

Suppose there are d_{iA} and $d_{iB} = d_i - d_{iA}$ events recorded at time t_i in treatment groups A and B, respectively, and denote the true unknown $d_i (>1)$ event times in the interval $(t_{i-1}, t_i]$ by $t_{i,1} < \cdots < t_{i,d_i}$. Both of the GLR extensions for tackling tied event

TABLE 7.1: Example with $d_i = 3$ events at t_i ($d_{iA} = 2$, $d_{iB} = 1$).

	Number at Risk in Group (A,B) Just Before $t_{i,j}$		
Possible Orderings	$t_{i,1}$	$t_{i,2}$	$t_{i,3}$
A→A→B	(n_{iA}, n_{iB})	$(n_{iA} - 1, n_{iB})$	$(n_{iA} - 2, n_{iB})$
A→B→A	(n_{iA}, n_{iB})	$(n_{iA} - 1, n_{iB})$	$(n_{iA} - 1, n_{iB} - 1)$
B→A→A	(n_{iA}, n_{iB})	$(n_{iA}, n_{iB} - 1)$	$(n_{iA} - 1, n_{iB} - 1)$
Average # at risk	(n_{iA}, n_{iB})	$\left(n_{iA} - \frac{2}{3}, n_{iB} - \frac{1}{3}\right)$	$\left(n_{iA} - \frac{4}{3}, n_{iB} - \frac{2}{3}\right)$
Nuisance parameter	$p_{i,1}$	$p_{i,2}$	$p_{i,3}$

times at t_i involve breaking the ties, averaging over all possible orderings of the unknown true d_i event times, and replacing E_{iA} and V_{iA} in the GLR statistic given by Equation 7.31 with versions of $\bar{E}_{iA}$ and $\bar{V}_{iA}$, respectively. The two extensions, GLR^{KP} and GLR^{E}, differ in how $\bar{E}_{iA}$ and $\bar{V}_{iA}$ are calculated. To illustrate, consider the example shown in Table 7.1.

For GLR^{KP}, $\bar{E}_{iA} \equiv \bar{E}_{iA}^{\text{KP}}$ is calculated by averaging E_{iA} over the three possible orderings separately at each of the three unobserved true time points in Table 7.1 and then summing these averages across the three time points, so that

$$\bar{E}_{iA}^{\text{KP}} = \frac{1}{3}[3E_{iA}(n_{iA}, n_{iB}, \theta, \tilde{p}_{i,1})] + \frac{1}{3}[2E_{iA}(n_{iA}-1, n_{iB}, \theta, \tilde{p}_{i,2}) + E_{iA}(n_{iA}, n_{iB}-1, \theta, \tilde{p}_{i,2})]$$

$$+ \frac{1}{3}[2E_{iA}(n_{iA}-1, n_{iB}-1, \theta, \tilde{p}_{i,3}) + E_{iA}(n_{iA}-2, n_{iB}, \theta, \tilde{p}_{i,3})]$$

$$\bar{V}_{iA}^{\text{KP}} = \frac{1}{3}[3V_{iA}(n_{iA}, n_{iB}, \theta, \tilde{p}_{i,1})] + \frac{1}{3}[2V_{iA}(n_{iA}-1, n_{iB}, \theta, \tilde{p}_{i,2}) + V_{iA}(n_{iA}, n_{iB}-1, \theta, \tilde{p}_{i,2})]$$

$$+ \frac{1}{3}[2V_{iA}(n_{iA}-1, n_{iB}-1, \theta, \tilde{p}_{i,3}) + V_{iA}(n_{iA}-2, n_{iB}, \theta, \tilde{p}_{i,3})].$$

$E_{iA}(\cdot)$ and $V_{iA}(\cdot)$ in the above two expressions are calculated using Equations 7.26 and 7.27, respectively; the calculation of $\tilde{p}_{i,j}$ is discussed later in this section. In general, for GLR^{KP}, $\bar{E}_{iA}^{\text{KP}}$ and $\bar{V}_{iA}^{\text{KP}}$ are calculated using the following expressions:

$$\bar{E}_{iA}^{\text{KP}} = \frac{\sum_{x=0}^{d_{iA}} \sum_{y=0}^{d_{iB}} I_{x+y} \binom{x+y}{x} \binom{d_i - x - y}{d_{iA} - x} E_{iA}(n_{iA} - x, n_{iB} - y, \theta, \tilde{p}_{i,x+y+1})}{\binom{d_i}{d_{iA}}}$$

(7.35)

and

$$\bar{V}_{iA}^{\text{KP}} = \frac{\sum_{x=0}^{d_{iA}} \sum_{y=0}^{d_{iB}} I_{x+y} \binom{x+y}{x} \binom{d_i - x - y}{d_{iA} - x} V_{iA}(n_{iA} - x, n_{iB} - y, \theta, \tilde{p}_{i,x+y+1})}{\binom{d_i}{d_{iA}}},$$

(7.36)

where $I_{x+y} = 0$ if $x + y = d_i$ and 1 otherwise.

For GLR^{E}, $\bar{E}_{iA} \equiv \bar{E}_{iA}^{\mathrm{E}}$ is determined by first calculating E_{iA} as a function of the margins of the average 2×2 table separately at each of the three unobserved true time points in Table 7.1 and then summing across the three time points, so that

$$\bar{E}_{iA}^{\mathrm{E}} = E_{iA}(n_{iA}, n_{iB}, \theta, \tilde{p}_{i,1}) + E_{iA}\left(n_{iA} - \frac{2}{3}, n_{iB} - \frac{1}{3}, \theta, \tilde{p}_{i,2}\right) + E_{iA}\left(n_{iA} - \frac{4}{3}, n_{iB} - \frac{2}{3}, \theta, \tilde{p}_{i,3}\right),$$

with $\bar{V}_{iA} \equiv \bar{V}_{iA}^{\mathrm{E}}$ being calculated analogously as

$$\bar{V}_{iA}^{\mathrm{E}} = V_{iA}(n_{iA}, n_{iB}, \theta, \tilde{p}_{i,1}) + V_{iA}\left(n_{iA} - \frac{2}{3}, n_{iB} - \frac{1}{3}, \theta, \tilde{p}_{i,2}\right) + V_{iA}\left(n_{iA} - \frac{4}{3}, n_{iB} - \frac{2}{3}, \theta, \tilde{p}_{i,3}\right).$$

In general, for GLR^{E}, $\bar{E}_{iA}^{\mathrm{E}}$ and $\bar{V}_{iA}^{\mathrm{E}}$ are calculated using the following expressions:

$$\bar{E}_{iA}^{\mathrm{E}} = \sum_{j=1}^{d_i} E_{iA}\left(n_{iA} - (j-1)\frac{d_{iA}}{d_i}, n_{iB} - (j-1)\frac{d_{iB}}{d_i}, \theta, \tilde{p}_{i,j}\right) \qquad (7.37)$$

and

$$\bar{V}_{iA}^{\mathrm{E}} = \sum_{j=1}^{d_i} V_{iA}\left(n_{iA} - (j-1)\frac{d_{iA}}{d_i}, n_{iB} - (j-1)\frac{d_{iB}}{d_i}, \theta, \tilde{p}_{i,j}\right). \qquad (7.38)$$

In Equations 7.35 through 7.38, the estimated nuisance parameters, $\tilde{p}_{i,j}$, are obtained by replacing the elements in Equation 7.30 with the corresponding elements of the average 2×2 table over all possible orderings of events at $t_{i,j}$, as shown in Table 7.2. Accordingly,

$$\tilde{p}_{i,j} \equiv \tilde{p}_{i,j,\theta} = \frac{h_i - \sqrt{h_i^2 - 4(n_{iA} + n_{iB} - j + 1)\theta}}{2(n_{iA} + n_{iB} - j + 1)\theta}, \qquad (7.39)$$

where

$$h_i = \theta\left[n_{iA} + \frac{d_{iB}}{d_i} - (j-1)\frac{d_{iA}}{d_i}\right] + n_{iB} + \frac{d_{iA}}{d_i} - (j-1)\frac{d_{iB}}{d_i}.$$

It is easily established that $\mathrm{GLR} = \mathrm{GLR}^{\mathrm{KP}} = \mathrm{GLR}^{\mathrm{E}}$ when there are no ties.

TABLE 7.2:   Average 2×2 table at $t_{i,j}$.

	Failed	Survived	Total
Group A	$\frac{d_{iA}}{d_i}$	$n_{iA} - j\frac{d_{iA}}{d_i}$	$n_{iA} - (j-1)\frac{d_{iA}}{d_i}$
Group B	$\frac{d_{iB}}{d_i}$	$n_{iB} - j\frac{d_{iB}}{d_i}$	$n_{iB} - (j-1)\frac{d_{iB}}{d_i}$
Total	1	$n_i - j$	$n_i - (j-1)$

7.4   Link between the Cox Model and the GLR Methods

It can be shown that the score statistic, $U^C(\beta_0)$, based on the Cox partial likelihood in Equation 7.12 can be expressed in terms of $\theta_0 = e^{\beta_0}$ as

$$U^C(\theta_0) = \frac{\left[\sum_{i=1}^{k} \{d_{iA} - E_{iA}(\theta_0, p_i = 0)\}\right]^2}{\sum_{i=1}^{k} V_{iA}(\theta_0, p_i = 0)}. \tag{7.40}$$

The Cox maximum partial likelihood estimator of θ, $\tilde{\theta}_C = e^{\tilde{\beta}_C}$, is the iterative solution for θ in $U^C(\theta) = 0$. Hence it follows from Equations 7.31, 7.32, and 7.40 that the Cox model estimate of θ, either without ties or based on the Cox [1] partial likelihood for handling ties, can be obtained by explicitly replacing each $\tilde{p}_{i,\theta}$ with zero in the GLR approach, i.e.,

$$\text{GLR}[\tilde{\theta}_C, \underline{0}] = \inf_{\theta} \text{GLR}[\theta, \underline{0}]. \tag{7.41}$$

Put another way, Equation 7.41 reveals that the Cox model approach implicitly sets each $p_{i,\theta}$ to zero when viewed through the GLR framework. Note that when the number at risk (n_i) at each t_i is large, Equations 7.30 and 7.39 reveal that $\tilde{p}_{i,\theta_0}$ and $\tilde{p}_{i,j,\theta_0}$ are ≈ 0; this shows that the estimator based on the GLR test is asymptotically similar to the Cox-model estimator. However, with small samples, setting each $p_{i,\theta}$ (or $p_{i,j,\theta}$) to zero in lieu of using $\tilde{p}_{i,\theta}$ (or $\tilde{p}_{i,j,\theta}$) will result in a less efficient estimator of θ. Both of these theoretical results are supported by the simulations reported in Mehrotra and Roth [2].

A similar argument to that in the preceding paragraph reveals that GLR^{KP} and GLR^E are asymptotically similar to the score statistics $U^{KP}(\beta_0)$ and $U^E(\beta_0)$, but they can differ meaningfully for small samples. Specifically, note that setting each $\tilde{p}_{i,j}$ to zero first in Equations 7.35 and 7.36 and then in Equations 7.37 and 7.38 leads approximately to the Kalbfleisch and Prentice score statistic based on Equations 7.19 and 7.20 and exactly to the Efron score statistic based on Equations 7.22 and 7.23, respectively.

7.5   Illustrative Examples

7.5.1   Example with No Tied Event Times

Table 7.3 displays survival times of 30 patients with cervical cancer who were recruited to a larger randomized trial in which patients received either radiotherapy alone (group A) or radiotherapy with the addition of a radiosensitiser (group B). Of these 30 patients, 16 were randomized to group A and 14 to group B. Note that 14/30 (47%) of the survival times are right censored, and there are no tied observations.

TABLE 7.3:   Survival times (in days) of 30 patients with cervical cancer.

Group A (control therapy, $N_A = 16$)
90, 142, 150, 269, 291, 468+, 680, 837, 890+, 1037, 1090+, 1113+, 1153, 1297, 1429, 1577+

Group B (new therapy, $N_B = 14$)
272, 362, 373, 383+, 519+, 563+, 650+, 827, 919+, 978+, 1100+, 1307, 1360+, 1476+

Source: Mehrotra, D.V. and Roth, A.J., *Statist. Med.*, 20, 2099, 2001. With permission.
Note: + denotes censored observation.

For these data, the value of $\theta(=e^\beta)$ that maximizes the Cox partial likelihood in Equation 7.1 is $\tilde{\theta}_C = 1.997$, with a 95% Wald-based confidence interval of (0.688, 5.798), and a score-based confidence interval of (0.665, 5.990). The corresponding estimator based on the GLR test is $\tilde{\theta}_{GLR} = 1.881$, with a 95% confidence interval of (0.691, 5.304), with $k^* = 16$ in Equations 7.33 and 7.34. While the two point estimates of θ are quite close, note that the Wald-based and score-based confidence intervals from the Cox model are 11% and 15% wider than the confidence interval based on the GLR method.

Figure 7.1 shows the profile of GLR$[\theta, \tilde{p}(\theta)]$ as a function of θ. Of note, as discussed in Section 7.4, if each $\tilde{p}_{i,\theta}$ is explicitly set to zero in the GLR method, a profile with similar shape but slightly less concavity emerges, with the minimum occurring at $\theta = 1.997$, the Cox maximum partial likelihood estimator.

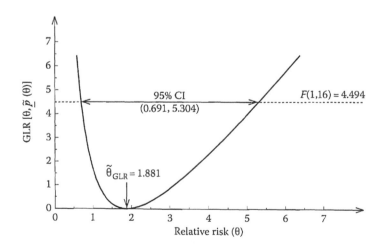

FIGURE 7.1:   Profile of the GLR statistic as a function of the relative risk for the cervical cancer data. (From Mehrotra, D.V. and Roth, A.J., *Statist. Med.*, 20, 2099, 2001. With permission.)

TABLE 7.4: Time (in weeks) to a particular adverse event in a hypothetical clinical trial.

Group A ($N_A = 20$)
2, 2, 4+, 8, 8+, 12, 12, 12, 12, 12+, 12+, 16+, 16+, 20+, 24+, 24+, 28+, 28+, 36, 36
Group B ($N_B = 20$)
4+, 4+, 4+, 4+, 8, 12+, 12+, 16+, 16+, 16+, 16+, 20+, 20+, 24+, 28+, 28+, 32+, 32+, 36, 36+

Note: +denotes censored observation.

TABLE 7.5: Relative risk estimates and 95% confidence intervals.

Kalbfleisch and Prentice	7.95	(1.04, 60.85)	GLR^{KP}	4.71	(1.05, 25.01)
Efron	5.12	(1.10, 23.86)	GLR^{E}	3.76	(1.03, 18.01)

7.5.2 Example with Tied Event Times

Table 7.4 shows times (in weeks) between randomization and a particular adverse event of interest for 40 patients in a hypothetical two-group clinical trial. Note that there are many tied event times, and 29/40 (73%) of the survival times are right censored.

Point estimates and 95% Wald-based confidence intervals for the relative risk based on the Kalbfleisch and Prentice [3] and Efron [4] partial likelihoods for the proportional hazards model with ties are shown in Table 7.5, along with corresponding entries for GLR^{KP} and GLR^{E}. Here, unlike the previous example, we see a notable difference in both the point estimates and the confidence intervals; the GLR^{KP} and GLR^{E} estimates are smaller than their Cox-model counterparts, and their confidence intervals are considerably narrower.

Of note, if each $\tilde{p}_{i,j}$ is explicitly set to zero in the GLR^{KP} and GLR^{E} methods, the resulting estimates of the relative risk are 5.81 (closer to the Kalbfleisch and Prentice estimate) and 5.12 (identical to the Efron estimate), respectively.

7.6 Efficiency Comparisons Using Simulations

Mehrotra and Roth [2] quantified the efficiency advantages of GLR relative to the Cox model using simulated time-to-event trials of 10 to 100 per group, with both censored and uncensored untied event times. Their simulations revealed that the estimators of $\beta = \ln(\theta)$ based on the GLR and Cox methods have similar biases (if any); both are essentially unbiased when β is zero, and both have small absolute

TABLE 7.6:   Mean squared errors (MSEs) and relative efficiencies (RE); K and P = Kalbfleisch and Prentice [3] method; %RE = $100 \times (MSE_{K \text{ and } P}/MSE_{GLR^{KP}})$; and 2000 simulations.

N/Group	$\beta = \ln(\theta)$	No Censoring			50% Censoring		
		K and P	GLR^{KP}	%RE	K and P	GLR^{KP}	%RE
20	0.0	.131	.110	120	.231	.202	114
	1.6	.210	.168	125	.351	.265	132
40	0.0	.055	.049	112	.111	.104	107
	1.6	.092	.081	114	.151	.135	112
100	0.0	.021	.020	106	.042	.041	103
	1.6	.035	.033	105	.054	.052	105

percent biases (typically <5%) for nonzero β. However, in every case studied, the relative efficiency (RE) based on MSEs, computed as %RE = $100 \times (MSE_{Cox}/MSE_{GLR})$, was greater than 100%, ranging from 103% to 146%.

Table 7.6 shows the efficiency of the GLR^{KP} estimator relative to the estimator based on Kalbfleisch and Prentice [3] in simulations with tied events times; results were very similar for the analogous comparison of GLR^E versus Efron [4] and are omitted for brevity. To generate ties, continuous survival times were simulated as described in Mehrotra and Roth [2] and then rounded to the nearest 0.10, which is approximately equivalent to rounding to the nearest month when the mean trial time is a year. The simulations studied each of the 24 possible cases obtainable by selecting one of four values for β (0, 0.6, 1.2, or 1.6), one of three values for N, the number of subjects per group (20, 40, or 100), and one of two levels of censoring (none or 50%).

The simulation results for the cases where β is 0 or 1.6 are summarized in Table 7.6. They reveal that β can be estimated with a consistently smaller MSE using GLR^{KP} than with the Kalbfleisch and Prentice [3] method, notably so for small trials, with RE ranging from 103% to 132%. The bias is approximately zero for both methods when $\beta = 0$, and the absolute percent bias for $\beta \in [0.6, 1.2, 1.6]$ ranges from 0.1% to 6.7% for the Kalbfleisch and Prentice [3] method and from 0.7% to 5.2% for GLR^{KP}.

7.7   Concluding Remarks

The GLR, GLR^{KP}, and GLR^E methods for relative risk estimation and inference discussed in this chapter are more efficient than their counterparts based on the Cox model; the gains in efficiency are quite remarkable for trials with up to 100 subjects per group. Further gains in efficiency are possible based on better estimation of the nuisance parameters discussed in Section 7.4 and by not invoking the approximation $1 - e^{-p_i} \approx p_i$ noted immediately below Equation 7.24. Research on such enhancements is ongoing.

Note that we have discussed only the case of a single binary covariate, namely a treatment indicator. However, extensions to trials with categorical covariates (e.g., stratified trials) can be easily derived using a conceptually similar framework. A SAS program to implement the GLR, GLR^{KP}, and GLR^E methods is available upon request from the first author.

References

[1] Cox, D. R. 1972: Regression models and life-tables (with discussion). *Journal of the Royal Statistical Society; Series B*; 34:187–220.

[2] Mehrotra, D. V. and Roth, A. J. 2001: Relative risk estimation and inference using a generalized logrank statistic. *Statistics in Medicine*; 20:2099–2113.

[3] Kalbfleisch, J. D. and Prentice, R. L. 1973: Marginal likelihood based on Cox's regression and life model. *Biometrika*; 60:267–278.

[4] Efron, B. 1977: Efficiency of Cox's likelihood function for censored data. *Journal of the American Statistical Association*; 72:557–565.

[5] Mantel, N. 1966: Evaluation of survival data and two new rank order statistics arising in its consideration. *Cancer Chemotherapy Reports*; 50:163–170.

[6] Tsiatis, A. A. 1981: A large sample study of Cox's regression model. *Annals of Statistics*; 9:93–108.

[7] Andersen, P. K. and Gill, R. D. 1982: Cox's regression model for counting processes: A large sample approach. *Annals of Statistics*; 10:1100–1120.

[8] Breslow, N. E. 1974: Covariance analysis of censored survival data. *Biometrics*; 30:89–99.

[9] Hertz-Picciotto, I. and Rockhill, B. 1997: Validity and efficiency of approximation methods for tied survival times in Cox regression. *Biometrics*; 53:1151–1156.

[10] DeLong, D. M., Guirguis, G. H., and So, Y. C. 1994: Efficient computation of subset selection probabilities with application to Cox regression. *Biometrika*; 81:607–611.

[11] Parmar, M. K. B. and Machin, D. 1995: *Survival Analysis: A Practical Approach*. John Wiley & Sons: Chichester.

Chapter 8

Estimation and Testing for Change in Hazard for Time-to-Event Endpoints

Rafia Bhore and Mohammad Huque

Contents

8.1   Introduction

A new treatment in a patient population may decrease or escalate the risk of one or more serious adverse events (SAEs) over time. Escalation of such a risk in particular is very important to detect as quickly as possible for the patients' safety sake. Risk may remain constant over a relatively short period of time but then suddenly it may start to take a wrong turn, that is, start to escalate over time. On the other hand, a new effective treatment may completely stop or decrease the progression of a serious disease, such as cancer, over time. Such a drug can be a lifesaver for many patients. In drug development it is important to learn about such treatment-related benefits and harm that are time dependent. This is usually best understood through randomized controlled clinical trials (RCTs). RCTs invariably collect efficacy and safety information on treatments under study through the so-called time-to-event endpoints. A time-to-event endpoint is a measurement of time for an event from the start of the treatment until the time that event occurs while the patient is in the clinical trial. Some examples

TABLE 8.1:   Examples of time-to-event endpoints with changes in hazard.

Reference	Time-to-Event Endpoint	Risk	Time Point(s) of Change in Risk
[1,2]	Thrombotic cardiovascular event(s)	Increases	8 months, 18 months
[3,4]	Invasive breast cancer	Increases	4 years, 6 to 7 years
[5]	Increase in serum creatinine, hypophosphatemia	Increases	48 weeks
[6]	Neuropathy	Increases	6 months
[7]	Pericardial effusion (cardiac toxicity)	Decreases	18 months
[8,9]	Cessation of pain	Decreases	24 days, 110 days
[10]	Survival in small cell lung cancer	Decreases	2 years

of time-to-event endpoints on this topic are summarized in Table 8.1 and discussed in detail below.

An example of a safety time-to-event endpoint is the thrombotic cardiovascular event endpoint which can be the first occurrence of any one of the events of myocardial infarction, unstable angina, cardiac thrombus, resuscitated cardiac arrest, sudden or unexplained death, ischemic stroke, or transient ischemic attacks. The vioxx gastrointestinal outcomes research (VIGOR) trial [1], a clinical trial evaluating Vioxx^{TM} (rofecoxib) in arthritis patients, raised the issue that the use of this drug may escalate the risk of such a safety event over time. In this case, the safety event is a composite of several related cardiovascular events. The adenomatous polyp prevention on vioxx (APPROVe) trial [2], a second clinical trial evaluating rofecoxib in colorectal polyp prevention confirmed that the risk of cardiovascular events escalates over time. Another example of a safety time-to-event endpoint is invasive breast cancer, found in a landmark clinical study by the Women's Health Initiative designed to clarify the risks and benefits of combination hormone replacement therapy of estrogen plus progestin [3]. This study was originally designed to evaluate the treatment benefits of prevention of coronary heart disease over a period of 8.5 years. However, the study was stopped prematurely in May 2002 after mean follow-up of 5.2 years because the study data showed that postmenopausal women receiving combined estrogen plus progestin had an increased risk of invasive breast cancer compared with placebo. Some argue that the critical points where this risk increases is around 4 years after treatment and again around 6–7 years after treatment [4].

In many clinical trials, safety events are not observable directly for several reasons; the length of follow-up in a trial is relatively short, the sample size too small, or the event is rare enough to be observed in the planned sample of the clinical trial. Often RCTs make conclusions about the safety of new treatments based on clinical judgments and by indirect means given the limited number of exposed patients in clinical trials.

Signals of a potentially serious adverse event (SAE) may be detected through biochemical markers such as abnormal elevations in laboratory tests. An example in this regard is the safety event of renal toxicity which can be detected through abnormalities in serum creatinine levels and serum phosphate levels. A randomized placebo-controlled clinical trial evaluating adefovir dipivoxil at a high dose of 120 mg for treatment of HIV infection showed that after 24 weeks of adefovir 120 mg treatment there was an increasing incidence of toxicity to the kidneys manifested by elevations in serum creatinine levels and by decrease in phosphorus levels called hypophosphatemia [5]. Survival analysis of time to increase in serum creatinine from baseline greater than 0.5 mg/dL indicated that this event can be expected in 35% of patients at 48 weeks and in 50% of patients at 72 weeks. Similar increase in risk over time was observed for time to phosphate level reduction endpoint. The potential for renal toxicity at high doses resulted in a nonapproval by the FDA for use of adefovir in treatment of HIV infection.

The biologic derivatives of thalidomide, a once banned drug in the United States, are now indicated for treatment for multiple myeloma, a type of cancer. One of thalidomide's major toxicities is neuropathy which limits the ability to continue longer treatment. A clinical study evaluating the relationship between the time course of occurrence of neuropathy and the length of treatment with thalidomide in patients with multiple myeloma, reported that the risk of peripheral neuropathy escalated from 38% at 6 months to 73% at 12 months [6]. A final example of a safety event is the risk of radiation injury when treating cancer. Radiation therapy is routinely used and is beneficial in combination with chemotherapy for treatment of many types of cancers. However, radiation therapy for treatment of malignant tumors in the thoracic region can put adjacent healthy organs such as the heart at risk. A study evaluating the time to cardiac toxicity in patients with esophageal cancer found that after radiation therapy ended, patients were at initially high risk of pericardial effusion (a cardiac toxicity) [7]. The rate of patients with this toxicity increased rapidly to 48% in the first 18 months after radiation therapy ended. After 18 months the risk leveled off.

An example of a time-to-event efficacy endpoint is time-to-cessation of pain associated with herpes zoster (commonly known as shingles), a viral disease characterized by painful skin rash with blisters. Although the rash heals in 2–4 weeks, acute pain may be followed by chronic pain known as postherpetic neuralgia (PHN) which could persist for months. To evaluate the effect of a treatment to alleviate zoster-associated pain, it was important to determine the transition times for each phase of pain and whether the rates of pain resolution remain constant or change over the phases. In an analysis of two clinical trials evaluating efficacy of antiviral therapy with acyclovir and valacyclovir it was estimated that the transition time from acute pain phase to subacute pain phase was 24 days and from subacute phase to chronic pain phase was 110 days [8,9]. In the acute phase of pain, the rate of pain cessation/ day with antiviral therapy was rapid and the rate decreased in the subsequent phases over time.

In another example of a efficacy endpoint, long-term survival was of great interest in the treatment of small cell lung cancer (SCLC). A literature review reported that the definition of long-term survival varied from 18 months to greater than 5 years [10]. Upon further examination of the survival data on 2196 patients in six randomized clinical trials, the review reported a hazard of 0.0035 during the first 2 years from randomization, followed by a transitional period, and a subsequently reduced hazard of 0.00035 from 3 year onward. It was suggested that 3 years should be adopted as the standard definition of long-term survival in SCLC.

These and many other examples indicate that statistical methodology of modeling the hazard function can be effectively used for understanding treatment-related efficacy and safety phenomena that are time dependent. The hazard function (also known as hazard rate) is a fundamental statistical concept. It is a frequently used function for modeling and evaluating the time course of events. The hazard function is a function of time, t, and is defined as the instantaneous risk of an event occurring in a small time interval after time t, given that the patient has not experienced that event ("survived") until time t. In traditional survival analysis, hazard simply defines the risk of dying in the next instant of time where the event of interest is death. In clinical trials, events do not necessarily have to be death, but may be other safety events such as occurrence of a SAE or occurrence of less serious laboratory abnormalities that may signal a serious event later. The hazard function, $h(t)$, equals minus the derivative of the natural logarithm of $S(t)$ with respect to time t, i.e., $h(t) = -\mathrm{d}\log S(t)/\mathrm{d}t$, where $S(t)$ is the survivor function. $S(t)$ is the probability of time-to-event being greater than t, i.e., $S(t) = \Pr(T > t)$. For time-to-event analysis, one usually works with the survivor function. Then the ordinary distribution function is $F(t) = \Pr(T \leq t) = 1 - S(t)$, and the density function is $f(t) = \mathrm{d}F(t)/\mathrm{d}t = -\mathrm{d}S(t)/\mathrm{d}t$. Interrelations between these functions are discussed in Section 8.3.

Time-to-event safety endpoints could be time to cardiovascular event, time to breast cancer, time to increase from baseline in liver function tests such as alanine transaminase (ALT) greater than three times upper limit normal, or time to increase in serum creatinine levels from baseline above a threshold. Time-to-event efficacy endpoints, for example, may be time to onset of response, time to relapse after remission, time to cessation of pain, and many more depending on the disease being treated. Thus an event of interest is always based on what is clinically meaningful for a given situation, but it can be mathematically defined to match clinical specifications.

An important goal of clinical researchers is to find whether the risk of an event remains constant, increases, or decreases over time after long-term exposure to treatment. Second, if the risk/benefit of a treatment does change abruptly over time then where does the change occur? The former problem relates to whether the hazard rate remains constant, increases, or decreases over time. All of the examples above illustrated that in clinical trial settings the hazard rate of an event can increase or decrease over time. For the latter problem, the time point at which an abrupt change occurs in the risk/benefit due to a treatment is defined as the "change-point." The hazard function may have one or more change points, or it remains constant. In clinical trials, however, the change-point(s) for an event of clinical interest is generally unknown and must be estimated. Testing for the existence of a change-point(s) and its estimation can be addressed through modeling of the survival data (or hazard function) using change-point methodology.

The goal of this chapter is to discuss methodology for estimation and testing of changes in hazard (function) with regard to its increase, decrease, or remaining constant for a time-to-event endpoint in the context of a single treatment group. In this regard, we have emphasized the piecewise hazard modeling approach. This is a compromise between fitting the simple parametric models and the complete nonparametric models. This is in the interest of gaining more efficiency and robustness for safety analysis.

Section 8.2 provides motivation for addressing the problem of increase in hazard in the context of drug safety evaluation. The same methodology can be applied to time-to-event endpoint data on drug efficacy assessment. Section 8.3 includes a statistical definition of the change point problem, in particular, based on semiparametric survival models. Section 8.4 is an overview of relevant change-points inferential methods. Sections 8.5.4 and 8.5.5 summarize methods for estimation, and testing of change in hazard along with goodness-of-fit of the model selected using the likelihood ratio test (LRT), respectively. Finally, Section 8.6 includes some discussion.

8.2   Escalation of Hazard in Drug Safety Evaluation

The motivation for the change point problem in the context of time-to-event endpoints comes from Robert O'Neill, CDER, FDA. In his book chapter, O'Neill [11] describes approaches for the assessment of safety of a drug product during its development and marketing stages with emphasis on statistical considerations for planning, analysis, and interpretation. He discusses considerations related to clinical trials (both controlled and uncontrolled) as well as for observational studies necessary for postmarketing surveillance of drug safety.

O'Neill observes that the assessment and characterization of drug safety in clinical trials has not received the same level of attention nor reached the same level of sophistication as the assessment of efficacy. He argues that even though medical literature has improved, for the most part it has been a sporadic and heterogenous improvement characterized by confusion in the way adverse event rates are reported and compared. Clinical trials have often used descriptive statistics such as crude proportions, while epidemiologic studies including cohort and case-control studies have used more sophisticated measures such as average occurrences per unit time and rate ratios (e.g., relative risk or odds ratios) to characterize adverse event rates.

The appropriateness of the statistical measures for estimating adverse event rates depends on (1) whether the disease being treated is *acute* or *chronic*, (2) the *type* of adverse events, and (3) the *pattern* of adverse events. Types of adverse events can be of two kinds: (1) either of *serious* nature causing withdrawal of a patient from treatment, hospitalization, and sometimes death, or (2) of *less serious* type such as nausea, headache, dry mouth, or constipation. These two types of adverse events may depend on the dose, duration of drug exposure, preexisting conditions of the subject, or presence of concomitant medications. As illustrated by O'Neill (in a presentation; 1988) in Figure 8.1, patterns of adverse events may be of three kinds: (1) in pattern 1, most of the adverse events are *acute* and occur early; (2) in pattern 2, the adverse events are spread out, occurring at a *constant* rate over the entire period of follow-up; and (3) in pattern 3, most of the events occur after a *delay*, with increased duration of exposure.

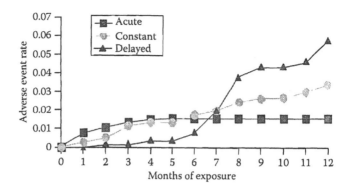

FIGURE 8.1:   Cumulative adverse event rates for three patterns of adverse event occurrence. (From O'Neill, R.T., Assessment of safety, in Peace, K.E., editor, *Biopharmaceutical Statistics for Drug Development*, Marcel Dekker Inc., New York, 543–604, 1988.)

The patterns of adverse events may also depend on the drug, disease treated, and use of the drug. For example, an acute event may be anaphylactic-type reaction to an anti-inflammatory drug occurring soon after drug exposure, a constant event may be headache, and a delayed event may be rhabdomyolysis and kidney failure occurring after increased duration of exposure to cerivastatin, a cholesterol-lowering drug. Many adverse events observed in clinical studies and postmarketing studies occur in patients who remain under treatment and thus are at risk for subsequent adverse events of the same or different type (serious or less serious). Certain mild adverse events occuring early may predict more SAEs later on (delayed pattern). Of particular interest is the role of time and duration of drug exposure in the estimation of adverse event rates. In this section, the events of interest are adverse events of serious type that occur with a delayed pattern. Such events will be underestimated if crude proportions are used instead of measures that account for time-dependency of the pattern.

Given the variety of scenarios for occurrences of adverse events, it is important to take into account above considerations in deciding which measure should be used to convey risk. O'Neill [11] reports that the following four measures have been used to estimate rates of occurrence of adverse events.

1. The *crude incidence rate* $R = X/N$ is the proportion of patients with an adverse event which is defined as the number of patients X experiencing a certain event, divided by the number of patients N initially exposed to the drug, regardless of the duration of drug use. The crude rate is based on a binary (Yes/No) variable. It is frequently used in medical literature because of its simplicity. However, it is misused for both short-term and long-term exposure with different time-dependent patterns. This measure is most appropriate to describe adverse events occurring with short-term drug use, or when all

patients are treated and followed for the same period of time, or when there is an acute pattern of events that occur close in time after exposure.

2. *Occurrences per unit time of exposure* could be defined in many ways, e.g., as average number of events per 100 patient-years, or number of events divided by number of prescriptions, etc. The denominator could be an unit of either time of exposure, or of number of prescriptions, or another surrogate of total exposure time.

   Such a measure assumes that the risk per unit of time exposed is constant during the entire period of treatment exposure and it is the same for each patient or subject. For example, a patient's risk in the first month of exposure is assumed to be the same as the risk in the ninth month of exposure, given that the patient is unaffected through month 8.

3. The *cumulative life table rate, H(t)*, at a given time t is calculated using the actuarial life table method [12,13]. This is one of the oldest methods for analyzing survival (failure time) data. It was popularized by demographers and actuaries to study the longevity of human populations. Actuarial life table is a preferred method when sample sizes and number of events is quite large, compared with the classic Kaplan–Meier product-limit method which can get lengthy.

   To compute the cumulative life table rate for estimating incidence of adverse events, the time interval of total drug exposure is divided into k nonoverlapping subintervals $[0 = \tau_0, \tau_1), [\tau_1, \tau_2), \ldots, [\tau_{k-1}, \tau_k)$. The intervals are almost always, but not necessarily, of equal lengths, for example, 1 month, 3 months, 6 months, or 1 year. Cumulative life table rate is then estimated as the cumulative sum across intervals of the number of events in a given interval divided by the effective sample size for that interval. The effective sample size for an interval is the effective number of patients at risk of experiencing an event in that interval. Using Klein and Moeschberger's [13] notation, we can formulate the cumulative life table rate as

$$\hat{H}(t) = \sum_{i=1}^{j} \frac{d_i}{\left(Y_i' - \frac{W_i}{2}\right)}, \quad \tau_{j-1} \le t < \tau_j, \quad j = 1, \ldots, k,$$

where
   d_i is the number of patients who experienced an event in the ith interval $[\tau_{i-1}, \tau_i)$,
   Y_i' is the number of patients entering the ith interval who have not yet experienced an event,
   W_i is the number of patients censored in that interval, and
   $Y_i = Y_i' - \frac{W_i}{2}$ is the effective sample size.

The life table method assumes that the censoring times are uniformly distributed over the interval. If the number of patients at risk at time went from Y_i' at time τ_{i-1} to $Y_i' - W_i$ at time τ_i, then it is reasonable to assume that the number at risk during the interval $[\tau_{i-1}, \tau_i)$ is the average of these two values (thus the division of W_i by 2) [12]. $Y_i = Y_i' - \frac{W_i}{2}$ is therefore known as the effective sample size.

Confidence intervals for the cumulative hazard rate can be obtained by taking minus the natural logarithm of the confidence intervals for the survival function, $S(t)$ [13]. The 95% confidence intervals for the survival function given by Kalbfleisch and Prentice [14] ensure that the limits are within $(0, 1)$ and are given by

$$\left(\hat{S}(t)^{\exp[1.96\hat{s}(t)]}, \hat{S}(t)^{\exp[-1.96\hat{s}(t)]}\right), \quad \tau_{j-1} \leq t < \tau_j, \quad j = 1, \ldots, k.$$

Here $\hat{s}(t) = \widehat{var}[\log \hat{S}(t)]/[\log \hat{S}(t)]^2$ is the standard error of $\hat{S}(t)$ and $\widehat{var}[\log \hat{S}(t)]$ is obtained from Greenwood's formula. For the life table method, the estimates of the survival function, $\hat{S}(t)$, and $\widehat{var}[\log \hat{S}(t)]$ are given below [13,14].

$$\hat{S}(t) = \prod_{i=1}^{j} \left(1 - \frac{d_i}{Y_i}\right) \quad \text{and}$$

$$\widehat{var}[\log \hat{S}(t)] = \sum_{i=1}^{j} \frac{d_i}{Y_i(Y_i - d_i)} \quad \text{for } \tau_{j-1} \leq t < \tau_j, \quad j = 1, \ldots, k.$$

Therefore, the 95% confidence limits of the cumulative hazard rate are

$$\left(-\log\{\hat{S}(t)^{\exp[-1.96\hat{s}(t)]}\}, -\log\{\hat{S}(t)^{\exp[1.96\hat{s}(t)]}\}\right).$$

Note that although it is convenient to think of cumulative hazard rate as a probability, it is not really a probability as it can exceed 1.0 because of the division by the time interval length.

Because the exact time of occurrence of adverse events is not always known, the life table method can be useful as it allows grouping of events and subjects at risk within intervals of time, e.g., 3 month intervals, 6 month intervals, etc. The cumulative rate can account for differential duration of drug exposure among an exposed group of patients as well as the time pattern of when, during exposure, the events occur relative to the number of patients at risk.

Unlike the measure of occurrences per unit time, cumulative life table rate also accounts for censored data.

O'Neill [11] illustrates how a crude rate (crude proportion) unadjusted for time of exposure can grossly underestimate the adverse event rate as compared to using the cumulative life table rate measure.

4. The *hazard rate*, $h(t)$, is a measure that is also conditional on the the time of exposure (similar to cumulative rate). Hazard rate is intended to quantify the instantaneous risk that an adverse event will occur in a small but specified interval after time t, conditioned on the fact that the patient has not had an event (i.e., survived) until time t. The condition is imposed because if the patient has already had an event, then they are clearly no longer at risk of that event. Hazard rate also known as *hazard function* is defined as

$$h(t) = \lim_{\Delta t \to 0} \frac{\Pr(t \le T < t + \Delta t | T \ge t)}{\Delta t},$$

where

T is the random variable for the event time and

Δt is a small increment in time.

Note that hazard rate is not really a probability because it can be greater than 1.0, just as cumulative rate can be.

In pattern 1 discussed above, where adverse events occur early in the exposure interval, the hazard rate is decreasing; in pattern 2, where the adverse events are spread out, the hazard rate is constant; and in pattern 3, where the adverse events occur after a delay in exposure, the hazard rate is increasing. Thus, the hazard rate may decrease, remain constant, or increase, or follow more complex patterns. The measure average occurrences per unit time assumes that the hazard rate is constant. Hazard rate measures the risk of an adverse event per unit of time over the duration of exposure and it complements the cumulative rate which is always a nondecreasing function of time. Cumulative rate is related to hazard rate through the relationship $H(t) = \int_0^t h(t)dt$ for continuous data or $H(t) = \sum_{t_i \le t} h(t)$ for discrete data.

For time-to-event data, the hazard rate or hazard function is the most popular way of describing the distribution of a time-to-event variable. A popular method for estimating the survival function and cumulative hazard function is the Kaplan–Meier method [15] which is now considered the classic in survival analysis.

8.3 Change Point Problem

Let $T_1, \ldots, T_n$ be independent and identically distributed (*iid*) event times with distribution function F, for n patients in a clinical trial. Also let $C_1, \ldots, C_n$ be *iid* with distribution G, where C_i is the censoring time associated with T_i. We can only observe the pairs (Y_i, δ_i), $i = 1, \ldots, n$ where

$$Y_i = \min(T_i, C_i) = T_i \wedge C_i \quad \text{and}$$

$$\delta_i = I(T_i \le C_i) = \begin{cases} 1 & \text{if } T_i \le C_i, \text{ that is } T_i \text{ is observed,} \\ 0 & \text{if } T_i > C_i, \text{ that is } T_i \text{ is censored.} \end{cases}$$

In clinical trials, the type of censoring is assumed to be random censoring, due to different patient entry times and different times of drop-outs. Under random censoring it is often assumed that T_i and C_i are independent, although this is not always the case, for example, if the reason for dropping out is related to the course of treatment, there may well be dependence between T_i and C_i.

The probability distribution of the random variable T can be specified in several ways; three of which are commonly used in survival applications: the survival function $S(t)$, the probability density function $f(t)$, and the hazard function $h(t)$. Interrelations between the functions can be described in many ways as follows:

$$S(t) = \Pr(T > t) = 1 - F(t) = \int_t^\infty f(u)du, \tag{8.1a}$$

$$f(t) = \frac{dF(t)}{dt} = F'(t) = -\frac{dS(t)}{dt} = -S'(t), \quad \text{and} \tag{8.1b}$$

$$h(t) = \frac{f(t)}{1 - F(t)} = \frac{f(t)}{S(t)} = \frac{-S'(t)}{S(t)} = -\frac{d \log S(t)}{dt}, \tag{8.1c}$$

which implies

$$S(t) = \exp\left(-\int_0^t h(u)du\right) = \exp[-H(t)] \quad \text{and} \tag{8.2a}$$

$$f(t) = h(t) \cdot S(t) = h(t) \cdot \exp\left(-\int_0^t h(u)du\right). \tag{8.2b}$$

A change-point is defined as the time point when a change in hazard occurs. In clinical trials, for example, the risk of a delayed SAE may increase after long-term exposure to a drug. In this case, the hazard rate is low initially and the hazard rate rapidly increases after some time. Similarly, the efficacy of a drug may show improvement in a disease condition after the treatment is in place for some time. In this case, the hazard rate of the disease condition may be high initially and the hazard rate declines after some time. Then, the change point problem is to make inference of where the change in hazard occurs, that is estimation and testing for change-point(s), and estimate the magnitude of change in hazard rate. To address this problem, often one assumes the following simple change-point model of the hazard function [16,17].

$$h(t) = \begin{cases} \lambda_1, & t \leq \tau, \\ \lambda_2, & t > \tau. \end{cases}$$

In this model, the hazard rate is assumed to be piecewise constant, i.e., constant hazard rate λ_1, until the jump occurs at the change-point, τ, and then the hazard rate changes to λ_2. Assuming a parametric model of the hazard function, the change point problem is to estimate the change point τ, and also estimate the hazard rates λ_1 and λ_2 before and after the time point of change.

8.4   Review of Change-Point Methods for Hazard Functions

The problem of change in distribution of a response variable at an unknown time point has been studied extensively in the area of statistical quality control. However, a related problem of assessing change in the hazard function for evaluating risk/benefit of a treatment over time is new to clinical trials. Published literature on change-points in a hazard function—which may occur in medical follow up studies—is emerging since the 1980s. Müller and Wang [18] give a nice overview of literature through 1994 on inferential methods for parametric models with change-points in hazard function. They also discuss their proposed nonparametric model of a kernel smoothing technique for change-point estimation and estimation of the hazard function. Since 1994, additional relevant literature on change point methodology for hazard functions has emerged. Most of the published work, with some exceptions, developed theory for the case of observed data without censoring. Completely observed time to event endpoints with no censoring is rarely the case in clinical trials. In the published applications, the censored observations were either discarded or were included in the likelihood function.

Although change point methodology could be useful and should be a commonly used tool to check for changes in hazard over time—for example, in many clinical trials submitted in New Drug Applications—these methods are not programmed for routine application to clinical data due to their mathematical complexity. Also, no systematic comparisons and recommendations of the relevant inferential methods have been made. For the purpose of application to clinical studies, the most relevant literature reviewed in this chapter are methods that discuss inference (including estimation, hypothesis testing, and properties of the estimators) on change points for hazard functions.

Matthews and Farewell [16] were the first to proposed a hypothesis test for survival data to determine whether hazard rate has changed. This was motivated by the survival analysis of a study in leukemia patients where the endpoint was *time-to-relapse after remission induction*. Physicians were interested in knowing whether a constant relapse rate is evident for some period after induction, but subsequently a reduction in relapse rate (i.e., change in hazard) occurs with the new treatment. The time point at which a reduction in the relapse rate occurs will be the change point. Assuming the following change point model for the hazard function,

$$h(t) = \begin{cases} \lambda_1, & t \leq \tau, \\ \rho\lambda_1, & t > \tau, \end{cases} \tag{8.3a}$$

which can be reparametrized as

$$h(t) = \begin{cases} \lambda_1, & t \leq \tau, \\ \lambda_2, & t > \tau, \end{cases} \quad \text{where } \lambda_2 = \rho\lambda_1. \tag{8.3b}$$

Matthews and Farewell proposed a LRT to determine the existence of a change point, τ, by comparing the null hypothesis of a simple exponential survival model (hazard rate is constant, i.e., $H_0 : \lambda_1 = \rho\lambda_1$ or $(\rho = 1, \tau = 0)$ versus the alternative hypothesis of a 2-piece PWE model (hazard rates are different before and after change point, i.e., $H_1 : \lambda_1 \neq \rho\lambda_1$, or $(\rho \neq 1, \tau > 0)$). Under the alternative hypothesis H_1, the likelihood function has a discontinuity at the change point, τ, due to which standard asymptotic likelihood inference on parameters is not possible. Therefore,

Matthews and Farewell showed that maximum likelihood estimates (MLEs) $\hat{\lambda}_1$, $\hat{\rho}$, and $\hat{\tau}$ of the parameters can be estimated by a direct search of the log-likelihood function $\log L(\lambda_1, \rho, \tau)$. However, they did not develop standard errors or confidence limits of the change point estimate, $\hat{\tau}$. Furthermore, through simulations they showed that the log-likelihood ratio (LLR) statistic for testing the existence of a change point, τ, given by

$$\text{LLR} = 2\{\log L(\hat{\lambda}_1, \hat{\rho}, \hat{\tau}) - \log L'(\hat{\lambda}, \hat{\lambda}, 0)\}, \tag{8.4}$$

where L and L' are the log-likelihood functions for 2-piece and simple exponentials, respectively, has approximately the same upper tails as the chi-square distribution with two degrees of freedom, χ_2^2. Significance levels for the LRT were obtained through simulations by comparing the percentiles of the distribution of the LLR statistic to the percentiles of the χ_2^2 distribution. Matthews and Farewell also compared, through simulation, the power of the LRT to the score tests based on Weibull or log gamma alternatives and showed that the LRT is generally as good as or better than the score tests in distinguishing between constant and nonconstant hazard. Note that the hypothesis test proposed above is only based on observable failure times and hence in the application data on leukemia, Matthews and Farewell dropped the 24 censored observations and analyzed the data for only 60 observed times.

Matthews, Farewell, and Pyke [19] continued their previous work with the piecewise exponential change point model and developed a score test to test the alternative hypothesis of the existence of a change point. They considered a variant of the three parameter model in Equation 8.3a by reparametrizing (λ_1, ρ, τ) with (λ, ξ, τ) where $\lambda_1 = \lambda$, and $\rho = 1 - \xi$ as follows

$$h(t) = \begin{cases} \lambda, & 0 \le t < \tau, \\ (1 - \xi)\lambda, & t \ge \tau, \end{cases}$$

and testing the hypotheses $H_0 : \xi = 0$ versus $H_1 : 0 < \xi < 1$. Let $\log L(\lambda, \xi, \tau)$ denote the log-likelihood function. The normalized score statistic for a given τ and λ is given by

$$Z_n(\tau, \lambda) = \frac{\partial \log L/\partial \xi}{[E(-\partial^2 \log L/\partial \xi^2)]^{1/2}} \bigg|_{\xi=0}$$

$$= n^{-1/2} \sum_{i=1}^{n} e^{\lambda \tau/2} [(T_i - \tau)\lambda - 1] I(T_i \ge \tau).$$

If τ is restricted to an interval $[0, b]$, $b < \infty$, Matthews et al. proved that for a given λ the score statistic process $\{Z_n(\tau, \lambda) : 0 \le \tau \le b\}$ converges weakly under the null hypothesis to an Ornstein–Uhlenbeck (O-U) process $\{Z(\tau, \lambda) : 0 \le \tau \le b\}$ with mean 0 and covariance $\exp\{-\frac{1}{2}\lambda|\tau_1 - \tau_2|\}$ which is a Brownian motion process normalized to constant variance 1. Then a suitable test for H_0 is one which rejects large values of statistics of the form $M_n(a, b, \lambda) := \sup_{a \leq \tau \leq b} Z_n(\tau, \lambda)$ which asymptotically tends to $M(a, b, \lambda) = \sup_{a \leq \tau \leq b} Z(\tau, \lambda)$ as $n \to \infty$. For some $c > 0$, reject H_0 if $M(a, b, \lambda) \geq c$ or equivalently if $T(c \cdot \lambda) \leq b - a$, where $T(c, \lambda) = \inf\{\tau \geq a : Z(\tau) \geq c\}$ is the first passage time of the O-U process. The asymptotic significance level is $\Pr\{M(a, b, \lambda) \geq c\} = \Pr\{T(c, \lambda) \leq b - a\}$. Approximates of c are discussed in Refs. [19,18]. Thus, the asymptotic significance level of the score test for no decrease in the hazard rate is shown to be the solution to a first passage time problem for this O-U process.

When λ is unknown, then the normalized score statistic $Z_n(\tau, \lambda)$ is replaced by

$$\hat{Z}_n(\tau) = \frac{\partial l/\partial \xi}{\partial^2 l/\partial \xi^2 - (\partial^2 l/\partial \xi \partial \lambda)^2/(\partial^2 l/\partial \lambda^2)}\bigg|_{\xi=0,\, \lambda=\hat{\lambda}_n}$$
$$= (1 - e^{-\lambda \tau})^{-1/2} Z_n(\tau, \lambda)\big|_{\lambda=\hat{\lambda}_n},$$

where $\hat{\lambda}_n = n/\sum T_i$ is the MLE of λ under the null. Using a transformation, Matthews et al. show that for the case of unknown λ, the test statistic is a Brownian bridge (compared with a Brownian motion for known λ) normalized to have a constant variance and thus asymptotic significance levels for the score test can also be obtained. The weak convergence results of this score test can be unreliable compared with a LRT and their small sample properties can be quite different [17].

Nguyen, Rogers, and Walker [20] noted that the likelihood function for change-point model in Equation 8.3b is unbounded and therefore the global maximum likelihood estimator does not exist, except when $\lambda_1 \geq \lambda_2$. When $\lambda_1 \geq \lambda_2$, the MLEs for λ_1, λ_2, and τ can be computed using the numerical algorithm of Matthews and Farewell. Otherwise, they proposed a consistent but pseudo-MLE of τ. First the MLEs, $\hat{\lambda}_1$ and $\hat{\lambda}_2$ are obtained for a fixed τ. Nguyen, Rogers, and Walker (NRW) proved that the alternative estimator $\hat{\tau} = \arg\max_{a \leq \tau \leq b} \log L(\hat{\lambda}_1, \hat{\lambda}_2, \tau)$, obtained by maximizing the log-likelihood over a restricted interval $[a, b]$ is consistent. However, they do not derive its distribution. Basu, Ghosh, and Joshi 1988 [21] provided alternative estimators of τ and also derived the asymptotic distribution of NRW estimate of τ.

Yao [22] derived restricted maximum likelihood estimators of τ, λ_1, and λ_2 and studied their distribution theory. In particular, Yao used $a = 0$ and $b = T_{(n-1)}$, and showed that the estimator $\hat{\tau}$ that maximizes $\log L(\lambda_1, \lambda_2, \tau)$ under the restriction $\tau \leq T_{(n-1)}$, is a consistent estimator. Here λ_1, and λ_2 for a fixed τ are

$$\lambda_1 = \frac{R}{\sum_{i=1}^{R} T_{(i)} + (n - R)\tau} \quad \text{and} \quad \lambda_2 = \frac{n - R}{\sum_{i=R+1}^{n} [T_{(i)} - \tau]},$$

where $R := R(\tau) = $ the number of $T_i \leq \tau := \sum_{i=1}^{n} I(T_i \leq \tau)$, that is number of events observed up to time τ. The MLEs $\hat{\lambda}_1$ and $\hat{\lambda}_2$ are obtained by substituting R with $\hat{R} = R(\hat{\tau})$. Pham and Nguyen [23] proved the strong consistency of the estimator $\hat{\tau}$ from which strong consistency of $\hat{\lambda}_1$ and $\hat{\lambda}_2$ follows. Both Yao, and Pham, and Nguyen derived the limiting distributions of these estimators.

Loader's [17] was an important inferential paper on change point because it addressed hypothesis testing as well as estimation of the change point. He further explored the Matthews and Farewell change-point model with or without censoring for the *iid* event times $T_1, \ldots, T_n$, namely,

$$h(t) = \begin{cases} \lambda_1, & 0 \leq t < \tau, \\ \lambda_2, & t \geq \tau, \end{cases} \tag{8.5}$$

where λ_1 and λ_2 are the hazard rates before and after the change point, τ. Using the associated counting process $X(t) = \sum_{i=1}^{n} I(T_i \leq t)$, and its transformation specified by $s(t) = \sum_{i=1}^{n} T_i \wedge t$ and $Y(s) = X(t)$ (Y is shown to be a Poisson process with rate λ_1 if there is no change point), Loader derived a likelihood-ratio test and the corresponding likelihood-ratio based approximate confidence regions for the change point. The LLR statistic for testing $H_0 : \lambda_1 = \lambda_2$ versus $H_0 : \lambda_1 \neq \lambda_2$, is given by

$$\mathrm{LLR} = X(\tau) \ln \left[\frac{X(\tau) \sum T_i}{n \sum (T_i \wedge \tau)} \right] + [n - X(\tau)] \ln \left\{ \frac{[n - X(\tau)] \sum T_i}{n \sum [T_i - (T_i \wedge \tau)]} \right\}.$$

The resulting confidence region of the change point may be a union of disjoint intervals because the underlying log likelihood is not a smooth function and has local peaks at the failure time points. Loader's method does not take into account the nature of the likelihood. In addition, Loader derived a joint confidence region for the change point, τ, and the size of the change in hazard measured by $\delta = \log(\lambda_2/\lambda_1)$.

Pham and Nguyuen [24] cautioned against applying bootstrapping naïvely for estimating the change-point. They instead recommend parametric boostrapping for obtaining the distribution of the change-point estimator and showed an estimator obtained through parametric bootstrapping is consistent and hence asymptotically valid. However, ordinary nonparametric bootstrapping is inconsistent. Jeong [25] later developed a parametric bootstrap method to compute confidence intervals for the change point for a Weibull model. Gardner [26] and Bhore and Gardner [27] extended Jeong's work incorporating a secondary level of bootstrapping to obtain percentile type bootstrap confidence intervals for the change point for the Matthews and Farewell model. The bootstrap confidence intervals can be an alternative to Loader's confidence regions. Details of these methods are covered in Sections 8.5.4 and 8.5.5.

Liang, Self, and Liu [28] proposed a semiparametric extension of the Matthews and Farewell change-point model by incorporating covariates. This model can also be viewed as an extension of the Cox-proportional hazards model with a change-point. The model was defined as

$$h(t; Z, \mathbf{x}) = \begin{cases} \lambda_0(t) \exp[(\beta + \theta)Z + \gamma' \mathbf{x}], & t \leq \tau, \\ \lambda_0(t) \exp[\beta Z + \gamma' \mathbf{x}], & t > \tau, \end{cases} \tag{8.6}$$

where
$a \leq \tau \leq b$, τ is the change point with range $[a, b]$ with both a and b known,
Z is a 1×1 scalar, and
$\mathbf{x}$ is a $p \times 1$ vector of covariates that vary from subject to subject.

Z differs from **x** in that the effect of Z on the hazard is time dependent, even though Z itself is not time dependent. The authors were concerned with inference on the parameter estimates of the extended Cox model, namely, β, θ, and γ for a fixed change point, τ, rather than inference on the change point itself. The authors proposed an extension of the score test [19] for the change point for testing $H_0 : \theta = 0$ by computing the maximum value of the Cox partial likelihood score for a fixed and known τ and choosing the largest of those maxima in a direct search over the values of τ. Confidence intervals for β, θ, and γ are computed assuming that the maximizing value of τ is the true one and ignoring the possible variability in the estimate of τ.

Müller and Wang [29] proposed a nonparametric alternative to the piecewise exponential model for analyzing changes in hazard rate. They proposed to detect the point of most rapid change (i.e., inflection point) in a smooth hazard function by finding the zero of the kernel smoothing estimator of the second derivative hazard function. Let H_n be Nelson's empirical estimator of the cumulative hazard function, and let $\hat{h}^{(\nu)}(x) = \frac{1}{b^{\nu+1}} \int K_\nu\left(\frac{x-u}{b}\right) dH_n(u)$ be the kernel estimator of the νth derivative of the hazard function, h, where K_ν is the kernel function and b is the bandwidth. Then $\hat{h}^{(\nu)}(x)$ is an asymptotically normally distributed estimate of $h^{(\nu)}(x)$ and the inflection point or change point, τ, of $h(x)$ is estimated by $\hat{\tau} = $ zero of $\hat{h}^{(2)}(x)$, which an asymptotically normal unbiased estimate of τ. Therefore, asymptotic confidence intervals can be constructed for the point of most rapid change in hazard. Müller and Wang proposed that the nonparametric approach can be used to assess the potential goodness-of-fit of parametric change point modeling as well as to determine whether there is more than one change point. However, a nonparametric approach will require larger sample sizes than a well-fitting parametric model for the purpose of inference.

Qin and Sun [30] explored generalizations of the one change-point model where the hazard function may follow a parametric form before a change point and is nonparametric after the change point. They proposed a maximal LRT statistic for testing existence of a change-point for which the distribution is very hard to find. Hence bootstrapping was used to find the critical values of the test statistic. Chang, Chen, and Hsiung [31] present an estimator of the change point based on a functional of the Nelson–Aalen estimator of the cumulative hazard function. Gijbels and Gürler [32] modified the change-point estimator based on a least squares estimator of the functional of the Nelson–Aalen estimator. The functional can be viewed as the slope (average hazard) of the cumulative hazard function estimator. A change point is estimated when the slope of Nelson–Aalen estimator of the cumulative hazard function changes (increases or decreases). Goodman, Li, and Tiwari [33] assume a piecewise linear model incorporating covariates and developed an asymptotic Wald type test to sequentially test for existence of multiple change points (no change versus one change point, one change point versus two change points, and so on until the appropriate number of change points is identified). The Wald-type statistic needs numerical methods for approximation as it requires differentiation of the log likelihood. Point estimates of the change point(s) can be obtained with this method but confidence intervals cannot be calculated. The authors also give multiple comparison adjustment of Type 1 error for model selection, however, it is not necessary as the testing is sequential whereby a model with fewer parameters has to be rejected before testing for the next higher model with one additional change point.

Additional literature reviewed on the PWE model and change points were by Friedman [34], Kim and Proschan [35], Worsley [36], Karrison [37], and Zelterman et al. [38]; all of which were not concerned with inference on change points.

Friedman, although not concerned with estimation of change points, proved the formal existence and asymptotic uniqueness of the MLEs of the parameters of a PWE model with multiple change points and covariates for individuals. Kim and Proschan's objective was not to identify real change points, rather it was to get a continuous estimator of the survival function and compare it with the Kaplan–Meier estimator. They do not assume a real PWE model with a fixed number of unknown change points to be estimated. Instead, their model assumes the change points to be successive uncensored failure times. Worsley considered a different problem which was not for survival data. They considered time between successive coal mine explosions with the hazard function over calendar time and this does not translate well into time until events for different patients in a clinical trial. Karrison described a way of dividing the time line so that a PWE model with covariates can be fit and median survival times (and confidence intervals) can be estimated. Zelterman et al. studied the 2-piece PWE model in which the two hazard rates, λ_1 and λ_2, are two constants shared by all the subjects but where the change point, τ, is an unobservable random variable, unique to each subject but *iid* from some distribution G across the population. They assume that although the hazard rate may change abruptly at the individual level, there is no abrupt change in the survival function at the population level.

8.5   Change-Point Models for Hazard Function

8.5.1   Piecewise Exponential Model

A commonly used parametric model for failure time data is the one-parameter *exponential* model. The exponential model assumes the hazard function to be constant over the range of t. The hazard function, survival function, and density function of the exponential model, are respectively,

$$
\begin{aligned}
h(t) &= \lambda, & t &\geq 0, \\
S(t) &= \exp(-\lambda t), & t &\geq 0, \\
f(t) &= \lambda \exp(-\lambda t), & t &\geq 0.
\end{aligned}
$$

The 2-piece PWE model is a generalization of the one-parameter exponential model. It is piecewise constant in two intervals of time with two constant hazard rates, λ_1 and λ_2, and one change point, τ. The hazard function for the 2-piece PWE model is defined as

$$h(t) = \begin{cases} \lambda_1, & 0 \le t \le \tau, \\ \lambda_2, & t > \tau. \end{cases} \tag{8.7}$$

In general, a k-piece PWE model will have k constant hazard rates, $\lambda_1, \ldots, \lambda_k$, and $k-1$ change points, $\tau_1, \ldots, \tau_{k-1}$. The hazard function for a k-piece PWE model is defined as

$$h(t) = \begin{cases} \lambda_1, & 0 = \tau_0 \le t \le \tau_1 \\ \lambda_2, & \tau_1 < t \le \tau_2 \\ \vdots & \vdots \\ \lambda_j, & \tau_{j-1} < t \le \tau_j \\ \vdots & \vdots \\ \lambda_k, & t > \tau_{k-1} \end{cases} \tag{8.8}$$

From Equations 8.2a and 8.2b, it follows easily that the survival function and density function for the k-piece PWE model are, respectively,

$$S(t) = \begin{cases} \exp(-\lambda_1 \tau_1), & 0 \le t \le \tau_1 \\ \exp(-\lambda_1 \tau_1 - \lambda_2(t - \tau_1)) & \tau_1 < t \le \tau_2 \\ \vdots & \vdots \\ \exp\left(-\sum_{i=1}^{j-1} \lambda_i(\tau_i - \tau_{i-1}) - \lambda_j(t - \tau_{j-1})\right), & \tau_{j-1} < t \le \tau_j \\ \vdots & \vdots \\ \exp\left(-\sum_{i=1}^{k-1} \lambda_i(\tau_i - \tau_{i-1}) - \lambda_k(t - \tau_{k-1})\right), & t > \tau_{k-1} \end{cases},$$

$$f(t) = \begin{cases} \lambda_1 \exp(-\lambda_1 \tau_1), & 0 \le t \le \tau_1 \\ \lambda_2 \exp(-\lambda_1 \tau_1 - \lambda_2(t - \tau_1)) & \tau_1 < t \le \tau_2 \\ \vdots & \vdots \\ \lambda_j \exp\left(-\sum_{i=1}^{j-1} \lambda_i(\tau_i - \tau_{i-1}) - \lambda_j(t - \tau_{j-1})\right), & \tau_{j-1} < t \le \tau_j \\ \vdots & \vdots \\ \lambda_k \exp\left(-\sum_{i=1}^{k-1} \lambda_i(\tau_i - \tau_{i-1}) - \lambda_k(t - \tau_{k-1})\right), & t > \tau_{k-1} \end{cases}.$$

8.5.2 Piecewise Weibull Model

Leung [39] illustrated through an example of time-to-recurrence data in colon cancer patients that when a change point is present, an exponential distribution alone or Weibull distribution alone does not fit the data. Therefore, piecewise models need to be considered.

In general, consider a piecewise constant hazard function (i.e., change point model) with one change point, τ, such as

$$h(t) = \begin{cases} h_1(t), & 0 \leq t \leq \tau, \\ h_2(t), & \tau < t < \infty. \end{cases}$$

Then it follows from Equations 8.2a and 8.2b that the survival function and density function, respectively, are

$$S(t) = \begin{cases} S_1(t), & 0 \leq t \leq \tau, \\ S_1(\tau)S_2(t - \tau), & \tau < t < \infty, \end{cases} \quad \text{and} \qquad (8.9)$$

$$f(t) = \begin{cases} f_1(t), & 0 \leq t \leq \tau, \\ S_1(\tau)f_2(t - \tau), & \tau < t < \infty. \end{cases} \qquad (8.10)$$

Similar to a 2-piece PWE model, a 2-piece piecewise Weibull model will consist of two separate Weibull models. The first piece will have $h_1(t)$ as the hazard function of a Weibull distribution with first set of parameters and the second piece will have $h_2(t)$ as the hazard function of a Weibull with second set of parameters. In their example data on time-to-recurrence in colon cancer, Leung [39] observed through survival plots and density plots that a change point exists. In the first stage, the density function comprised of a skewed (to the right side) bell-shaped peak and in the second stage, the pattern was random. Hence, Leung [39] proposed a change point model that was a composite of Weibull distribution before the change point, τ, and an exponential distribution after the change point:

$$h(t) = \begin{cases} \alpha\beta(\beta t)^{\alpha-1}, & 0 < t \leq \tau, \\ \lambda, & \tau < t < \infty. \end{cases}$$

Here $\alpha > 0$ is a scale parameter and $\beta > 0$ is a shape parameter of the Weibull distribution which represents the piece before the change point occurs. In the second piece after the change point occurs, the distribution is exponential with constant hazard λ, not necessarily related to either α or β from the first piece. The Weibull distribution is flexible enough to accomodate either increasing hazard ($\alpha > 1$), decreasing hazard ($\alpha < 1$), or constant hazard rate ($\alpha = 1$). It is well known that the exponential distribution is a special case of the Weibull distribution when the scale parameter $\alpha = 1$.

The survival and density functions of such a composite piecewise model can be easily derived from Equation 8.9. However, as described in Section 8.5.3, the hazard function is fully sufficient to derive the log-likelihood function which will be useful for maximum likelihood estimation of the parameters. Hazard functions, survival functions, and density functions of some common parametric models for survival data are nicely tabulated in Klein and Moeschberger [13].

8.5.3 Likelihood Function

Using the notations of Miller [40], Kalbfleisch and Prentice [14], and Cox and Oakes [41] we show how the MLEs of the unknown change point(s) and the hazard rates of a PWE model can be obtained by formulating the likelihood in terms of the hazard function. As noted in Section 8.3, we only observe the data (Y_i, δ_i), $i = 1, \ldots, n$, where Y_i is the observed event time or the censoring time, and δ_i is the indicator of whether an event has occurred or not, respectively, for the ith patient. It is known that the likelihood function for the the ith observation, (Y_i, δ_i), is

$$L(Y_i, \delta_i) = \begin{cases} f(Y_i) & \text{if } \delta_i = 1 \text{ (uncensored)}, \\ S(Y_i) & \text{if } \delta_i = 0 \text{ (censored)}, \end{cases}$$
$$= f(Y_i)^{\delta_i} S(Y_i)^{1-\delta_i}.$$

Actually, under random censoring, the likelihood function for (Y_i, δ_i) and therefore the full sample $(Y_1, \delta_1), \ldots, (Y_n, \delta_n)$ can be written as

$$L(Y_i, \delta_i) = \begin{cases} f(Y_i)[1 - G(Y_i)] & \text{if } \delta_i = 1, \\ g(Y_i)S(Y_i) & \text{if } \delta_i = 0, \end{cases} \quad \text{and}$$

$$L(Y_1, \ldots, Y_n; \delta_1, \ldots, \delta_n) = \left(\prod_u f(Y_i) \right) \left(\prod_c S(Y_i) \right) \left(\prod_c g(Y_i) \right) \left(\prod_u [1 - G(Y_i)] \right),$$

where

    g and G are density and cumulative distribution functions for censored observations only and

    $\prod_u$ and $\prod_c$ denote products over uncensored and censored observations, respectively.

Under the assumption that the censoring time, C_i, is independent of the event time, T_i, the last two products in the likelihood $\prod_c g$ and $\prod_u [1 - G]$, do not involve the unknown lifetime parameters and can be treated as constants when maximizing the likelihood. Therefore, $L(Y_1, \ldots, Y_n; \delta_1, \ldots, \delta_n) \propto \left(\prod_u f(Y_i) \right) \left(\prod_c S(Y_i) \right)$. It is easier to write the likelihood function fully in terms of the hazard function using Equations 8.2a and 8.2b, as follows:

$$L(Y_1, \ldots, Y_n; \delta_1, \ldots, \delta_n) \propto \left(\prod_u f(Y_i) \right) \left(\prod_c S(Y_i) \right)$$

$$= \left(\prod_u h(Y_i) \right) \left(\prod_{i=1}^n S(Y_i) \right)$$

$$= \left(\prod_u h(Y_i) \right) \exp \left(- \sum_{i=1}^n \int_0^{Y_i} h(t)dt \right).$$

For a parametric model of a hazard function, let $\underset{\sim}{\theta} = (\theta_1, \ldots, \theta_p)'$ be the vector of parameters. Then, the likelihood function is expressed as

$$L(\underset{\sim}{\theta}) \propto \prod_u h(Y_i, \underset{\sim}{\theta}) \cdot \exp\left(-\sum_{i=1}^{n} \int_0^{Y_i} h(t, \underset{\sim}{\theta}) \, dt \right). \tag{8.11}$$

Finding the MLE of $\underset{\sim}{\theta}$ is equivalent to finding the solution $\hat{\underset{\sim}{\theta}}$ to the likelihood equations $\frac{\partial}{\partial \theta_j} \log L(\underset{\sim}{\theta}) = 0$ for $j = 1, \ldots, p$. Therefore, under fairly mild assumptions of the censoring times, the log-likelihood function is

$$\log L(\underset{\sim}{\theta}) = \sum_u \log h(Y_i, \underset{\sim}{\theta}) - \sum_{i=1}^{n} \left(\int_0^{Y_i} h(t, \underset{\sim}{\theta}) dt \right). \tag{8.12}$$

8.5.4   Estimation of Hazard Rates and Change Points

It follows from Equation 8.12 that the log-likelihood function for an exponential model with one parameter, λ, is

$$\log L(\lambda) = \sum_u \log \lambda - \sum_{i=1}^{n} \lambda Y_i = d \log \lambda - \lambda \sum_{i=1}^{n} Y_i,$$

where
  d is the total number of events (uncensored observations) and
  $\sum Y_i$ is the total of censored and uncensored event times.

Similarly, the log-likelihood functions for a 2-piece PWE model and 3-piece PWE model, respectively, are as follows:

$$\log L(\lambda_1, \lambda_2; \tau) = (d_1 \log \lambda_1 + d_2 \log \lambda_2) - \lambda_1 \sum_{i=1}^{n} (Y_i \wedge \tau) - \lambda_2 \sum_{i=1}^{n} (Y_i - \tau)^+,$$

$$\log L(\lambda_1, \lambda_2, \lambda_3; \tau_1, \tau_2) = \left(\sum_{j=1}^{3} d_j \log \lambda_j \right) - \lambda_1 \sum_{i=1}^{n} [(Y_i \wedge \tau_1) - 0]^+$$
$$- \lambda_2 \sum_{i=1}^{n} [(Y_i \wedge \tau_2) - \tau_1]^+ - \lambda_3 \sum_{i=1}^{n} (Y_i - \tau_2)^+$$

$X \wedge Y$ means $\min(X, Y)$, and X^+ means $X^+ = (X$, if $X > 0$; and 0, if $X \leq 0)$. This was the notation used by Loader [17] for a 2-piece PWE model.

In general, we write the log-likelihood function for a k-piece piecewise exponential model described in Equation 8.8 as

$$\log L(\underset{\sim}{\lambda}; \underset{\sim}{\tau}) = \left(\sum_{j=1}^{k} d_j \log \lambda_j \right) - \sum_{j=1}^{k-1} \lambda_j \sum_{i=1}^{n} \left[(Y_i \wedge \tau_j) - \tau_{j-1} \right]^+$$
$$- \lambda_k \sum_{i=1}^{n} (Y_i - \tau_{k-1})^+, \tag{8.13}$$

where

d_j is the number of events observed in the jth interval $(\tau_{j-1}, \tau_j]$

the sum $\sum \left[(Y_i \wedge \tau_j) - \tau_{j-1} \right]^+$ represents the total time at risk in the jth interval $(\tau_{j-1}, \tau_j]$

For fixed and known change-points $\underset{\sim}{\tau} = (\tau_1, \ldots, \tau_{k-1})$, we generalize the MLEs of the hazard rates $\underset{\sim}{\lambda} = (\lambda_1, \ldots, \lambda_k)$ by differentiating the log likelihood (Equation 8.13), giving

$$\hat{\lambda}_j = \frac{d_j}{\displaystyle\sum_{i=1}^{n} \left[(Y_i \wedge \tau_j) - \tau_{j-1} \right]^+}, \quad j = 1, \ldots, k-1,$$

and

$$\hat{\lambda}_k = \frac{d_k}{\displaystyle\sum_{i=1}^{n} (Y_i - \tau_{k-1})^+}.$$

In real clinical data, however, the change points are unknown and must be estimated. For a 2-piece PWE model, an estimate $\hat{\tau}$ of τ can be obtained by substituting the MLE of the hazard rates $\hat{\lambda}_1$ and $\hat{\lambda}_2$ into the log-likelihood function (Equation 8.13) and maximizing $\log L(\hat{\lambda}_1, \hat{\lambda}_2; \tau)$ with respect to τ over a restricted interval $[\tau_a, \tau_b]$, $0 \leq \tau_a < \tau_b < \infty$. Let $Y_{(1)}, \ldots, Y_{(n)}$ be the order statistics of observed times $Y_1, \ldots, Y_n$. Yao [22] suggests using $\tau_a = 0$ and $\tau_b = Y_{(n-1)}$. Usually, we take the lower limit of restricted interval $\tau_a > 0$ since a small number of early events can cause a spuriously large likelihood [17]. Second the upper limit of the restricted interval τ_b must be smaller than the largest observed time $Y_{(n)}$ because the likelihood function is unbounded [20,22] at the last observed time, i.e., $\tau_b \leq Y_{(n-1)}$. The value of τ in the grid search that maximizes the profile log likelihood is an estimate of the unknown change point, i.e.,

$$\hat{\tau} = \arg \sup_{\tau_a \leq \tau \leq \tau_b} \log L(\hat{\lambda}_1, \hat{\lambda}_2; \tau), \quad \text{where } \tau \in \left\{ Y_{(1)}^-, Y_{(1)}, \ldots, Y_{(n-1)}^-, Y_{(n-1)} \right\}.$$

Because of the discontinuity of the log-likelihood function at the change point, it is sufficient to evaluate the log likelihood at the $2(n-1)$ time points given above. These time points are the $n-1$ event times, $Y_{(1)}, \ldots, Y_{(n-1)}$, and the $n-1$ time points of the infimums from below of the event times, $Y_{(1)}^-, \ldots, Y_{(n-1)}^-$. Yao [22] studied the distribution theory of the estimators and showed that $\hat{\tau}$ converges to τ in probability under the restriction $\tau \leq Y_{(n-1)}$ stated above. An alternative estimator of τ is given by Nguyen et al. [20] which is consistent but the distribution theory is unknown.

An approximate confidence region for the change point, τ, given by Loader [17] has the form:

$$I = \left\{ t : \log L(t) \geq \sup_{\tau_a \leq u \leq \tau_b} \log L(u) - c \right\}, \tag{8.14}$$

where L is the likelihood function of a 2-piece PWE model and c is related to the confidence level $(1 - \alpha)$ by the equation $1 - \alpha = (1 - e^{-c})[1 - v(\hat{\delta})e^{-c}]$.

$\hat{\delta} = \log(\hat{\lambda}_2/\hat{\lambda}_1)$ is the estimated size of change in hazard, and $v(\hat{\delta})$ is a function of the estimated change in hazard given by

$$v(\hat{\delta}) = \frac{1 - \left[|\hat{\delta}|/\left(e^{|\hat{\delta}|} - 1\right)\right]}{\left[|\hat{\delta}|/\left(1 - e^{-|\hat{\delta}|}\right)\right] - 1}.$$

For details regarding the above derivations see Loader [17]. The confidence region (Equation 8.14) may be a union of disjoint intervals because the underlying likelihood function is not a smooth function of τ, but is a jagged function with local peaks at the failure times. Jeong [25], however, recommends parametric boostrapping as a method of estimating a confidence interval for the change point. Gardner [26] illustrated that the ordinary nonparametric bootstrapping (sampling with replacement) and jacknife sampling are not appropriate for estimating a confidence interval for the change point because these methods are heavily influenced by whether the observed times are included in the bootstrap sample. Therefore, Gardner [26] developed an efficient parametric bootstrapping algorithm to estimate a confidence interval for the change point. With the parametric bootstrapping method, B bootstrap samples of size N are randomly generated from the assumed PWE distribution using the estimates $\hat{\tau}$, $\hat{\lambda}_1$, and $\hat{\lambda}_2$ from the original data. The mean and standard deviation of the B bootstrap samples are

$$\hat{\theta}^*(\cdot) = \sum_{b=1}^{B} \hat{\theta}^*(b)/B,$$

$$\widehat{se}_B = \sqrt{\frac{\sum_{b=1}^{B}\left[\hat{\theta}^*(b) - \hat{\theta}^*(\cdot)\right]^2}{B - 1}},$$

where $\hat{\theta}^*(b)$ is the estimate of the change point τ at the maximum of the profile log likelihood for a given restricted search interval $[\tau_a, \tau_b]$. The resulting algorithm gives four types of $100(1 - \alpha)\%$ confidence intervals described in Efron and Tibshirani [42], namely, (1) Z confidence interval: $\hat{\theta}^*(\cdot) \pm z_{1-\alpha/2}\widehat{se}_B$, (2) bootstrap-$t$ interval, (3) percentile interval with $\alpha/2$ and $(1 - \alpha/2)$ percentiles as the lower and upper confidence limits, and (4) bias corrected and accelerated (BC_a) confidence interval. Gardner's comparison of these four confidence intervals showed that the percentile bootstrap estimates perform well in terms of coverage of the interval. The percentile bootstrap estimates can be improved by adjusting for the observed bias in the bootstrap mean, i.e., $\hat{\tau} - \hat{\theta}^*(\cdot)$. Thus, $100(1 - \alpha)\%$ percentile confidence intervals for the change point estimate, $\hat{\tau}$, can be calculated by using the $\alpha/2$ and $(1 - \alpha/2)$ percentiles of B bootstrap estimates $\hat{\theta}^*(b)$. Furthermore, these interval estimates can be adjusted by subtracting the observed bias.

Example 1

To explore how sample size and effect size of change in hazard (i.e., λ_2/λ_1) affect the length and coverage of the confidence interval for the estimate of the

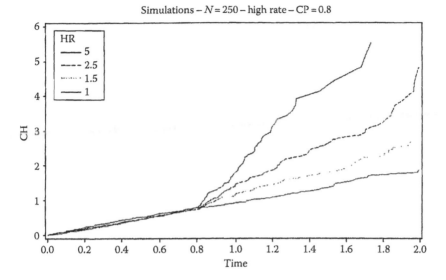

FIGURE 8.2: Simulated time-to-event data showing increasing hazard and one change point.

change point, Bhore and Gardner [27] simulated time-to-event data from 2-piece PWE models for various parameters of $\lambda_1 = 1$, $\lambda_2 = 1$, 1.5, 2.5, 5, $\tau = 0.8$, and $N = 250$ subjects. Figure 8.2 shows cumulative hazard plots for the simulated data. Note that as the late hazard, λ_2, increases the change point becomes more visible at 0.8. Table 8.2 summarizes the point estimates and confidence regions or confidence intervals of the change point using Loader's method and the Boostrapping method. The two methods are compared in terms of length and coverage of the confidence intervals in Table 8.3.

Both methods are computationally difficult but similar in terms of length and coverage. The bootstrapping confidence interval has shorter length than the length of Loader's confidence region. This may be due to the disjoint nature of the confidence region. Loader's method needs many iterations to get good coverage and may need improvement in terms of the initial estimate of c to get accurate coverage.

TABLE 8.2: Estimates of change point and 95% confidence region/interval.

λ_2	τ	Loader's Method Point and Confidence Region Estimates ($\hat{\tau}$)	Gardner's Bootstrap Method (Percentile) Point and 95% Confidence Intervals ($\hat{\tau}$)
1.5	0.8	0.748(0.059, 3.382)	0.748(0.390, 1.14)
2.5	0.8	0.811(0.561, 1.009)	0.811(0.638, 0.990)
5.0	0.8	0.785(0.734, 0.897)	0.785(0.765, 0.810)

$N = 250$ subjects, $\lambda_1 = 1$, change point $\tau = 0.8$.

TABLE 8.3:   Length and coverage of confidence
region/interval of change point.

	Loader's Method		Gardner's Bootstrap Method (Percentile)	
λ_2	Length	Coverage	Length	Coverage
1.5	0.744	90.3%	0.665	97.5%
2.5	0.486	98.6%	0.299	94.7%
5.0	0.115	100.0%	0.054	94.5%

$N = 250$ subjects, $\lambda_1 = 1$, change point $\tau = 0.8$.

Bootstrapping is relatively easy. Both methods could be useful for estimation of the time point of change in hazard and the hazard rates before and after the change.

8.5.5   Testing of Change Points and Model Selection

There are three commonly known hypothesis testing procedures, namely, (1) *likelihood ratio tests* based on the maximum likelihood itself, (2) *score* or *Rao tests* based on the first and second derivatives of the log likelihood, and (3) *Wald tests* based on the large-sample distribution of the maximum likelihood estimator [13]. A hypothesis testing method for the existence of a change point could be based on one of these procedures.

Let Y denote the data, $\theta = (\theta_1, \ldots, \theta_p)$ be the parameter vector, $\log L(\theta; Y)$ be the log-likelihood function, and $\hat{\theta}$ be the maximum likelihood estimator that maximizes the log likelihood. Then the statistics for testing the simple null hypothesis $H_0 : \theta = \theta_0$ are given as follows:

$$\text{Likelihood ratio test: } \chi^2_{\text{LR}} = 2\left[\log L(\hat{\theta}; Y) - \log L(\theta_0; Y)\right],$$

$$\text{Score test: } \chi^2_{\text{S}} = U(\theta_0)I^{-1}(\theta_0)U'(\theta_0),$$

$$\text{Wald test: } \chi^2_{\text{W}} = (\hat{\theta} - \theta_0)I(\hat{\theta})(\hat{\theta} - \theta_0)'.$$

Here $U(\theta)$ is the efficient score vector with elements $U_j(\theta) = \frac{\partial}{\partial \theta_j} \log L(\theta; Y)$ for $j = 1, \ldots, p$ and $I(\theta)$ is the observed Fisher's information matrix with elements $I_{j,k}(\theta) = -\frac{\partial^2}{\partial \theta_j \partial \theta_k} \log L(\theta; Y)$ for $j, k = 1, \ldots, p$. All three test statistics above have an asymptotic chi-squared distribution with p degrees of freedom when the null hypothesis is true. In this chapter, we focus on the LRT.

Testing for change point(s), τ, is actually a problem of testing composite (not simple) hypotheses, because the hazard rate parameter(s), λ, are considered to be nuisance parameters. All the above three test statistics can be refined for testing a composite hypothesis, i.e., for testing a subset of parameters. Suppose the parameter θ is divided into two vectors as $\theta = (\psi, \phi)$ with ψ being a parameter vector of interest of length p_1 and ϕ a nuisance parameter vector of length p_2. Then the likelihood ratio statistic for testing $H_0 : \psi = \psi_0$ is given by

$$\chi^2_{LR}(\tau) = 2\left[\log L(\hat{\psi}, \hat{\phi}; Y) - \log L\left(\psi_0, \hat{\phi}(\psi_0); Y\right)\right]$$

and has an asymptotic chi-squared distribution with p_1 degrees of freedom. The degrees of freedom are computed as number of parameters under the alternative hypothesis minus number of parameters under the null.

Therefore, the LRT statistic for testing the hypothesis of no change point, i.e., $H_0 : \tau = 0$ versus the alternative $H_1 : \tau \neq 0$ assuming a 2-piece PWE model is given by

$$\chi^2_{LR} = 2\left[\log L(\hat{\lambda}_1, \hat{\lambda}_2, \hat{\tau}) - \log L(\hat{\lambda}, \hat{\lambda}, 0)\right],$$

where

$\hat{\lambda}$ is the MLE under the null hypothesis of a simple exponential model and $(\hat{\lambda}_1, \hat{\lambda}_2, \hat{\tau})$ are the MLEs under the 2-piece PWE model given in Section 8.5.4.

Although a naïve application of the likelihood ratio theory may lead one to conclude that the above test statistic should have χ^2 distribution with two degrees of freedom, this is not quite accurate because the likelihood function has a discontinuity at the change-point τ under the alternative hypothesis H_1. However, Matthews and Farewell simulated the critical regions for the LRT and showed that the percentiles of $\chi^2_{(2)}$ appear to approximately agree. Thus, the derivation of a significance level for the LRT statistic for testing exisitence of a change point is more complicated than using the chi-square distribution.

Loader [17] derived the following restricted LRT statistic for testing $H_0 : \tau = 0$ (or $\lambda_1 = \lambda_2$) versus $H_1 : \tau \neq 0$ (or $\lambda_1 \neq \lambda_2$) by using the pseudo (or restricted) MLEs $(\hat{\lambda}_1, \hat{\lambda}_2, \tau)$ discussed in Section 8.5.4.

$$l(\hat{\tau}) = X(\hat{\tau}) \log\left\{\frac{X(\hat{\tau})\sum Y_i}{N\sum(Y_i \wedge \hat{\tau})}\right\} + [N - X(\hat{\tau})]\log\left\{\frac{[N - X(\hat{\tau})]\sum Y_i}{N\sum[Y_i - (Y_i \wedge \hat{\tau})]}\right\},$$

where

$X(\hat{\tau})$ (also denoted by d_1) is the number of events (uncensored observations) observed up to time $\hat{\tau}$,

$[N - X(\hat{\tau})]$ (also denoted by d_2) is the number of events after the change point $\hat{\tau}$, and N is the total number of events.

Note that $X(t)$ is a counting process. Using a time scale transformation of $s = \sum(Y_i \wedge t)$ and $Z(s) = X(t)$, Loader showed that Z follows a Poisson distribution with rate λ_0 under the null hypothesis of no change point. Therefore, the LRT statistic can be rewritten in terms of the time transformation and the significance level of the LRT test can be derived by approximating the boundary crossing probabilities of a Poisson process [17]. The revised LRT statistic is invariant under the time transformation and is given by

$$l_Z(s) = Z(s) \log\left\{\frac{Z(s)S}{Ns}\right\} + [N - Z(s)]\log\left\{\frac{[N - Z(s)]S}{N(S - s)}\right\},$$

H_0 is rejected if $l_Z(s) > \frac{1}{2}c^2$ for some $c > 0$ which is related to the significance level of the test by the following equations.

Lower tail probability :

$$\Pr[Z(u_0) \le np(u_0)] + ce^{-\frac{1}{2}c^2} \int_{u_0}^{u_1} \frac{[1 - p(s)]\,[p\prime(s) - p(s)/s]}{(1 - s)\frac{c}{\sqrt{n}}\sqrt{2\pi p(s)[1 - p(s)]}}\,ds.$$

Upper tail probability:

$$\Pr[Z(u_0) \ge nq(u_1)] + ce^{-\frac{1}{2}c^2} \int_{u_0}^{u_1} \frac{[1 - q(s)]\{q\prime(s) - [1 - q(s)]/(1 - s)\}}{(1 - s)\frac{c}{\sqrt{n}}\sqrt{2\pi q(s)[1 - q(s)]}}\,ds.$$

Significance level:

$$\alpha \approx \text{Lower tail probability} + \text{Upper tail probability.}$$

To complete the equations, one needs $Z(u_j) \sim Bin(n - 1, u_j), j = 0, 1$; as well as find the solutions $p(s)$ and $q(s)$ in x of $[x \log(x/s)] + (1 - x)\log[(1 - x)/(1 - s)] = \frac{1}{2}(c^2/n)$. Loader [17] recommends that we choose the constants $u_0 = 1 - u_1 = 0.05$ for large data sets and 0.10 for small data sets.

Gardner [26] explored the distribution of the likelihood ratio statistic through bootstrapping by simulating the distribution of the LRT statistic under various one change point models. To test for the existence of one change point we assume a 2-piece PWE model and use the bootstrapping algorithm [26, pp. 49–52] for a LRT as follows:

1. For the observed data, calculate the MLE $\hat{\lambda}_0$ of the hazard rate for a simple exponential model and restricted MLEs $(\hat{\lambda}_1, \hat{\lambda}_2, \hat{\tau})$ discussed earlier for a one change point model (i.e., 2-piece PWE model). Then, compute the LRT statistic $2[\log L(\hat{\lambda}_1, \hat{\lambda}_2, \hat{\tau}) - \log L(\hat{\lambda}_0, \hat{\lambda}_0, 0)]$ for the observed data.

2. Next generate B bootstrap samples under the null hypothesis of a simple exponential model with parameter $\hat{\lambda}_0$ from the previous step. Assuming one change point model, compute $(\hat{\lambda}_{1b}, \hat{\lambda}_{2b}, \hat{\tau}_b)$ for each bootstrap sample with $b = 1, \ldots, B$, and the associated log likelihood. Similarly, assuming a simple exponential model compute $\hat{\lambda}_{0b}$, for $b = 1, \ldots, B$, and the associated log likelihood. This will give an empirical distribution of the LRT statistic, $2[\log L(\hat{\lambda}_{1b}, \hat{\lambda}_{2b}, \hat{\tau}_b) - \log L(\hat{\lambda}_{0b}, \hat{\lambda}_{0b}, 0)]$ from B bootstrap samples.

3. Finally map the observed LRT statistic to a percentile in the empirical distribution of LRT values (distribution under null hypothesis) from the second step. If observed LRT statistic is greater than the 95th percentile of the empirical distribution (for a one-sided p-value of 0.05), then reject H_0 and conclude that a change point exists.

The computer programs for implementing this boostrapping algorithm can be found in Gardner's dissertation [26]. Furthermore, Gardner also addressed the problem of estimation and testing for two change points through bootstrapping.

Changes in hazard can sometimes be visually observed by plotting the cumulative hazard function (cumulative incidence) against time. Visual checks of data are not confirmatory as to whether a change point exists, and if the hazard does change, whether there is one change point or two change points. As discussed earlier, researchers have debated whether the hazard changes at more than one time points. Therefore, goodness-of-fit of the change-point model selected is an issue.

Hammerstrom and Bhore [43] addressed the accuracy of the likelihood ratio in choosing the correct distribution for the times among exponential, PWE with one change point, PWE with two change points, and Weibull. The authors simulated time-to-event data under different scenarios given in the example below. They concluded that the LRT provides an effective way to distinguish among Weibull and 1-piece, 2-piece, and 3-piece PWE models for sample sizes over 150. Even with sample sizes of 40, the test could separate Weibull from exponential and exponential from PWE if hazard ratio at least doubled.

Example 2

Hammerstrom and Bhore [43] simulated time-to-event data from 15 two-piece PWE models (one change point) with varying parameters of $\lambda_1 = 1$, $\lambda_2 = 0.2$, 0.5, 1, 2, 5, and $\tau = $ 30th, 50th, 70th percentiles of the prechange exponential. λ_1 is the early hazard rate, λ_2 is the late hazard rate, and τ is the change point. Decreasing hazard is represented by values for which $\lambda_2 < \lambda_1$, constant hazard rate by $\lambda_1 = \lambda_2 = 1$, and increasing hazard rate by $\lambda_2 > \lambda_1$. Assuming the 2-piece PWE to be the true model, Figure 8.3 shows five panels of the LRT statistics for pairwise comparisons of fitting simple exponential, 2-piece PWE, 3-piece PWE, and Weibull models. Here each group of disjoint graphs represent comparisons of one pair of

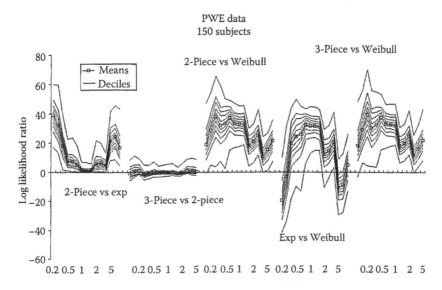

FIGURE 8.3: Change point model selection based on LRT.

models: 2-PWE:exponential, 3-PWE:2-PWE, 2-PWE:Weibull, exponential:Weibull, 3-PWE:Weibull. Each connected graph summarizes 15 true models. Late to early hazard ratios vary more slowly from 0.2 to 0.5, 1, 2, 5 and are marked on the x-axis. Three choices of time of change-point are within each ratio: 30th, 50th, 70th percentiles of early hazard. In the first panel, as one goes from left to right, one has the quantiles of the likelihood ratio statistics comparing 2-piece to exponential for data drawn from a 2-piece PWE model with late: early means $= 0.2$, 0.5, 1, 2, 5 successively.

In this example, the LRT rejects exponential and Weibull models in favor of 2-piece and 3-piece PWE models for sample size of 150 subjects. Here one can see that even the lowest 10th percentile of LRT statistic selects 2-PWE over exponential or Weibull (except when the hazard rates are constant at $\lambda_1 = \lambda_2 = 1$) and that the overfitted 3-PWE is not preferred even by the most extreme 10th decile of LRT statistic.

8.6   Discussion

The primary objective of many RCTs in Phases II and III of drug development is to evaluate efficacy for a predetermined duration. Typically, after the blinded phase of the RCT ends and the efficacy of the new treatment group is established compared to the control group, the trial is continued into an uncontrolled, often open-label, phase. During the latter phase all patients switch to a single treatment group to receive open label treatment. As such, longer-term safety data continues to accumulate for a single treatment group. In other cases, a clinical trial may be designed at the outset to collect uncontrolled safety data on a test drug for long periods of time.

As O'Neill [11] notes uncontrolled or open-label clinical trials provide a major source of long-term safety data for a single treatment group. In particular, SAEs associated with long-term drug exposure are usually found through analysis of time-to-event data in clinical trials. Uncommon adverse events such as liver injury, cardiovascular injury, renal failure, or other types of abnormalities may begin to appear in longer-term data, implying a temporal relationship between drug exposure and occurrence of adverse events. Crude proportions will grossly underestimate the incidence of such adverse events and it is recommended that time-to-event methods be used to understand the treatment-related phenomena of harm. Similarly, temporal relationship between treatment-related benefit and drug exposure are best understood through time-to-event methods.

Several examples of time-to-event safety and efficacy endpoints from the medical literature were provided where the hazard does not remain constant. Most time-to-event analyses, however, assume that the hazard (risk of an event, either safety or efficacy) remains constant throughout the time of drug exposure. As discussed in this chapter, the constancy assumption of the hazard can be tested by modeling the hazard function as a piecewise constant function. If a plot of a cumulative hazard function visually shows an abrupt change in hazard around one time point, then a

2-piece PWE model for the hazard function can be fit. Change in hazard (whether increasing or decreasing) can be tested by testing for the existence of a single change point and unknown change point can be estimated. The choice of piecewise models does not have to be limited to a 2-piece PWE model, but can be extended to a k-piece PWE model. This chapter has shown how to generalize the maximum likelihood estimation of $k - 1$ change points and corresponding k hazard rates. Although, the focus of this chapter was on the PWE model which is a generalization of the simple exponential model, other choice of models could include piecewise Weibull models or combinations of PWE and piecewise Weibull. Model selection for choosing the best-fitting model may be done using the LRT as discussed in Section 8.5.5. Müller and Wang's nonparametric method is an alternative to the semiparametric models such as PWE model. However, the nonparametric approach will require larger sample sizes than a well-fitting parametric model for the purpose of inference. A semiparametric model such as a 2-piece PWE model provides ease of interpretation to a medical colleague. For example, a well-fitting 2-piece PWE model may show that the hazard of a safety event increases after 18 months of drug exposure, or the hazard of relapse decreases 4 months after surgery.

Mathematical complexity of even the simplest 2-piece PWE model and the presence of censoring has possibly prevented routine application of the change point methodology to testing for changes in hazard. However, application of change point models can easily be overcome by modern computing (including bootstrapping) if the theory is well understood. This chapter has attempted to simplify the theory given in the literature and shown how applicable change point methodology can be for evaluating and testing for abrupt time-dependent changes in treatment efficacy and safety data collected in clinical trials. The hope is that change point methodology will become a routinely used statistical tool to check for changes in hazard over time, for example, in long-term clinical trial data submitted in New Drug Applications to the FDA.

References

[1] Bombardier, C., Laine, L., Reicin, A., Shapiro, D., Burgos-Vargas, R., Davis, B., Day, R., et al. (2000): Comparison of upper gastrointestinal toxicity of rofecoxib and naproxen in patients with rheumatoid arthritis. *New England Journal of Medicine* 343(21): 1520–1528.

[2] Bresalier, R., Sandler, R., Quan, H., Bolognese, J., Oxenius, B., Horgan, K., Lines, C., et al. (2005): Cardiovascular events associated with rofecoxib in a colorectal adenoma chemoprevention trial. *New England Journal of Medicine* 352(11): 1092–1102.

[3] Writing Group for the Women's Health Initiative Investigators (2002): Risks and benefits of estrogen plus progestin in healthy postmenopausal women.

Principal results from the Women's Health Initiative randomized controlled trial. *Journal of American Medical Association* 288(3): 321–333.

[4] McDonough, P. G. (2002): The randomized world is not without its imperfections: Reflections on the Women's Health Initiative study. *Fertility and Sterility* 78(5): 951–956.

[5] Kahn, J., Lagakos, S., Wulfsohn, M., Cherng, D., Miller, M., Cherrington, J., Hardy, D., et al. (1999): Efficacy and safety of adefovir dipivoxil with antiretroviral therapy. *Journal of the American Medical Association* 282(24): 2305–2312.

[6] Mileshkin, L., Stark, R., Day, B., Seymour, J., Zeldis, J., and Prince, H. M. (2006): Development of neuropathy in patients with myeloma treated with thalidomide: Patterns of occurrence and the role of electrophysiologic monitoring. *Journal of Clinical Oncology* 24(27): 4507–4514.

[7] Wei, X., Liu, H. H., Tucker, S., Wang, S., Mohan, R., Cox, J., Komaki, R., and Liao, Z. (2008): Risk factors for pericardial effusion in inoperable esophageal cancer patients treated with definitive chemoradiation therapy. *International Journal of Radiation Oncology, Biology, Physics* 70(3): 707–714.

[8] Arani, R. B., Soong, S. -J., Weiss, H. L., Wood, M. J., Fiddian, P. A., Gnann, J. W., and Whitley, R. (2001): Phase specific analysis of herpes zoster associated pain data: A new statistical approach. *Statistics in Medicine* 20(16): 2429–2439.

[9] Desmond, R. A., Weiss, H. L., Arani, R. B., Soong, S. -J., Wood, M. J., Fiddian, P. A., Gnann, J. W., and Whitley, R. (2002): Clinical applications for change-point analysis of herpes zoster pain. *Journal of Pain and Symptom Management* 23(6): 510–516.

[10] Stephens, R. J., Bailey, A. J., Machin, D., and Medical Research Council Lung Cancer Working Party (1996): Long-term survival in small cell lung cancer: The case for a standard definition. *Lung Cancer* 15: 297–309.

[11] O'Neill, R. T. (1988): Assessment of Safety. In Peace, K. E., editor, *Biopharmaceutical Statistics for Drug Development*, pp. 543–604. Marcel Dekker Inc., New York, USA.

[12] Cantor, A. (1997): *Extending SAS Survival Analysis Techniques for Medical Research*. SAS Institute Inc., Cary, North Carolina, USA.

[13] Klein, J. P. and Moeschberger, M. L. (1997): Survival Analysis: Techniques for Censored and Truncated Data. Springer-Verlag Inc., New York, USA.

[14] Kalbfleisch, J. D. and Prentice, R. L. (2002): The Statistical Analysis of Failure Time Data. John Wiley & Sons., Hoboken, New Jersey, USA.

[15] Kaplan, E. L. and Meier, P. (1958): Nonparametric estimation from incomplete observations. *Journal of the American Statistical Association* 53: 457–481.

[16] Matthews, D. E. and Farewell, V. T. (1982): On testing for a constant hazard against a change-point alternative. *Biometrics* 38: 463–468.

[17] Loader, C. R. (1991): Inference for a hazard rate change point. *Biometrika* 78: 749–757.

[18] Müller, H. -G. and Wang, J. -L. (1994): Change-point models for hazard functions. In Carlsten, E. G., Müller, H. -G., and Siegmund, D., editors, *Change-Point Problems*, vol. 23 of *IMS Lecture Notes and Monograph Series*, pp. 224–241. Institute of Mathematical Statistics, Hayward, California, USA.

[19] Matthews, D. E., Farewell, V. T., and Pyke, R. (1985): Asymptotic score-statistic processes and tests for constant hazard against a change-point alternative. *The Annals of Statistics* 13: 583–591.

[20] Nguyen, H. T., Rogers, G. S., and Walker, E. A. (1984): Estimation in change-point hazard rate models. *Biometrika* 71: 299–304.

[21] Basu, A. P., Ghosh, J. K., and Joshi, S. N. (1988): On estimating change point in a failure rate. In Gupta, S. S. and Berger, J. O., *Statistical Decision Theory and Related Topics IV*, in two volumes, Vol. 2, pp. 239–252. Springer-Verlag Inc., New York, USA.

[22] Yao, Y. -C. (1986): Maximum likelihood estimation in hazard rate models with a change-point. *Communications in Statistics: Theory and Methods* 15: 2455–2466.

[23] Pham, D. T. and Nguyen, H. T. (1990): Strong consistency of the maximum likelihood estimators in the change-point hazard rate model. *Statistics* 21: 203–216.

[24] Pham, D. T. and Nguyen, H. T. (1993): Bootstrapping the change-point of a hazard rate. *Annals of the Institute of Statistical Mathematics* 45: 331–340.

[25] Jeong, K. M. (1999): Change-point estimation and bootstrap confidence regions in Weibull distribution. *Journal of the Korean Statistical Society* 28(3): 359–370.

[26] Gardner, S. (2007): Change point models for discontinuation rates of pneumocystis carinii pneumonia prophylaxis in an Ontario HIV patient population. PhD thesis, University of Toronto, Toronto, Canada.

[27] Bhore, R. and Gardner, S. (2006): Analyzing change in hazard for time-to-event endpoints in clinical trials. In *ASA Proceedings of the Joint Statistical Meetings*, pp. 526–529. American Statistical Association, Alexandria, Virginia, USA.

[28] Liang, K. -Y., Self, S. G., and Liu, X. (1990): The Cox proportional hazards model with change point: An epidemiologic application. *Biometrics* 46: 783–793.

[29] Müller, H. -G. and Wang, J. -L. (1990): Nonparametric analysis of changes in hazard rates for censored survival data: An alternative to change-point models. *Biometrika* 77: 305–314.

[30] Qin, J. and Sun, J. (1997): Statistical analysis of right-censored failure-time data with partially specified hazard rates. *The Canadian Journal of Statistics/ La Revue Canadienne de Statistique* 25: 325–336.

[31] Chang, I. -S., Chen, C. -H., and Hsiung, C. A. (1994): Estimation in change-point hazard rate models with random censorship. In Carlsten, E. G., Müller, H. -G., and Siegmund, D., editors, *Change-Point Problems*, vol. 23 of *IMS Lecture Notes and Monograph Series*, pp. 78–92. Institute of Mathematical Statistics, Hayward, California, USA.

[32] Gijbels, I. and Gürler, U. (2003): Estimation of a change point in a hazard function based on censored data. *Lifetime Data Analysis* 9(4): 395–411.

[33] Goodman, M. S., Li, Y., and Tiwari, R. C. (2006): Survival analysis with change point hazard functions. Working paper 40, Harvard University Biostatistics Working Paper Series, http://www.bepress.com/harvardbiostat/paper40.

[34] Friedman, M. (1982): Piecewise exponential models for survival data with covariates. *The Annals of Statistics* 10: 101–113.

[35] Kim, J. S. and Proschan, F. (1991): Piecewise exponential estimator of the survival function. *IEEE Transactions on Reliability* 40(2): 134–139.

[36] Worsley, K. J. (1986): Confidence regions and tests for a change-point in a sequence of exponential family random variables. *Biometrika* 73: 91–104.

[37] Karrison, T. (1996): Confidence intervals for median survival times under a piecewise exponential model with proportional hazards covariate effects. *Statistics in Medicine* 15: 171–182.

[38] Zelterman, D., Grambsch, P. M., Le, C. T., Ma, J. Z., and Curtsinger, J. W. (1994): Piecewise exponential survival curves with smooth transitions. *Mathematical Biosciences* 120: 233–250.

[39] Leung, S. -H. S. (1993): A change point model to evaluate the patterns of recurrence and survival for patients with operable colon cancer. Master's thesis, University of Pittsburgh, Pittsburgh, PA.

[40] Miller, R. G. Jr., Gong, G., and Munoz, A. (1981): *Survival Analysis*. John Wiley & Sons., New York, USA.

[41] Cox, D. R. and Oakes, D. (1984): *Analysis of Survival Data*. Chapman & Hall Ltd., Boca Raton, Florida, USA.

[42] Efron, B. and Tibshirani, R. (1993): *An Introduction to Bootstrap*. Chapman & Hall Ltd., Boca Raton, Florida, USA.

[43] Hammerstrom, T. and Bhore, R. (2006): Confidence intervals and goodness-of-fit in piecewise exponential models. In *ASA Proceedings of the Joint Statistical Meetings*, pp. 570–574. American Statistical Association, Alexandria, Virginia, USA.

Chapter 9

Overview of Descriptive and Graphical Methods for Time-to-Event Data

Michael O'Connell and Bob Treder

Contents

9.1   Introduction and Methods

Graphical summaries of time-to-event data are a critical component in the analysis and reporting of results from many clinical studies. The event can be death, or more likely some other nonfatal event such as disease diagnosis or recurrence. This chapter summarizes key features of graphical methods for time-to-event data.

Our presentation includes a review of recent journal articles with graphical summaries of time-to-event data, and an analysis of graphical output from statistical software. Our software analysis includes relevant graphical output from the statistical software S-PLUS, and extensions to this software to promote focused comparisons of results from the graphical presentations.

9.2   Applications and Analysis

There are several methods for descriptive analysis and presentation of time-to-event data. The most common presentation of time-to-event data is the Kaplan–Meier survival plot [1] which graphs a nonparametric estimate of survival versus time. Graphical methods are also used for model diagnostics such as review of the proportional hazards assumption [2]. In what follows, we provide examples of graphical displays of the Kaplan–Meier survival plot and diagnostics for the proportional hazards model.

9.2.1   Survival Plots

9.2.1.1   Example of Graphical Presentation

Figure 9.1 shows a Kaplan–Meier survival plot, created using the S-PLUS function survfit(), comparing survival by sex from a study of advanced lung cancer [2,3]. The solid line is the Kaplan–Meier survival function estimate for males, and the dashed line for females. Dotted lines are 95% confidence bands around the two estimates.

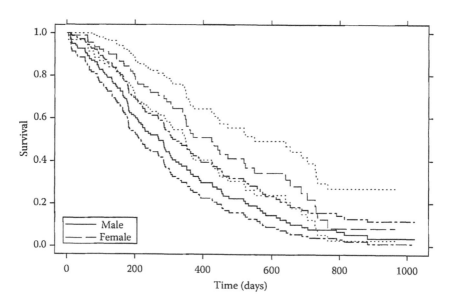

FIGURE 9.1:   Kaplan–Meier survival plot comparing survival by sex from a study of advanced lung cancer. The solid line is the Kaplan–Meier survival function estimate for males, and the dashed line for females. Dotted lines are 95% confidence bands around the two estimates.

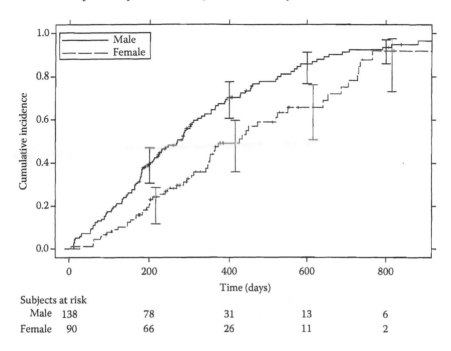

Subjects at risk				
Male	138	78	31	13	6
Female	90	66	26	11	2

FIGURE 9.2: Kaplan–Meier cumulative incidence plot comparing cumulative death (1 – survival) by sex from a study of advanced lung cancer. The solid line is the Kaplan–Meier cumulative incidence function estimate for males, and the dashed line for females.

There are several items that can be improved on Figure 9.1; a new graph is provided in Figure 9.2. The updates comprise the following:

- Confidence bands are replaced with confidence intervals at the major tick mark locations

- Graph is turned upside-down to form a cumulative incidence plot

- Censored observations are marked on the survival curves

- Number of subjects at risk have been added to the plot margin, at the major tick mark locations on the *x*-axis

- Survival estimates are truncated at the last observed event

- Feint, dotted reference lines have been added at the major tick marks on the *y*-axis

The updates in Figure 9.2 are described in more detail below. Some of these updates in Figure 9.2 are discussed by Pocock et al. [4].

9.2.1.2   Measures of Uncertainty

Confidence intervals are displayed in Figure 9.2 at the major tick marks. Alternate displays include error bars, half error bars, half confidence intervals, or confidence bands around the survivor functions as shown in Figure 9.1. Confidence bands often overlap, leading to a confusing display, e.g., as in Figure 9.1. The error bars or confidence intervals are best shown at a small subset of specific time-points, such as the major tick marks. It is also convenient to display the number-at-risk at these same locations (see below). Confidence intervals and/or error bars can overlap across treatments when treatment survivor function estimates are not widely separated. This may be resolved with treatment offsets as shown in Figure 9.2, where the confidence intervals for females are slightly offset to the right of those for males.

Error or confidence bands can provide an attractive display when the survivor functions are well separated. Bands may use a lighter line-style to differentiate from the survivor functions themselves. Bands without shading are confusing when survivor curve estimates are not well separated, with odd-shaped rectangles being formed by the bands and the survivor function. Shading can help reduce such confusion; however in many cases error bars or confidence intervals are preferred.

9.2.1.3   Survival versus Cumulative Incidence

A Kaplan–Meier or survival plot displays the proportion of subjects that are free of the event of interest, e.g., death. A cumulative incidence plot displays the cumulative proportion of subjects that experience the event of interest.

Both survival and cumulative incidence plots provide excellent comparative information on survival and incidence. The respective use of these two plots is largely a matter of preference and situation. Pocock et al. [4] prefer the cumulative incidence plot; we submit that other layout considerations, especially the *y*-axis scale and the aspect ratio or banking of the plot [11] are more important. Pocock et al. [4] argue that in cases of low event rates that the curves do not separate very well. However, the example they provide has a poorly chosen scale for the *y*-axis, resulting in the curves being unsatisfactorily banked. In particular, when the origin is shown on a survival plot (0 time, 0 survival) and the survival is high, then the curves are not banked to show differences between the curves.

We submit that the interpretability of the survival and cumulative incidence plots is directly related to the banking and aspect ratio of the plot. Banking is discussed in detail by Cleveland [5]; and banking to 45° enables maximal interpretation of separation between the survival or incidence curves. We illustrate this by Trellising the curves in Figure 2 by an additional variable, the patient-reported Karnofsky score [6]. We provide two plots to illustrate; both are banked to 45°, the default in the S-PLUS Trellis implementation. Figure 9.3 shows the lung data grouped on sex and Trellised on Karnofsky score; subjects with Karnofsky score greater than 80 (normal activity) are shown in the right-hand panel and subjects with Karnofsky score less than or equal to 80 (normal activity with effort, or unable to do normal activity) on the left-hand panel. Figure 9.4 shows the same plots for cumulative incidence.

Statistical graphics are typically read from the lower left to the upper right. In Trellis graphics this is also true for the ordering of the panels. Both the cumulative incidence plot (Figure 9.3) and the survival plot (Figure 9.4) can be read quickly in

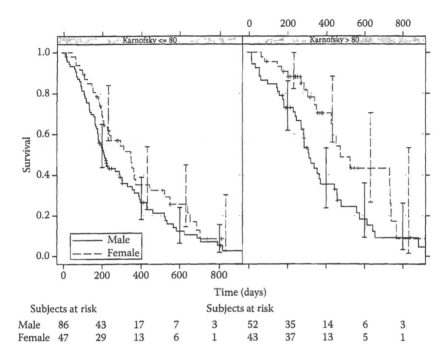

FIGURE 9.3: Kaplan–Meier survival plot comparing survival by sex and patient-reported Karnofsky score from a study of advanced lung cancer. The solid line is the Kaplan–Meier survival function estimate for males, and the dashed line for females. The left-hand panel shows subjects with Karnofsky score less than or equal to 80 (normal activity with effort, or unable to do normal activity) and the right-hand panel shows subjects with Karnofsky score greater than 80 (normal activity).

this way. The cumulative incidence plot has its origin (0 time, 0 incidence) in the lower left-hand corner and the curves always start in this lower left-hand corner. Indeed, as noted by Pocock et al. [4], the (0, 0) origin can always be shown in a cumulative incidence plot; whereas in cases where survival is high across the board, the survival plot may have no data for low survival rates, even for long time exposures. As such, in some cases, the (0, 0) origin (0 time, 0 survival) may not be included in a survival plot with suitable interpretive banking of the curves. However, the survival plots read well from lower left to upper right; such a directed eye-scan can actually accentuate differences between the curves as it is approximately perpendicular to survival curves that are banked to 45°.

In summary, both the survival and cumulative incidence plots display comparative information, provided they are banked appropriately, i.e., banked to approximately 45°.

9.2.1.4   Censored Observations

Figures 9.2 through 9.4 show censored observations as small vertical lines on the survival curve. This provides useful additional information in both the Trellis and non-Trellis plots. In the Trellis plots the additional panel makes the censored

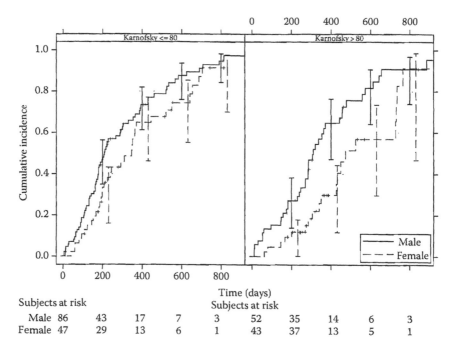

FIGURE 9.4: Kaplan–Meier cumulative incidence plot comparing cumulative incidence (death) by sex and patient-reported Karnofsky score from a study of advanced lung cancer. The solid line is the Kaplan–Meier cumulative incidence function estimate for males, and the dashed line for females. The left-hand panel shows subjects with Karnofsky score less than or equal to 80 (normal activity with effort, or unable to do normal activity) and the right-hand panel shows subjects with Karnofsky score greater than 80 (normal activity).

observations more distinct and useful in the comparisons across the group and Trellis covariables.

9.2.1.5 Follow-Up and Number at Risk

As discussed above, error bars, confidence intervals, or confidence bands provide useful uncertainty information around the survival or cumulative incidence curves. In the same vein, the addition of the number of subjects at risk helps to guide interpretation of the estimated survival or cumulative incidence functions. This is particularly important at the right-hand end of the graph where small numbers at risk should be a deterrent to overinterpretation of differences between the survivor curves.

For the lung data in Figures 9.2 through 9.4, the right-hand end of the survival and cumulative incidence curves are not supported by much data. This is especially the case in the Trellis plots of Figures 9.3 and 9.4. Pocock et al. [4] recommend that survival and cumulative incidence plots be truncated "once the proportion of patients free of an event, but still in follow-up, becomes unduly small." They suggest truncating the plot when 10%–20% or less are still in follow-up. We prefer to include confidence intervals and number at risk in the plots and to extend the curves through the last observed event. This view is in alignment with one of Tufte's [7] key graphics principles, i.e., show all the data.

We do, however, take the position that in most circumstances, survival and cumulative incidence functions can be truncated to suppress estimates from time-points following the last observed event. This has been done in Figures 9.2 through 9.4. This is preferred to the alternative display in Figure 9.1 where estimates are shown up to the end of the study, via horizontal lines extending from the right-hand points shown on the graph. This is not a big issue for the lung dataset since the last observed event is fairly close to the end of the study. It can be misleading however in cases where the study follow-up time extends well after the last observed event. In this case, if the extension is really wanted in the display, the inclusion of (large) error bands and (small) subjects at risk is important since there are no observed data providing support.

9.2.2   Graphics for Proportional Hazards Models

Apart from the graphical representation of the survival through the survival or cumulative incidence plot, the other major use of graphics in the analysis of time-to-event data is the graphical assessment of the proportional hazards assumption.

To examine the proportional hazards assumption graphically, for covariables with a small number of levels one can plot the Kaplan–Meier survival curves. If the proportional hazards assumption is true, the curves drift steadily apart [2]. When there are more than a few levels, or when the covariable is continuous, plotting the survival curves for different variable levels is not helpful. In this situation, one may plot the scaled Schoenfeld residuals versus some function of time, e.g., time, log(time). Such a plot helps distinguish between proportional hazards and time-dependent covariables. For example, if a treatment loses its effect over time, its coefficient may decrease with time. The utility of this plot for detecting such departures from proportional hazards is based on the work of Grambsch and Therneau [9].

Figure 9.5 shows a diagnostic proportional hazards plot using the S-PLUS function plot.cox.zph(). The plot shows the scaled Schoenfeld residuals versus km(time) for Karnofsky score in the analysis of the Veterans Administration lung cancer data from Kalbfleisch and Prentice [8, p. 223] as shown in Therneau and Grambsch [2, p. 135]. The plot includes a least squares regression line and a smooth spline curve with error band, along with the residuals.

There have been several statistical tests proposed for detecting departure from the proportional hazards assumption. Therneau and Grambsch [2] show that these can all be visualized as a trend test applied to the plot of scaled residuals versus $g(t)$. The graphical representation is extremely important, as is the case with any trend test, by enabling the viewer to see all of the data points and ensure that the (linear) departure captured in the test is driven by the body of the data and not a few isolated points.

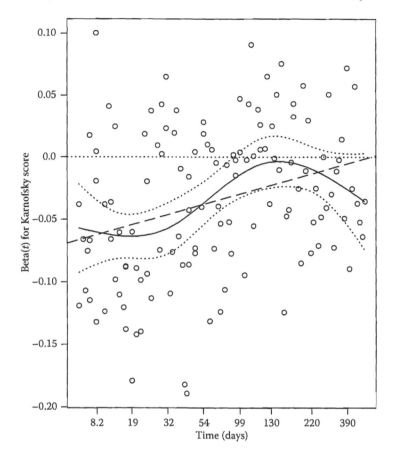

FIGURE 9.5: Graphical diagnostic for proportional hazards assumption: scaled Schoenfeld residuals versus km (time) for Karnofsky score in the analysis of the Veterans Administration lung cancer data from Kalbfleisch and Prentice [8, p. 223] as shown in Therneau and Grambsch [2, p. 135]. The dashed line is the least squares regression line, the solid line is a smooth spline curve, and the dotted line is the smooth spline error band.

The spline smooth provides additional character to the relationship beyond the linear departure captured in the test. In the veterans data we see that early on, a low Karnofsky score is protective; this effect diminishes over time and is effectively over after about 100 days. At that point the initial Karnofsky score, then 3–4 months old, is no longer clinically relevant.

In Figure 9.5, we chose "km" for the time transformation. This spreads the residuals fairly evenly across the plot from left to right, thus avoiding potential problems with outliers distending the x–y relationship. This is fine for the body of the curve, but may give a somewhat misleading representation at the right-hand end of the time scale. It is also a little difficult to interpret, since it uses a left-continuous

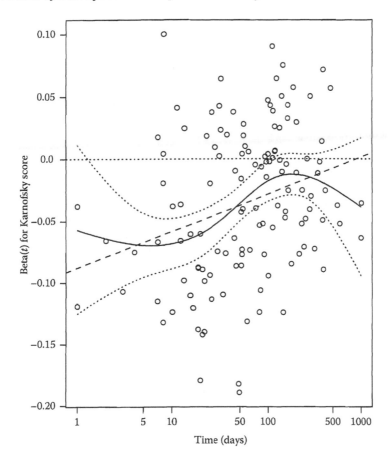

FIGURE 9.6: Graphical diagnostic for proportional hazards assumption: scaled Schoenfeld residuals versus log(time) for Karnofsky score in the analysis of the Veterans Administration lung cancer data from Kalbfleisch and Prentice [8, p. 223] as shown in Therneau and Grambsch [2, p. 135]. The dashed line is the least squares regression line, the solid line is a smooth spline curve, and the dotted line is the smooth spline error band.

version of the Kaplan–Meier survival curve to scale the time axis. Figure 9.6 shows the scaled residuals versus log(time). In this plot it is clearer that the downturn at the right-hand end of the curve may be an artifact of the small numbers at this time, and that the downturn goes away if the last handful of points are removed. Other time transformations available in the S-PLUS function are "identity" ($g(t) = t$) and "rank" for the rank of event times.

The plot given by the S-PLUS function plot.cox.zph() is the default plot for the summary of output of a Cox regression. Following Therneau and Grambsch [2], the sequence is to first fit the model, then summarize the results, and then do the proportional hazards diagnostic plot(s).

```
> fit.vet <- coxph(Surv(futime, status) ~ trt + celltype +
    karno + months + age + prior.rx, data = veteran)
> zph.vet <- cox.zph(fit.vet, transform = 'km')
> plot(zph.vet[3])
```

Note that the object zph.vet is of class cox.zph so that plot(zph.vet[3]) invokes the plotting function plot.cox.zph. In the plot in Figure 9.5, we actually slightly modified the function plot.cox.zph to enable custom axis labels and the reference lines.

9.2.3   Software Analysis and Output

The basic descriptive analysis of time-to-event data may be obtained from the LIFETEST procedure in SAS or the survfit() function in S-PLUS. These analyses produce estimates of the survival curve and/or survivor function using a variety of options including the Kaplan–Meier method described above.

The S-PLUS survfit() function [9] computes an estimate of a survival curve for censored data using either the Kaplan–Meier [1] or the Fleming–Harrington method [10]; or computes the predicted survivor function for a Cox proportional hazards model [2].

The error bars and confidence intervals around the survival curve are computed using the Greenwood formula for the variance. This is a sum of terms $d/(n \times (n - m))$, where d is the number of deaths at a given time point, n is the sum of weights for all individuals still at risk at that time, and m is the sum of weights for the deaths at that time. The justification is based on a binomial argument when weights are all equal to one; extension to the weighted case is ad hoc. Tsiatis [11] proposes a sum of terms $d/(n \times n)$, based on a counting process argument which includes the weighted case.

When the dataset includes left censored or interval censored data (or both), then the expectation-maximization (EM) approach of Turnbull [12] is used to compute the overall curve. When the baseline method is the Kaplan–Meier, this is known to converge to the maximum likelihood estimate. Based on the work of Link [13], the log transform is expected to produce the most accurate confidence intervals; this is used in Figures 9.1 through 9.4.

S-PLUS objects produced by the survfit() function may be graphed automatically by the classed method plot.survfit(). This plot function may be extended as shown in Figures 9.1 through 9.4. The extensions to the plot may be described as arguments to an S-PLUS function, e.g., my.plot.survfit() as follows:

- A "group" argument can be set to allow separate colors and line-styles to be used for the different treatment groups. Different line styles enable the grouping to be apparent if the graph is rendered in black and white.

- A "Trellis" argument can be set to allow different panels to be set for levels of an additional covariable.

- An "n.risk" argument can be set to allow the number of subjects at risk to be displayed at selected times. These times are conveniently displayed below the *x*-axis and aligned with the axis tick labels, and using the same colors as the group variables.

- An "error" argument can be set to allow error bars or confidence intervals to be included on the plot.

- A "truncate" argument can be set to allow truncation of the display at the last observed event or continuation of the plot through the follow-up period.

- A "gridlines" argument can be set to display light horizontal gridlines that help interpret values of the survival functions.

- A "cum.incid" flag can be set for the graph to display cumulative incidence ($= 1 -$ survival) rather than survival, as in Figure 9.2. This results in scaling the *y*-axis to an appropriate upper *y*-axis limit (less than 1) for the cumulative incidence graph rather than setting the lower limit of the *y*-axis to a value greater than 0 for the survival graph.

The extensions listed above require a fundamental rewrite of plot.survfit() to incorporate the Trellis mechanisms of paneling and grouping within panels. These are accomplished by setting up the plot using the setup.2d.trellis function and writing a panel function that computes and plots the survival or cumulative incidence curves by the groups defining the panels and the within panel groups. By using existing Trellis machinery much work is saved. For example, creating panels, drawing axes for each panel and associating different colors and line styles with different levels of grouping is all handled by internal Trellis functions. The creation of the subjects at risk table below the graph is accomplished using non-Trellis graphics commands. The table is written underneath the *x*-axis with mtext(), and the margin space at the bottom of the graph is expanded using par(fig $= \ldots$) to dynamically accommodate the table space.

9.3   Discussion

We have presented graphical analyses for basic presentation of time-to-event data and exploration of assumptions in Cox modeling of time-to-event data. Our graphical analyses extend the usual presentations in current statistical software offerings, SAS and S-PLUS. S-PLUS is generally considered to be the state of the art for graphical analysis and presentation of time-to-event data; and we used S-PLUS software for our extensions.

Our extensions to survival graphics primarily involve providing care and insurance for comparisons being made from the survival plots. Such comparisons are typically made through grouping the plot, i.e., by including multiple survival lines on the plot. We also show how the survival plots may be Trellised to show comparisons across additional covariables. The comparative-care that we introduce includes the addition of confidence intervals or error bars on the plot itself and the addition of the number at risk along the bottom of the x-axis. Both of these additions provide a measure of statistical uncertainty to the survival curves that is especially useful when comparisons are made between covariables on an ongoing basis across the duration of the trial. We also recommend truncating the curves at the last observed event(s) rather than extending the x-axis across the entire follow-up period

We present grouped and Trellised survival and cumulative incidence plots. We recommend both of these forms for the survival plot. Cumulative incidence plots provide a convenient way of anchoring a graph at the (0, 0) origin in the lower-left corner. Both survival and cumulative incidence plots Trellis well across (multiple) covariables provided the curves are banked suitably, e.g., to 45°.

Our graphics for investigation of the proportional hazards model focus on a plot of scaled Schoenfeld residuals versus g(time). This highlights departures from proportional hazards assumption for the case of time-dependent coefficients. Our extensions to standard S-PLUS software are fairly minimal in this case, including the customization of labels and ready addition of lines and curves across time to show the pattern of nonproportional behavior.

For both of cases considered, i.e., survival v time and investigation of proportional hazards assumptions, the use of graphical methods is central to the analysis and presentation of the study and modeling results. We recommend care in the use of graphics for analysis of time-to-event data, so that comparisons of interest are accurately displayed and featured in the presentation.

Acknowledgment

Some of this work was done in collaboration with GSK as part of the Insightful S-PLUS graphics implementation at GSK in 2006–2007. The authors acknowledge the excellent collaborative insight provided by the GSK staff Peter Lane, Shi–Tao Yeh, and Michael Durante in this work. The graphical software contributions of Peter McKinnis, Robert Collins, and Sven Knudsen from Insightful are also acknowledged.

References

[1] Kaplan EL and Meier P (1958): Nonparametric estimation from incomplete observations. *J Am Stat Assoc* 53: 457–481.

[2] Therneau T and Grambsch P (2000): *Modeling Survival Data: Extending the Cox Model*. Springer-Verlag, New York.

[3] Loprinzi CL, Laurie JA, Wieand HS, Krook JE, Novotny PJ, Kugler JW, Bartel J, et al. (1994): Prospective evaluation of prognostic variables from patient-completed questionnaires. *J Clinical Oncol* 12: 601–607.

[4] Pocock SJ, Clayton TC, and Altman DG (2002): Survival plots of time-to-event outcomes in clinical trials: Good practice and pitfalls. *Lancet* 359: 1686–1689.

[5] Cleveland WS (1994): *The Elements of Graphing Data*. Hobart Press, Summit, NJ.

[6] Schag CC, Heinrich RL, and Ganz PA (1984): Karnofsky performance status revisited: Reliability, validity, and guidelines. *J Clinical Oncol* 2: 187–193.

[7] Tufte ER (1984): *Visual Display of Quantitative Information*. Graphics Press cheshire, CT.

[8] Kalbfleisch JD and Prentice, RL (1980): *The Statistical Analysis of Failure Time Data*. Wiley, New York.

[9] TIBCO Spotfire (2006): *S-PLUS* 8: *Guide to Statistics*, vol. 2. Seattle, WA.

[10] Fleming TH and Harrington DP (1984): Nonparametric estimation of the survival distribution in censored data. *Commun Stat* 13: 2469–2486.

[11] Tsiatis A (1981): A large sample study of the estimate for the integrated hazard function in Cox's regression model for survival data. *Ann Stat* 9: 93–108.

[12] Turnbull BW (1974): Nonparametric estimation of a survivorship function with doubly censored data. *J Am Stat Assoc* 69: 169–173.

[13] Link CL (1984): Confidence intervals for the survival function using Cox's proportional hazards model with covariates. *Biometrics* 40: 601–610.

Chapter 10

Design and Analysis of Analgesic Trials

Akiko Okamoto, Julia Wang, and Surya Mohanty

Contents

10.1   Introduction

Pain is the most common symptom for which patients seek medical attention. According to the International Association for the Study of Pain (IASP), pain is defined as an unpleasant sensory and emotional experience associated with actual or potential tissue damage or described in terms of such damage [1]. Pain is always subjective. The subject may experience pain regardless of actual existence of any stimuli, and inability to communicate the pain does not mean that it does not exist. The cause of pain may be underlying disease, injury, surgery, or simply unknown. Pain can be categorized based on its duration as well as mechanisms.

10.1.1   Types of Pain Based on Duration

The diagnosis of pain varies based on the duration, the origin of pain, intensity, pain mechanism, and location of the body. Based on the duration, pain may be categorized to acute and chronic pain. If pain disappears after a period without any medical intervention, it is defined as "acute" pain [2]. The common definition of acute pain is "the normal, predicted physiological response to a noxious chemical, thermal or mechanical stimulus and typically associated with invasive procedures, trauma and disease. It is generally time-limited [3]." For example, a subject undergoes surgery, and immediately after the surgery, the pain is quite severe and requires medical intervention. As the wounds heal, the pain subsides and eventually disappears. This type of pain is considered acute pain. In contrast, if pain persists without medical intervention and/or resolution of the underlying disease condition that causes pain, it is considered "chronic" pain. The common definition of chronic pain is [4] "a state in which pain persists beyond the usual course of an acute disease or healing of an injury or that may or may not be associated with an acute or chronic pathologic process that causes continuous or intermittent pain over months or years." The etiology of acute pain is known (injury/surgery), but the etiology of chronic pain in many cases is unknown. Chronic pain may have no apparent cause. The examples of chronic pain include low back pain and pain due to osteoarthritis and diabetic polyneuropathy.

10.1.2   Mechanism of Pain

Pain is an experience and cannot be separated from the patient's mental state, including his or her environment and cultural background. These factors can be so critical that they can actually cause the brain to trigger or abolish the experience of pain, independent of what is occurring elsewhere in the body. Therefore, when considering pain, it is important to appreciate the appropriate mental and environmental factors.

Pain experts have divided the physical causes of pain into two types: nociceptive and neuropathic pain. The differences are important for understanding the nature of the pain problem.

Examples of nociceptive pain include sprains, bone fractures, burns, bumps, bruises, inflammation (from an infection or arthritic disorder), obstructions, and myofascial pain (which may indicate abnormal muscle stresses).

Nociceptors are the nerves that sense and respond to parts of the body that suffer from damage. The stimulation to the nociceptor due to damage of the tissue is called nociceptive pain. Nociceptors signal tissue irritation, impending injury, or actual injury. When activated, they transmit pain signals (through the peripheral nerves and the spinal cord) to the brain. The pain is typically well localized, constant, and often with an aching or throbbing quality. Visceral pain is the subtype of nociceptive pain that involves the internal organs. It tends to be episodic and poorly localized. Visceral pain may be caused by surgery or injury to the organ itself.

Somatic pain is due to prolonged activation of nociceptive receptors in places such as bone, joint, muscle, or skin. Based on the location of somatic pain, the pain types and intensity may vary. Somatic pain due to an injury to skin or just below the skin, such as minor cuts, may be sharp because of a high concentration of nerve endings. On the other hand, somatic pain due to ligaments, tendons, and bones, such as sprains or broken bones, may be prolonged and dull pain.

Nociceptive pain is usually time-limited, meaning that when the tissue damage heals, the pain typically resolves. (Arthritis is a notable exception in that it is not time-limited.) Another characteristic of nociceptive pain is that it tends to respond well to treatment with opioids.

Examples of neuropathic pain include postherpetic (or postshingles) neuralgia, reflex sympathetic dystrophy/causalgia (nerve trauma), components of cancer pain, phantom limb pain, entrapment neuropathy (e.g., carpal tunnel syndrome), and peripheral neuropathy (widespread nerve damage). Among the many causes of peripheral neuropathy, diabetes is the most common, but the condition can also be caused by chronic alcohol use, exposure to other toxins (including chemotherapy), vitamin deficiencies, and a large variety of other medical conditions—it is not unusual for the cause of the condition to go undiagnosed.

Neuropathic pain is frequently chronic and tends to have a less robust response to treatment with opioids but may respond well to other drugs such as antiseizure and antidepressant medications. Usually, neuropathic problems are not fully reversible, but partial improvement is often possible with proper treatment. Neuropathic pain is defined as pain initiated or caused by the area corresponding to the nervous system [4]. There are two types of neuropathic pain, peripheral and central neuropathic pain. Peripheral neuropathic pain is caused by damage to the nerves. When the damage is caused in the brain, the subsequent pain caused by the damage is considered central neuropathic pain. One of the most frequent classifications of neuropathic pain is based on its etiology [5]. The etiology can vary significantly and include metabolic (e.g., diabetic polyneuropathy), traumatic, infectious, hereditary, and toxic causes. In contrast to nociceptive pain, these persistent pain syndromes offer no biological advantage such as a protective role.

In some conditions the pain appears to be caused by a complex mixture of nociceptive and neuropathic factors. An initial nervous system dysfunction or injury may trigger the neural release of inflammatory mediators and subsequent neurogenic inflammation. For example, migraine headaches probably represent a mixture of neuropathic and nociceptive pain. Myofascial pain is probably secondary to nociceptive input from the muscles, but the abnormal muscle activity may be the result of neuropathic conditions.

10.1.3   Treatment of Pain

The primary objective of pain treatment is to manage pain level not necessarily to alleviate an underlying disease condition. There are no pain treatments that work for all conditions. Pain management can differ based on the pain type. As described here, acute pain is caused by a known trauma to the tissue and considered to heal after a period. Thus, the treatment of acute pain starts immediately. The treatment of chronic pain may differ based on the diagnosis. Though there are no analgesic medications specific for visceral or somatic pain, some medications are approved for specific types of pain such as neuropathic pain [6]. Management of pain can extend beyond standard medications and may include physical therapies and alternative medicines such as traditional Chinese medicines and nutritional supplements. There are several types of medications that are considered for the management of pain. According to the American Pain Society, the medications for acute pain and chronic cancer pain can be classified into three categories: (a) nonopioid analgesics including acetaminophen and nonsteroidal anti-inflammatory drugs (NSAIDs), (b) opioid analgesics, and (c) coanalgesics [7]. These medications can also be taken by patients with chronic pain of nonmalignant origin.

10.1.3.1   Nonopioid Analgesics

The types of nonopioid analgesics include many over-the-counter analgesic medications: acetylsalicylic acid (aspirin), acetaminophen, and NSAIDs. They are all considered effective analgesics to treat mild to moderate pain with different tolerability profiles.

Aspirin is one of the oldest nonopioid oral analgesics. The drug has also been used for cardiac prophylaxis. The common side effect includes gastric bleeding, and it has been considered to have a possible association with Reye's syndrome.

Acetaminophen has analgesic potency similar to that of aspirin but a different side effect profile. Acetaminophen also has a reduced risk of gastric complications such as ulcers compared with nonselective NSAIDs. Though it is safe and effective at the therapeutic dose, it is known to cause severe hepatic damage if overdosed. In acute overdose of acetaminophen, hepatic failure may occur. Since acetaminophen is a common ingredient in many cold medicines and other nonprescription drugs, patients may unknowingly overdose.

In addition to analgesic effects, NSAIDs are useful for pain involving inflammation because of their anti-inflammatory property. The common side effects of the NSAIDs are gastrointestinal effects such as dyspepsia (e.g., indigestion) and in more severe cases, gastric ulcers. Selective NSAIDs such as COX-2 inhibitors have an improved gastric side effect profile but are considered to have increased cardiac side effects in prolonged use. Some NSAIDs such as ketorolac may cause renal insufficiency in patients.

10.1.3.2   Opioid Analgesics

Depending on the pain level and conditions, nonopioid analgesics do not provide sufficient pain control in some subjects. In these situations, opioid analgesics may provide additional pain relief. Opioid analgesics are also the basis of management of postoperative pain. Many of the opioid medications are μ-opioid agonists. All μ-agonists provide similar analgesia and side effects though individual patients respond differently to different opioids. Opioid analgesics have multiple formulations such as oral, intravenous, transdermal, subcutaneous, intramuscular, and intraspinal, and their uses are specific to the condition and location of pain and surgical procedures applied. The most common side effects of opioid analgesics are nausea, vomiting, and constipation. For prolonged use of opioids, physical dependence on the drug and increased tolerability may become a problem. When the medication is suddenly stopped, the patient may experience symptoms related to withdrawal. The symptoms may include anxiety, irritability, and physical conditions such as chills and hot flashes. When it is necessary to discontinue opioids, doses should be decreased gradually to avoid withdrawal symptoms.

10.1.3.3 Coanalgesics

Coanalgesics are the medication that may enhance the effects of acetaminophen, opioids, or NSAIDs or have independent analgesic activities. Certain types of pain do not respond to typical analgesics. For example, patients with neuropathic pain do not respond to NSAIDs [8]. In some patients with neuropathic pain or fibromyalgia, antidepressants such as tricyclics, selective norepinephrine reuptake inhibitors (SNRIs), or antiepileptics such as gabapentins have been shown to provide pain relief.

10.1.4 Drug Development in Pain

There were approved or draft guidelines by the Committee for Medicinal Products for Human Use (CHMP) in the European Medicines Agency for clinical medicinal products intended for the treatment of nociceptive pain and neuropathic pains [9]. There are no final guidelines available by the Food and Drug Administration for the development of medicines for pain. The guidelines for nociceptive pain by the CHMP describe that the development program should consist of pharmacokinetic studies, interaction studies, dose–response studies, and/or pivotal efficacy studies. They also state that additional pharmacokinetic studies should be conducted for medication with different routes of administration beyond those considered following the existing guidelines to assess the effect on absorption levels.

Since pain is associated with other underlying disease conditions, comorbidity is common, and interaction with other medications should be carefully assessed. Especially, common medication taken in the population intended to be studied in the pivotal efficacy and safety studies should be examined for the effect of potential drug–drug interaction. The guidelines also recommend that well-planned dose ranging studies should be carried out before confirmatory pivotal studies. Depending on the indication and degree of pain and management, appropriate doses should be used in clinical trials to minimize the adverse events, while producing a useful level of pain relief.

10.1.5   Assessment of Pain

Since pain is subjective, patients themselves must perform pain assessment. Inability to sufficiently communicate pain often results in undertreatment of the condition; it is critical to have the appropriate measurement tool to assess pain. Pain can be measured directly as pain intensity and pain relief but also using surrogate measures such as the use of rescue medication, time to first rescue medication, and physical functions. Pain intensity and pain relief scores are assessed on a scheduled interval. In chronic pain studies, the pain intensity may be measured daily or twice a day. In acute pain studies, the assessment of pain intensity is more frequent and often several pain scores are assessed relative to the intake of medication. Pain intensity is assessed in clinical studies in both chronic and acute pain studies, and the pain relief scale is commonly assessed in clinical studies in acute pain. The pain relief scale is not strongly correlated with changes between pre- and posttreatment pain intensities. In some patients, pain relief scores indicate some level of pain reduction, whereas the changes in pain intensity indicate no reduction or increase in pain level compared to the pretreatment level. This may be due to difficulty recalling the original pain level after a period of treatment.

Pain intensity can be assessed using the visual analog scale (VAS), numerical rating scales (NRS), and verbal rating scales (VRS). No one scale was shown to be superior to the other scales in detecting treatment effect in a consistent manner [10]. The VASs usually show higher failure rates than NRSs and VRSs, and NRSs tend to show higher failure rates than VRS when there are differences. VRSs and NRSs tend to be preferred over VASs by patients [11]. Increased age and amount of opioid intake are associated with more difficulty completing the VAS [11]. NRS was also shown to be correlated with patients' ratings of global impression of change (CGIC)—which has been validated and is commonly used as a measure of the overall condition [12].

10.2   Confirmatory Trial Designs

Clinical trials of analgesics for chronic pain often have difficulty showing the treatment effect against placebo even in situations in which the effect of the medication is known. A review of 29 clinical trails in opioid analgesics examined the effect of study designs and use of concomitant analgesic medications. It showed that flexible-dose designs were associated with the positive outcome of the studies. Though it was not clear from the review that the use of concomitant analgesic medication affected the study outcome, it affects pain intensity assessments if the medication is taken before the pain assessment [12].

10.2.1   Study Design

The design of many confirmatory trials is the double-blind controlled randomized design (CRD) (if single center) or controlled randomized balanced design (CRBD) (if multicenter), in which patients are randomly assigned to parallel groups. The groups would reflect at least one dose level of the drug under development and a control—either placebo and/or, in many cases, an active comparator. The subjects undergo a screening period to assess their eligibility for participation. Upon completion, eligible patients assess the pain intensity (baseline pain) and are randomized to receive either the active treatment or the control. During the treatment period, the patient continues to assess the pain level on an ongoing basis.

Other trial designs used are the randomized withdrawal design. This uses the enriched population that has shown response to the treatment. Patients undergo a screening period and assess baseline pain intensity. Then they start receiving the active treatment for a period of time. At the end of the treatment period, patients are assessed for their eligibility to continue. The eligibility criteria may include tolerability (no severe or serious AEs) and efficacy (shown response to the medication) aspects. Only patients who meet the criteria are randomized to receive active treatment or placebo. The randomized patients continue assessing the pain intensity. Additional caution must be exercised in the case of analgesics that may cause withdrawal effects, because it is difficult to distinguish the worsening of pain condition from the symptom of withdrawal. A clinical trial in an enriched population is acceptable as a confirmatory study; however, if the medication is intended to treat patients in general population with pain, a trial in a nonenriched population must be conducted to show efficacy in the intended population.

10.2.2 Duration

For acute pain studies, the duration of the study is short due to the nature of pain. In a single-dose study such as dental surgery study, the duration of the treatment period is 8–12 h. Even in multiple-dose studies, the duration of the treatment period is 1–10 days long. In chronic pain studies, the treatment duration is often 12 weeks. If the dosing regimen requires titration, the required duration for the titration should be added to the overall treatment duration.

10.2.3 Doses

Previously, trials in acute pain may have included single-dose studies. In these studies, patients are randomized to receive active treatment or placebo. After randomization, they receive one dose of the medication and continue assessing the intensity of pain until study completion or intake of rescue analgesic medications. Since a single dose does not provide information on accumulating effects and usually the medication is intended to be taken more than once, confirmatory trials usually require multiple doses.

Many confirmatory studies use a fixed-dose study design. Subjects were randomized to drug (under development) or control. If more than one dose of drug is studied, patients are randomized to the dose groups or to the control. The patients are not allowed to change doses during the treatment period. If the intake of medication is more than once a day, the frequency of intake may or may not vary depending on the intended dosing regimen of the study medication. For example, if the medication is intended to be given every 4–6 h (such as acetaminophen), the study may be conducted by fixing the regimen to every 4 h to allow maximum exposure or by applying the intended dosing regimen.

Flexible dosing may also be applied in confirmatory clinical trials. Subjects are randomized to the drug group or to a placebo group (if that is the control). Medication would be packaged for various dose levels to maintain blinding. Typically, patients begin study medication on the lowest dose. During the treatment period, the dose may be titrated upward or downward based on the response (or lack thereof) to the current dose. These designs may be preferred in a situation when patients' pain levels vary often and when they may not achieve adequate pain control at a fixed dose. If the flexible-dose design is used in a confirmatory trial, additional analyses examining the patterns of changes in doses may be required.

10.2.4   Primary Endpoint

In many pain studies, the primary endpoint is based on pain intensity. Daily or weekly average pain intensity may be calculated from the individual pain intensities assessed by subjects and used as the primary endpoint. In acute pain studies, the sum of pain intensity and the sum of pain relief are also commonly used. Sum of Pain Intensity Difference (SPID) is defined as the weighted sum over all changes from baseline in pain intensity (PID) to a specified time point with the actual time elapsed from the previous pain assessment as the weight. Similarly, Total Pain Relief (TOTPAR) is defined as the weighted sum over all pain relief with the actual time elapsed from the previous pain relief assessment as the weight. Sum of SPID and TOTPAR is called Sum of TOTPAR and sum of Pain Intensity Difference and Relief (SPRID). Any one of these endpoints may be considered as a primary endpoint.

Using pain intensity, percent change from baseline can be calculated. This score is often considered a useful clinical endpoint. The percent change of 30% or 50% in pain intensity is considered clinically meaningful, and analysis of these endpoints is often performed. In an acute breakthrough cancer pain study, a change score of -2.0 and a percentage change of -33% on the NRS (an 11-point NRS with 0 being no pain and 10 being the worst it could be) were shown to be associated with the clinically important outcome defined as a patient's need to take additional medication to treat pain [13].

In an enriched study, additional criteria of time to treatment failure can also be considered as a primary endpoint. The treatment failure will be determined based on the predefined criteria depending on pain intensity or use of rescue medication. Time to treatment failure is defined as time between randomization and the time the criteria for the treatment failure were met. If the patient does not meet the criteria during the treatment period after randomization, time to treatment failure is censored at the time of discontinuation or completion of the treatment.

If pain intensity is used in the study, it is critical to understand the use of concomitant or rescue analgesic medication. In many studies, rescue analgesic medications were discouraged to reduce the confounding effect. However, in some situations, the use of rescue analgesic medication may be required to ensure that patients remain in the study. Use of concomitant or rescue analgesic medication may affect the pain intensity scores and ultimately influence the primary endpoint.

Especially in acute pain clinical studies, the treatment duration is quite short, pain intensity is severe, and the assessments of pain intensity are frequent; the use of rescue medications can influence many of the pain intensity scores. In order to reduce the effect of rescue analgesic medications, the pain scores may be imputed or ignored until the time when the effect of rescue analgesic is no longer impacted. Since pain is subjective, the effect of analgesic medication on pain intensity varies from patient to patient. Thus, completely distinguishing the effect of the study medication and the rescue analgesic medications may not be possible. In these situations, different endpoints that take into account the use of rescue medication may be needed.

The following sections focus on the time to rescue medication as a surrogate endpoint to pain intensity in acute pain clinical trials.

10.3 Surrogate Endpoints and Time to Rescue

Surrogate endpoints such as intermediate endpoints or biomarkers have been used for possible reduction in sample size or trial duration. Such endpoints are evaluated before the true clinical endpoints are observed. An intermediate endpoint occurs sometime between a given exposure or intervention that affects the disease process and the time of clinical diagnosis of the disease. A biomarker is a characteristic that is objectively measured and evaluated as an indicator of normal biological processes, pathogenic processes, or pharmacologic responses to a therapeutic intervention. A valid surrogate endpoint is expected to predict clinical benefit and allows correct inference to be drawn regarding the effect of an intervention on the often unobserved true clinical endpoint of interest.

In analgesic trials, reduction in painful sensation has been the primary objective, which naturally leads to pain relief and current pain intensity scores being the true clinical endpoints of interests. However, subjects need rescue with other analgesics due to insufficient pain relief that leads to missing pain relief and intensity scores. On the other hand, the time to rescue is either fully observed or censored at the end of observation period scheduled for the study. Unlike the commonly used surrogate endpoints, the time to rescue is observed at the same time these true clinical endpoints are being collected. It will not lead to reduction in trial duration. However, it will lead to a statistical inference unhampered by missing value imputation strategies. In the event that a most conservative imputation strategy has to be adopted for the calculations of primary variables such as TOTPAR or SPID, the use of time to rescue as a primary variable often leads to reduction in sample size.

For time to rescue to reach a correct inference regarding the analgesic effect of the tested compound, it needs to function as a full surrogate endpoint for the primary variables based on the longitudinally collected pain relief/intensity profiles, such as TOTPAR or SPID, as governed by Prentice criterion.

According to the Prentice criterion [14], a surrogate for a true endpoint should yield a valid test of the null hypothesis of no association between treatment and the true response. This criterion essentially requires the surrogate variable to "capture" any relationship between the treatment and the true endpoint, a notion that can be operationalized by requiring the distribution of the true endpoint to be independent of treatment, given the value of the surrogate variable.

Let us assume V is the primary variable, S is the time to rescue, and X is the variable indicating study dose or treatment groups. For S to be a surrogate for V, we should have

$$P(V|X,S) = P(V|S) \tag{10.1}$$

Graphically, Equation 10.1 implies that at each level of S, the distributions of V look similar for all levels of X. From a modeling standpoint, when V is fitted as a function of X and S, the effect of X should be negligible.

For surrogate endpoint S to give a valid test of the null hypothesis of no association between treatment and the true response V, Condition A below should hold.

Condition A:

$$P(S|X) = P(S) \text{ leads to } P(V|X) = P(V)$$

This implies that when we reject the null hypothesis of no treatment effect based on S, we should also reject the null hypothesis of no treatment effect based on V. If we make a Type-I error using S, we also make a Type-I error using V.

On the other hand, an association between treatment and S should also lead to an association between treatment and V; therefore, Condition B below should also hold.

Condition B:

$$P(S|X) \neq P(S) \text{ leads to } P(V|X) \neq P(V)$$

or equivalently,

$$P(V|X) = P(V) \text{ leads to } P(S|X) = P(S)$$

When S is a surrogate of V and satisfies Equation 10.1, Condition A holds automatically, because

$$P(V|X) = \int P(V|X,S)*f(S|X)dS = \int P(V|S)*f(S|X)dS = \int P(V|S)*f(S)dS = P(V)$$

$$\tag{10.2}$$

On the other hand, when Condition B holds with $P(V|X) = P(V)$ and S is a surrogate of V, we have from Equation 10.2

$$\int P(V|S)*f(S|X)dS = \int P(V|S)*f(S)dS \tag{10.3}$$

For this to lead to $P(S|X) = P(S)$, we need additional assumptions. First, we should have

$$P(V|S) \neq P(V) \qquad (10.4)$$

since when $P(V|S) = P(V)$, we will have Equation 10.3 regardless of the relationship between S and X. This means that V and S should not be independent. Graphically, the distributions of V should be different at different levels of S. From the modeling perspective, when V is fitted as a function of S, the effect of S should not be negligible.

Still, there exist possible functions of $f(S|X)$ that satisfy Equation 10.3 but still invalidate Condition B. Prentice discussed restricting the functional forms of $f(S|X)$ so that Equation 10.3 leads to Condition B.

In the special case when Equation 10.4 holds and also $P(V|S)$ is monotonic in S, in the sense that V is stochastically larger for bigger S and $P(S|X)$ is either flat with no dose–response or monotonic in X with S stochastically higher with higher dose, Equation 10.3 will lead to Condition B.

Conditions A and B ensure that the statistical inferences on the effect of treatment group X on the true clinical endpoint V and the surrogate S are the same in terms of rejecting the null hypothesis. If the null hypothesis of no treatment effect is rejected using one of either V or S, the similar null hypothesis should also be rejected using one of either V or S. For an analgesic with demonstrable efficacy, the distributions of V and those of S should be discernibly different simultaneously at different levels of X graphically. This is made possible as V and S are both observable at the same time in the acute pain trials. From a modeling perspective, both a fitting of V as a function of X as well as a fitting of S as a function of X should demonstrate nonnegligible effect of X at the same time.

In the case of an analgesic with demonstrable efficacy using V or S where S acts as a surrogate for V, the effect of X should be nonnegligible when V is fitted as a function of X alone but negligible when V is fitted as a function of both X and S. Ideally, we would like to see the estimated treatment group difference change from highly significant without adjustment for S to vanishing small after adjustment for S. In the surrogate endpoint literature [15], the percent change in the magnitudes of effect in X from these two models, or proportion of treatment effect explained by the surrogate percentage of treatment effect (PTE), has been used to estimate the proportion of net effect of true endpoint, which is explained by the effect of the surrogate. For a perfect surrogate the true unobserved PTE should be 1 and the estimated PTE should be consistent with this fact. The estimation of PTE does not necessarily imply that the surrogate has caused a portion of the change in the true clinical endpoint.

In the discussions so far, vague terms such as "negligible" and "nonnegligible" effects have been used. These terms have meanings in a sense relative to each other. A relatively smaller effect becomes negligible in comparison to a relatively larger effect that is nonnegligible and vice versa. Due to the influence of sample sizes and Type-I errors of statistical tests, being "statistically significant" is not always a criterion for declaring a nonnegligible effect.

10.4   Examples

In this section, two examples are given to demonstrate the surrogacy of the time to rescue to the longitudinally collected pain relief and pain intensity scores. The first is an 8 h single-dose dental pain study, and the second is a 12 h multiple-dose bunionectomy study. In the first example, the time to rescue fully captured the treatment effect exhibited in the primary efficacy variable. The situation was not as ideal in the second example. However, this example exposed design considerations that need to be incorporated to ensure that the time to rescue acts as a full surrogate for the primary efficacy variable.

10.4.1   Single-Dose Dental Pain Study

An analgesic drug T was being developed for moderate to moderately severe acute pain. Eighty subjects experiencing pain from an oral surgical procedure were enrolled for each of the five treatment arms: placebo, 50, 100, 200, and 300 mg of drug T for a total of 400 subjects in the study. Following the administration of study medication, subjects evaluated current pain relief compared to baseline and current pain intensity at 30 min, and 1, 2, 3, 4, 5, 6, 7, and 8 h after medication. Pain relief was evaluated using a five-point categorical scale (0, none; 1, a little; 2, some; 3, a lot; 4, complete) where higher scores indicate greater pain relief and 0 indicates no pain relief. Pain intensity was evaluated using an 11-point NRS ranging from $0 =$ no pain to $10 =$ most severe pain. Subjects were encouraged to wait for at least 1 h after study drug intake and until current pain intensity returned to the baseline level before requesting a rescue analgesic, after which the pain relief and pain intensity scores were no longer collected. These missing scores were imputed using last-observation-carried-forward (LOCF) in the planned analysis for the study. The 8 h TOTPAR score was selected as the primary efficacy variable.

10.4.1.1   Time to Rescue

Subjects started to request rescue analgesics at 1 h after study drug administration. For subjects who withdrew or completed the study without taking rescue medication, their times to rescue were censored at the last observation time point.

For those subjects who took rescue analgesics, their last pain relief score before rescue are summarized in Table 10.1. Nearly all subjects (96.6%) who took rescue had pain relief scores of 0 (no pain relief), and all except one subject of the rest had pain relief scores of 1 (a little pain relief). Either these subjects did not experience any pain relief from treatment or the treatment effect had worn out. Therefore, the time to rescue was related to the temporal analgesic profile of the treatment and was clearly driven by the lack of efficacy at the time of rescue request.

The distribution of the time to rescue for each treatment group was estimated by Kaplan–Meier survival curves and compared across groups using the log-rank statistics, as shown in Figure 10.1.

Except for the tail portion of the 50 mg dose group, there is a clear monotonic dose–response observed at almost all time points. Time to rescue has captured the

TABLE 10.1: Distribution of last pain relief scores before taking rescue.

	Pain Relief Score				
Group	0	1	2	3	4
Placebo (N = 73)	71 (97.3%)	2 (2.7%)	0	0	0
50 mg (N = 58)	56 (96.6%)	2 (3.4%)	0	0	0
100 mg (N = 67)	63 (94.0%)	3 (4.5%)	0	0	1 (1.5%)
200 mg (N = 55)	54 (98.2%)	1 (1.8%)	0	0	0
300 mg (N = 42)	41 (97.6%)	1 (2.4%)	0	0	0
Total (N = 295)	285 (96.6%)	9 (3.1%)	0	0	1 (0.3%)

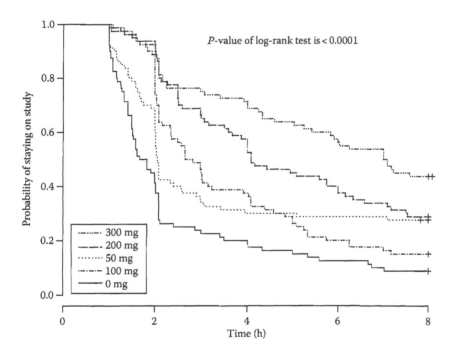

FIGURE 10.1: Estimated distribution of time to rescue.

highly statistically significant treatment effect. Based on Figure 10.1, it is reasonable to assume that underlying unobserved survival distribution follows monotonic dose–response at all time points.

10.4.1.2 Pain Profiles Stratified by Time to Rescue

To examine how much of the treatment effect has been captured by the time to rescue, jittered individual pain relief profiles over time were plotted for the five treatment groups, stratified by the time to rescue and presented in Figure 10.2. Subjects who rescued between the same two successive observation time points

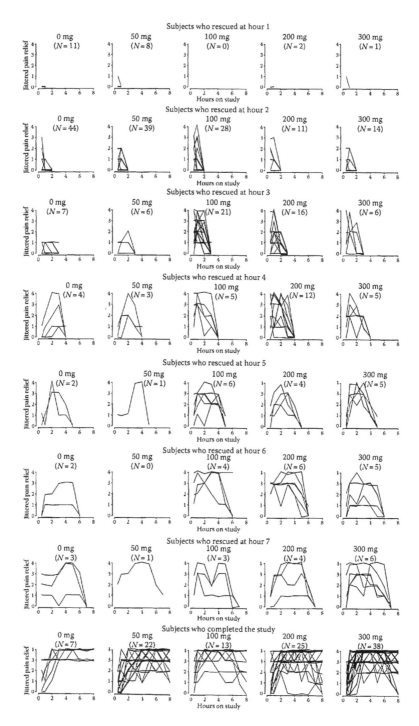

FIGURE 10.2: Individual pain relief profile over time.

were grouped together, and their pain relief scores collected just before taking rescue were entered for the next scheduled observation time point.

We observe from Figure 10.2 that the subjects who rescued at the same time had very similar pain relief profiles regardless of treatments, meaning that conditional on the time to rescue, there is very little treatment effect left to be captured by the pain relief scores. In addition, rescue intake was clearly efficacy-driven. Pain relief scores remained or returned to 0 before rescue, while almost all subjects who completed the study had continued to receive pain relief from study treatment at hour 8. Subjects who rescued at hour 1 experienced none or minimal pain relief from treatment. The longer it took subjects to rescue, the longer they experienced pain relief. Moreover, more placebo subjects rescued early and more actively treated subjects rescued later or completed the study in a dose–response fashion. Lastly, the temporal profiles of pain relief and time to rescue obviously were not independent.

In Figure 10.3, the mean pain relief profiles over time are plotted for the five treatment groups stratified by the time to rescue. The stratified mean temporal profiles form patterns that are remarkably similar across the five dose groups. The calculation of the primary efficacy variable, TOTPAR, requires imputation for the missing pain relief scores after rescue. Since 96.6% of the pain relief scores just before rescue were zeros, all of the LOCF imputations (as well as the baseline-observation-carried-forward [BOCF] and worst-observation-carried-forward [WOCF] imputations) for these subjects were zeros. Therefore, the stratified mean TOTPARs should also form similar patterns across the five dose groups.

The TOTPARs calculated using LOCF imputation were plotted in Figure 10.4, stratified by the time to rescue. For subjects who rescued around the same time, their

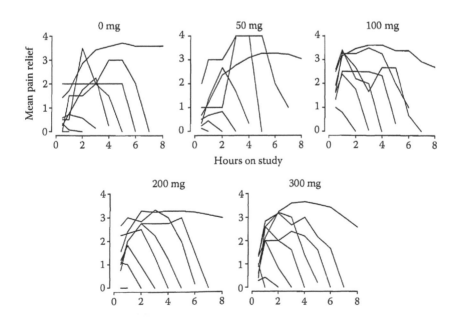

FIGURE 10.3: Mean pain relief profile over time.

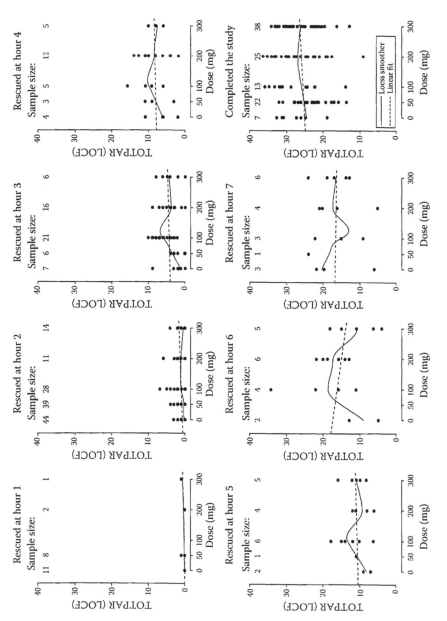

FIGURE 10.4: Individual TOTPAR over dose, stratified by time to rescue.

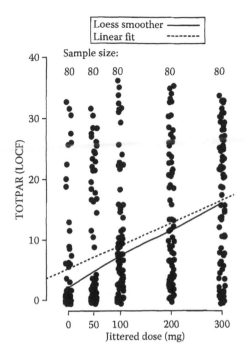

FIGURE 10.5: Individual TOTPAR over jittered dose.

TOTPARs were plotted again dose. By visual examination, TOTPARs do not seem to capture any monotonic dose–response within each panel. Both a Loess smoother and a linear line were fitted in each panel, and they are very similar, suggesting a plausible flat linear relationship.

The TOTPARs were also plotted against doses regardless of time to rescue and are presented in Figure 10.5. Both the loess smoother and the linear fit showed an upward dose–response. This monotonic dose–response was driven by that exhibited by time to rescue, as the overall mean TOTPAR for each dose group is a weighted average of the mean TOTPARs in each rescue strata, and the weights are determined by the distribution of time to rescue.

10.4.1.3 Percentage of Treatment Effect Explained

We have seen graphically that the monotonic dose–response in TOTPAR seemed to have disappeared once conditioning on the distribution of time to rescue, which also exhibited a monotonic dose–response. Judging from Figures 10.4 and 10.5, it is reasonable to assume a linear dose–response relationship within the studied dose range. Two linear models were fitted to estimate the PTE explained. In the first model, TOTPAR was fitted as a linear model of dose and time to rescue. Time to rescue was treated as a factor of eight levels at hours 1–8. In the second model, TOTPAR was fitted as a linear model of dose only.

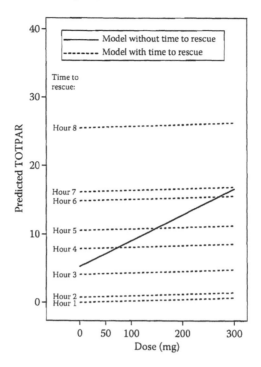

FIGURE 10.6:   Predicted dose–response of TOTPAR.

Both models can be valid representations of the unobserved reality. In the first model, time to rescue was included explicitly to account for the variability observed in the data, whereas in the second model, this portion of the variability was unexplained and absorbed into the residual error. The individual TOTPAR may not be following a normal distribution with identical variances in these two models. Therefore, variability estimates and test statistics are ignored.

PTE explained will be estimated using the following recipe. It will be estimated as the percent change of the coefficients of the dose variable from the second model to the first model. Its statistical properties can be estimated with the bootstrap technique.

The coefficients of dose in the first and second models are 0.229 (very negligible) and 3.769 per 100 mg dose, respectively. PTE is estimated as 93.9% with a 95% bootstrap percentile confidence interval of (84%, 100.0%) based on 10,000 bootstrap simulations.

The predicted linear dose–responses of TOTPAR from both models are presented in Figure 10.6. Time to rescue is a highly statistically significant covariate. Its effect can be seen in Figure 10.6.

10.4.2   Repeated-Dose Bunionectomy Study

An analgesic drug V was being developed for moderate to moderately severe acute pain. Around 80 subjects experiencing pain from a bunionectomy surgical procedure were enrolled for each of the four treatment arms: placebo, 50, 100, and

200 mg of drug T for a total of 316 subjects in the study. A total of three doses were given at 4 h intervals each. Subjects evaluated current pain relief compared to baseline (0, none; 1, a little; 2, some; 3, a lot; 4, complete) and current pain intensity at 30 min, and 1, 2, 3, 4, 5, 6, 7, 8, 10, and 12 h after the first dose. A VAS ranging from $0 =$ no pain to $100 =$ most severe pain was used to measure current pain intensity. Subjects were allowed to take rescue analgesic 90 min after study drug intake, after which the pain relief and pain intensity scores were no longer collected. These missing scores were imputed using LOCF in the planned analysis for the study. The 12 h TOTPAR score was selected as the primary efficacy variable.

10.4.2.1 Time to Rescue

Subjects started to request for rescue analgesics at 90 min after study drug administration. For subjects who withdrew or completed the study without taking rescues, their times to rescue were censored at the last observation time point.

Unlike the first example, subjects were not required to wait until their pain relief returned to baseline before requesting rescue. For those subjects who took rescue analgesics, their last pain relief scores before rescue are summarized in Table 10.2. Only 47% of the subjects who took rescue had no pain relief compared to baseline. There were 14% of the subjects, all in the actively treated groups, with a considerable degree of or complete pain relief requesting rescue analgesics. Lack of efficacy is no longer the main reason for taking rescues.

The distribution of the time to rescue for each treatment group was estimated by Kaplan–Meier survival curves and compared across groups using the log-rank statistics, as shown in Figure 10.7.

Figure 10.7 demonstrates a clear monotonic dose–response observed at all time points. The higher the dose, the fewer the subjects who took rescues at any given time point. Time to rescue has captured the highly statistically significant treatment effect. Based on Figure 10.7, it is also reasonable to assume that the underlying unobserved survival distribution follows monotonic dose–response at all time points.

10.4.2.2 Pain Profiles Stratified by Time to Rescue

Again, to examine how much of the treatment effect had been captured by the time to rescue, jittered individual pain relief profiles over time were plotted for the four

TABLE 10.2: Distribution of last pain relief scores before taking rescue.

	Pain Relief Score				
Group	0	1	2	3	4
Placebo ($N = 72$)	44 (61%)	16 (22%)	12 (17%)	0	0
50 mg ($N = 58$)	24 (41%)	12 (21%)	11 (19%)	9 (16%)	2 (3.4%)
100 mg ($N = 43$)	18 (42%)	11 (26%)	5 (12%)	6 (14%)	3 (7%)
200 mg ($N = 41$)	14 (34%)	12 (29%)	5 (12%)	6 (15%)	4 (9.8)
Total ($N = 214$)	100 (47%)	51 (24%)	33 (15%)	21 (9.8%)	9 (4.2%)

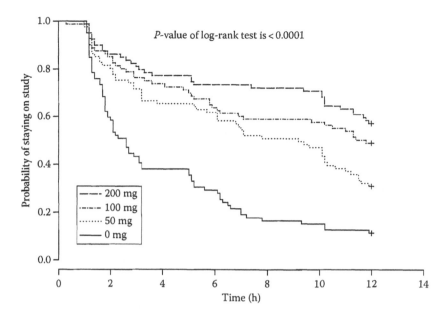

FIGURE 10.7:   Estimated distribution of time to rescue.

treatment groups stratified by the time to rescue. These plots for the six selected time points are presented in Figure 10.8. Subjects who rescued between the same two successive observation time points were grouped together, and their pain relief scores were collected just before taking rescue and were entered for the next scheduled observation time point.

From Figure 10.8, we again observe that the subjects who rescued at the same time had very similar pain relief profiles regardless of treatments, meaning that conditional on the time to rescue, there is very little treatment effect left to be captured by the pain relief scores. However, rescue intake was no longer clearly efficacy-driven. Pain relief scores did not remain or return to 0 before rescue for all subjects. Subjects who rescued at hour 1 experienced none or minimal pain relief from treatment. The longer it took subjects to rescue, the longer they had experienced pain relief. More placebo subjects rescued early and more actively treated subjects rescued later or completed the study in a dose–response fashion. The temporal profiles of pain relief and time to rescue were not independent.

The mean pain relief profiles over time were plotted for the four treatment groups stratified by the time to rescue (Figure 10.9). The stratified mean temporal profiles form patterns that still look roughly similar across the four dose groups. The calculation of the primary efficacy variable, TOTPAR, when using any of the imputation strategies, such as LOCF, BOCF, or WOCF, that are based solely on the observed pain relief scores to fill in the missing pain relief scores after rescue, will remain similar within each rescue strata. Therefore, the stratified mean TOTPARs should also form similar patterns across the four dose groups.

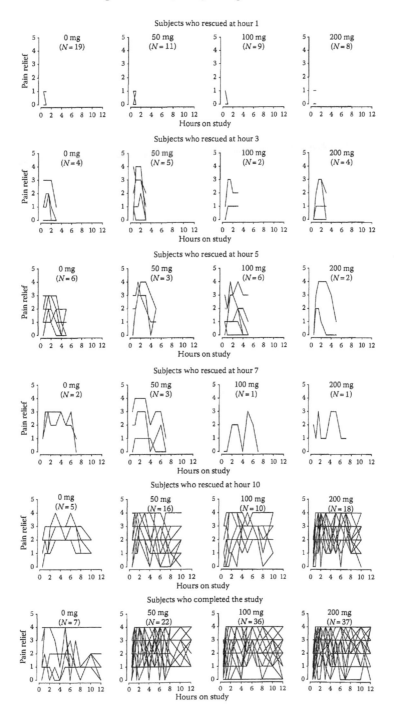

FIGURE 10.8: Individual pain relief profile over time.

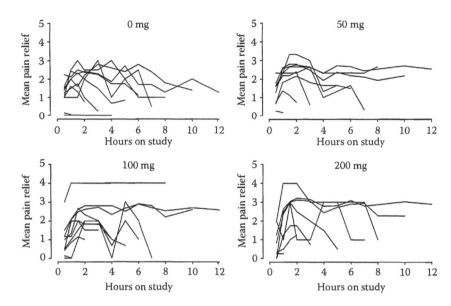

FIGURE 10.9:   Mean pain relief profile over time.

The TOTPARs calculated using LOCF imputation are plotted in Figure 10.10, stratified by the time to rescue. Since subjects were scheduled to take the second dose of study medication at hour 4 and the third dose at hour 8, there were respectively only three and six subjects who requested rescue analgesic before hours 4 and 8, and these are not presented. For subjects who rescued around the same time, their TOTPARS were plotted against dose. By visual examination, TOTPARs do not seem to capture any monotonic dose–response within each panel except the last two. Both a loess smoother and a linear line were fitted in each panel, and they are very similar, suggesting a linear relationship.

In contrast to Figure 10.4, there was a clear dose–response captured by the pain relief scores among the subjects who completed the study. Since the third dose was given at hour 8, there was sufficient treatment effect remaining at hour 12 not captured by time to rescue, which was censored at that point. It is possible that this would not have been an issue had time to rescue been captured beyond hour 12.

There was a clear dose–response captured by the pain relief scores among the subjects who took rescue by hour 10 as well. As seen from Figure 10.8, many of these subjects were still experiencing pain relief from the third dose when they took rescue. It was suspected that these subjects wanted to leave the study earlier as it was quite late in the night, and this phenomenon affected all treatment groups equally. It is also possible that this would not have been an issue had time to rescue been captured beyond hour 10 for these subjects.

The plot of TOTPAR against dose regardless of time to rescue is presented in Figure 10.11. Both the loess smoother and the linear fit showed an upward dose–response. As explained in the last example, this monotonic dose–response was

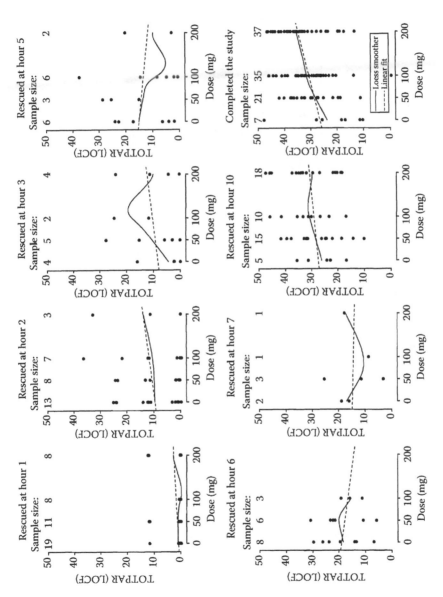

FIGURE 10.10: Individual TOTPAR over dose. stratified by time to rescue.

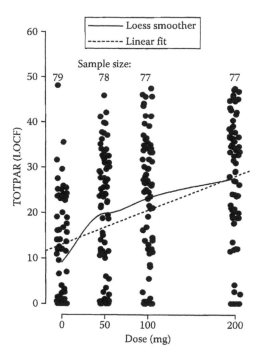

FIGURE 10.11: Individual TOTPAR over jittered dose.

chiefly driven by that exhibited by time to rescue. In addition, it was also driven by the remaining dose–response in pain relief scores not captured by time to rescue.

10.4.2.3   Percentage of Treatment Effect Explained

As before, two linear models were fitted to estimate the PTE explained. In the first model, TOTPAR was fitted as a linear model of dose and time to rescue. Time to rescue was treated as a factor of 10 levels at hours 1–8 and hours 10 and 12. In the second model, TOTPAR was fitted as a linear model of dose only.

PTE explained was estimated as the percent change of the coefficients of the dose variable from the second model to the first model. The coefficients of dose in the first and second models are 2.25 and 7.43 per 100 mg dose, respectively. PTE is estimated as 69.7% with a 95% bootstrap percentile confidence interval of (57.8%, 91.9%) based on 10,000 bootstrap simulations.

Ideally, a perfect surrogate should have a PTE as close to 100% as possible. Time to rescue only explained an estimated 69.7% of the efficacy in TOTPAR in this example. There are two major reasons for this. The first is that the subjects were not required to wait until their pain had returned to baseline before remedicating with rescue, and therefore, a significant portion of the subjects took rescue without having the need. This practice severed the transfer of efficacy signal from the pain scores to time to rescue because the act of rescue taking was no longer entirely driven by lack

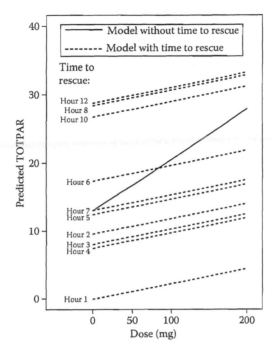

FIGURE 10.12: Predicted dose–response of TOTPAR.

of efficacy. The second reason is the failure of documenting rescue intake beyond the analgesic duration of the last study dose. Both of these drawbacks can be easily rectified. The predicted linear dose–responses of TOTPAR from both models are presented in Figure 10.12.

10.5 Discussion

In controlled clinical trials involving acute pain, efficacy variables such as pain relief/intensity scores are collected over time. The time course of these variables is vital for understanding the analgesic effect of the test compound. The treatment group comparisons, as well as the estimation of the onset and duration of analgesic activities, are closely related to and dependent on these profiles. The primary variables in these studies, such as TOTPAR, are typically time-weighted summary variables derived from the longitudinally collected pain relief/intensity scores.

One complicating factor in the design and analysis of acute analgesic trials is the intake of rescue analgesics when subjects experience insufficient pain relief from study medication before the end of the evaluation period. Pain relief/intensity scores collected after the rescue intake no longer reflect the sole analgesic activities of the study medication. As it is unethical to deny subjects adequate analgesic treatment, it has been a common practice to stop collecting pain relief/intensity scores after rescue and withdraw the patient from the study. Variations of this practice exist, which produce a similar outcome: missing pain relief/intensity scores caused by intake of rescue analgesics.

Missing pain relief/intensity scores pose difficulties for statistical analysis. Analysis based on completers has been known to be biased. In order to include all randomized subjects in the analysis, imputation methods have to be used to fill in the missing scores. Historically, the LOCF has been the prevailing method of choice for its ease of use and also for a lack of a gold-standard imputation strategy. Other imputation strategies routinely used in analgesic trials include BOCF and WOCF. Missing value imputation is a notoriously difficult statistical problem due to the inherent assumptions being untestable. Statistical analyses and conclusions are influenced by how missing data are imputed. Missingness in the data may be due to different reasons, and thus various patterns of missingness can occur in the data. Aggregate effect of the imputation is dependent on the differential missing patterns in various treatment groups. Prespecification of an imputation strategy is quite challenging because it is extremely difficult to predict these patterns of missingness within each treatment group in a double-blind trial.

Having missing value imputation strategy affecting statistical inference is not the ideal situation. The LOCF has been used across almost all analgesic trials without much deliberation. This practice has served to standardize the imputation aspect of statistical analysis across all trials from all sponsors and helped to exempt this issue from intense regulatory scrutiny. More recently, this has changed, and regulatory agencies have been requesting sponsors to justify their imputation strategies and conduct sensitivity analyses using various other methods of imputation. The most conservative method often ends up to be the one used to support the efficacy claim, raising the regulatory hurdles for drug approval and leading to a larger study than that was acceptable in the past.

In analgesic trials, patients need rescue with other analgesics because of insufficient pain relief from study medications. The predominant reason for early discontinuation—a reason for missing scores—is the inadequate pain relief from study medication. Subjects with less analgesic pain relief tend to rescue earlier. When designed properly, secondary endpoints such as "time to rescue," defined as the duration between "times of study drug administration" and "time of rescue intake," capture this aspect of treatment benefit. Time to rescue is either fully observed or predominantly censored at the end of the observation period scheduled for the study. The observation period for time to rescue should be made sufficiently long to cover the analgesic duration of the last study dose. Early censoring for other reasons such as adverse events is very rare in short-term pain trials. The analysis of time to rescue is not plagued by the imputation issue discussed earlier caused by missing pain relief/intensity scores. We have presented our observation from acute pain studies to illustrate and demonstrate that time to rescue fully captures the analgesic efficacy information of the study medication and serves as a surrogate for the longitudinally collected pain relief/intensity scores when the act of rescue taking is efficacy-driven. Time to rescue should be adopted as a primary efficacy variable in acute analgesic trials.

The validation of a surrogate endpoint is a difficult problem. Our effort is much less than all-inclusive and all confirming. Our major objective has been to bring to the public awareness that the time to rescue acts as a full surrogate to the longitudinally collected pain relief/intensity scores in a properly designed study and therefore facilitate the adoption of time to rescue as a primary efficacy variable in acute analgesic trials of short duration. There have been many such trials conducted during the past 20 years or more, and consistent results as those presented here will definitely serve to validate the surrogacy of time to rescue convincingly, as long as the time to rescue is designed to be efficacy-driven and is observed beyond the analgesic duration of the last dose.

References

[1] IASP Authors (2008): Definition of Pain. International Association for the Study of Pain. Available at http://www.iasp-pain.org/AM/Template.cfm?Section = Home&template =/ CM/HTMLDisplay.cfm& ContentID = 6017#Pain (accessed July 2008).

[2] Carr D and Goudas L (1999): Acute pain. *Lancet* 353: 2051–2058.

[3] Federation of State Medical Boards of the United States Inc. (2004): *Model Policy for the Use of Controlled Substances for the Treatment of Pain*. Dallas, TX: Federation of State Medical Boards of the United States Inc.

[4] Jensen TS, Gottrup H, Sindrup SH, and Bach FW (2001): The clinical picture of neuropathic pain. *Eur. J. Pharmacol.* 429: 1–11.

[5] Sindrup SH and Jensen TS (1999): Efficacy of pharmacological treatments of neuropathic pain: An update and effect related to mechanism of drug action. *Pain* 83: 389–400.

[6] Finnerup NB, Otto M, McQuay HJ, Jensen TS, and Sindrup SH (2005): Algorithm for neuropathic pain treatment: An evidence based proposal. *Pain* 118: 289–305.

[7] Various authors (2003): *Principles of Analgesic Use in the Treatment of Acute Pain and Cancer Pain*, 5th edn. Glenview, IL: American Pain Society.

[8] The European Agency for the Evaluation of Medicinal Products Committee for Medicinal Products for Human Use (2002): Note for Guidance on Clinical Investigation of Medicinal Products for Treatment of Nociceptive Pain, CPMP/EWP/612/00. Available at: http://www.emea.europa.eu/pdfs/human/ewp/061200en.pdf

 [9] The European Agency for the Evaluation of Medicinal Products Committee for Medicinal Products for Human Use (2002): Guideline on Clinical Medicinal Products Intended for the Treatment of Neuropathic Pain, CPMP/EWP/252/03. Available at: http://www.emea.europa.eu/pdfs/human/ewp/025203enfin.pdf

[10] Jensen MP and Karoly P (2001): *Self-report Scales and Procedures for Assessing Pain in Adults*, Turk DC and Melzack R (eds.). New York: Guilford Press, pp. 15–34.

[11] Jenssen MP (2003): The validity and reliability of pain measures in adults with cancer. *J. Pain* 4(1): 2–21.

[12] Farrar JT, Youg JP Jr, Lemoreaux L, Werth JL, and Poole RM (2001): Clinical importance of changes in chronic pain intensity measured on an 11-point numerical pain rating scale. *Pain* 94: 149–158.

[13] Farrar JT, Portenoy RK, Berlin JA, Kinman J, and Strom BL (2000): Defining the clinically important difference in pain outcome measures. *Pain* 88: 287–294.

[14] Prentice RL (1989): Surrogate endpoints in clinical trials: Definition and operational criteria. *Stat. Med.* 8: 431–440.

[15] Lin DY, Fleming TR, and De Gruttola V (1997): Estimating the proportion of treatment effect explained by a surrogate marker. *Stat. Med.* 16: 1515–1527.

Chapter 11

Design and Analysis of Analgesic Trials with Paired Time-to-Event Endpoints

Zhu Wang and Hon Keung Tony Ng

Contents

11.1 Introduction

The word "analgesic" originates from Greek meaning without-pain. An important application of analgesic trials is to help develop pain killers, which influence the peripheral and central nervous systems, such as the nonsteroidal anti-inflammatory drugs (NSAIDs). Therefore, pain treatment and research have attracted many clinical specialists and pharmaceutical companies. The related analgesic trials have been conducted in many disease categories, toward improving the understanding of the pain mechanisms or providing more efficient interventions for pain control. Sheiner et al. [50] list some typical clinical designs for new analgesic drugs: a pain-inducing procedure is undertaken for medical indications, usually a surgical procedure; when anesthesia has worn off, the patient asks an analgesic; the patient receives a randomly assigned treatment with either placebo or drug; at prespecified times after drug administration, the patient's pain status is recorded after questioning the patient. An introduction to the history, design, and analysis of analgesic trials can be found in [39]. Depending on the aims of such trials, there can be different types of data and time-to-event data are commonly collected in analgesic trials.

In this chapter, we explore the statistical methods to analyze paired time-to-event data from analgesic trials. In Section 11.2, we discuss the issues in designing clinical trials with time-to-event endpoints and matched pairs design for both situations with complete and censored data. In Section 11.3.1, we review some statistical methods for testing the equality of mean time-to-event endpoints of two treatments based on complete paired data. These methods include parametric methods based on normality distributional assumption, conditional Weibull distributional assumption, and gamma frailty models as well as nonparametric methods. Note that these methods are also applicable to data which are not time-to-event endpoints, for example, they are useful for comparing mean self-reported pain scores in matched paired studies. For censored time-to-event data, nonparametric rank-based tests are discussed in Section 11.3.2. Then, in Section 11.3.3, we focus on the estimation of the dependence by using copula models. In Section 11.4, examples are used to illustrate the methodologies present in the previous sections. Some concluding remarks are given in Section 11.5.

11.2   Design of Trials with Paired Time-to-Event Endpoints

In analgesic trials, the experimenters often deal with measurement in time units. For example, the investigators can measure the effect of a pain reliever by defining the origin of the timescale for a patient as the time that the patient is taking an analgesic, then the event of interest is the time at which the patient reported that the pain is relieved. In designing clinical trial for an analgesic involving time-to-event measurement, the time origin and the event of interest need to be defined explicitly before the trials. For instance, in studying an analgesic for a particular stimulus, one can define the time origin as the time that the stimulus applied to the patient and the event of interest can be the time at which the patient cannot tolerate the pain and requests an analgesic. Another example of time-to-event data from analgesic trials is the use of crying time of infants as an outcome measure (pain related to venipuncture) [12]. Since it is difficult to identify pain in young infants, crying time was checked and recorded from the infant's first cry after venipuncture until that vocalizations were sustained.

In clinical trials, we often want to compare treatments or groups of treatments. Ideally, one should always try to control other factors besides the experimental conditions. Matched pairs design, a study design that employs matched pairs or one-to-one matching that assume a certain uniqueness of each member of the pair, is one of the approaches to control other factors in the design stage. The rationale for matching resembles that of blocking in statistical design, in that each stratum formed by the matching pair is essentially the same with respect to the factors being controlled. By using a matched pairs design, the trials can be more efficient to detect a difference (i.e., gains in power), compared to independent two sample studies. Twin study, in which one twin is compared to the other, offers one of the best examples of matched pairs study, in that each twin pair is indeed unique with respect to their genes and their shared environment in general. In some situations, readily determined factors like age, gender, and ethnicity are used to ensure that each member of a particular pair is identical in these respects. Other instances such as "before" and "after" treatment on the same subject, measurements for left eye and right eye, and measurements from left hand and right hand, naturally give two correlated observations in the form of a pair. Nevertheless, the potential costs for a matched pairs design are finding appropriate matching variable(s) which may need some pretests to measure the matching variable(s).

Design issues for complete data and incomplete (censored) data are discussed separately in this section. After identifying the research question in analgesic trials and defining the time origin and the event of interest, one of the objectives in designing clinical trials is to find out a suitable size of sample to achieve a certain power to detect a clinically meaningful difference. Usually, the determination of sample size depends on the procedure or model that has been chosen for the analysis. For complete data, we will briefly review two commonly used statistical procedures, namely the paired t-test and the Wilcoxon signed rank test. Note that some other statistical methods for analysis of paired time-to-event endpoints are discussed further in Section 11.3. We also discuss scenarios in which censoring may occur in the paired design. For more technical details in sample size determination in clinical trials, readers may consult a standard reference, such as [8].

Suppose the observed paired time-to-event endpoints of n subjects are denoted by (T_{i1}, T_{i2}), $i = 1, \ldots, n$. For example, two infants having similar age and weight are matched as a pair; one of them received sucrose before venipuncture (treatment group) and the other did not (control group). Their crying times are recorded as T_{i1} and T_{i2}, where T_{i1} is the crying time of the infant in the ith pair receiving the treatment and T_{i2} is the crying time of the infant in the ith pair without the treatment. We are interested in comparing the two time-to-event distributions and testing their differences if any.

11.2.1   Sample Size: Noncensored Time-to-Event Endpoints

We denote the population means of the time-to-event (e.g., average crying times) for "treatment" and "control" groups by μ_1 and μ_2, respectively. In many situations, we are interested in comparing the mean differences within the pairs. More formally, we would claim a new treatment is as good as or not worse than a known effective treatment at level of significance α^* by testing

$$H_0 : \mu_1 - \mu_2 = 0 \quad \text{versus} \quad H_1 : \mu_1 - \mu_2 \neq 0. \tag{11.1}$$

In this section, we describe two commonly applied sample size formulas used to test the hypotheses in Equation 11.1 based on parametric and nonparametric frameworks.

11.2.1.1   Using Paired *t*-Test

A widely used method is the paired *t*-test based on the normality assumption. The sample size calculations are routinely conducted with the major statistical software. The related formula can be found, for instance, in [8]. Although the *t*-test is robust for nonnormal distributions, the sample size required to achieve such robustness may be not large enough in the design of trials. Therefore, it might be useful to consider transformations, for instance, logarithmic transformation assuming $T_{ij} > 0$ or square-root transformation, so that the transformed data will be more close to the normal distributions. We illustrate such a transformation-based method. Denote $D_i = \ln(T_{i1}) - \ln(T_{i2})$,

$$\bar{D} = \frac{1}{n} \sum_{i=1}^{n} D_i, \quad s_\mathrm{d} = \sqrt{\frac{1}{n-1} \sum_{i=1}^{n} (D_i - \bar{D})^2},$$

and $\mu_\mathrm{d} = \ln(\mu_1) - \ln(\mu_2)$, then the paired *t*-test based on log-transformed data is given by

$$t_n^{(L)} = \frac{\sqrt{n}\bar{D}}{s_\mathrm{d}}.$$

Under the null hypothesis $H_0 : \mu_\mathrm{d} = 0$, $t_n^{(L)}$ has a Student's *t*-distribution with $(n - 1)$ degrees of freedom. Thus, the null hypothesis in Equation 11.1 is rejected if

$$|t_n^{(L)}| > t(n - 1, \alpha^*/2),$$

where
   $| \cdot |$ denotes the absolute value function
   $t(n - 1, c)$ is the *c*-th upper percentile of the *t*-distribution with $n - 1$ degrees of freedom

We now consider sample size required for the above test in testing the differences based on log-transformed data. Suppose one wants to have type-I error α^* and the power of paired *t*-test to be at least $1 - \beta$ in testing the null hypothesis versus the two-sided alternative in Equation 11.1 and assume that the true difference between the two means of the log-transformed time-to-event endpoints is $\delta = \ln(\mu_1) - \ln(\mu_2)$ and the standard deviation of D_i is σ_d, then the sample size required to achieve this task can be approximated by

$$n = \frac{(z_{\alpha*/2} + z_\beta)^2 \sigma_d^2}{\delta^2},$$

where z_c is the cth upper percentile of the standard normal distribution. In practice, since the values of δ and σ_d (or simply the ratio of the two) is unknown, therefore, σ_d/δ is often estimated from previous studies or from a clinically meaningful estimate [29].

11.2.1.2 Using Wilcoxon Signed Rank Test

The hypotheses in Equation 11.1 can be tested with nonparametric test procedures, especially when the distributional assumptions are violated or the distributions of the time-to-event endpoints are uncertain. As an alternative to the paired t-test, Wilcoxon signed rank test (Wilcoxon paired-sample test) is one of the commonly used nonparametric test procedures for this purpose. The test procedure can be described as follows: First, we rank the absolute values $|D_i|$ in ascending order by assigning rank 1 to n. Then, we compute the sum of ranks for positive D_i and denote this sum as W_+. The null hypothesis in Equation 11.1 is rejected if the value of W_+ is too large or too small. For specific values of the significance level $\alpha*$ and small sample size $n \leq 50$, the critical values of Wilcoxon signed rank test can be found in many standard nonparametric textbooks [25] or major statistical software. For large sample sizes, asymptotic normal approximation of the null distribution can be used, that is,

$$\frac{W_+ - E(W_+|H_0)}{\sqrt{\text{Var}(W_+|H_0)}} \xrightarrow{L} N(0, 1),$$

where

$$E(W_+|H_0) = \frac{n(n+1)}{4} \quad \text{and} \quad \text{Var}(W_+|H_0) = \frac{n(n+1)(2n+1)}{24}.$$

Under a specific alternative hypothesis H_1 in Equation 11.1 with type-I error $\alpha*$ and the minimum power value $1 - \beta$, the required sample size can be approximated by [40]

$$n = \frac{(z_{\alpha*/2} + z_\beta)^2}{3(p - 0.5)^2},$$

where $p = \Pr(D + D' > 0)$ with D and D' being two independent differences. The quantity p can be obtained based on previous studies or a clinically meaningful estimate. For other approaches to approximate the sample size required for the Wilcoxon signed rank test, one may refer to [51] for a concise review.

11.2.2   Sample Size: Censored Time-to-Event Endpoints

One of the main features for time-to-event endpoints is that often the observed data are not complete by the end of the clinical trials due to time and financial constraints as well as ethical reasons. For example, in studying the effect of a pain reliever, the subjects are allowed to terminate the study and receive an effective dose of an established analgesic at any time due to ethical reasons. As a result, we may only have the information that the exact time-to-event endpoint is greater or smaller than an observed value but not the exact value itself. If the time-to-event endpoints to the right are missing (i.e., the exact time-to-event endpoints are greater than the observed value), then the resulting data are called right censored data. Similarly, if the observed time-to-event endpoints are greater than the true times, then the resulting data are called left censored data. We are interested in testing the hypotheses in terms of the survival functions for the two populations:

$$H_0 : S_1(t) = S_2(t), \text{ for all } t \quad \text{versus} \quad H_1 : S_1(t) \neq S_2(t), \text{ for some } t. \quad (11.2)$$

As the log-rank test is commonly applied to censored time-to-event data, some methods have been suggested to determine the appropriate sample sizes. Gangnon and Kosorok [18] proposed a simple sample size formula based on a weighted log-rank statistic applied to clustered time-to-event data. With cluster size of 2, their formula can be applied to paired time-to-event data. In a special case where the paired time-to-event endpoints are independent, their formula reduces to Schoenfeld's formula [48] for the proportional hazards model. We briefly illustrate their sample size formula for the log-rank test statistic. Suppose we have n pairs of time-to-event endpoints subject to censoring. Let (T_{i1}, C_{i1}) and (T_{i2}, C_{i2}), $i = 1, \ldots, n$ be independent random vectors, where T_{i1} and T_{i2} represent the time-to-event endpoints and C_{i1} and C_{i2} represent the censoring times for the first and second members of the ith pair, respectively. T_{i1} and T_{i2} may represent time-to-event for treatment 1 and treatment 2, respectively. We assume that (T_{i1}, T_{i2}) and (C_{i1}, C_{i2}) are independent. Denote $X_{ij} = \min(T_{ij}, C_{ij})$ for the ith pair and $k_{ij} = I(T_{ij} < C_{ij})$, for $j = 1, 2$, where $I(\cdot)$ is the indicator function. We further use counting process notation. Define the at-risk processes

$$Y_{ij}(t) = I\{X_{ij} \geq t\}, \quad \bar{Y}_j = \sum_{i=1}^{n} Y_{ij}.$$

The log-rank test statistic for paired data proposed in [18] is

$$H_n = \frac{1}{n} \int_0^{\infty} \frac{\bar{Y}_1(s)\bar{Y}_2(s)}{\bar{Y}_1(s) + \bar{Y}_2(s)} \left\{ \frac{d\bar{N}_1(s)}{\bar{Y}_1(s)} - \frac{d\bar{N}_2(s)}{\bar{Y}_2(s)} \right\},$$

where

$$N_{ij} = I\{X_{ij} \leq t, k_{ij} = 1\}, \quad i = 1, \ldots, n, \quad \bar{N}_j = \sum_{i=1}^{n} N_{ij}, \quad j = 1, 2$$

are the counting processes of observed events. Let

$$\hat{M}_{ij}(t) = N_{ij}(t) - \int_0^t Y_{ij}(s)d\bar{N}_j(s)/\bar{Y}_j(s).$$

Under mild regularity conditions, the test statistic H_n has a limiting normal distribution, which may be used to test the null hypothesis versus the two-sided alternative in Equation 11.2. Denote Δ the ratio of the hazard function of the first member in the pair given treatment 1 to second member given treatment 2. To test the null hypothesis $S_1(t) = S_2(t)$ versus the treatment effect Δ with type-I error α^* and power $1 - \beta$, a required number of events is

$$n = \frac{2(z_{1-\alpha^*/2} + z_\beta)^2(1 - \eta)}{(\ln \Delta)^2},$$

where η is the intraclass correlation coefficient between $\int_0^\infty d\hat{M}_{i1}(s)$ and $\int_0^\infty d\hat{M}_{i2}(s)$. The intraclass correlation coefficient η may be determined by a clinical meaningful parameter. Alternatively, if the data from the previous studies are available, η may be conveniently estimated, since the quantities $\int_0^\infty d\hat{M}_{ij}(s)$ can be obtained as martingale residuals from the Cox regression procedures in SAS, S-Plus, and R.

11.3 Analysis of Trials with Paired Time-to-Event Endpoints

As we discussed in Section 11.2.1, for the matched pairs design, we need to consider the dependencies within pairs (T_{i1}, T_{i2}), $i = 1, \ldots, n$ and take them into account in the statistical analysis. There are different approaches to analyze such data. In this section, we will focus on the discussion of nonregression type methods. For regression methods on time-to-event endpoints, for example, proportional hazard models, one may refer to [30].

For complete paired time-to-event data, we will discuss the parametric methods to test the null hypothesis versus the two-sided alternative in Equation 11.1 based on the normal distributional assumption, the conditional Weibull distributional assumption and the gamma frailty models in Section 11.3.1. In contrast, we will also discuss the nonparametric methods and provide a comparison between these methods. For censored paired time-to-event data, test procedures for testing hypotheses in Equation 11.1 are discussed in Section 11.3.2. Besides testing of hypothesis, we also discuss the estimation of dependence using copula models in Section 11.3.3.

11.3.1 Analysis of Complete Paired Time-to-Event Endpoints

Following the notation in Section 11.2.1, we discuss procedures to test the null hypothesis versus the two-sided alternative in Equation 11.1 based on parametric and nonparametric frameworks.

11.3.1.1   Parametric Methods Based on Normal Distribution

For paired time-to-event data, we can consider to apply the paired t-test to the data. We focus on the log-transformed data. To test hypotheses in Equation 11.1, under the assumption that the difference within the pair $D_i = \ln(T_{i1}) - \ln(T_{i2})$ is normally distributed with mean $\mu_d = \ln(\mu_1) - \ln(\mu_2)$ and variance σ_d^2, the paired t-test is the most powerful test [33]. The paired t-test based on log-transformed data can be conducted as described in Section 11.2.1.1.

11.3.1.2   Parametric Methods Based on Conditional Weibull Distribution

The Weibull distribution was originally invented by Waloddi Weibull for estimating machinery lifetime in 1937 and he claimed that this statistical distribution can be applied to a wide range of problems [57]. Nowadays, the Weibull distribution is a broadly used statistical model in lifetime data analysis. Due to its flexibility to model distributions with either nonincreasing or nondecreasing hazard rates, it is particularly useful in time-to-event data.

For paired time-to-event data, it is well-known that the difference of the log-transformed observations within the pair can be modeled by a logistic distribution if the conditional distributions of time-to-event endpoints are modeled by particular Weibull distributions [4,31,46]. Specifically, assume that the conditional distribution of the time-to-event endpoint T_{ij}, given an unobservable positive random variable Θ (frailty), is Weibull with scale parameter $\eta_j\theta$ and common shape parameter ρ, that is, the probability density function (PDF) of T_{ij} is

$$f_j(t; \rho, \eta_j) = \rho(\theta\eta_j)^\rho t^{\rho-1} e^{-(\theta\eta_j t)^\rho}, \quad t > 0,$$

$i = 1, \ldots, n, j = 1, 2$. Frailty is a random effect which describes unexplained heterogeneity or the influence of unobserved risk factors. More discussion will be given in Section 11.3.1.3. We further assume that the two time-to-event endpoints, T_{i1} and T_{i2}, are conditionally independent, given $\Theta = \theta$. Then $D_i = \ln(T_{i1}) - \ln(T_{i2})$ follows a logistic distribution with PDF

$$f_D(d) = \frac{e^{\left(\frac{d-\gamma}{1/\rho}\right)}}{1/\rho\left[1 + e^{\left(\frac{d-\gamma}{1/\rho}\right)}\right]^2}, \quad -\infty < d < \infty,$$

where
$\gamma = \ln(\eta_1/\eta_2)$ is the location parameter
$1/\rho$ is the scale parameter

Since the PDF of D_i is independent of the value of θ, the D_i's can be used to test

$$H_0^*: \gamma = 0 \quad \text{versus} \quad H_1^*: \gamma \neq 0, \tag{11.3}$$

which is equivalent to testing Equation 11.1. It is clear that any test procedures for testing the location parameter $\gamma = 0$ in logistic distribution will be applicable here to test the null hypothesis versus the two-sided alternative in Equation 11.3. Owen et al. [46] proposed two pivotal tests and Wang [54] studied the asymptotic versions of these tests.

11.3.1.2.1   Q-Test   The test statistic has the exact same form as the paired t-test, namely,

$$Q_n = \frac{\sqrt{n}\bar{D}}{s_d},$$

where

$$\bar{D} = \frac{1}{n}\sum_{i=1}^{n}D_i, \quad s_d = \sqrt{\frac{1}{n-1}\sum_{i=1}^{n}(D_i - \bar{D})^2}.$$

However, because the Q-test is an exact test, a critical value for the test is based on Monte Carlo simulations for a given value of ρ and level of significance α^*. Note that this test is asymptotically equivalent to the paired t-test based on log-transformed time-to-event endpoints and the asymptotic version of the Q-test, namely LQ-test, is a test using the same test statistic Q_n but calibrated by a standard normal distribution.

11.3.1.2.2   Test Based on Maximum Likelihood Estimators (MLEs)   Owen et al. [46] also proposed a test based on MLEs of γ and ρ. The MLEs, $\hat{\rho}$ and $\hat{\gamma}$, can be obtained by solving the system of nonlinear equations

$$\begin{cases} \dfrac{2}{n}\displaystyle\sum_{i=1}^{n}\dfrac{\exp\left(\frac{d_i-\gamma}{1/\rho}\right)}{1+\exp\left(\frac{d_i-\gamma}{1/\rho}\right)} = 1, \\[3ex] \dfrac{2}{n}\displaystyle\sum_{i=1}^{n}\dfrac{(d_i-\gamma)\exp\left(\frac{d_i-\gamma}{1/\rho}\right)}{1+\exp\left(\frac{d_i-\gamma}{1/\rho}\right)} = 1/\rho - \gamma + \dfrac{1}{n}\displaystyle\sum_{i=1}^{n}d_i. \end{cases} \tag{11.4}$$

Note that numerical methods, such as the Newton-Raphson method, is required to solve the above equations. The test statistic is

$$M_n = \frac{\sqrt{n}\hat{\gamma}}{1/\hat{\rho}}. \tag{11.5}$$

For a given value of level of significance α^*, the critical value of the test can be simulated. This exact test procedure is named as *M*-test. An asymptotic version of the *M*-test, namely *LM*-test, is proposed in [54], where it is shown that

$$\lim_{n \to \infty} n \text{Var}(\hat{\gamma}) = 3/\rho^2,$$

and

$$\frac{\sqrt{n}(\hat{\gamma} - \gamma)}{\sqrt{3}/\rho} \xrightarrow{L} N(0, 1).$$

The *LM*-test statistic is given by

$$LM_n = \frac{M_n}{\sqrt{3}},$$

which has a limiting standard normal distribution $N(0, 1)$ under the null hypothesis H_0^*. In this case, LM_n is not only an asymptotic pivotal test but also an exact pivotal test [46].

11.3.1.2.3 Likelihood Ratio Test Based on Logistic Distribution Likelihood ratio test (LRT) relies on a test statistic that is the ratio of the maximum value of the likelihood function under the constraint of the null hypothesis to the maximum likelihood with that constraint relaxed. Based on the logistic model, the log-likelihood function is

$$\ln L(\rho, \gamma) = \sum_{i=1}^{n} \frac{d_i - \gamma}{1/\rho} - n \ln(1/\rho) - 2 \sum_{i=1}^{n} \ln \left[1 + \exp \left(\frac{d_i - \gamma}{1/\rho} \right) \right].$$

The maximum likelihood under the whole parameter space $\Omega = \{\rho, \gamma | \rho > 0, -\infty < \gamma < \infty\}$ is $L(\hat{\rho}, \hat{\gamma})$ where the MLEs, $\hat{\rho}$ and $\hat{\gamma}$, can be obtained as before. Under the null hypothesis $H_0^* : \gamma = 0$, the maximized likelihood under the restricted parameter space $\Omega^* = \{\rho, \gamma | \rho > 0, \gamma = 0\}$ is $L(\hat{\rho}, 0)$. Therefore, the log-likelihood ratio is

$$\ln \Lambda = \ln \frac{\sup_{(\rho, \gamma) \in \Omega^*} L(\rho, \gamma)}{\sup_{(\rho, \gamma) \in \Omega} L(\rho, \gamma)} = \ln L(\hat{\rho}, 0) - \ln L(\hat{\rho}, \hat{\gamma}).$$

The LRT statistic is then given by $-2 \ln \Lambda$. Under the null hypothesis H_0^*, $-2 \ln \Lambda$ asymptotically follows a χ^2 distribution with one degree of freedom. Therefore, for a given level of significance α^*, we reject H_0^* in Equation 11.3 when $\chi_1^2(-2 \ln \Lambda) < \alpha^*$, where $\chi_1^2(\cdot)$ is the cumulative distribution function of the chi-square distribution with one degree of freedom. As the chi-square approximation for the LRT statistic may be poor for small sample sizes, resampling procedure such as parametric bootstrap method [16] can be used to obtain the *p*-value of the test for small sample size [55].

11.3.1.3 Parametric Methods Based on Gamma Frailty Model

The test procedures discussed in Section 11.3.1.2 are based on models where the bivariate dependence is eliminated. A potential impact of such elimination is that if frailty is not taken into account when it should be, misleading inference may result [27]. Frailty model is used to model multivariate time-to-event data, where the time-to-event endpoints are conditionally independent, given the frailty, which is an individual random effect. In clinical trials, it is ideal to study a homogeneous population such as the paired data in which the two members within the pair are under the same risk (e.g., risk of death, risk of disease recurrence). However, even for the matched pairs, still there exist genetic and environment variations. Therefore, a more practical assumption is that the matched pairs are from a heterogeneous population, that is, with different hazards within the pair. To account for heterogeneity caused by unmeasured covariates, a frailty model assumes a multiplicative effect on the baseline hazard function. Hence, frailty models are extensions of the proportional hazards model. For a recent review on frailty models, see [15].

To test the null hypothesis versus the two-sided alternative in Equation 11.1, Wang [54] introduced three parametric testing procedures based on the assumptions that the frailty distribution is gamma with PDF

$$g(z) = \frac{1}{\Gamma(\alpha)} z^{\alpha-1} e^{-z}, \quad \text{for } z > 0,$$

where $\Gamma(\cdot)$ is the complete gamma function, and the baseline distribution is assumed to be the Weibull distribution described as below, which has a different parameterization compared with the Weibull PDF in Section 11.3.1.2.

$$f_j(t; \rho, \lambda_j) = \rho z \lambda_j t^{\rho-1} e^{-z\lambda_j t^{\rho}}, \quad t > 0,$$

$i = 1, \dots, n, j = 1, 2$. Given $Z = z$, the conditional joint survival function of the paired time-to-event endpoints is

$$S(t_1, t_2|z) = \Pr(T_1 > t_1, T_2 > t_2|Z = z) = \exp\{-z(\lambda_1 t_1^{\rho} + \lambda_2 t_2^{\rho})\}.$$

The bivariate model based on gamma frailty was initialized in [10] and has been studied in [9,42,43]. Other works include [32,34–37]. This model also belongs to the Archimedean copulas [20] which we will have further discussion in Section 11.3.3. The unconditional joint distribution of T_1 and T_2 is a bivariate Burr distribution [11] with joint survival function

$$S(t_1, t_2) = E_z[S(t_1, t_2|z)] = (1 + \lambda_1 t_1^{\rho} + \lambda_2 t_2^{\rho})^{-\alpha},$$

and the Kendall's τ correlation between T_1 and T_2 is given by [27]

$$\tau = 1/(1 + 2\alpha). \tag{11.6}$$

Letting $\gamma = \ln(\lambda_1/\lambda_2)$, it is clear that testing hypothesis Equation 11.1 is equivalent to testing

$$H_0^{**} : \gamma = 0 \quad \text{versus} \quad H_1^{**} : \gamma \neq 0. \tag{11.7}$$

Based on the gamma frailty model, utilizing the asymptotic results for the MLE of γ, Wang [54] proposed a procedure for testing Equation 11.7. It can be shown that the MLE $\tilde{\gamma} = \ln(\tilde{\lambda}_1/\tilde{\lambda}_2)$ has an asymptotic normal distribution

$$\sqrt{n}(\tilde{\gamma} - \gamma) \xrightarrow{L} N(0, \sigma_\gamma^2),$$

where $\sigma_\gamma^2 = B/A$, and A and B are given below:

$$A = 2(\alpha + 2)[\psi'(2)(3\alpha^4 + 9\alpha^3 + 10\alpha^2 + 4\alpha) + \psi'(\alpha)(3\alpha^4 + 6\alpha^3 + 4\alpha^2)$$
$$+ (\alpha^4 + 5\alpha^3 + 5\alpha^2 - 4)],$$

$$B = (\alpha + 3)\left[\frac{2A}{\alpha + 2} + \gamma^2(3\alpha^4 + 12\alpha^3 + 16\alpha^2 + 8\alpha)\right],$$

where $\psi(\cdot)$ denotes the trigamma function.

Consistent estimator of σ_γ^2, such as the MLE $\tilde{\sigma}_\gamma^2$ can be used to construct the Wald test statistic:

$$W_n = \frac{\sqrt{n}\tilde{\gamma}}{\tilde{\sigma}_\gamma}, \tag{11.8}$$

which has a limiting standard normal distribution $N(0, 1)$ under the null hypothesis H_0^{**} in Equation 11.7.

Based on the large sample theory, a LRT is proposed in [54] along the same line in Section 11.3.1.2.3.

11.3.1.4 Nonparametric Methods

Nonparametric methods based on ranks or permutation distribution can be used to test the null hypothesis versus the two-sided alternative in Equation 11.1 as alternatives to the parametric procedures when the model of the time-to-event endpoints is uncertain. The Wilcoxon signed rank test described in Section 11.2.1 is a commonly used nonparametric procedure based on ranks.

A permutation test is one of the procedures which utilize the exchangeability of data under the null hypothesis. The sampling distribution of the test statistic under the null hypothesis is computed by forming all or many of the permutations (which are typically chosen by a Monte Carlo method), calculating the test statistic for each permutation and considering all these values as equally likely [23]. For paired time-to-event data, a permutation test for testing the hypotheses in Equation 11.1 is explained in [55].

11.3.1.5   Comparison of Test Procedures for Tests of Two Means

The aforementioned test procedures for testing the hypotheses in Equation 11.1 are compared by means of Monte Carlo simulation studies. In summary, here are the test procedures considered in the comparative study:

t-test: paired *t*-test for data with/without log-transformation
Q-test: *Q*-test, calibrated with simulated critical values
M-test: *M*-test, calibrated with simulated critical values
LQ-test: *Q*-test, calibrated with normal distribution
LM-test: *M*-test, calibrated with normal distribution
LRTL: LRT based on logistic model, calibrated by bootstrap method
WALD: Wald test based on gamma frailty model
LRTG: LRT based on gamma frailty model
WSRT: Wilcoxon signed rank test for data with/without log-transformation
PERM: permutation test for data with/without log-transformation

The settings for Monte Carlo simulation studies can be found in [54,55]. From the simulation results, we observed that the *LM*-test has larger power values than *LQ*-test, similar to the performances of their counterparts, the *M*-test and *Q*-test, respectively, as reported in [45]. The *LM*-test can be used to approximate the *M*-test, with a slightly larger inflation of the type-I error rate for small samples. The *LQ*-test also can be used to approximate the *Q*-test, although with the similar disadvantage of inflation of type-I error rate. The *t*-test, WSRT, PERM and the *M*-test, *Q*-test and LRTL have similar type-I error rates and power values for log-transformed data. We also found that LRTG and WALD outperform other tests, when the conditional marginal distributions of the time-to-event endpoints are moderate or less skewed. When the conditional distribution is highly skewed, the log-transformation-based tests (*t*-, *Q*-, *M*-, *LQ*-, *LM*-tests, and LRTL) have better performances. When data are highly skewed, the *t*-test, WSRT, PERM can perform very poorly for data without log-transformation. In summary, for moderate and less skewed lifetime data, particularly when sample size is large, the LRTG and WALD are recommended to use while for highly skewed data, the tests based on log-transformed data are preferred.

11.3.2   Analysis of Censored Paired Time-to-Event Endpoints

In censored time-to-event paired data, suppose we have n pairs of time-to-event endpoints subject to censoring. Let (T_{i1}, C_{i1}) and (T_{i2}, C_{i2}) $i = 1, \ldots, n$ be independent random vectors, where T_{i1} and T_{i2} represent the time-to-event endpoints and C_{i1} and C_{i2} represent the censoring times for the first and second members of the ith pair, respectively. We assume that (T_{i1}, T_{i2}) and (C_{i1}, C_{i2}) are independent. The observed values are $X_{i1} = \min(T_{i1}, C_{i1})$ and $X_{i2} = \min(T_{i2}, C_{i2})$ for the ith pair and we further denote $k_{i1} = I(T_{i1} < C_{i1})$ and $k_{i2} = I(T_{i2} < C_{i2})$ where $I(\cdot)$ is the indicator function. Nonparametric rank-based tests for survival differences have been studied extensively. In general, the rank-based tests are based on a score assigned to each individual derived from the observed data $\xi(X_{ij}, k_{ij})$, $i = 1, \ldots, n$, $j = 1, 2$. Two frequently used score systems proposed by Prentice [47] and Akritas [1,2], respectively, are reviewed and the related test procedures are discussed. For more details on nonparametric rank-based tests with paired data under censoring and comparisons among different procedures, one may refer to [3,13,14,38,44,59,60].

11.3.2.1   Paired Prentice–Wilcoxon Test

A scoring system suggested by Prentice [47] for censored data is a generalization of the Wilcoxon signed rank test. Assume there are no ties in the observations. The score ξ can be obtained as follows:

1. Pool the paired observations X_{i1} and X_{i2}, $i = 1, \ldots, n$ into a single sample of size $2n$.

2. Rank the pooled observations in ascending order and denote $n(l)$ as the number of observations in the pooled sample with values greater than or equal to the lth distinct ordered value, $l = 1, \ldots, 2n$.

3. Assign the score $\xi(X_{i1}, k_{i1}) = 1 - \tilde{S}(X_{i1}) - k_{i1}\tilde{S}(X_{i1})$ to observation (X_{i1}, k_{i1}), where

$$\tilde{S}(X_{i1}) = \prod_{l=1}^{i} \frac{n(l)}{n(l) + 1}.$$

The scores for $\xi(X_{i2}, k_{i2})$, $i = 1, \ldots, n$ can be obtained in a similar manner. The paired Prentice–Wilcoxon on (PPW) test proposed in [44] compares the difference between the scores in the pairs. With $\Delta_i = \xi(X_{i1}, k_{i1}) - \xi(X_{i2}, k_{i2})$, O'Brien and Fleming [44] showed that the test statistic $Z = \sum_{i=1}^{n} \Delta_i / (\sum_{i=1}^{n} \Delta_i^2)^{1/2}$, has a limiting standard normal distribution $N(0, 1)$ and thus the p-value of the test can be computed.

In the case when ties exist, for example, if m_l events are observed at X_l, we can arbitrarily rank these times by assigning them distinct values infinitesimally less than X_l. Repeat this procedure for all tied event times, then compute the scores as displayed above. Finally, each of the m_l individuals with an observed event at X_l is assigned the average score for the associated m_l individuals.

11.3.2.2   Akritas Test

Another score system for nonparametric rank-based test for equality of two time-to-event distribution is studied in [1,2]. The score can be obtained as follows:

1. Compute the Kaplan–Meier estimates from (X_{i1}, k_{i1}) and (X_{i2}, k_{i2}), $i = 1, \ldots, n$ for the first and second members in the pairs and denote them as $\hat{S}_1(\cdot)$ and $\hat{S}_2(\cdot)$, respectively.

2. Assign the score

$$\xi(X_{ij}, k_{ij}) = 1 - \frac{1}{2}\bar{S}(X_{ij}) - \frac{1}{2}k_{ij}\bar{S}(X_{ij})$$

to observation (X_{ij}, k_{ij}), for $i = 1, \ldots, n$, $j = 1, 2$, where

$$\bar{S}(\cdot) = \frac{1}{2}\left[\hat{S}_1(\cdot) + \hat{S}_2(\cdot)\right].$$

The Akritas test is to apply the paired t-test to the paired scores $(\xi(X_{i1}, k_{i1})$, $\xi(X_{i2}, k_{i2}))$, for $i = 1, \ldots, n$.

11.3.3 Estimation of Dependence with Copula Models

With paired time-to-event data, we might be interesting in the dependence relationship between the pairs. The patterns and strength of dependencies in paired studies can provide empirical evidence on the generic and environmental contributions to the diseases. A correlation coefficient has been extensively applied to indicate the strength and direction of a linear relationship between two random variables. For instance, Pearson's product correlation can completely determine the dependence structure when the paired data have a bivariate normal distribution. Instead, Kendall's τ is a nonparametric estimation of correlation which can be extended to censored data [6,41,58]. However, Kendall's τ cannot be used in situations where covariates need to be incorporated. In this subsection, we provide an overview of a parametric approach, called copula models, to estimate dependence for paired time-to-event data. Starting from univariate marginal distributions, with a fixed copula dependence structure, a bivariate copula model can be constructed [49] as follows: Let u_1 and u_2 be two (possibly correlated) uniform random variables on $(0, 1)$ and their relationship is described through their joint distribution function

$$C(u_1, u_2) = \Pr(U_1 \leq u_1, U_2 \leq u_2).$$

The function C is called a copula, which means a "link" or "tie" in Latin. With selected marginal distribution functions $F_1(t_1)$, $F_2(t_2)$, the function

$$C(F_1(t_1), F_2(t_2)) = F(t_1, t_2)$$

defines a bivariate distribution function, evaluated at t_1, t_2, with marginal distributions F_1, F_2, respectively.

An important copula is Archimedean copula [20] which has been studied extensively due to its simple form, nice statistical properties, and advantages for estimation [22,53]. Denote a generator function as $\phi_\alpha : [0, \infty] \to [0, 1]$ which is a strictly decreasing convex function such that $\phi(0) = 1$. The dependence parameter α in the subscript is omitted without confusion. An Archimedean copula can be generated as

$$C(u_1, u_2; \alpha) = \phi[\phi^{-1}(u_1) + \phi^{-1}(u_2)].$$

TABLE 11.1: Some archimedean copulas.

Family	Parameter Space	Generator ϕ	Bivariate Copula	Kendall's τ
Gumbel	$\alpha \geq 1$	$(-\ln t)^\alpha$	$\exp\{-[(-\ln u_1)^\alpha + (-\ln u_2)^\alpha]^{1/\alpha}\}$	$\frac{\alpha-1}{\alpha}$
Clayton	$\alpha > 0$	$t^{-\alpha} - 1$	$\left(u_1^{-\alpha} + u_2^{-\alpha} - 1\right)^{-1/\alpha}$	$\frac{\alpha}{\alpha+2}$
Frank	$\alpha \neq 0$	$-\ln\left[\frac{\exp(-\alpha t)-1}{\exp(-\alpha)-1}\right]$	$-\frac{1}{\alpha}\ln\left[1 + \frac{(\exp(-\alpha u_1)-1)(\exp(-\alpha u_2)-1)}{\exp(-\alpha)-1}\right]$	$1 - \frac{4}{\alpha}\left\{1 - \frac{1}{\alpha}\int_0^\alpha \frac{t}{\exp(t)-1}dt\right\}$

We denote $c(u_1, u_2; \alpha)$ the joint density function derived from $C(u_1, u_2; \alpha)$. Genest and Mackay [19] showed that the expected Kendall's τ correlation is

$$\tau = 4\int_0^1 \frac{\phi(t)}{\phi'(t)}dt + 1.$$

We present here three Archimedean copula families including the Gumbel [24], Clayton [10], and Frank [17] copulas in Table 11.1. Their corresponding expected Kendall's τ correlations are also presented. There are several approaches to estimate the parameters of copula models: (i) the full maximum likelihood approach by maximizing $c(t_1, t_2; \alpha)$ based on the observed data (T_{i1}, T_{i2}), $i = 1, 2, \ldots, n$; (ii) a two-step approach, where in the first step, estimation of marginal parameters is conducted based on parametric or nonparametric methods assuming independence [26,52]. In the second step, the estimates from the first step is substituted into $c(u_1, u_2; \alpha)$ to estimate the remaining dependence parameter α based on usual maximum likelihood method; and (iii) a semiparametric approach, where we estimate the dependence structure without specifying the marginal distributions. In this approach, we use the empirical distribution function of each marginal distribution to transform the observations (T_{i1}, T_{i2}) into pseudo-observations with uniform margins (u_{i1}, u_{i2}) and then estimate the dependence parameter as in step 2 in (ii). Many authors have studied the estimation problem for censored data with covariates by using the copula models [28,52,53].

11.4   Illustrative Examples

Due to lack of public accessible time-to-event analgesic data in paired studies, in particular, with complete data, we use two real data sets in other research areas to demonstrate the testing and estimation procedures described in this chapter for analyzing paired time-to-event data.

11.4.1   Example 1: Parkinson's Disease

The data are related to experiments with old people having Parkinson's disease, which causes pain on neuropathic, muscle, joints, and tendons, attributable to tension, dystopia, rigidity, joint stiffness, and injuries associated with attempts at

TABLE 11.2: Bivariate observations (T_1, T_2).

T_1	0.159	0.173	0.195	0.243	0.100	0.219	0.217	0.214	0.089	0.172	0.139	0.139
	0.565	0.162	0.227	0.080	0.256	0.216	0.140	0.226	0.132	0.118	0.240	0.086
	0.248	0.183	0.143	0.150	0.143	0.157	0.165	0.185	0.268	0.212	0.334	0.258
	0.250	0.172	0.184	0.124	0.166	0.162	0.166	0.143	0.163	0.193	0.152	0.162
	0.129	0.262	0.341	0.291	0.133	0.335	0.159	0.158	0.216	0.464	0.201	0.297
	0.170	0.264	0.105	0.222	0.142	0.155	0.179	0.218	0.231	0.208	0.129	0.456
T_2	0.081	0.077	0.085	0.209	0.065	0.056	0.073	0.078	0.118	0.355	0.189	0.225
	0.076	0.136	0.090	0.121	0.088	0.137	0.087	0.189	0.193	0.072	0.075	0.117
	0.106	0.094	0.111	0.130	0.198	0.106	0.126	0.117	0.095	0.122	0.110	0.221
	0.334	0.128	0.084	0.049	0.094	0.056	0.129	0.053	0.086	0.077	0.099	0.079
	0.062	0.093	0.124	0.116	0.091	0.172	0.075	0.120	0.084	0.162	0.198	0.155
	0.117	0.107	0.113	0.180	0.078	0.098	0.106	0.186	0.102	0.189	0.090	0.196

Source: Caroni, C. and Kimber, A., *J. Statist. Comput. Simul.*, 74, 15, 2004. With permission.

accommodation. Techniques developed in testing the equality of means and estimation of dependence in paired time-to-event data are applied to a data set from an experiment on the extent to which old people sway about when attempting to stand still [56]. There are 72 pairs of observations representing the root mean square of the sway amplitude over 1 min under two experiment conditions [7]. As we mentioned in Section 11.1, methods discussed in this chapter are applicable to paired data which are not time-to-event endpoints. The data set is presented in Table 11.2.

In testing the equality of two means sway amplitude under two experimental conditions, we consider the parametric tests based on normal distributional assumption, conditional Weibull distributional assumption and gamma frailty model and the nonparametric tests discussed in Section 11.2.1. For tests based on normal distributional assumption, the paired t-test statistic with and without log-transformed data are 8.75 and 6.974, respectively, both with p-values <0.001. Under the conditional Weibull distributional assumption, the MLE for the parameters of logistic distribution are $\hat{\gamma} = 0.533$ and $\hat{\rho} = 0.28$. The M-test and Q-test statistics are 15.98 and 8.75, respectively, both with p-values <0.005. Based on a gamma frailty model, the estimates of the parameters are given by $\hat{\alpha} = 3.356$, $\hat{\rho} = 2.825$, $\hat{\lambda}_1 = 27.08$, and $\hat{\lambda}_2 = 99$ and the log-likelihood is 198.46. The Wald test statistic is $W_n = 6.07$ and the LRT statistic is 50.2, both with p-values <0.001. It is interesting to note that the estimate of α corresponds to Kendall's $\tau = 0.13$ from Equation 11.6, which is similar to the observed value of Kendall's τ (0.137). For nonparametric tests, we found that both the p-values of Wilcoxon signed rank tests and the permutation test are <0.001. We can see that all the tests procedures considered here conclude that the data provide enough evidence to reject the null hypothesis that the two means are equal.

Now we use this data set to illustrate the methodologies to estimate dependence with copula models. The three approaches described in Section 11.3.3 are used to estimate parameters of Gumbel, Clayton, and Frank copula models. For the first two approaches, the marginal Weibull distributions are assumed. The estimates are presented in Table 11.3. When using the two-stage estimation method, all the marginal distribution estimates are the same for the three copula families. For

TABLE 11.3: Estimation of copula models based on methods discussed in Section 11.3.3.

Family	Method	Dependence	Shape 1	Scale 1	Shape 2	Scale 2
Gumbel	(i)	1.00	2.43	37.05	2.22	80.90
	(ii)	1.00	2.43[a]	37.05[b]	2.22[c]	80.90[d]
	(iii)	1.11	—	—	—	—
Clayton	(i)	1.19	2.31	31.67	2.08	64.80
	(ii)	1.04	a	b	c	d
	(iii)	0.23	—	—	—	—
Frank	(i)	2.23	2.43	36.15	2.20	120.67
	(ii)	2.18	a	b	c	d
	(iii)	1.21	—	—	—	—

[a] Denotes the same estimation results for the corresponding marginal distribution parameters in the two-stage approach (ii).

[b,c] and [d] are defined similar to [a] denotes nonavilable results since the marginal distribution is not specified in the semiparametric approach (iii).

the semiparametric approach, no marginal distribution is assumed, therefore, there is no estimates shown in Table 11.3. We can see that the first two methods give similar estimates of the dependence parameters while the third approach gives a different estimate for Clayton and Frank copulas. This suggests that further analysis is needed to check whether the assumption of Clayton copula and Frank copula are valid, with the techniques such as goodness-of-fit [21].

11.4.2   Example 2: Survival Time of Skin Grafts for Burn Patients

In this example, we consider the data from [5] in which each of the burn patients received both a closely and a poorly matched graft and the days of survival of skin grafts are recored. A skin graft is to remove and transplant healthy skin from one area of the body (donor site) to another area where the skin has been damaged. The source sites most commonly used for skin grafts include the inner thigh and leg. A skin graft can cause pain of varying intensity and duration, even in the postoperative period. Therefore, pain in the graft donor site may be the primary concern of patients in the postoperative period. The main goal of skin graft is the fast recovery of the donor site, which can reduce pain and infection.

The matched paired skin graft data are presented in Table 11.4. There are two right censoring observations in the close match group which are denoted by "+". To test the equality of the two survival distributions for close match and poor match skin grafts, the paired Prentice–Wilcoxon test statistic is $4.524/\sqrt{4.568}$ and the corresponding p-value is 0.017. With Akritas test, the test statistic is 2.568 and the corresponding p-value is 0.028. In conclusion, the data provide enough evidence to reject the null hypothesis that the close match and poor match skin grafts have the same survival distributions.

TABLE 11.4: Days of survival of skin grafts on burn patients.

Close match	37	19	57+	93	16	22	20	18	63	29	60+
Poor match	29	13	15	26	11	17	26	21	43	15	40

+ denotes the right censored data.

11.5 Concluding Remarks

Paired data analysis has been an active topic in the statistical research and applications. With time-to-event paired data, statistical procedures based on normal assumptions may not be appropriate. In addition, it is common to have censored data. We provide an overview on design and analysis of time-to-event paired data. Parametric and nonparametric methods for analyzing both noncensored and censored paired data are reviewed. Estimation of dependence in paired observations based on copula models is also discussed. All the methods considered in this chapter can be applied to paired data arising from analgesic studies. Since the literature in this field is rich, there are many other methods for analyzing paired data are not covered in this chapter. For example, there are methods for competing risk and models for difference types of dependence structure, such as early/late dependence, instantaneous dependence, and short/long-term dependence. Statistical research and applications for paired time-to-event data have provided fruitful solutions in analyzing such data, despite it is still an active research area. Among other development for paired time-to-event endpoints, we expect more progress for the methodologies with high-dimensional data, such as the high-throughout gene expression microarray data.

References

[1] M. G. Akritas. The rank transform method in some two-factor designs. *Journal of the American Statistical Association*, 85:73–78, 1990.

[2] M. G. Akritas. Rank transform statistics with censored data. *Statistics and Probability Letters*, 13:209–221, 1992.

[3] W. Albers. Combined rank tests for randomly censored paired data. *Journal of the American Statistical Association*, 83:1159–1162, 1988.

[4] N. Balakrishnan. *Handbook of the Logistic Distribution*. Marcel Dekker Inc., New York, 1991.

[5] J. R. Batchelor and M. Hackett. HL-A matching in treatment of burned patients with skin allografts. *Lancet*, 2:581–583, 1970.

[6] W. B. Brown, M. Hollander, and R. M. Korwar. *Nonparametric Tests of Independence for Censored Data with Applications to Heart Transplant Studies*, pp. 327–354. SIAM, Philadelphia PA, 1974.

[7] C. Caroni and A. Kimber. Detection of frailty in Weibull lifetime data using outlier tests. *Journal of Statistical Computation and Simulation*, 74:15–23, 2004.

[8] S. C. Chow, J. Shao, and H. Wang. *Sample Size Calculations in Clinical Research*, 1st edn. CRC Press, Boca Raton FL, 2003.

[9] D. Clayton and J. Cuzick. Multivariate generalizations of the proportional hazards model (C/R: p108-117). *Journal of the Royal Statistical Society, Series A, General*, 148:82–108, 1985.

[10] D. G. Clayton. A model for association in bivariate life tables and its application in epidemiological studies of familial tendency in chronic disease incidence. *Biometrika*, 65:141–152, 1978.

[11] M. Crowder. A multivariate distribution with Weibull connections. *Journal of the Royal Statistic Sociey, Series B*, 51:93–107, 1989.

[12] S. J. Curtis, H. Jou, S. Ali, B. Vandermeer, and T. Klassen. A randomized controlled trial of sucrose and/or pacifier as analgesia for infants receiving venipuncture in a pediatric emergency department. *BMC Pediatrics*, 7:27, 2007.

[13] D. M. Dabrowska. Signed-rank tests for censored matched pairs. *Journal of the American Statistical Association*, 85:478–485, 1990.

[14] M. J. Dallas and P. V. Rao. Testing equality of survival functions based on both paired and unpaired censored data. *Biometrics*, 56:154–159, 2000.

[15] L. Duchateau and P. Janssen. *The Frailty Model*, 1st edn. Statistics for Biology and Health. Springer, New York, 2007.

[16] B. Efron and R. J. Tibshirani. *An Introduction to the Bootstrap*. Chapman & Hall, New York, 1993.

[17] M. J. Frank. On the simultaneous associativity of $f(x, y)$ and $x + y - f(x, y)$. *Aequatioins Mathematicae*, 19:194–226, 1979.

[18] R. E. Gangnon and M. R. Kosorok. Sample-size formula for clustered survival data using weighted log-rank statistics. *Biometrika*, 91:263–275, 2004.

[19] C. Genest and J. MacKay. The joy of copulas: Bivariate distributions with uniform marginals (Com: 87V41 p248). *The American Statistician*, 40:280–283, 1986.

[20] C. Genest and R. J. MacKay. Archimedean copulas and bivariate families with continuous marginals (French). *The Canadian Journal of Statistics/La Revue Canadienne de Statistique*, 14:145–159, 1986.

[21] C. Genest, J. -F. Quessy, and B. Remillard. Goodness-of-fit procedures for copula models based on the probability integral transformation. *Scandinavian Journal of Statistics*, 33:337–366, 2006.

[22] C. Genest and L. Rivest. Statistical inference procedures for bivariate Archimedean copulas. *Journal of the American Statistical Association*, 88:1034–1043, 1993.

[23] P. Good. *Permutation, Parametric, and Bootstrap Tests of Hypotheses*, 3rd edn. Springer, New York, 2005.

[24] E. J. Gumbel. Bivariate exponential distributions. *Journal of the American Statistical Association*, 55:698–707, 1960.

[25] M. Hollander and D. A. Wolfe. *Nonparametric Statistical Methods*, 2nd edn. John Wiley & Sons, Inc., New York, 1999.

[26] P. Hougaard. A class of multivariate failure time distributions (Corr: V75 p. 395). *Biometrika*, 73:671–678, 1986.

[27] P. Hougaard. *Analysis of Multivariate Survival Data*. Springer, New York, 2000.

[28] W. J. Huster, R. Brookmeyer, and S. G. Self. Modelling paired survival data with covariates. *Biometrics*, 45:145–156, 1989.

[29] S. A. Julious, M. J. Campbell, and D. G. Altman. Estimating sample sizes for continuous, binary, and ordinal outcomes in paired comparisons: Practical hints. *Journal of Biopharmaceutical Statistics*, 9:241–251, 1999.

[30] J. D. Kalbfleisch and R. L. Prentice. *The Statistical Analysis of Failure Time Data*. John Wiley & Sons, New York, 2002.

[31] J. F. Lawless. *Statistical Models and Methods for Lifetime Data*, 2nd edn. John Wiley & Sons, Inc., New York, 2002.

[32] L. Lee. Multivariate distributions having Weibull properties. *Journal of Multivariate Analysis*, 9:267–277, 1979.

[33] E. L. Lehmann and J. P. Romano. *Testing Statistical Hypotheses*, 3rd edn. Springer, New York, 2005.

[34] J. C. Lu. Weibull extensions of the Freund and Marshall-Olkin bivariate exponential models. *IEEE Transactions on Reliability*, 38:615–619, 1989.

[35] J. C. Lu and G. K. Bhattacharyya. Some new constructions of bivariate Weibull models. *Annals of the Institute of Statistical Mathematics*, 42:543–559, 1990.

[36] J. C. Lu and G. K. Bhattacharyya. Inference procedures for a bivariate exponential model of Gumbel based on life test of component and system. *Journal of Statistical Planning and Inference*, 27:383–396, 1991.

[37] J. C. Lu and G. K. Bhattacharyya. Inference procedures for bivariate exponential model of Gumbel. *Statistics & Probability Letters*, 12:37–50, 1991.

[38] N. Mantel and J. L. Ciminera. Use of logrank scores in the analysis of litter-matched data on time to tumor appearance. *Cancer Research*, 39:4308–4315, 1979.

[39] M. Max, R. Portenoy, and Laska E., eds. *The Design of Analgesic Clinical Trials*, volume 18 of *Advances in Pain Research and Therapy*. Raven Press, New York, 1991.

[40] G. E. Noether. Sample size determination for some common nonparametric tests. *Journal of the American Statistical Association*, 82:645–647, 1987.

[41] D. Oakes. A concordance test for independence in the presence of censoring. *Biometrics*, 38:451–455, 1982.

[42] D. Oakes. A model for association in bivariate survival data. *Journal of the Royal Statistical Society, Series B, Methodological*, 44:414–422, 1982.

[43] D. Oakes. Bivariate survival models induced by frailties. *Journal of the American Statistical Association*, 84:487–493, 1989.

[44] P. C. O'Brien and T. R. Fleming. A paired Prentice-Wilcoxon test for censored paired data. *Biometrics*, 43:169–180, 1987.

[45] W. J. Owen. A power analysis of tests for paired lifetime data. *Lifetime Data Analysis*, 11:233–243, 2005.

[46] W. J. Owen, D. Sinha, and M. H. Capozzoli. A paired-data analysis for a lifetime distribution. *The American Statistician*, 54:252–256, 2000.

[47] R. L. Prentice. Linear rank tests with right censored data (Corr: V70 p. 304). *Biometrika*, 65:167–180, 1978.

[48] D. A. Schoenfeld. Sample-size formula for the proportional-hazards regression model. *Biometrics*, 39:499–503, 1983.

[49] B. Schweizer and A. Sklar. *Probabilistic Metric Spaces*. Elsevier/North-Holland [Elsevier Science Publishing Co., New York; North-Holland Publishing Co., Amsterdam], 1983.

[50] L. B. Sheiner, S. L. Beal, and A. Dunne. Analysis of nonrandomly censored ordered categorical longitudinal data from analgesic trials (C/R: pp. 1245–1255). *Journal of the American Statistical Association*, 92:1235–1244, 1997.

[51] G. Shieh, S. L. Jan, and R. H. Randles. Power and sample size determinations for the wilcoxon signed-rank test. *Journal of Statistical Computation and Simulation*, 77:717–724, 2007.

[52] J. H. Shih and T. A. Louis. Inferences on the association parameter in copula models for bivariate survival data. *Biometrics*, 51:1384–1399, 1995.

[53] W. Wang and M. T. Wells. Model selection and semiparametric inference for bivariate failure-time data (C/R: pp.73–76). *Journal of the American Statistical Association*, 95:62–72, 2000.

[54] Z. Wang. Tests for paired lifetime data with frailty models. *Submitted for publication*, 2008.

[55] Z. Wang and H. K. T. Ng. A comparative study of tests for paired lifetime data. *Lifetime Data Analysis*, 12:505–522, 2006.

[56] J. A. Waterston, M. B. Hawken, S. Tanyeri, P. Jantti, and C. Kennard. Influence of sensory manipulation on postural control in Parkinson's disease. *Journal of Neurology, Neurosurgery & Psychiatry*, 56:1276–1281, 1993.

[57] W. Weibull. A statistical distribution function of wide applicability. *Journal of Applied Mechanics*, 18:293–297, 1951.

[58] D. R. Weier and A. P. Basu. An investigation of Kendall's τ modified for censored data with applications. *Journal of Statistical Planning and Inference*, 4:381–390, 1980.

[59] R. F. Woolson and P. A. Lachenbruch. Rank tests for censored matched pairs (Corr: V71 p. 220). *Biometrika*, 67:597–606, 1980.

[60] R. F. Woolson and T. W. O'Gorman. A comparison of several tests for censored paired data. *Statistics in Medicine*, 11:193–208, 1992.

Chapter 12

Time-to-Event Endpoint Methods in Antibiotic Trials

Karl E. Peace

Contents

12.1 Introduction

Two efficacy endpoints of primary interest in the clinical development of antibiotic drugs for the treatment of infections are microbiological cure and clinical cure. Microbiological cure is typically defined as eradication of the infecting pathogen by the end of treatment and at the posttreatment follow-up visit. Similarly, clinical cure is defined as complete abatement of signs and symptoms of the infection by the end of treatment and at the posttreatment follow-up visit.

Categorical methods, such as Fisher's exact test, Cochran–Mantel–Haenszel tests, or tests deriving from logistic regression are commonly performed comparing treatment groups in terms the proportions of patients achieving cure status. Such methods ignore the time at which cure begins (onset of cure). This chapter presents an example in the area of chronic urinary tract infections, in which time-to-event methods were used to compare treatment groups in terms of the patterns of onset of cure.

12.2 Background

Suppose that a prospective randomized clinical trial with a parallel design is conducted to compare the effectiveness of two regimens in the treatment of a particular chronic disease; e.g., chronic urinary tract infections. In such trials, after satisfying entry criteria, patients are randomized to the two treatment groups. Then patients in Group I receive treatment A (say) for a particular length of time, and patients in Group II receive treatment B for the same length of time. Usually, both groups are treated on an outpatient basis and patients are instructed to return for follow-up at various times within the treatment period, at the end of the treatment period, and at least once posttreatment. Measures of efficacy are the proportions of patients in the treatment groups achieving microbiological or clinical "cure" status.

The definition of either type of cure involves observations made during the treatment period and at the first posttreatment follow-up. That is, a patient is considered microbiologically cured if the infecting pathogen shows negative by the end of the treatment period and also at the first posttreatment follow-up. Similarly, a patient is considered clinically cured if a complete abatement of signs and symptoms (of the disease) is observed by the end of the treatment period and at the first posttreatment follow-up.

In such trials, it is common practice to perform univariate analyses of microbiological cure and clinical cure using endpoint categorical data methodology. For various reasons (absence of pathogens specified by the protocol, patient withdrawal due to adverse reactions, losses to follow-up, inadequate culture, etc.), data on only a subset (e.g., the modified intent-to-treat population) of the individuals originally enrolled in the trial may be included in such analyses. Additionally, such analyses do not reflect different types of "cure patterns" over the treatment period. For example, a patient who experienced a complete abatement of signs and symptoms within the treatment period, at the end of the treatment period and at the first posttreatment follow-up and a patient who experienced a complete abatement at the end of the treatment period and at the first posttreatment follow-up would contribute the same information (both would be clinical cures) in the analysis of the clinical efficacy data. Time-to-event analyses of the efficacy data would, however, allow for the different cure patterns to be reflected. Additionally, losses to follow-up may be appropriately weighted, and thus potentially contribute information for as long as patients were known to be in the trial.

Since the definition of cure requires a posttreatment observation, prospectively it is not possible to classify a patient as being cured during the treatment period. Hence in applying survival analysis methodology to the efficacy data, the onset of cure would be retrospectively located (the earliest time during the treatment period at which abatement began and was observed thereafter). Then time to "cure" is synonymous with time to "failure" (in the usual survival analysis nomenclature).

Thus, the two treatment regimens may be compared by first investigating baseline comparability, then using an appropriate method (e.g., [1–3]) to estimate "noncure" probability curves, and test the null hypothesis of no difference between the two treatment regimens by an appropriate method: e.g., Cox [3] (regressing on important prognostic variables) or Mantel–Haenszel [4–6]; adjusting for important prognostic variables.

12.3 Notation and Methods

Let S_I denote the "noncure function" (survival function in the usual nomenclature) of the target population represented by those patients in Group I, and S_{II} denote the noncure function of the target population represented by those patients in Group II. The efficacy comparison of the two regimens may be formalized as H_0: $S_I = S_{II}$ versus a suitable alternative hypothesis, H_a (noninferiority, for example). The notation which follows is more amenable to the Kaplan–Meier [2] procedure and to the Mantel–Haenszel [4–6] procedure than to the actuarial method or method of Cox [3]. Prognostic (or concomitant) information available on patients at the time of randomization is not notated (Refs. [3–6] may be seen for utilization of such information). Further, except in the discussion of the Mantel–Haenszel statistic, the notation is not indexed by the particular treatment group.

12.3.1 No Withdrawals, or Withdrawals Unweighted

Let N_0 denote the number of patients evaluated for efficacy (microbiological or clinical) at the first posttreatment follow-up (N_0 would be the number at entry if there were no protocol violations and/or no withdrawals). Let t_0 denote the time at which treatment began ($t_0 = 0$). Let t_i, $i = 1, 2, \ldots, v$, denote the times at which cures are located (t_i could represent scheduled times or times of actual follow-up during the treatment period: the choice depending upon the size of v, the spacing of the scheduled times, and patient follow-up compliance; t_v denotes the end of the treatment period). Let t_{v+1} denote the time (nominal) of the first scheduled posttreatment follow-up. Let C_i denote the number of cures at time t_i; nC_i, the number not cured at time t_i; N_i, the number not cured just prior to time t_i; q_i, the proportion cured at time t_i of those not cured just prior to time t_i ($q_i = C_i/N_i$); $p_i = 1 - q_i$, the proportion noncured at t_i of those not cured just prior to time t_i; $\hat{S}_i = \pi P_j$ (product over $j \leq i$), the proportion noncured at at least time t_i; and $F_i = 1 - S_i$, the cumulative proportion cured at time t_i. For illustration, suppose that $v = 3$. The location of the cures may be facilitated by a map of possible patient activity such as that given in Figure 12.1.

A table such as Table 12.1 would then provide a summary of the proportions noncured. The estimated noncure probability curves could then be constructed from the information in Table 12.1.

A table such as Table 12.2 provides a convenient summary of the computations necessary for the value of the Mantel–Haenszel [4–6] statistic.

The Mantel–Haenszel statistic may be written as

$$\chi^2 = \frac{\left(\left| \sum_i c_{1i} - \sum (EC_{1i}) \right| - 1/2 \right)^2}{\sum_i V(C_{1i})} \tag{12.1}$$

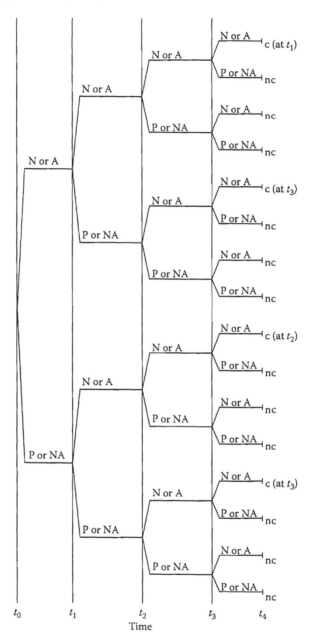

FIGURE 12.1:   Map of possible patient activity for $v = 3$; N denotes negative, P denotes positive, A denotes abated, and NA denotes nonabated.

TABLE 12.1: Typical table for summarizing estimated noncure rates, when no withdrawals occur or when withdrawals are unweighted.

t_i	N_i	C_i	nC_i	q_i	p_i	$\hat{S}_i$	$\hat{F}_i$
$t_o = 0$	N_o	0	N_o	0	1	1	0
t_1	N_1	c_1	nc_1	c_1/N_1	$1-q_1$	p_1	$1-\hat{S}_1$
t_2	N_2	c_2	nc_2	c_2/N_2	$1-q_2$	$p_1 p_2$	$1-\hat{S}_2$
t_3	N_3	c_3	nc_3	c_3/N_3	$1-q_3$	$p_1 p_2 p_3$	$1-\hat{S}_3$
t_4							

TABLE 12.2: Typical table for summarizing the computations necessary for the value of the Mantel–Haenszel statistic.

t_i	Group	C_i	nC_i	N_i	C_{1i}	$E(C_{1i})$	$V(C_{1i})$
t_o	I	0	N_{10}	N_{10}	0	0	0
	II	0	N_{20}	N_{20}			
t_1	I	c_{11}	nc_{11}	N_{11}	c_{11}	$E(C_{11})$	$V(C_{11})$
	II	c_{21}	nc_{21}	N_{21}			
t_2	I	c_{12}	nc_{12}	N_{12}	c_{12}	$E(C_{12})$	$V(C_{12})$
	II	c_{22}	nc_{22}	N_{12}			
t_3	I	c_{13}	nc_{13}	N_{13}	c_{13}	$E(C_{13})$	$V(C_{13})$
	II	c_{23}	nc_{23}	N_{23}			
t_4	I	0	nc_{13}		0	0	0
	II	0	nc_{23}				
	Total				$\sum_{i=1}^{3} C_{1i}$	$\sum_{i=1}^{3} C_{1i}$	$\sum_{i=1}^{3} C_{1i}$

where the first subscript (one) references Group I, c_{1i} denotes the number of cures in Group I at time t_i, $E(C_{1i})$ denotes the expected value of C_{1i} at time t_i, and $V(C_{1i})$ denotes the variance of C_{1i} at time t_i. Both $E(C_{1i})$ and $V(C_{1i})$ are computed from 2×2 tables (Group I, Group II; cure–noncure) constructed at each t_i utilizing the appropriate moment formulae for the hypergeometric distribution. Under the hypothesis H_o: $S_I = S_{II}$, χ^2 is distributed asymptotically as chi-square with 1 degree of freedom.

It is noted that the hypothesis above is equivalent to the hypothesis H_o: $F_I = F_{II}$. (The test based upon the Mantel–Haenszel statistic could not be applied utilizing the cumulative numbers cured due to correlated observations. There is however no problem in applying the test utilizing the numbers cured at a particular time obtained from the tables summarizing the noncure rates. Note that in such tables the number of cures, c_i, at a particular time, t_i, is removed from the number, N_i, possible to be cured at t_i before obtaining the number possible to be cured at time t_{i+1}).

12.3.2   Withdrawals Due to Loss to Follow-Up Weighted

Let N_o denote the number of patients entering the study. Let t_i, C_i, c_i, nC_i, nc_i, q_i, p_i, $\hat{S}_i$, and $\hat{F}_i$ be defined as in Section 12.2.1. Let W denote withdrawals, W_{fi} denote the number of withdrawals due to loss to follow-up just after time t_i, and W_{oi} the number of withdrawals due to other causes just after time t_i, $i = 0, 1, \ldots, v$. Further, let $W_{fi} = \sum j W_{fij}$. Note that for $i > 0$, W_{fi} may consist of patients of at least two "types"—the maximum number of types being 2^i, and dependent on the observed response (negative or positive, abated or not abated) at time t_i. Let N_{i+1} denote the number possible to be cured at time t_{i+1}, $i = 0, \ldots, v - 1$ $(N_{i+1} = N_i - C_i - W_{fi} - W_{oi})$. Let $N(\text{nc})$ denote the number observed noncured at the first posttreatment follow-up: $N(\text{nc}|n_1)$, denote the number observed noncured at the first posttreatment follow-up of those observed negative (microbiological; abated, if clinical) at time t_1; $N(|n_1)$, denote the number observed negative (abated) at time t_1; etc. Let P_{f1j}^*, denote the conditional proportion noncured from the data when tracing the number evaluated for efficacy at the first posttreatment follow-up, from entry as though there were no withdrawals; e.g., $P_{fo1}^* = N(\text{nc})/N_o$, $P_{f11}^* = (\text{nc}|n_1)/N(|n_1)$, etc. Let N'_{i+1} denote the effective number exposed to the "risk" of being cured $(N'_{i+1} = N_{i+1} + \sum j P_{fij}^* W_{fij})$. Finally let q_i denote the proportion cured at time t_i given noncured at time t_{i-1} $(q_i = c_i/N'_i)$.

Again for the purpose of illustration, suppose $v = 3$. Figure 12.2 and Table 12.3 are the analogues of Figure 12.1 and Table 12.1.

A table for summarizing the computations necessary for the value of the Mantel–Haenszel statistic would be the same as Table 12.2 with N'_i replacing N_i.

12.4   Example

As an example* suppose that a trial, as discussed in Sections 12.1 and 12.2 was conducted with a treatment period of 10 days and that patients had intratreatment follow-up on each day. Further suppose: (1) that 100 patients in each treatment group were evaluated for efficacy at the first posttreatment follow-up; (2) that the groups of 100 each were comparable at baseline with respect to possible prognostic variables (e.g., sex, age, weight, height, race, number of previous UTIs, localization of present UTI, and signs and symptoms total) and their incidences of adverse experiences were

---

* The data in this example are contrived. Real data, the nature of which is confidential, have been analyzed by the author by the methods (including weighting withdrawals) described.

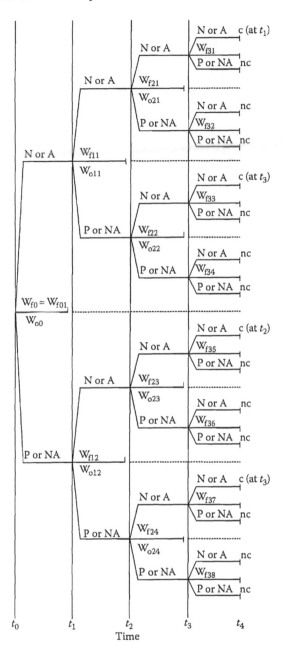

FIGURE 12.2: Map of possible patient activity for $v = 3$; when withdrawals due to loss to follow-up are weighted. Notation is explained in the text.

TABLE 12.3: Typical table for summarizing estimated noncure rates, when withdrawals due to loss to follow-up are weighted.

t_i	N_i	W		C_i	nC_i	N_i	q_i	$p_i{}^{a}$	$\hat{S}_i{}^{b}$	$\hat{F}_i{}^{c}$
		W_{fi}	W_{oi}							
t_o	N_o	0	0	0	N_o	N_o	0			
		W_{f0}	W_{o0}							
t_1	N_1			c_1	nc_1	N_1	c_1/N_1			
		W_{f1}	W_{o1}							
t_2	N_2			c_2	nc_2	N_2	c_2/N_2			
		W_{f2}	W_{o2}							
t_3	N_3			c_3	nc_3	N_3	c_3/N_3			
		W_{f3}	W_{o3}							
t_4										

Notation is explained in the text.
a $p_i = 1 - q_i$.
b $\hat{S}_i = \pi p_j$.
  $j \le i$
c $\hat{F}_i = 1 - \hat{S}_i$.

low and roughly the same; (3) that 90 cures (clinical, say) were among each of the 100 patients; and (4) that the therapy days (and frequencies) from which patients experienced an abatement of signs and symptoms through the first posttreatment follows-up were

Group I: 1(40), 2(14), 3(14), 4(12), 5(4), 6(3), 7(3)

Group II: 3(3), 4(3), 5(4), 6(2), 7(4), 8(4), 9(20), 10(50)

No difference between the two treatments using the proportion cured (or non-cured) in each treatment group as the response variable is observed. Consequently, no analysis of endpoints ignoring the times at which clinical cure began would detect a treatment difference.

Estimating the noncure probabilities as suggested in Table 12.1 and plotting gives the "noncure" patterns in Figure 12.3. Certainly the noncure patterns suggest that treatment A is the superior treatment.

The Mantel–Haenszel procedure strongly detects this difference with a χ^2 value of 78.11 (Table 12.4).

Some modifications in the observed cure patterns would also lead to the endpoint analyses failing to detect a treatment difference and survival analyses detecting a difference; e.g., if at day 10 there were 41, 42, ..., 49 cures in Group B. These examples are similar to those (in the usual survival nomenclature) alluded to by Mantel [6].

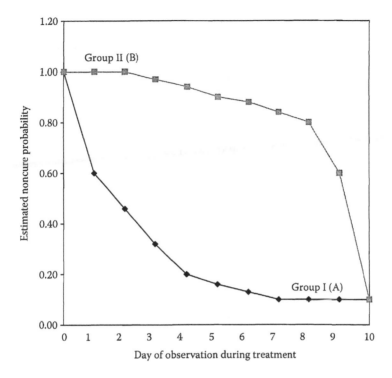

FIGURE 12.3: Estimated noncure probability curves utilizing the data in the example of Section 3.

12.5 Discussion

Data generated in a setting such as that described in Sections 12.1 and 12.2 are commonly analyzed by endpoint contingency table methods. Analyses of the survival data type have been suggested as alternative methods [7,8]. Such analyses utilize the data more fully than do endpoint ones. The reasons for this are (1) such analyses reflect the cure (noncure) patterns over the treatment period—leading to identification of the onset of cure, and (2) such analyses allow for withdrawals due to loss to follow-up to be incorporated.

Endpoint analyses may be applied more easily to test the hypothesis of no treatment difference than may the survival type analyses. However, there are situations (such as the example(s) presented) which are design and/or data dependent in which a survival-type analysis may be the analysis of choice. Even if one performs an endpoint analysis to test the hypothesis of no treatment difference, accompanying the result with graphs of the estimated noncure curves is useful information.

TABLE 12.4: Summary of computations necessary for the value[a] of the Mantel–Haenszel statistic for the example data.

t_i	Group	C_{ji}	nC_{ji}	N_{ji}	C_{1i}	$E(C_{1i})$	$V(C_{1i})$
	I	40	60	100			
1	II	0	100	100	40	20.00	8.04
		40	160	200			
	I	14	46	060			
2	II	0	100	100	14	5.25	3.01
		14	146	160			
	I	14	32	046			
3	II	3	97	100	14	5.36	3.26
		17	129	146			
	I	12	20	32			
4	II	3	94	97	12	3.72	2.49
		15	114	129			
	I	4	16	20			
5	II	4	90	94	4	1.40	1.09
		8	106	114			
	I	3	13	16			
6	II	2	88	90	3	0.75	0.62
		5	101	106			
	I	3	10	13			
7	II	4	84	88	3	0.90	0.74
		7	94	101			
	I	0	10	10			
8	II	4	80	84	0	0.43	0.37
		4	90	94			
	I	0	10	10			
9	II	20	60	80	0	2.22	1.55
		20	70	90			
	I	0	10	10			
10	II	50	10	60	0	7.14	1.77
		50	20	70			
		Total			90	47.17	22.94

[a] $\chi^2 = (90 - 47.17 - 0.5)^2/22.94 = 78.11$.

References

[1] Berkson J and Gage RP (1950): Calculations of survival rates for cancer. *Proceedings of Staff Meetings; Mayo Clinic* 25(11): 270–286.

[2] Kaplan EL and Meier P (1958): Nonparametric estimation from incomplete observations. *Journal of the American Statistical Association* 53: 457–481.

[3] Cox DR (1972): Regression models and life tables. *Journal of the Royal Statistical Society; Series B* 32: 187–220.

[4] Mantel N and Haenszel W (1959): Statistical aspects of the analysis of data from retrospective studies of disease. *Journal of the National Cancer Institute* 22(4): 719–748.

[5] Mantel N (1963): Chisquare tests with one degree of freedom: Extension of the Mantel-Haenszel procedure. *Journal of the American Statistical Association* 58: 690–700.

[6] Mantel N (1966): Evaluation of survival data and two new rank order statistics arising in its consideration. *Cancer Chemotherapy Reports* 50(3): 163–170.

[7] Peace KE (1979): Performing a survival analysis instead of an endpoint analysis. *Biometrics* 35(4): 892–893.

[8] Peace KE (2007): A survival analysis instead of an endpoint analysis for antibiotic data. *The Philippine Statistician* 56(1–2): 9–18.

Chapter 13

Design and Analysis of Cardiovascular Prevention Trials

Michelle McNabb and Andreas Sashegyi

Contents

13.1 Introduction

The combination of disease state, patient population, and types of endpoints considered in a clinical outcomes trial determine the commonly used classification of such studies as either treatment or prevention trials. This chapter will focus specifically on the prevention paradigm and examine design and analytical issues particularly for cardiovascular outcomes trials.

This chapter will explore in some detail issues relating to definition of study endpoints and event rate estimation; further discussion will focus on exposure considerations as well as the analysis of composite endpoints and accommodating the possibility of multiple events per patient. Each of these broad topics present a number of practical challenges that warrant careful consideration. In the latter part of the chapter, topics of interest that all relate to prevention trials more generally are discussed as well. In Section 13.3, the Raloxifene Use for The Heart (RUTH) study will be used to illustrate concepts.

Prevention trials typically focus on individuals with a chronic condition in which the goal of intervention is to prevent an undesirable event for which this population is at risk, but which may take years to develop. The chosen terminology emphasizes the most desirable outcome of risk elimination, though in practical terms the context in which the term "prevention" is used is often synonymous with "risk reduction," and in some cases this is essentially tantamount to a significant delay in event onset. This contrasts with the treatment trial paradigm, which focuses on interventions for the amelioration of acute conditions, or the management of sequelae of acute injury. The above notwithstanding, a patient in the prevention setting may in some cases be subclassified as belonging to a secondary versus a primary prevention population, depending on whether or not he/she has already experienced a key event of interest at some point previously and is at risk for subsequent events, as opposed to being at risk for the first occurrence. This distinction illustrates that the division between prevention and treatment trials is not necessarily a sharp one. Furthermore, both types of trials may be designed to provide information on the same kind of measure, such as a risk reduction or relative hazard. Nonetheless, the following key differences are noteworthy. Patient populations in prevention trials tend to be more broadly defined, healthier, and experience lower event rates than those typical of pure treatment trials. As a consequence, these trials tend to be larger, and/or involve longer exposure durations. An added challenge may be faced in the definition and complexity of a suitable primary endpoint, which will invariably constitute a composite of numerous relevant components as opposed to a single clinical event type.

13.2   Methods

Due to the size and duration of cardiovascular prevention trials, study design requires particularly careful attention to detail. While it is possible to modify a study design after study initiation, in practice many modifications can be avoided with careful planning and realistic estimates of parameters defining the sample size and study duration.

13.2.1   Defining Appropriate Study Endpoints

Trials designed to demonstrate reductions in risk of cardiovascular events with a therapeutic intervention typically focus on primary study endpoints defined as composites of two or more specific event types [1]. One common definition of such an endpoint is the occurrence of myocardial infarction, stroke, or cardiovascular death [2–4]. A patient is then counted as having reached a primary study endpoint if he or she experiences any of the specific event types that contribute to the definition. Numerous methods for analyzing composite endpoints are available, and are addressed further in Section 13.2.5. The choice of a composite primary endpoint has a dual motivation. First, cardiovascular events themselves imply any of a number of clinical outcomes or syndromes that lie in the pathophysiology of cardiovascular disease. Where to draw the line in terms of which particular components to include in defining an appropriate study endpoint is itself an important question, and is discussed further below. Second, from a practical but no less relevant perspective, designing a prevention trial with a single event type such as myocardial infarction (MI) as the primary outcome would be infeasible because, for the most part, cardiovascular event rates in the prevention setting are confined to percentages per annum in the very low single digits [2–5]. In terms of a study well-powered to demonstrate a clinically meaningful risk reduction, this would essentially necessitate a prohibitively large sample size (quite possibly tens of thousands of patients) and many years of follow-up to generate the number of events required for analysis, thus rendering the value proposition from the perspective of both cost and practical clinical benefit unacceptable.

13.2.2   Considerations Impacting Sample Size

Due to the long-term nature of cardiovascular trials, sample size estimation can be influenced by many factors. Throughout this chapter we largely focus on survival analysis examining time-to-event, arguably the most common choice for the primary analysis, although as indicated other methods for analyzing event data are also available. In addition to the usual need for an estimated treatment effect, sample size estimation for time-to-event analyses in long-term cardiovascular trials often relies upon good estimates of event rates (taking into account the impact of event adjudication), patient accrual patterns, treatment-benefit lag, carry-over effects, as well as drop-out and drop-in rates, i.e., the impact of treated patients discontinuing therapy and control patients commencing some form of active treatment, respectively.

13.2.2.1   Event Rate Estimation

The problem of accurately estimating a background event rate for the control arm of a clinical outcomes trial is challenging at best. For cardiovascular prevention trials this issue is likely to be exacerbated:

- Although methods for analyzing multiple endpoints per subject are readily available [6] (see also Section 13.2.5.), examination of the time-to-first-event in subjects is ostensibly a primary analysis standard for outcomes trials. Use of a composite primary endpoint with two or more components thus requires consideration of the degree of overlap between the individual components in estimating the composite event rate—the prevalence of patients who experience more than one component over the course of the trial, but whose first event is the only one counted in the analysis.

- Heterogeneity in the patient population adds additional uncertainty to event rate estimation. Prevention trials may enroll both primary and secondary prevention patients which may, or may not be controlled during randomization. Additionally, enrollment and exclusion criteria may lead to unexpected enrollment patterns, especially in a multinational trial.

- Cardiovascular health is a quickly evolving field. During long duration prevention trials, new treatments and diagnostics often emerge having the potential to impact event rates over time.

- Given the importance of endpoint adjudication in cardiovascular outcomes trials [7,8] it follows that the primary analysis and most, if not all, secondary analyses are typically performed on adjudicated events. Depending on the process of confirming definitive events in a particular trial, adjudicated outcomes may exceed or fall short of investigator-reported events. In any case, a difference in adjudicated and investigator-reported event rates is to be expected and must also be considered in estimating event rates.

13.2.2.2   Patient Accrual

Duration and patterns of patient accrual are influenced by many factors. Enrollment criteria, exclusion criteria, number of investigative sites, and sample size are direct contributors to duration of patient accrual. Enrollment and exclusion criteria should be carefully assessed to ensure that they are not unduly restrictive. For example, enrollment of a trial examining secondary prevention patients would be dependent upon the prevalence of existing disease (e.g., prior coronary event, prior stroke) in the population being studied. A compromise is often a combination of secondary prevention patients supplemented with inclusion of primary prevention patients at high risk of cardiovascular disease or the specific event being studied [4,5].

Some factors influencing accrual patterns can be anticipated during study development. For example, investigative sites may initiate enrollment in stages. Examples of factors that may not be anticipated include delays in ethical review board (ERB) approval or limited availability of study drug.

13.2.2.3   Treatment Lag and Carry-Over Effects

Preventive therapies may require a lead-in period before they achieve necessary plasma concentrations of the test drug or patient exposure to become effective. Lagtimes delay treatment effects and thus, while increasing overall pooled event rates (assuming that treatment effect delay results in event rates among treated patients closer to the higher placebo rate), they decrease observed treatment differences, with the net effect of requiring larger sample sizes. Similarly carry-over effects may extend treatment effects even after therapy is discontinued such that carry-over time can be considered as a contributor to exposure. Pharmacokinetic and pharmacodynamic research can provide information to assist with estimates, but often lag and carry-over effect estimates are founded on expert clinical judgment.

13.2.2.4 Study Duration: Time-Driven versus Endpoint-Driven Designs

In view of potentially high variability inherent in estimating event accrual, the importance of a trial design which defines study termination in terms of the achievement of a specified number of primary endpoints (more accurately, number of patients each having experienced at least one primary endpoint) is well-motivated. Such endpoint-driven designs offer greater flexibility than fixed-termination designs in terms of the ability to balance sample size and follow-up duration for a given trial, and provide considerable insulation to misjudgment in the control group event rate—over-estimation simply leads to a longer trial, and vice versa. At the same time, these advantages must be appreciated in the context of other constraints that may apply, as discussed further in Section 13.3.2. For example, follow-up duration in a prevention trial must fall within a reasonable window. Average follow-up that is too short—say, less than 12–24 months, depending on whether secondary or primary prevention is the focus—does not allow for assessment of long-term treatment effects, a hallmark of the prevention paradigm. On the other hand, if even with a reasonable sample size an unduly long follow-up period is necessary to achieve the required number of events, the absolute magnitude of the implied treatment is likely to be too small to be clinically meaningful.

13.2.2.5 Sample Size Estimation

If nothing else, this chapter highlights the great (and on the periphery perhaps not immediately apparent) complexity of cardiovascular prevention trials. Each of the issues discussed here has the potential to impact the determination of an appropriate sample size to a greater or lesser extent. Given the differences and uncertainty in distributional assumptions regarding survival times, and in the numerous other important factors that should ideally be taken into account, there is no single approach that can be proposed as a universal standard for estimating sample size for clinical outcomes studies. Nonetheless the literature offers numerous reasonable starting points (see, for example, [9–13]), and software packages for clinical trial design have made it relatively easy to investigate the impact on sample size of varying assumptions in a wide range of parameters, such as compliance with treatment, drop-ins, varying accrual rates, and a lag in onset of treatment effect.

As the simplest first pass at the initial trial planning stage, one can gain an idea of the approximate number of patients required by treating the outcomes data not as survival or censoring times, but as dichotomous responses, simply indicating whether a subject has experienced an event or not. If the proportions of subjects experiencing events in the control and active treatment arms of a study are given by p_C and p_T for instance, and assuming n patients in each group, then letting $\bar{p} = (p_C + p_T)/2$, Z_q the upper-q quantile of the standard normal distribution, and α and $1 - \beta$ the size and power for a two-tailed test, the binomial sample size formula

$$n = \frac{2\left(Z_{\alpha/2}\sqrt{2\bar{p}(1-\bar{p})} + Z_{\beta}\sqrt{p_C(1-p_C) + p_T(1-p_T)}\right)^2}{(p_C - p_T)^2}$$

can be used to determine the total number of patients required for a two-tailed test. The impact of other design features and anticipated trial operating characteristics can be accounted for, at least crudely, by making an educated guess at their impact on p_C and p_T. Nonetheless it would be inappropriate to dwell on the binomial formula if the intent were indeed to use survival methods for analyzing the data, which is more typically the case. In this setting sample size is commonly determined by considering first the number of events required to meet assumptions about effect size and error rates, and calculating from this the number of patients needed. Freedman [10] derives these values for use of the logrank test; assuming a constant hazard ratio over time and expressing this as $\theta = \log(1 - p_T)/\log(1 - p_C)$, the total number of events d required for the analysis is

$$d = \left(Z_{\alpha/2} + Z_{\beta}\right)^2 \left(\frac{1+\theta}{1-\theta}\right)^2,$$

from which the sample size can be determined as $n = 2d/(p_C + p_T)$. Freedman [10] also gives the extension for these formulae in cases where randomization is not 1:1. Lakatos [12] extends this work by presenting a general framework for sample size determination which does not assume proportional hazards and accommodates realistic trial conditions such as staggered entry, noncompliance, or lag times in treatment effect. Survival curves are modeled using stochastic processes in which states are defined according to the various classifications desired to describe a patient's condition at any given point during the study. Less restrictive approaches to sample size calculation may be particularly beneficial in dealing with a common phenomenon in treatment, but also certain secondary prevention trials, in which event rates are often markedly higher in the early weeks or months after randomization, but taper off thereafter [14,15]. Clearly this impacts not only selection of an appropriate follow-up duration, but also depending on the nature of the anticipated treatment effect, may lead to very different (in particular, nonproportional) patterns of event accrual in the control and active treatment groups.

The work of these and other authors has been incorporated into software products such as SAS® and East® [16,17] to provide a great deal of flexibility in helping the practitioner choose an appropriate sample size. It is important to bear in mind, however, that an estimate of sample size is always just that—an estimate. In cardiovascular prevention trials, the numerous assumptions that must be made at the planning stage are likely to render this estimate much less reliable than the sample size for a smaller, shorter study in which experimental conditions are more tightly controlled. A sensible approach in light of this is to explore several methods for determining sample size before settling on the most reasonable one, and then investigate the robustness of the results to departures from key assumptions in a series of sensitivity analyses. Clinical trial simulation tools that assess operating characteristics of particular trial designs under realistic assumptions about enrollment patterns, drop-out patterns, etc. could be very useful in this regard.

In any case, the calculation of sample size should reflect as closely as possible the intended analysis population and method. We highlight two points in this regard: first, the treatment of noncompliant patients, including those who may have permanently discontinued the experimental therapy, is a particularly important consideration. In an intent-to-treat survival analyses, such patients typically remain in the risk set until the occurrence of an event, as though they had never discontinued study drug. This helps approximate realistic conditions anticipated in clinical practice, thus supporting the estimate of a practical treatment effect that takes expected noncompliance into account. For patients who are lost to follow-up or drop out of the study through deliberate withdrawal of consent, the date of last contact may be used to censor their time in the study.

Secondly, insofar as sample size is calculated by a derivation from what drives it—the number of events required (specifically, the number of patients having at least one event in a time-to-first-event analysis), it often makes most sense to also define the termination of the study in an event-driven manner, as the time at which the required number of endpoints have been observed, as opposed to fixing the study duration in advance. As discussed also in Section 13.2.2.4., this may offer an important protection against misspecification of event and accrual rates, as well as other parameters impacting the occurrence of endpoints; although such misspecification will impact the follow-up time required to observed the required number of events, it may be feasible to accommodate the resulting (typically longer) follow-up time and continue to run the study to its end without a protocol amendment. When departures from parameter assumptions are more extreme, some sort of intervention is likely to be required in any case.

13.2.3   Trial Monitoring

Due to the long-term nature of cardiovascular prevention trials and the often serious nature of the outcomes being studied, ongoing monitoring of patient safety is mandatory. Data Monitoring Committees (DMCs) are generally used to perform this important duty. Additionally, trials may be monitored in a blinded fashion by those conducting the study. Both scenarios will be discussed.

13.2.3.1   Data Monitoring Committees

DMCs consist of a small group of experts who periodically review study data; see Ellenberg et al. [18] for a useful general reference. DMCs review partially or completely unblinded data. To reduce the risk of potential bias introduced by interim reviews of unblinded data, DMCs should be composed of individuals who are not directly involved with the day-to-day conduct of the study [19]. Typically, the primary purpose of a DMC is to monitor patient safety. A DMC may also review efficacy endpoints to determine whether a study should be stopped early for futility or outstanding efficacy. As adaptive study designs become more common, DMCs are being employed to execute and evaluate outcomes of adaptive algorithms to make recommendations to study sponsors regarding dosing, sample size, and other trial considerations. A DMC charter should be prepared with explicit guidelines for evaluating futility and efficacy. A DMC charter may also include guidelines for evaluating specific safety outcomes or risk–benefit scores. To that end, safety and efficacy monitoring are inextricably linked in cardiovascular outcomes trials, insofar as the outcomes of interest are all adverse by nature and the distinction between safety and efficacy is drawn according to whether a therapy increases or decreases the risk of an event. Therefore sensible monitoring rules are called for that effectively evaluate the risk–benefit balance of the accumulating data.

Rules for early stopping for either futility or efficacy should be stringent to ensure minimal risk of error. Early stopping for efficacy in particular is more problematic than futility. Interim efficacy tests inflate the trial-wise type-I error rate, the impact of which must be incorporated in the study design. Many methods exist to adjust significance levels to ensure trial-wise type-I error does not exceed 0.05. An excellent summary of such methods is offered in Jennison and Turnbull [20], and an example from the RUTH study is included in Section 13.3.3.1.

13.2.3.2 Blinded Monitoring

Although viewed as controversial by some, blinded monitoring of randomized trials by the study sponsor (in addition to the unblinded data monitoring carried out independently by a DMC) can be useful especially in the case of long-term trials as a means for assessing the accuracy of the assumed event rate specified in the protocol. In cardiovascular prevention, a typical treatment effect size used for planning trials is a 20% relative risk reduction or relative hazard with the experimental treatment versus control. Using the assumed effect size and a specified estimate of the event rate in the control group, a putative overall event rate (pooled across treatment groups) can be calculated. Large departures in the observed pooled event rate of an ongoing trial from this projected rate are unlikely to be driven by misjudgment in the magnitude of the treatment effect, particularly if the observed rate is much smaller than the putative rate. Blinded monitoring as described admits the possibility of protocol changes even to an ongoing study, such as the addition of other relevant components to the primary endpoint to increase the primary event rate. Specific examples of such changes and conditions under which these are acceptable are described in Section 13.2.4. This illustrates an advantage of utilizing an independent DMC. Because the individuals conducting the study remain blinded to study outcomes, they may make unbiased decisions to modify a study's design.

13.2.4 Modifying an Ongoing Study

In general terms, a number of questions must be considered when contemplating an intervention to more closely realign emerging event rates during the live phase of a trial with protocol-specified assumptions. First of all, given the effectiveness of the standard of cardiovascular care in many parts of the world, coupled with secular trends globally, undue underestimation of event rates is unlikely to ever present an issue. More commonly, event rates may be observed to fall short of design assumptions, as was the case in RUTH. As pointed out above, one must then consider whether compensation by means of extending the follow-up period or increasing sample size is feasible from a practical perspective, and in view of the implications this would have on the relevance of the treatment effect. The possibility of broadening the definition of the composite primary endpoint by adding an additional endpoint component should be considered and may be an attractive alternative to extending follow-up provided the following criteria are met:

- The new endpoint component is acceptable from a medical perspective in that it reflects a common outcome of the cardiovascular disease pathway.

- The new endpoint component is acceptable from a medical and a regulatory perspective in that it is sufficiently robust and unambiguous in its definition— this highlights the distinction between "hard" and "soft" endpoints, the latter referring to outcomes such as unstable angina that are more difficult to define precisely and over which there is typically more debate.

- The treatment effect assumed to have bearing on the events originally included in the primary endpoint can also be assumed to have a similar effect on the proposed new endpoint component.

- The addition of the new component has the potential to increase the rate of first occurrences of primary endpoints in the trial. In other words, the correlation between this and the original primary endpoint components is not so strong as to expect that occurrences of the new component will be observed primarily in patients who would also have experienced a primary endpoint under the original definition anyway. This would obviously not help in planning for a time-to-first-event analysis.

These criteria are quite stringent, and one might argue that any event identified as a potential candidate to expand the definition of a composite primary endpoint, which meets each of these criteria without qualifying caveats, should have been considered as part of the primary endpoint definition at the design stage. Design changes such as this in an ongoing trial, while not unmanageable, are fraught with challenges and are never to be considered as a matter of convenience. Section 13.3.2 highlights some of these challenges in specifically exploring events of the RUTH trial in more detail.

13.2.5   Analysis of Composite Endpoints and Multiple Events Per Patient

Although the analysis of time-to-first-event is a well-established regulatory standard for the primary analysis of an outcomes trial, it has obvious limitations and where appropriate should be augmented, in secondary or sensitivity analyses, by other approaches that account for the potential multiplicity of event occurrences in terms of type and number that may be observed in individual patients over the course of a study, especially one having a composite primary endpoint. Moreover, the analysis of multiple events per patient is particularly recommended for prevention trials, in which typically lengthy follow-up times may increase the likelihood of multiple events of interest per patient.

Consider a trial in which the primary endpoint is a composite of three event types of varying seriousness: Coronary death, nonfatal MI, or Acute Coronary Syndrome (ACS) other than MI—ordered here from most to least serious. Over the course of the study patients may experience multiple occurrences of MI and/or ACS; they may suffer none, any or all of the individual endpoints that form the composite. A time-to-first-event analysis does not distinguish between a patient who has an MI at time t_1 but remains event-free for the rest of the study and one who has an MI at time t_1, followed by two subsequent MIs at time t_2 and t_3; furthermore, based on the timing of the first event, with $t_1 < t_2 < t_3$ such an analysis would regard a patient outcome of a single occurrence of ACS at t_1 as less favorable than suffering an MI at t_2, followed by coronary death at t_3. This underscores the potential loss of information and misinterpretation of data that a time-to-first-event analysis may be prone to by not taking into account event multiplicity and/or severity. That said, whereas such examples motivate deliberate analysis of multiple events per patients, the multivariate models available for this purpose also imply a certain increased complexity in the analysis and interpretation of the data. Moreover, analysis of multiple events is not necessarily an effective means of increasing power, which is influenced by factors such as the proportion of patients experiencing multiple events, the correlation between time-to-first-event and time-to-subsequent-events, and the treatment effect on first versus subsequent events. Indeed, a number of univariate approaches may be considered that mitigate, at least in part, the pitfalls of a time-to-first-event analysis. One alternative would suggest analyzing time-to-most-serious-event, in cases where composite endpoint components can be ordered according to severity. This type of an analysis is clinically meaningful and easy to interpret, though it may still ignore information related to multiplicity; thus it makes sense to augment analysis of time-to-most-serious-event with a categorical analysis that does not distinguish between event types but addresses multiplicity by simply classifying patients as having experienced, for example, 0, 1, 2, or ≥ 3 events. Standard treatment group comparisons for this latter analysis are appropriate provided exposure duration and patterns are similar between the groups being compared. Secondary analyses commonly examine time to each composite endpoint component individually, to investigate consistency of effect. Such analyses have to be interpreted with great care, however; marginal analysis of an endpoint component of lesser severity is difficult to interpret without taking into account the more serious outcomes, especially when event types are related to a common pathophysiology. A more reasonable approach would be to begin with an analysis of time-to-most-serious event and broaden this to include additional event types in the composite endpoint one by one in order of decreasing severity; e.g., time-to-coronary death, followed by time-to-coronary death or nonfatal MI, followed by time-to-coronary death, nonfatal MI, or ACS other than MI. Finally, one may consider the construction of a score or count based on the composite endpoint that accounts for the possibility of multiple events per patient. This could be conceptually straightforward and make use of all available data, but may also be criticized for being arbitrarily chosen and therefore lacking robustness.

Despite the options above, and acknowledging the greater complexity of a comprehensive analysis of multiple events per patient, such investigation may nonetheless be a critical step in achieving a full understanding of the data. A number of approaches that apply Cox's proportional hazards analysis for modeling survival data to multiple events per patient have been proposed and are readily implemented [6,21–25]. Each of these approaches estimates regression coefficients from a model fit that ignores the correlation between the multiple observations (induced by multiple events) from a given subject, but applies a robust covariance matrix which corrects for this correlation. Andersen and Gill [23] describe a model based on independent increments in which a patient's observations correspond to interevent times (e.g., for a individual with three events: study entry to first event, first to second event, second to third, and third to censoring time). The intensity process for a given patient is nearly identical to the Cox model for single-event setting, the only difference being the fact that a patient is not removed from the risk set upon experiencing an event. This model is perhaps the most intuitive adaptation to accommodating multiple events per patient but makes the rather strong assumptions of a common underlying baseline hazard for each event and independence of observations within a subject—risk of a subsequent event follows the proportional hazards assumption and is not affected by earlier events. Moreover, the model does not differentiate between event types. In contrast Wei et al. [24] propose a marginal approach in which outcomes are analyzed like a competing risks problem. Unlike the Andersen and Gill model, this formulation is particularly suited to cases in which assessment of treatment effect on time-to-specific-event types is of interest such that patients' observations would correspond to time from study entry to each of type of event, e.g., study entry to ACS other than MI, entry to nonfatal MI, and entry to coronary death. A patient is at risk for the jth event type until the (first) occurrence of that type of event, barring censoring. The analysis is stratified by event type and admits a separate baseline hazard for each event, as well as event-specific regression coefficients. Finally, a conditional model proposed by Prentice et al. [25] offers a third alternative in which a patient is not at risk for the jth event until he or she has experienced event $j - 1$, and remains at risk until the jth event or censoring takes effect. Observations in the input to this model follow the counting process representation used in Andersen and Gill's model. Like the Andersen and Gill approach, this formulation does not distinguish between event types, but similar to the Wei, Lin, and Weissfeld model, it does allow for separate baseline hazards and coefficients for each event occurence. In fact, the latter two models have the same intensity process, differing only in the definition of the risk sets. Thus, Prentice, Williams, and Peterson's approach is appropriate in cases where interest lies primarily in assessing the effect of treatment not only on first event occurrences, but also on second and subsequent occurrences.

Whether or not to employ any of these (or other) approaches to address the issue of multiple events per patient, and if so, which ones, hinges on the prevalence of multiple events and the specific scientific questions of interest. The discussion above has focused on a range of approaches that take a variety of inferential perspectives. Importantly, this discussion has not addressed multiplicity in the sense of nominal significance level adjustments for hypothesis testing, to control type I error. But of course such considerations apply to this context as to any other in which multiple hypotheses are of interest; the nature of the adjustments required will depend on the number of tests to be performed and the intended purpose of the inferences.

13.3   Application: The RUTH Study

Raloxifene HCl is a selective estrogen receptor modulator exhibiting estrogen-agonist effects in the skeletal system and antiestrogenic effects in the breast and uterus. Clinical studies have demonstrated that raloxifene increases bone mineral density and reduces the risk of vertebral fractures, findings which formed the basis of its approval for indications for both prevention and treatment of osteoporosis in postmenopausal women. Animal studies evaluating the compound's potential cardiovascular efficacy showed reductions in serum cholesterol and regression of atherosclerosis. In clinical testing, significant positive effects on biochemical markers of cardiovascular risk were demonstrated in a 6 month study of raloxifene versus placebo or hormone therapy. These findings led to the planning of a Phase III confirmatory cardiovascular prevention trial sponsored by Eli Lilly and Company.

RUTH was a global, double-blinded, placebo-controlled, parallel study, originally designed to determine whether chronic treatment with 60 mg/day of raloxifene HCl reduces the incidence of the composite primary endpoint of coronary death or nonfatal MI, in postmenopausal women at risk for coronary events [26]. Secondary objectives of the study included assessment of whether chronic raloxifene treatment changes the incidence of a broader composite cardiovascular endpoint, defined as cardiovascular death, nonfatal MI, myocardial revascularization, and stroke. In addition, each of these endpoint components were assessed individually in secondary analyses. To be eligible for randomization, women had to be postmenopausal, at least 55 years of age, and at risk of a MI. This latter criterion was met if a score of at least 4 points was achieved on a cardiovascular risk assessment, which assigned 1 or more points to various conditions or risk factors that predispose to coronary events [26]. Essentially this meant that women had to have some combination of established coronary heart disease (CHD), peripheral arterial disease, diabetes, or multiple risk factors for CHD. Those with established CHD were classified as secondary prevention, whereas the remaining women were classified as primary prevention subjects. Women were asked to return to their investigator's office for follow-up at 3 months, 6 months, and every 6 months thereafter for clinical and laboratory assessments. At every visit, subjects were probed for the occurrence of study endpoints, insofar as these had not already been reported to the investigator. The RUTH study design is illustrated in Figure 13.1.

13.3.1   Study Endpoints and Sample Size

In the primary analysis of the RUTH data, the time-to-first-event curves of the two treatment groups were compared using the logrank test. The RUTH trial was

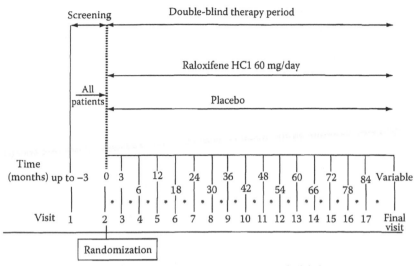

*Retention-related telephone contacts to occur between scheduled visits.

FIGURE 13.1:   Illustration of RUTH study design.

designed to be endpoint-driven: according to Lakatos' method for determining sample size [12,27,28], follow-up until 1670 women experienced at least one primary endpoint was required to achieve 90% power to show a 20% relative risk reduction. Thus the specific trial duration or number of postbaseline follow-up visits necessary was left unspecified at the design stage. It was projected, however, that approximately 10,000 women followed for an average of 6.25 years would yield the required number of events. This projection was based upon the following assumptions: (1) final analysis significance level (type 1 error): two-sided significance test at the $p = 0.0477$ level—reduced from the nominal 0.05 to allow for interim analysis; (2) power: 90%; (3) uniform patient accrual over 2.5 years; (4) annual placebo-group primary-endpoint event rate of 3.2% (no explicit assumptions were made as to event rates among primary versus secondary prevention patients separately); (5) raloxifene treatment benefit lag of 9 months; (6) after the lag period, 20% risk reduction with raloxifene; (7) annual loss to follow-up rate of 0.8% in each treatment group (incorporates loss rate due to documented noncardiovascular deaths); (8) drop-out rate (permanent discontinuation of raloxifene therapy) of 8% in the first year and 2% per year thereafter; and (9) among those assigned to placebo, an annual drop-in rate of 1% (subjects receiving a drug with efficacy assumed to be similar to that of raloxifene).

The study was designed with an intention-to-treat (ITT) analysis plan. In other words, data were analyzed by the treatment group to which a woman was randomized, even if she was inadvertently randomized, did not take the assigned treatment, did not receive the correct treatment, or otherwise did not follow the protocol or procedures. In situations where long-term therapy is being evaluated, ITT analyses are widely used because this design is considered more indicative of efficacy in actual clinical practice.

Specific definitions for the primary endpoint components were provided in the RUTH protocol. Investigators were instructed to report occurrences of all study endpoints to the sponsor along with appropriate supporting documentation. An external adjudication committee was convened to review, on a blinded basis, all reports of MI or coronary death. This committee was charged with determining definitively, according to prespecified criteria, whether or not a reported event was indeed classifiable as the particular endpoint in question. Such adjudication committees play a particularly important role in cardiovascular outcomes trials. The spectrum of ACS, ranging from unstable angina to sudden coronary death can be regarded as more or less continuous, and classification of events along this spectrum into specific categories involves expert medical judgment, despite definitions and guidelines published by cardiology societies. In RUTH in particular, rigorous adjudication of investigator-reported events was indispensable, given the fact that the investigators were not all cardiologists; internists and diabetologists, for instance, also participated. The work of the endpoint adjudication committee ensured that consistent criteria were applied throughout the trial in the assessment of study endpoints. This was a critical prerequisite for data quality in a study which generated outcomes from around the globe and over a span of several years. The primary analysis included only events confirmed by adjudication.

An independent DMC, without representatives from the sponsor, was convened and met regularly to review unblinded accumulating data from the study. The DMC was charged with monitoring the safety of study participants and with helping to ensure the scientific integrity of the trial. Furthermore, the DMC had the responsibility of conducting three interim analyses planned for this trial, offering the possibility of early termination for overwhelming evidence of efficacy or for futility. The timing of these analyses was designed to be event-driven as well, to occur at equal information fractions throughout the trial (that is, after observing one, two, and three quarters of the planned total of 1670 endpoints). An O'Brien–Fleming-type efficacy stopping boundary specified nominal significance levels for a two-sided test of 0.001, 0.005, 0.005, and 0.0477 for the three interim analyses and the final analysis, respectively, to control the overall type I error rate at 0.05. The statistical guideline for a conclusion of lack of efficacy for the coronary primary endpoint at the second and third interim analysis was an overall 99.99% confidence interval (CI) excluding a 15% treatment benefit, simply reflecting a very high futility threshold. Futility was not assessed at all at the first interim analysis.

13.3.2   Endpoint-Related Design Changes in RUTH

Patient accrual met expectations with 10,101 women enrolled in 2.5 years between 1998 and 2000. The proportion of primary and secondary prevention patients was not prespecified in the study design. Ultimately, approximately half of the subjects in RUTH had documented CHD and were thus considered "secondary prevention" patients, whereas the rest of the subjects had multiple coronary risk factors, but without a history of a prior event—the "primary prevention" patients whose risk for having an event during the trial was considerably lower. Figure 13.2 describes the

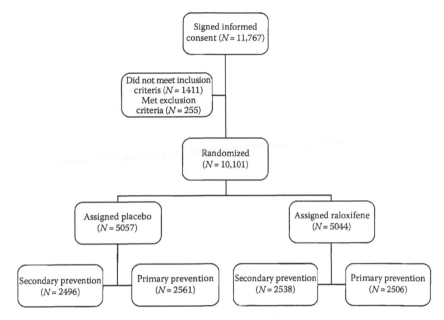

FIGURE 13.2:   Patient flow in the RUTH study.

flow of patients from the initial cohort screened to the final treatment group assignments, classified by prevention status.

The study team monitored key study metrics on a blinded basis from the outset of the trial. It became apparent almost at the outset of the trial that the overall primary endpoint event rate was considerably lower than that based upon the protocol assumptions. The reason for the lower event rate could not be determined with certainty, but the relative proportion of primary prevention patients in addition to a significantly higher than anticipated use of statins may have contributed. The high usage of statins is an example of how standard-of-care can evolve rapidly as additional benefits of concomitant medications are discovered or patient eligibility for alternative treatment increases as diagnostic criteria change.

Changes to the study design were undertaken in two major protocol amendments. Notably, the definition of the coronary primary endpoint of the study was expanded 2 years into the study to add hospitalized ACS as a third endpoint component. This change occurred following conversations between the sponsor and steering committee composed of external scientific advisors to discuss alternatives. The addition of a third component to the primary endpoint of coronary death or nonfatal MI, in an effort to increase event rates, was deemed to be the most attractive option. The fact that the sponsor, steering committee, and all parties that had contact with study sites or participants were blinded to treatment assignment paved the way for implementing this change to the protocol. This level of blinding (study subjects, investigators, sponsor personnel, and scientific advisors) was a fundamental regulatory prerequisite to entertaining postbaseline design changes, in an effort to avoid the inadvertent introduction of bias. Regulatory agencies offered no advice as to which cardiovascular event type would be most suited for incorporation in the definition of the composite primary endpoint, instead awaiting the sponsor's recommendation in this regard. Throughout the deliberations between the sponsor and the steering committee on this question, care was taken to ensure the DMC's disengagement from these discussions, precisely because of the Committee's unique position as the only group at that point having been privy to unblinded data from the trial.

Consideration was given to stroke, myocardial revascularization, and hospitalized ACS as potential additional endpoint components. Given a desire to focus the primary endpoint purely on coronary events, stroke was ruled out. Further, in consideration of the criteria described in Section 13.3.1, and recognizing the challenges that secular trends could bring with the addition of myocardial revascularization, particularly as relates to sociocultural differences in the urgency with which revascularization is performed in different regions of the world, hospitalized ACS was selected as the new endpoint component of choice. The criteria for meeting the definition of hospitalized ACS versus nonfatal MI were distinguished in such a way that for the purpose of endpoint accounting in RUTH, qualifying events were classified as one or the other, but not both.

A key challenge in including hospitalized ACS in the composite primary endpoint revolved around establishing crisp, unambiguous criteria for the adjudication committee to follow, in evaluating these relatively "soft" events reported by investigators. Given the complexity of cardiovascular disease, the multifaceted manifestation of the pathology, and changes over time in definitions of events and syndromes as declared by scientific societies, there is arguably no single, static definition appropriate for MI, and much less for a more elastic endpoint such as hospitalized ACS. It was more important, therefore, for the endpoint adjudication committee to agree to one reasonable definition and abide by it throughout the course of the trial. The addition of hospitalized ACS also raised the question of what to do about potentially eligible events that had been reported prior to the protocol amendment; the reports of hospitalization due to unstable angina were of particular interest in this regard. In addition to having investigators report potential hospitalized ACS events after the implementation of the first protocol amendment in 2000, as comprehensive a review as possible of all previously reported hospitalizations due to unstable angina was undertaken retrospectively, to determine whether any of these would have met the hospitalized ACS definition. The FDA agreed that events identified in this manner were also eligible to be included in the primary analysis. Numerous cases of hospitalized ACS were indeed confirmed through this review, though in many other cases it was not possible to obtain sufficient supporting documentation for the adjudication committee to make a definitive judgment. The consequent exclusion of certain potential events from the final analysis, while a shortcoming, was not however expected to bias the assessment of treatment effect.

A second fundamental design change implemented through the first major protocol amendment concerned breast cancer, originally one of the secondary endpoints in the RUTH trial. Although tangential in some sense to the topic of this chapter, we describe this change here since it greatly impacted RUTH, and also illustrates the latitude of design alterations that may be admissible. The Multiple Outcomes of Raloxifene Evaluation (MORE) trial [29], which supported the osteoporosis indications, also demonstrated a significant 76% reduction in the risk of newly diagnosed invasive breast cancer in a secondary analysis [30]. Although this finding was highly suggestive of a real effect of raloxifene, a compound known to target multiple organ systems, the MORE data alone were deemed insufficient to support a regulatory claim of breast cancer risk reduction; a confirmatory outcomes trial was deemed necessary. Debate between the sponsor and the RUTH steering committee, and further discussions with the FDA, resulted in the agreement that RUTH could serve as the required trial to definitively test the hypothesis that raloxifene reduces the incidence of invasive breast cancer. Although this study was designed as a cardiovascular prevention trial, enrolling postmenopausal women at risk of coronary events, these subjects (by virtue of their age, for instance) were ostensibly also at some appreciable risk of developing breast cancer. Breast cancer had already been specified a secondary endpoint of the trial at the design stage. The substantive change formalized by the protocol amendment involved elevating invasive breast to a second primary endpoint in the study. Notably, the coronary and invasive breast cancer endpoints were not regarded as coprimary, in the sense of requiring significant results on both to enable any claim. Rather, each endpoint was to be evaluated independent of the results on the other. The only consequence of this change to the coronary endpoint was a slight reduction in the nominal significance level for testing, allowing for a test of the breast cancer endpoint with minimal alpha while still controlling the type I error rate for the trial at 0.05; the significance levels for the coronary and invasive breast cancer endpoints were set at 0.0423 and 0.008, respectively. Although the latter significance level appeared to be unduly strict in comparison to more typical thresholds, it was deemed to be acceptable in view of the strong anticipated treatment effect on invasive breast cancer, and desire to minimize erosion of alpha for the coronary endpoint. In fact, this alpha allocation preserved power of 89% for the coronary and 80% for the invasive breast cancer endpoint. Mammograms were to be collected at baseline and every 2 years thereafter, with an interim analysis for breast cancer planned after the collection of the 2 year mammograms. However, since no plans were made for early termination of the study due to breast cancer efficacy, a trivial alpha spend was assigned to this analysis, not impacting the final significance level of 0.008. Minor alpha spend for the coronary interim analyses, reduced even from the original levels given in Section 13.3.1., resulted in a final significance level of 0.0417 for this endpoint.

A key difference in the treatment of the coronary and the invasive breast cancer endpoints was the fact that the final breast cancer analysis was not designed to be endpoint-driven, but rather planned to be performed after collection of the scheduled 4 year mammograms was complete. The practical feasibility of performing final analyses for the two primary endpoints of the RUTH study at differing times relied on numerous operational provisions, as well as the key assumption that the analysis time points would not differ by more than approximately 1 year. However, despite the expanded definition of the coronary primary endpoint, event rates still fell significantly short of protocol projections. Whereas a placebo event rate of 3.2% per annum in conjunction with a 20% risk reduction with raloxifene, as assumed at the design stage, would have suggested a pooled event rate of 2.88% in a trial with equal allocation to treatment groups, a pooled rate closer to 2.0% was actually observed. It became clear that follow-up until 1670 women experienced a coronary primary endpoint would extend well beyond a realistic time frame for the study. In a second attempt to realign the trial more closely with the original projections about its duration, the protocol was amended once more to reduce the required number of women experiencing a coronary endpoint from 1670 by approximately a quarter, to 1268. This new endpoint target implied a reduction in power for the coronary endpoint to 80%, leaving the power for the invasive breast cancer endpoint unchanged. Yet even this modification was not sufficient to avoid an inevitably approaching conflict between the protocol and the informed consent document (ICD), with the former not specifying a fixed follow-up time for the coronary endpoint and the latter stipulating a follow-up duration between 5 and 7.5 years. After thorough deliberations by the sponsor and steering committee of the merits of continuing the study as well as an assessment of the impact of early study termination to patients and the integrity of the study, and after hearing no objections to the sponsor's proposed plan from the DMC, the RUTH study was terminated in December 2005. At that point patients had already been followed for an average of 6.25 years. A total of 1086 women had experienced a coronary primary endpoint.

13.3.3   Outcomes of the RUTH Study

Figure 13.3 shows the cumulative incidence of events over time and reports the inferential statistics of the coronary primary analysis. The RUTH study failed to demonstrate a significant reduction in the risk of major coronary events, yielding similar event rates in the two treatment groups [5]. As expected based on the results of the MORE trial, the RUTH study did demonstrate a significant reduction in the risk of invasive breast cancer, on the basis of incidence rates of 0.27% and 0.15% in placebo and raloxifene-treated patients, respectively (HR $= 0.56$ (0.38, 0.83), $p = 0.003$).

Table 13.1 displays the results of the coronary primary analysis as well as the analysis of individual endpoint components. Similar event rates in the two groups were also noted when examining time-to-first-component for each of the three components of the coronary primary endpoint. Of course such marginal analyses are difficult to interpret, especially when analyzing event types of differing severity in the same disease continuum. Analysis of an event type of lesser severity is of limited meaning without explicit accounting for the possibility that a patient may also have experienced related but more serious events. Nonetheless one can conclude from Table 13.1 that beyond the lack of effect on the composite endpoint, the incidence of the individual endpoint components was also similar; thus, for instance, compared to placebo, women on raloxifene did not avoid substantially more coronary deaths or nonfatal MIs in favor of, say, a higher incidence of hospitalized ACS. Note, however, that while Table 13.1 offers an indirect appreciation of the extent to which patients experienced multiple event types in each treatment group (compare counts of the composite endpoint to the sums of counts across the individual components), it says nothing directly about multiple occurrences, particularly of the same event type, in a patient. (Table 13.2 presents a general analysis accounting for multiple events per patient, regardless of type.)

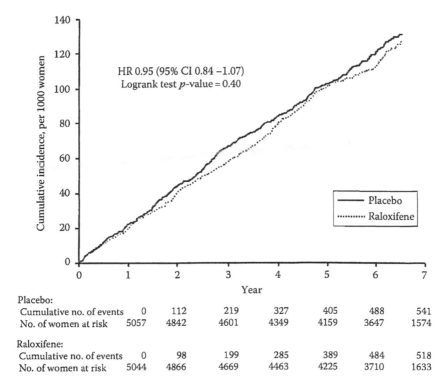

FIGURE 13.3: Cumulative incidence of coronary events in the RUTH study. (From Barrett-Connor, E., Mosca, L., Collins, P., Geiger, M.J., Grady, D., Kornitzer, M., McNabb, M., Wenger, N.K., for the RUTH Trial Investigators. *N. Engl. J. Med.* 355(2), 127, 2006. With permission.)

TABLE 13.1: Incidence and hazard ratios: Primary coronary endpoint and individual components.

	No. of Events (Annualized Rate,%)			
	Placebo ($N = 5057$)	Raloxifene ($N = 5044$)	Hazard Ratio (95% CI)	*p*-Value
Composite coronary endpoint	553 (2.16)	533 (2.06)	0.95 (0.84–1.07)	0.40
Coronary death	273 (1.03)	253 (0.95)	0.92 (0.78–1.09)	0.31
Nonfatal MI	208 (0.80)	183 (0.69)	0.87 (0.71–1.06)	0.16
Hospitalized ACS	185 (0.71)	169 (0.64)	0.90 (0.73–1.11)	0.34

TABLE 13.2: Time-to-event analysis accounting for multiple events per patient.

	No. of Events (Percent of Randomized Patients)		Hazard Ratio (95% CI)	p-Value[a]	Mean Years between Events[b]	
	Placebo (N = 5057)	Raloxifene (N = 5044)				
Most serious coronary event[c]	553(10.94)	533(10.57)	0.95(0.84, 1.07)	0.40		
Recurrent coronary event						
First event	553(10.94)	533(10.57)	0.95(0.84, 1.07)	0.40	0.81	0.94
Second event	122(2.41)	92(1.82)	0.80(0.61, 1.05)	0.10	1.00	0.66
Third event	28(0.55)	17(0.34)	0.61(0.33, 1.12)	0.11	0.67	0.77
Fourth event	7(0.14)	2(0.04)	0.24(0.05, 1.17)	0.08	0.28	0.23
Fifth event	2(0.04)	1(0.02)	N/A	N/A	0.00	0.09
Sixth event	0(0.00)	1(0.02)	N/A	N/A		

[a] p-Value is obtained from a logrank test for most serious event, from a PWP-GT model for recurrent events.

[b] Mean years between the first and second events, the second and third events, the third and fourth events, and the fourth and fifth events for each treatment arm.

[c] Coronary death is considered the most serious event, followed by nonfatal MI, with hospitalized ACS other than MI being considered the least serious.

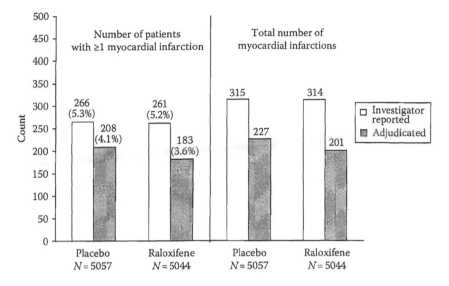

FIGURE 13.4: Number of investigator reported and adjudicated myocardial infarctions.

Figure 13.4 explores the occurrence of nonfatal MI in particular in more detail, by examining differences in results when focusing on adjudicated versus investigator-reported events, and when focusing on incidence (patients with at least one event) versus total event numbers. Whether counting patients with an event or all event occurrences, the numbers reported demonstrate the substantial attrition in formally analyzable outcomes when investigator-reported events pass through the adjudication process. In the RUTH study, this loss amounted to between one-quarter and one-third of investigator-reported events. Factors that affect the extent of attrition one can expect in general include the strictness of the adjudication criteria and to some extent the profile of expertise in cardiology among investigators. In any case, the impact of filtering events through adjudication that do not meet a consistent, prespecified definition should clearly not be assumed to be negligible. When comparing total (adjudicated) event counts to counts of patients with at least one event, an increase of 10%–20% was noted for nonfatal MI, and this difference must be appreciated in the context of the average follow-up time for patients. Arithmetic rearrangement of the values in Table 13.2 shows that a total of 1358 events, across all types, were experienced by the 1086 women who had at least one event, an increase of 25%. This raises some interest in an exploratory analysis accounting for multiple events per patient, and such an analysis is discussed below. Finally, Figure 13.5 illustrates the degree of heterogeneity in event rates observed in RUTH by providing the analysis of women with at least one investigator-reported nonfatal MI for secondary and primary prevention patients separately. Event rates for the secondary prevention patients were nearly twofold higher than for the healthier primary prevention cohort, confirming the critical importance of basing overall event rate assumptions at the trial

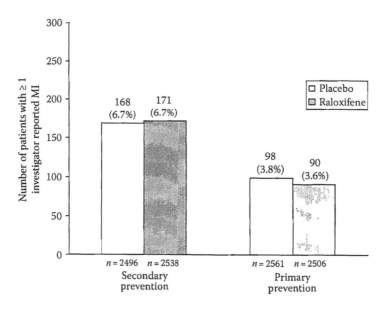

FIGURE 13.5:   Number of investigator reported myocardial infarctions by prevention subgroup.

design stage on a very thoughtful consideration of the anticipated blend of patient characteristics and risk factors in the study population. (A similar analysis for the adjudicated events could not be produced here at the time of writing, due to pending publication of these data in another venue.)

Note that the detailed examination of nonfatal MI in Figure 13.4 could not be applied directly to the other coronary endpoint components. Coronary death, for example, was not reported as such by investigators. Instead, adjudicators examined all reported deaths and determined the cause to be either cardiovascular or noncardiovascular, and, if cardiovascular, whether the death was specifically coronary or noncoronary. Moreover, the issue of multiple events per patient obviously does not apply to fatal outcomes. Hospitalized ACS was also less amenable to analyzing in the same fashion as in Figure 13.4, given that this endpoint was not specified at the outset of the study, but rather added as a third component part way through and augmented, where possible, by the retrospective assessment of reported cases of unstable angina.

Table 13.2 provides a time-to-event analysis, accounting for the possibility of multiple events per patient. This is an application of the conditional model proposed by Prentice, Williams, and Peterson, discussed in Section 13.2.5. Recall that this particular model does not distinguish between the event types making up the definition of the composite primary endpoint, but aims to assess the effect of treatment not only on the first occurrence of one of these events in a patient, but also on second and subsequent occurrences. The hazard ratio for time-to-first-event is of course just that for the primary analysis reported in Table 13.1. Patients having had one event are then at risk for a second one, and in fact 214 patients did experience a second event. The hazard ratio of 0.80 for time-to-second-event is consistent with the previous one, though its p-value of 0.10 might lead some to speculate whether there might be a trend toward reduction of risk of recurrent events. A total of 45 and 9 third and fourth events, respectively, were observed, with corresponding hazard ratios of 0.61 ($p = 0.11$) and 0.24 ($p = 0.08$). These two results make it more tempting still to entertain the possibility of a protective effect of raloxifene in reducing the risk of multiple events. Clearly, however, one has to be careful to avoid over-interpreting the data. It would be difficult to conceive of a mechanism whereby the risk of an initial event is unchanged but that of subsequent events is reduced. The data-based evidence to support this conjecture, while sufficient to raise the question, is slim at best. One might test whether the overall event intensity between the two treatment groups differs, but even if a particular test suggested it does, it would be difficult from a practical perspective to make that argument convincingly without a corresponding difference in the incidence of patients with at least one event (i.e., the analysis of first events). Another line of reasoning might argue that each of the hazard ratios in Table 13.2, including that for first events, is consistent with a common, modest, but real reduction in the risk of coronary events—too small, unfortunately, to be clinically meaningful. This may well be the case, and would be in keeping with the overall conclusion for the trial based on just the analysis of time-to-first-event. Hence time-to-first-event, while on the one hand far from offering a complete analysis solution for survival data, as discussed previously, is nonetheless not an unreasonable primary analysis from the perspective of its simplicity and a certain practically oriented gate-keeping quality: the examples motivating analysis of multiple events per patient in Section 13.2.5. notwithstanding, in most cases if the analysis of time-to-first-event fails to show a significant effect, it is at least far less likely that more sophisticated analyses accounting for multiple events per patient will offer additional information changing the conclusion from the primary analysis. Conversely, if a significant effect is seen on examining time-to-first-event, this does invite richer, more detailed analysis such as that discussed in Section 13.2.5., and also makes the interpretation of these analyses more natural and straightforward.

13.4 Discussion

Rather than presenting a comprehensive overview of appropriate statistical methodology, the aim of this chapter was to highlight several tiers of challenges practitioners face in the conduct of cardiovascular prevention trials, and to discuss practical approaches to dealing with these challenges in the context of numerous relevant experiences from a recent landmark trial. In very general terms, these studies require the same careful attention to the design, execution, and analysis as any clinical outcomes studies would mandate. The prevention setting in particular, however, adds a unique layer of complexity. We have discussed the impact of studying healthier, broader patient populations, in terms of leading to larger, longer trials, and the range of considerations which arise as a result. An increased, deliberate focus on the risk/benefit balance for patients in interpreting study results is inevitable in the prevention paradigm. In trials testing interventions to treat acute conditions, patients normally require, by definition, some form of therapy. And, whether implicit or explicit, this entails a parallel tolerance of a certain risk threshold, in terms of acceptable side effects. If the safety profile of a particular intervention does not exceed this threshold, formal risk/benefit analyses may receive less emphasis, provided the intervention demonstrates the desired improvement in efficacy over the control. Moreover, as the seriousness of the condition requiring treatment increases, so does tolerance for adverse effects. In the prevention setting, there is no perceived comparable urgency for patients to adopt a particular treatment for their condition. Cardiovascular disease is a prime example where risk factors can intensify over years with no or minimal symptomatic impact to the afflicted individual. Hence the proposition to begin therapy, inevitably incurring the risk of adverse side effects, is a more difficult argument. Moreover, what is an acceptable risk threshold for a patient in this context is made more challenging by the fact that he or she often cannot tangibly feel the intervention work, which naturally gives rise to skepticism. Some doubt may be alleviated through the demonstration of reduction in relevant, measurable disease markers. But in the end the problem of dealing with the unknown counterfactual remains: the patient in whom an efficacious intervention has prevented an event will never know whether the event would have occurred or not in the absence of treatment.

The cardiovascular therapeutic area is among the most demanding for conducting prevention trials. A multitude of effective medicines and procedural interventions have become available for managing heart health, offering a host of alternatives to patients for reducing risk levels and raising the bar for new entrants to this therapeutic space. These challenges all had bearing on the investigation of raloxifene as to its effectiveness in reducing the risk of coronary events. An advantage of pursuing this added indication for a drug already approved for the prevention and treatment of osteoporosis was the recognition that significant numbers of postmenopausal women would be able to derive both benefits from using the drug. Pitted against this were the risks associated with raloxifene use—an increase in the incidence of hot flashes, particularly in younger postmenopausal women, and an increase in the risk of venous thromboembolism, including pulmonary embolism. Despite the potential for added benefits and in light of the overall profile of the drug, as the years of follow-up in the RUTH study increased, the question of whether a meaningful outcome in terms of coronary risk reduction was at all achievable anymore became more and more pressing. In hindsight one might fairly ask whether stopping rules for futility were considered thoroughly enough. Undoubtedly, settling at the design stage on the trade-off between rules that offer meaningful protection against pursuing a path that is highly unlikely to lead to a conclusion of efficacy, and ones that effectively control Type II error, can be harrowing indeed. Considering Bayesian approaches to assessing predictive probability of success (see, for instance, Trzaskoma and Sashegyi [31]) is helpful in this regard. Nonetheless, even without having specified more stringent futility rules in RUTH, other circumstances eventually led quite naturally to an appropriate decision to terminate the trial. In any case, what was not anticipated at the outset of the trial was the fact that in the end this study was able to support two important conclusions: Raloxifene does not in fact significantly decrease the risk of coronary events, but was confirmed to be efficacious in reducing the risk of invasive breast cancer.

Finally, for all the design work, preparation and contingency planning for the conduct of a cardiovascular prevention trial, the unexpected is almost sure to arise in one form or another over the long course of follow-up. Good, transparent communication with regulators, a close working relationship with scientific advisory committees, and leveraging the unique advantages afforded by an independent DMC all serve to maximize the potential for changes in course correction during the conduct of the trial, should the need arise. This is critical in view of the fact that a cardiovascular prevention trial is among the largest and costliest of clinical investigations, and thus practically not a repeatable experiment. The delivery of high-quality, definitive clinical outcomes data relies most heavily on numerous groups and hundreds of competent individuals tasked with the myriad of activities required to conduct, monitor, and analyze the trial. Close coordination and cooperation between these groups are essential and a great responsibility.

References

[1] Lauer M and Topol E. Clinical trials—multiple treatments, multiple endpoints, and multiple lessons. *JAMA* 289(19), 2575–2577, 2003.

[2] Steg G, Bhatt DL, Wilson P, D'Agostino R, Ohman EM, Röther J, Liau C-S, et al. for the REACH Registry Investigators. One-year cardiovascular event rates in outpatients with atherothrombosis. *Journal of the American Medical Association* 297, 1197–1206, 2007.

[3] Heart Outcomes Prevention Evaluation Study Investigators. Effects of an angiotensin-converting-enzyme inhibitor, ramipril, on cardiovascular events in high-risk patients. *New England Journal of Medicine* 342(3), 145–153, 2000.

[4] Bhatt DL, Fox K, Hacke W, Berger PB, Black HR, Boden WE, Cacoub P, et al. for the CHARISMA Investigators. Clopidogrel and aspirin versus aspirin alone for the prevention of atherothrombotic events. *New England Journal of Medicine* 354(16), 1706–1717, 2006.

[5] Barrett-Connor E, Mosca L, Collins P, Geiger MJ, Grady D, Kornitzer M, McNabb M, and Wenger NK, for the RUTH Trial Investigators. Effects of raloxifene on cardiovascular events and breast cancer in postmenopausal women. *New England Journal of Medicine* 355(2), 127–137, 2006.

[6] Therneau TM and Grambsch P. Modeling survival data: Extending the Cox model. New York: Springer-Verlag, 2000.

[7] Mahaffey K, Harrington R, Akkerhuis M, Kleiman N, Berdan L, Crenshaw B, Tardiff B, et al. for the PURSUIT Investigators. Systematic adjudication of myocardial infarction end-points in an international clinical trial. *Current Controlled Trials in Cardiovascular Medicine*. 2(4), 180–186, 2001.

[8] Kirwan B, Lubsen J, de Brouwer S, Danchin N, Battler A, de Luna A, Dunselman P, et al. on behalf of the ACTION Investigators. Diagnostic criteria and adjudication process both determine published event-rates: The ACTION trial experience. *Contemporary Clinical Trials*. 28, 720–729, 2007.

[9] Schoenfeld D. The asymptotic properties of nonparametric tests for comparing survival distributions. *Biometrika* 68, 316–319, 1981.

[10] Freedman LS. Tables of the number of patients required in clinical trials using the logrank test. *Statistics in Medicine* 1, 121–129, 1982.

[11] Schoenfeld D. Sample-size formula for the proportional-hazards regression model. *Biometrics* 39, 499–503, 1983.

[12] Lakatos E. Sample sizes based on the log-rank statistic in complex clinical trials. *Biometrics* 44, 229–241, 1988.

[13] Lakatos E and Lan KKG. A comparison of sample size methods for the logrank statistic. *Statistics in Medicine* 11, 179–191, 1992.

[14] The Clopidogrel in Unstable Angina to Prevent Recurrent Events Trial Investigators. Effects of clopidogrel in addition to aspirin in patients with acute coronary syndromes without ST-segment elevation. *New England Journal of Medicine* 345, 494–502, 2001.

[15] Wiviott SD, Braunwald E, McCabe CH, Montalescot G, Ruzyllo W, Gottlieb S, Neumann FJ, et al. for the TRITON-TIMI 38 Investigators. Prasugrel versus clopidogrel in patients with acute coronary syndromes. *New England Journal of Medicine* 357, 2001–2015, 2007.

[16] SAS®. SAS Institute Inc., Cary, NC. http://www.sas.com/

[17] East®. Cytel Inc., Cambridge, MA. http://www.cytel.com/

[18] Ellenberg SS, Fleming TR, and DeMets DL. *Data Monitoring Committees in Clinical Trials: A Practical Perspective*. Wiley, West Sussex, U.K., 2002.

[19] Ellenberg SS and George SL. Should statisticians reporting to data monitoring committees be independent of the trial sponsor and leadership? *Statistics in Medicine* 23, 1503–1505, 2004.

[20] Jennison C and Turnbull BW. *Group Sequential Methods with Applications to Clinical Trials*. Boca Raton, FL: Chapman & Hall/CRC, 2000.

[21] Wei LJ and Glidden DV. An overview of statistical methods for multiple failure time data in clinical trials. *Statistics in Medicine* 16, 833–839, 1997.

[22] Lin DY. Cox regression analysis of multivariate failure time data: the marginal approach. *Statistics in Medicine* 13, 2233–2247, 1994.

[23] Andersen PK and Gill RD. Cox's regression model for counting processes: a large sample study. *Annals of Statistics* 10, 1100–1120, 1982.

[24] Wei LJ, Lin DY and Weissfeld L. Regression analysis of multivariate incomplete failure time data by modeling marginal distributions. *Journal of the American Statistical Association* 84, 1065–1073, 1989.

[25] Prentice RL, Williams BJ, and Peterson AV. On the regression analysis of multivariate failure time data. *Biometrika* 68, 373–379, 1981.

[26] Mosca L, Barrett-Connor E, Wenger NK, Collins P, Grady D, Kornitzer M, Moscarelli E, Paul S, Wright TJ, Helterbrand JD, and Anderson PW. Design and methods of the Raloxifene Use for The Heart (RUTH) study. *American Journal of Cardiology* 88(4), 392–395, 2001.

[27] Lakatos E. Sample size determination in clinical trials with time-dependent rates of losses and non-compliance. *Controlled Clinical Trials* 7, 189–199, 1986.

[28] Shih J. Sample size calculation for complex clinical trials with survival endpoints. *Controlled Clinical Trials* 16, 395–407, 1995.

[29] Ettinger B, Black DM, Mitlak BH, Knickerbocker RK, Nickelsen T, Genant HK, Christiansen C, et al. Reduction of vertebral fracture risk in postmenopausal women with osteoporosis treated with raloxifene. Results from a 3-year randomized clinical trial. *Journal of the American Medical Association* 282, 637–645, 1999.

[30] Cummings SR, Eckert S, Krueger KA, Grady D, Powles TJ, Cauley JA, Norton L, et al. The effect of raloxifene on risk of breast cancer in postmenopausal women. *Journal of the American Medical Association* 281, 2189–2197, 1999.

[31] Trzaskoma BL and Sashegyi A. Predictive probability of success and the assessment of futility in large outcomes trials. *Journal of Biopharmaceutical Statistics* 17, 45–63, 2007.

Chapter 14

Design and Analysis of Antiviral Trials

Anthony C. Segreti and Lynn P. Dix

Contents

14.1 Introduction

The development of antiviral therapy is a recent phenomenon that has accelerated dramatically since the mid-1980s. The investigation of agents for treating viral disease began in the 1950s as an outgrowth of the search for antitumor compounds and the resultant interest in drugs that affected DNA synthesis *in vivo*. A number of these drugs were shown to inhibit viral DNA synthesis in laboratory settings as well [1]. In the 1960s, Kaufman used topical idoxuridine to treat herpes keratitis [2] and Bauer employed thiosemicarbazone to prevent smallpox in patients exposed to this disease [3]. However, these successes were limited and it remained difficult to identify agents which could inhibit viral replication without affecting host cells and producing unacceptable toxicity in patients. There was a perception in the scientific community that it would be difficult to develop antiviral chemotherapy that was appropriately selective. Since viral replication occurs intracellularly and uses host cell mechanisms, the task of identifying effective and safe antiviral compounds was seen as nearly impossible. In the early 1980s, the successful development and marketing of acyclovir [4] for treating a wide variety of herpes virus infections in a number of different patient populations changed the way antivirals were viewed and encouraged the subsequent development of numerous compounds. The AIDS epidemic has highlighted the continued need for antiviral chemotherapy and the last two decades have seen a plethora of new compounds developed for AIDS as well as other viral diseases.

This chapter addresses the specific elements of the design and analysis of clinical trials most relevant to the development of antiviral agents. While this discussion is relevant to all antiviral chemotherapy, it focuses on the diseases caused by the human immunodeficiency virus (HIV), the hepatitis B virus, and the hepatitis C virus. These diseases are the ones most studied and have the largest body of clinical and statistical research. Since they are manifested as chronic diseases, the assessment of their potential therapies will require the use of time-to-event endpoints. In contrast, treatment for other infectious diseases, such as skin infections in healthy individuals, is often assessed by a "cure/no cure" endpoint which requires statistical method- ology appropriate to binary outcomes.

14.1.1   Key Clinical Issues

The search for new therapy for any disease is dynamic and dependent to some degree on the existing standard of care, but this general principle is manifested most clearly in the development of antivirals where the standard of care can change dramatically over the course of a few years. We see this in the development of treatments for the AIDS epidemic where the first effective treatment, zidovudine, was marketed in 1987. As of 2008, there were more than 20 FDA-approved antiretroviral drugs available in the United States for this disease [5]. The best available current therapy will affect the choice of a control group as well as the objectives for any new trial. Likewise, the type of study, whether superiority or noninferiority, and the patient population are affected by the standard of care. Nevertheless, the discussion of this chapter should be relevant to the development of new antivirals and especially for those diseases that we address here.

Two key interrelated aspects of antiviral therapy are the development of drug resistance and viral latency. Viruses have the ability to replicate at high rates in host cells and can mutate quickly and those with an error-prone replication process tend to mutate rapidly [1]. Genetic mutation can quickly lead to viral resistance especially in individuals who are immunocompromised. Although the degree of concern will vary with disease, all antiviral development should be cognizant of this possibility and the assessment of resistance will generally be an important objective, especially for a long-term trial.

Viral latency refers to the ability of virus to reside in a host cell while not actively replicating. While treatment with an active agent may shorten the period of viral replication and promote healing, e.g., treating a herpes simplex infection with acyclovir, it does not prevent the virus from reactivating after the end of treatment. It also does not eliminate the virus while it is in the latent state. Latency often requires the use of prolonged therapy to achieve long-term therapeutic success. The use of chronic, even lifelong, antiviral therapy, although necessary for some diseases, can itself lead to the development of resistant virus particularly if the viral concentrations of the agent(s) are subinhibitory for a sufficient duration.

14.2 Design

14.2.1 Human Immunodeficiency Virus

The identification of the HIV [6,7] launched efforts to develop effective antiretroviral therapy for this disease. The introduction of zidovudine in 1987 marked the first agent to show therapeutic activity. It soon became clear that HIV possessed an ability to mutate quickly and become resistant especially to a single agent. Other antiretrovirals were developed at a rapid pace and these provided alternatives as well as the potential for combinations with additional benefit. However, it was not until the initiation of highly active antiretroviral therapy (HAART) in the late 1990s that patients began to see dramatic increases in survival [8]. HAART combined two antiretrovirals with a protease inhibitor and revolutionized HIV therapy. Since then the pace of drug development has intensified as new drugs and new classes of agents continue to be introduced on a regular basis. The standard of care has changed as rapidly in this therapeutic area as any other over the last 20 years and this fact has important implications for the design of clinical trials. Perhaps most importantly, the current focus of HIV development has been relatively short-term trials (24–48 weeks) and based on surrogate endpoints such as viral load rather than mortality or the occurrence of AIDS-defining events such as opportunistic infections. This paradigm allows patients to leave a trial and move on to an alternative regimen if they do not receive sufficient antiviral benefit from their assigned therapy or if that activity is of relatively short duration.

The HIV area is unique because of the speed of clinical development, the development of the pandemic over a relatively short time, the complex manifestations of this disease in terms of opportunistic infections, lymphomas and solid tumors, and the disparity between the needs of developing countries for AIDS treatment and the resources required for appropriate care.

14.2.1.1 Length of Trial and Endpoints

In the first controlled study of HIV therapy, the primary endpoint was mortality and the treatment effect was noteworthy with 19 deaths in the placebo group and only one in the zidovudine group [9]. Primarily because of the success of HIV therapy, surrogate endpoints have played an increasingly prominent role and clinical endpoints have retreated into the background. In the early 1990s, important trials such as Concorde [10] focused on the endpoints of opportunistic infections and AIDS-defining conditions. As new antivirals were developed and greater efficacy achieved, it became apparent that AIDS-defining events were becoming less common and focus on these endpoints would lead to increasingly larger, longer, and more expensive trials. Investigators were hesitant to enter patients in trials that had a long time horizon in the face of such a rapidly evolving therapeutic area. Instead, the CD_4 cell count rose to the fore as a surrogate endpoint that was easily measured, was predictive of opportunistic infections and mortality and was responsive to the initiation of therapy. By the late 1990s, CD_4 cell count had been "validated" as a surrogate endpoint [11]—not in the formal sense but informally as a primary endpoint that regulators would look toward when assessing the substantial evidence of efficacy required for marketing approval. Relatively soon after CD_4 cell count became the leading surrogate endpoint, it was superseded by plasma HIV viral RNA levels as a more powerful and sensitive predictor of therapeutic response. This endpoint has become more sensitive over time as the lower limit of detection has dropped from 400 to 50 copies/mL and it remains the primary endpoint in most key efficacy studies. Mortality, the development of AIDS-defining conditions, and CD_4 cell count continue as important secondary endpoints with the priority varying with the length of trial, patient populations, and trial duration. Time to loss of viral response (TLOVR) is an important secondary endpoint [12]. It measures the time from the initiation of antiviral therapy until that therapy begins to lose effectiveness: viral load reaches its nadir and begins to increase. Interestingly, viral RNA load is analyzed as a binary endpoint based on the value at the end of the treatment period and the time required to reach an undetectable value is not factored into the analysis. This variable functions as a composite endpoint that takes into account individuals who drop out because of unacceptable adverse experiences or lack of viral response and considers these individuals as treatment failures.

Most clinical trials enrolling treatment-experienced patients have duration of 24 weeks or more while treatment-naïve patients generally are treated for at least 48 weeks. Demonstration of efficacy and safety for trials of these durations is feasible and meets the regulatory requirement of being able to demonstrate superiority. Enrolling treatment-experienced patients in a trial of 24 weeks allows a reasonable path toward accelerated approval. These durations and the sample sizes used in these trials mean that the frequency of clinical endpoints (AIDS defining events) and mortality will be low and while, of interest, these endpoints cannot be relied upon for the assessment of efficacy.

14.2.1.2   Patient Populations

The major division in the HIV population for clinical trial purposes is between treatment-experienced and treatment-naïve patients. Of course, there are gradations among treatment-experienced patients and one important component of any trial enrolling these patients is to ensure, by means of inclusion/exclusion criteria, a relative homogeneity with respect to antiviral resistance. The longer a patient has been exposed to antivirals, the more likely a patient will have resistant virus and respond poorly or not at all to a new agent or combination. Because it is difficult to define a standard of care for heavily pretreated patients, it can be difficult to specify a control regimen when designing a randomized trial enrolling these patients. In addition, heavily retreated patients with few treatment options may not be good candidates for randomized trials since they may be reluctant to participate in a clinical trial for an extended period of time.

Treatment-naïve patients have not been exposed to any antiretroviral therapy. This group of patients should be relatively uniform with respect to resistant virus although the status of their immune system could vary widely.

14.2.1.3 Superiority, Noninferiority Trials

At one time, almost all controlled HIV studies fell into the category of classical superiority studies, that is, they had the objective of identifying if the experimental therapy was superior to the control arm based on a null hypothesis of no difference between the two arms. As combinations have become increasingly effective, showing superiority to the standard of care is a more difficult task and trials are more often focused on the issue of whether it is possible to achieve the same level of efficacy with fewer adverse experiences or with a simpler regimen which may promote better compliance. The latter objectives are generally addressed through a noninferiority design (or equivalence design) in which the null and alternative hypotheses are reversed and the objective is to determine if an experimental regimen is equivalent to or perhaps only slightly worse than a control arm. This objective is achieved by demonstrating that the confidence interval based on the difference between the experimental and control arms lies entirely outside of the region of inferiority. Since any study deficiencies will tend to bias toward the null hypothesis, a noninferiority study is often held to an even higher degree of scientific rigor than a superiority study.

Another important issue for the interpretation of noninferiority studies lies in the nature of the composite primary endpoints. These endpoints include both virologic failure as well as nonvirologic events. One useful analysis is to perform a supplemental analysis using only the virologic endpoints [13] to clearly compare the regimens with respect to the virologic endpoints which are arguably more clinically relevant than the endpoint of a patient withdrawing consent.

While the noninferiority design has become a staple of the HIV therapeutic area, the choice of a noninferiority threshold remains a challenge. While there are rules of thumb for choosing this margin, typically based on some proportion of a therapeutic effect, margins have been criticized as ad hoc, arbitrary and difficult to defend scientifically. For a defensible margin, the activity of the control regimen has to be meticulously defined for the population of interest and must be based on study data and clinical relevance [14].

14.2.1.4 Summary for HIV

The unusual characteristics of the HIV pandemic have posed striking challenges for the design and analysis of therapeutic trials. In this chapter, we have reviewed the customary approaches to these issues primarily in the context of those key trials intended to provide substantial evidence of efficacy as a basis for new drug approval. There has been notable progress in extending the life expectancy of individuals with HIV. At the same time, antiviral resistance remains a challenge as does the need for new agents and new strategies. Many important issues, both of efficacy and safety, cannot be addressed adequately within this conventional paradigm. Although this paradigm has remained stable over the last 10 years, it would not be reasonable to expect this stability to continue indefinitely. We should expect to see a greater diversity in randomized studies including a greater emphasis on outcome studies even if the therapeutic arms are defined by strategies or sequences of regimens rather than individual agents in the manner of ACTG 384 [15]. It will also be increasingly important to assess the long-term adverse effects of therapy, e.g., the long-term cardiovascular effect of protease inhibitors.

Viral load will continue in the foreseeable future as the primary endpoint for most controlled studies but we can expect to see this endpoint refined as assays become more sensitive. As our knowledge of the genetics of HIV resistance deepens, we will see this information incorporated more integrally into study design and analysis. The complexity of HIV combination therapy has increased since the first HIV treatment just over two decades ago. This trend will likely continue as new strategies are developed to deal with HIV resistance.

14.2.2   Chronic Hepatitis B

Chronic hepatitis B is a viral disease affecting over 350 million people worldwide [16]. It is most common in Southeast Asia where between 10% and 20% of the population are carriers while the carrier rate in North America is an order of magnitude lower. It can lead to a variety of long-term complications including cirrhosis, liver cancer, and liver failure. In recent years, a number of nucleoside analogues have been approved for marketing to treat this disease based on placebo-controlled trials. The therapeutic paradigm is shifting as investigators consider new endpoints, combination therapy and active-controlled trials.

14.2.2.1   Length of Trial/Endpoints

Historically, 1 year is seen as the minimum trial length needed to provide substantial evidence of effectiveness for a drug to treat hepatitis B. However, this duration has been considered by some to be inadequate since it is not long enough to observe the long-term sequelae of this disease. Instead trials of this duration must rely on the surrogate endpoint of histologic improvement as primary [17]. The relationship between histologic improvement as a candidate surrogate endpoint for the clinical complications of cancer, cirrhosis, and liver failure remains to be fully determined. The ideal trial would follow a large number of patients for extended periods of time in order to observe enough events to provide sufficient (80%–90%) power against the minimum clinically important difference. The idea of a large simple trial has proved useful in the cardiovascular therapeutic area. Although there are compelling reasons to consider this possibility, there are challenges as well. One important concern is the time and money needed to perform a large simple trial. It is not certain that a "simple" trial is feasible in a relatively complex, chronic disease. Another related issue concerns the sponsorship of such a trial. The government organizations that are the most likely sponsors would come from the countries of Southeastern Asia where this disease is endemic. These developing nations may have other health-care priorities now and it could be years before they can devote enough resources to support this type of research. Another issue is the rapid introduction of new therapies. The standard of care may continue to evolve raising the possibility that an expensive long-term trial may yield an answer to a therapeutic question that is no longer relevant.

14.2.2.2 Active Control versus Placebo Control

The two most recently approved drugs for treating hepatitis B infection, lamivudine and adefovir, were approved on the basis of placebo-controlled clinical trials of 1-year duration with a primary endpoint of histologic response (≥ 2 point increase in Knodell score) based on liver biopsy. Consequently, we should expect to see future pivotal trials use either of these agents as the active control. Three potential trial designs are feasible here:

1. A superiority design comparing a new compound to the active control.

2. A noninferiority design comparing a new compound to the active control.

3. A superiority design comparing the combination of a new compound used in conjunction with the active control to the active control alone.

14.2.2.3 Follow-Up beyond the Treatment Period

Since there is concern about the development of resistance when antivirals are continued indefinitely and these drugs are not intended for lifelong use in treating hepatitis B, it is typical to follow patients beyond the end of the treatment period to observe the duration of effect. A duration of off-drug follow-up of 3–6 months based on a trial of 1-year duration is customary. Based on current therapy, this period is sufficient to observe a potential rebound in viral replication after drug discontinuation as well as associated elevations of aminotransferase and the occurrence of severe liver decompensation.

14.2.2.4 Summary for Hepatitis B

Lin has argued that the recent development of lamivudine and adefovir may not be an effective guide to the development of new antiviral for treating hepatitis B [17]. If that is the case, future development programs will have to be longer and more expensive. Although it is apparent that more rigorous trials will provide a higher level of scientific and clinical evidence, it will be important for regulators to manage the greater level of societal cost. If the level of scientific evidence is such that no company can afford the development cost, this could dampen the development of new agents which remains an important need.

14.2.3   Hepatitis C

Chronic hepatitis C is a global problem affecting about 170 million people worldwide and 3–4 million more are infected each year [18]. Although the incidence of hepatitis C is decreasing, the manifestations of this infection such as cirrhosis, end-stage liver disease, and liver cancer continue to increase. Currently, it is the most common reason for liver transplantation. At the same time, there has been considerable progress since 1990 in developing therapies that eradicate the virus—the primary goal of chronic hepatitis C therapy. This improvement has been based on interferon therapies and is related to the employment of longer treatment duration, the addition of ribavirin, the use of pegylated interferon, weight-based dosing, and greater treatment adherence [19]. The future therapeutic needs include finding new oral agents which can replace interferon while eliciting less toxicity and to identify new therapies, either single agents or combinations, which can be used in treatment-experienced patients whose response to current therapy is less than optimal. Of course, with the recent availability of an effective vaccine, we would expect that this disease will decrease in incidence as the vaccine is more widely utilized.

14.2.3.1   Length of Trial/Primary Endpoint

Clinical trials to evaluate new therapies for CHC should include 48 weeks of active therapy for Genotypes 1 and 4 and 24 weeks of therapy for Genotypes 2 and 3 based on the current standard of care [19]. This represents an Industry/FDA consensus. The endpoint of sustained virologic response (SVR) is primary for regular and accelerated approval as defined by undetectable HCV RNA (<100 copies/mL) with 24 weeks of follow-up beyond the treatment period required to demonstrate that the response is sustained. Long-term follow-up may be needed for trials designed to evaluate the durability of SVR or to evaluate the complications of disease such as liver cancer or the need for transplantation.

14.2.3.2   Patient Populations

There are a number of important factors in hepatitis C disease which should be taken into consideration in designing clinical trials, either through the use of stratification or through patient selection: stage of disease, treatment experienced or treatment naïve, genotype, comorbidities including HIV and hepatitis B, pre- and post-liver transplantation, and racial and ethnic groups[19].

14.2.3.3   Control Regimen

For treatment-experienced patients, the combination of pegylated interferon and ribavirin is the current standard of care for treatment of chronic hepatitis C and should serve as a control regimen for studies of new active agents. These randomized studies should compare a new active agent to placebo added on to the above combination and should be powered to determine if the new agent plus the combination of pegylated interferon and ribavirin is superior to the combination alone [19]. For treatment naïve-patients at risk of progression, the control regimen is the same but these studies could be powered for noninferiority or for superiority depending on the context for the development of the agent.

14.2.3.4 Follow-Up beyond the Treatment Period

The current consensus is that viral replication should be monitored for 24 weeks after the end of therapy and that hepatitis C viral RNA must be undetectable (<100 copies/mL) to confirm SVR [19]. There is some controversy regarding the timing of this measurement as most patients who recur do so within 12 weeks after treatment discontinuation. SVR is confirmed as a surrogate for long-term (5–10 years) viral clearance for interferon-based therapies but only for 3 years for noninterferon-based treatment. It is appropriate to monitor patients with SVR at 4–5 year intervals for liver enzymes and liver biopsy as well as viral replication to ensure that the disease remains under control.

14.2.3.5 Summary for Hepatitis C

Despite the advances in chronic hepatitis C therapy in recent years and the advent of an effective vaccine, this disease continues to be a significant public health problem. Like other chronic diseases with effective but not optimal therapy, the patient population is heterogeneous. It includes treatment-naïve patients as well as heavily pretreated patients who have not responded to existing therapy or have responded but have seen disease recurrence, often accompanied by the development of viral resistance. The drug development process must address this diversity. Generally, specific studies are designed for each population, but in some cases, disparate populations can be included in the same study after using a stratified randomization to ensure balance for key covariates.

New treatments must build on the existing standard of care—pegylated interferon and ribavirin. Given the complexity of this disease and the potential for development of resistance, we should expect to see more complicated combinations emerge in the future as the standard of care, as in the development of HIV treatments. Treatment-experienced patients remain the greatest therapeutic need and the identification of an agent or agents that improves SVR in these patients represents the quickest path to regulatory approval, even perhaps accelerated approval. As with any antiviral for the treatment of a chronic disease, the development of resistance is a concern and this should be addressed in the drug development process, either pre- or post-approval.

14.3 Analysis and Interpretation

Whether evaluating therapy for HIV disease, chronic hepatitis B, chronic hepatitis C disease, or some other viral disease, basic principles of analysis apply.

1. For superiority studies, the primary inference should be based on the intention-to-treat (ITT) population or modified ITT population. Other populations such as per-protocol should be regarded as supportive or secondary in importance. However, regulators in Europe generally place more emphasis on the per-protocol population in superiority studies and less emphasis on the ITT population than does the FDA. Conversely, for noninferiority studies where regulators want the primary inference to have maximum sensitivity to discriminate new therapies from existing treatments, the per-protocol population will become primary and modified-ITT will be supportive.

2. Important covariates should be addressed when designing the study and either incorporated in the inclusion/exclusion criteria, or if not, implemented in the design and analysis strategy. In designing the study, we must decide if it is important to stratify the randomization (or perform an adaptive randomization) based on the factors under consideration. This decision will depend on a number of criteria:

   a. The predictive power of the covariate with respect to the primary or key secondary endpoints should be taken into account. The stronger the relationship, the more important it is to achieve balance.

   b. The size of the study is important. Smaller studies have a greater need to balance important covariates while larger studies can rely to a greater extent on randomization especially for less important covariates.

   c. The number of other important covariates is a limiting factor. There is a limit to the number of covariates that can be utilized in a stratified randomization and that issue becomes dramatically more challenging if we wish to stratify the randomization by center as well as is frequently the case. Using an adaptive randomization, we can incorporate a larger number of covariates at the risk of additional complexity and logistical challenges including the assessment of covariates in real time and dispensation of clinical trial material in accord with the randomization. Adaptive randomizations, while not the norm, can gain regulatory acceptance, if they include a stochastic element [20]. Algorithms that are deterministic are not acceptable.

3. In the analysis process, we should incorporate important covariates into our statistical model and these covariates should be identified in the protocol based on a review of the scientific literature and not based on statistical criteria related to their performance in the study at hand [21]. Selection of covariates based on current performance can increase the probability of type 1 error. In linear models, the omission of balanced covariates can lead to a loss of precision, especially in smaller studies, but this loss is generally modest. In some nonlinear models such as Cox regression and logistic regression, the omission of key covariates can result in bias toward acceptance of the null hypothesis and markedly decrease power [22]. As a general rule, key covariates should be specified in the protocol and statistical analysis plan for primary

and key secondary endpoints (such as mortality). Failure to do so will restrict any models that utilize different covariates to be secondary or supportive in nature. Certainly for regulatory purposes, these results will be considered ad hoc or worse post hoc. For publication in scientific literature, there may be more flexibility in utilizing other models as a basis for inference if the covariates are regarded as standard.

14.3.1 Censoring

In the analysis of time-to-event endpoints, we generally assume that the censoring mechanism is noninformative, that is, that individuals with censored responses are similar to and can be represented by the remaining individuals who have survival times beyond the censoring point. Although this assumption is reasonable in the context of many clinical trials, there are situations where we question the accuracy of this assumption. It may be then useful to explore one or more sensitivity analyses that are based on a different foundation than noninformative censoring. One option is to consider all censored observations as events at the time of censoring and this analysis may be useful as a sensitivity analysis in a regulatory context. Other more sophisticated analyses are also possible.

Robins [23] developed marginal structural models to adjust for time-dependent confounding variables. In the context of randomized trials, a time-dependent confounder is a time-dependent covariate that is a predictor of the event of interest and is also influenced by the randomized therapy. For example, if our endpoint is the occurrence of an AIDS-defining event, plasma HIV RNA levels could be a time-dependent covariate. It is affected by the randomized therapy, predicts the occurrence of an AIDS-defining event, and is associated with a patient leaving the trial and going on to some rescue therapy. Although these models can be used in both observational study and the randomized clinical trial (RCT) setting, we will discuss in the context of the RCT since it is most relevant to this chapter. In HIV trials, patients who fail to respond to randomized therapy or respond initially but lose this viral response before the end of the trial are treated as censored responses in time-to-event analyses. The effect of any subsequent therapy is effectively ignored in this analysis and this can cause bias in the estimation of treatment effects especially if one randomized arm is markedly more effective than another. This bias is an important reason why the analysis of proportions is used more frequently than a time-to-event analysis in AIDS trials. The marginal structural model allows for the estimation of the causal effects of randomized therapy after controlling for the confounding effects of rescue therapy. Rescue therapy may be a confounder since the need for rescue is related to the effectiveness of the randomized therapy.

The fitting of these marginal structural models is complex and beyond the scope of this book. They have been rarely used in the analyses of RCTs, partly because of their novelty, and partly because many applied statisticians are not familiar with these models which have been primarily used to analyze observational studies. Importantly, although progress has been made in adapting standard statistical software to employ these models, more work needs to be done in bridging the gap between the model developers and the applied statistician before these models can be used routinely.

14.3.2   Summarization of Time-to-Event Analyses

Estimation of the clinical effectiveness of any treatment is an important component of the statistical analysis. The summarization of time-to-event analyses is most often based on the hazard ratio. This arises because of the natural link with Cox's regression model based on proportional hazards [24] the most widespread model for survival analysis. This approach confers a number of advantages including

1. The ability to provide estimates of treatment effect while controlling for important covariates

2. Ease of computation of estimates, standard errors, and associated confidence intervals

However, the hazard ratio is not always ideal and other alternatives should be considered, either as a supplement to or a replacement for the hazard ratio. Although the use of the hazard ratio does not, strictly speaking, require proportional hazards, it is difficult to interpret the hazard ratio if the hazards are not proportional since this ratio is dependent on the length of follow-up. A more fundamental criticism lies in the difficulty of the clinician and patient in understanding and utilizing the hazard ratio. Spruance et al. [25] liken the hazard ratio to the odds of winning a race. While important, the margin of victory is a more important factor when assessing treatment effectiveness. The degree of patient benefit is a function of both the hazard ratio and the underlying population distribution. This distinction is most prominent in those time-to-event analyses where all patients will reach the endpoint of interest, except for censoring. For example, the time to resolution of influenza symptoms is such an endpoint. This distinction is less relevant to the situation where only a fraction of individuals will achieve the endpoint, for example, the time to loss of viral responsiveness over a period of time where many patients will continue to be responsive to the antiviral. If all patients achieve the endpoint, the difference in medians has been suggested as a more useful measure of patient benefit than the hazard ratio [26]. This summary, based on the Kaplan–Meier product-limit estimate, is straightforward and clinically relevant. Calculation of standard errors is readily available using standard statistical software and the calculation of confidence intervals on the treatment difference can be provided using bootstrap methods. It is not dependent on the assumption of proportional hazards but can be used if that assumption is reasonable. There are, however, disadvantages to this approach:

1. Focusing on one time point ignores differences that could be present at other points of the survival curve.

2. The hazard ratio is adjusted for important covariates in Cox's regression model. Medians are not adjusted for these covariates in the Kaplan–Meier

method. In large randomized trials, this is less of an issue but increases in importance for smaller, randomized trials, or in nonrandomized studies.

3. In cost-effectiveness analyses, medians are less useful than means since total cost is the key factor from an economic perspective.

14.4 Discussion

Patients with viral disease have far more therapies available that they did when the search for antiviral therapies began in the 1950s and the development of new therapies has increased exponentially since the onset of the AIDS epidemic. Antiviral chemotherapy is a dynamic situation and this means that the design and analysis of antiviral trials cannot remain static. Statisticians base their work on the design and analysis of a particular study on the key objectives associated with the study. As antiviral therapy evolves, key objectives will change as well and the design and analysis of novel studies must consequently respond to remain relevant to future medical need and the evolving standard of care.

Although it is not possible to predict the future perfectly, we can point to a number of developing trends which may influence antiviral therapy. The potential for an influenza pandemic has galvanized interest in the development of compounds for this disease. There are a limited number of drugs marketed to treat influenza and it is not clear how effective any of these would be against an emerging avian flu virus although laboratory studies suggest that zanamavir and oseltamivir would have some effectiveness. The catastrophic nature of a possible pandemic has led researchers to investigate possible therapies, especially agents with a different mechanism of action, institutions to sponsor this research, and for governments to consider stockpiling medication to deal with a pandemic. It is not clear how to establish the effectiveness of antiviral therapy when the virus has not emerged. At the same time, if therapy cannot be developed until the disease is widespread, it may be too late for any treatment to have optimal impact, even if highly effective. While there is no simple answer to this dilemma, it may be helpful to link efficacy in animal models of disease with testing in a limited number of patients coupled with a willingness on the part of regulators to relax their expectations regarding substantial evidence for the effectiveness of a new therapy. On a related note, the threat of biological warfare using orthopoxviruses such as smallpox has resulted in additional research in this area.

Another important area of research will be around utilizing combination chemotherapy. In any chronic viral disease where a single agent has limited effectiveness, we can expect to see combinations evaluated. The success of multiple agents used together to treat HIV disease will encourage the use of this same strategy for other viral disease. The rational exploration of effective combinations rests on three different but not mutually exclusive objectives: to improve efficacy compared to single-agent therapy, to reduce toxicity by using lower doses of the single agents which make up the combination and to reduce the development of drug resistance [1]—a key concern of any antiviral therapy. We would expect to see development strategies geared toward evaluating combinations as well as clinical trials designs with the objective of identifying the optimal dose of a combination with the expectation that this combination dose will be further evaluated in later phase of development.

At the same time, there are a number of viral diseases which currently have no safe and effective treatment. Examples of these diseases include the respiratory syncytial virus which commonly causes infections in pediatric patients and the West Nile virus [4]. The development of treatments for these diseases may spur progress in the design and analysis of antiviral trials and may entail new statistical methodology. Likewise as transplantation becomes more common, the treatment of opportunistic infections related to immunosuppression will become an increasingly important area of antiviral therapy. In the future, it would not be surprising to find new viral diseases akin to the HIV pandemic which would necessitate the development of new treatments and new methods to evaluate these treatments.

References

[1] Bean, B. (1992): Antiviral therapy: Current concepts and practices. *Clinical Microbiological Report*s 5:146–182.

[2] Kaufman, H. E., Martola, E. L., and Dohlman, C. (1962): Use of 5-iodo-2'-deoxyurindine (IDU) in treatment of herpes simplex keratitis. *Archives of Opthamology* 68:235–239.

[3] Bauer, D. J., St. Vincent, L., Kempe, C. H., and Downie, A. W. (1963): Prophylacytic treatment of smallpox contact with n-methyliatin beta-thiosemi-carbazone. *Lancet* ii:494–496.

[4] Rottinghaus, S. T. and Whitley, R. J. (2007): Current non-AIDS chemotherapy. *Expert Review of Anti-Infective Therapy* 5:217–230.

[5] Panel on Antiretroviral Guidelines for Adults and Adolescents. (2008): Guidelines for the use of antiretroviral agents in HIV-1-infected adults and adolescents. Department of Health and Human Services; http://www.aidsinfo.nih.gov/ContentFiles/adultandadolescentGL.pdf (accessed June 22, 2008).

[6] Barre-Sinousa, F., Chermann, J. C., Rey, F., et al. (1983): Isolation of a T-lymphotrophic retrovirus from a patient at risk for acquired immune deficiency syndrome (AIDS). *Science* 220:868–871.

[7] Gallo, R. C., Salahuddin, S. Z., Popovic, M., et al. (1984): Frequent detection and isolation of cytopathic retrovirues (HLTV-III) from patients with AIDS and at risk of AIDS. *Science* 224(4648):500–503.

[8] Bareta, J. C., Galai, N., Strathdee, S. A., et al. (2002): *International Conference on AIDS*. Jul 7–12; 14: abstract no. MoPeC3340. http://gateway.nlm.nih.gov/MeetingAbstracts/ma?f = 102254651.html (accessed June 23, 2008).

[9] Fischl, M. A., Richman, D. D., Grieco, M. H., et al. (1987): The efficacy of azidothymidine (AZT) in the treatment of patients with AIDS and AIDS-related complex. A double-blind, placebo-controlled trial. *The New England Journal of Medicine* 317 (4):185–191.

[10] Walker, A. S., Peto, T. E. A., Babiker, A. G., and Darbyshire, J. H. (1998): Markers of HIV infection in the concorde trial. *Quarterly Journal of Medicine* 91:423–438.

[11] Chuang-Stein, C. and DeMasi, R. (1998): Surrogate endpoints in AIDS drug development: Current status. *Drug Information Journal* 32:439–448.

[12] Antiretroviral drugs using plasma HIV RNA measurement—Clinical considerations for accelerated and traditional approval, FDA Guidance for Industry, October 2002.

[13] Hill, A. and Sabin, C. (2007): Developing and interpreting HIV noninferiority trials in naïve and experienced patients. *AIDS* 22:913–921.

[14] Note for Guidance on the Clinical Development of Medicinal Supplements for Treatment of HIV Infection 2004, European Agency for the Evaluation of Medical Products. Evaluation of Medicines for Human Use, Committee for Proprietary Medicinal Products (CPMP), March, 19, 2003.

[15] Smeaton, L. M., DeGruttola, V., Robbins, G. K., and Shafer, R. W. (2001): ACTG (AIDS Clinical Trials Group) 384: A strategy trial for comparing consecutive treatments for HIV-1. *Controlled Clinical Trials* 22:142–159.

[16] World Health Organization. Hepatitis B Fact Sheet Geneva: World Health Organization, October 2000, http://www.who.int/mediacentre/factsheets/fs204/en/print.html (accessed June 16, 2008).

[17] Lin, Y.-L. (2004): Clinical trials design issues for chronic hepatitis B. *Drug Information Journal* 38:287–291.

[18] World Health Organization. Hepatitis C Fact Sheet Geneva: World Health Organization, October 2000, http://www.who.int/mediacentre/factsheets/fs164/en/print.html (accessed June 16, 2008).

[19] FDA Antiviral Drugs Advisory Committee, October 19–20, 2006, http://www.fda.gov/ohrms/dockets/ac/06/transcripts/2006-4250T1-Part1.pdf (accessed June 18, 2008).

[20] International Conference on Harmonization E9—Statistical Principles for Clinical Trials. http://www.emea.europa.eu/pdfs/human/ich/036396en.pdf (accessed June 25, 2008).

[21] Raab, G. M., Day, S., and Sales, J. (2000): How to select covariates to include in the analysis of a clinical trial. *Controlled Clinical Trials* 21:330–342.

[22] Gail, M. H., Wieand, S., and Piantadosi, S. (1984): Biased estimates of treatment effect in randomized experiments with nonlinear regression and omitted covariates. *Biometrika* 71:431–444.

[23] Robins, J. M. (1998): Marginal structural models. In: *1997 Proceedings of the Section on Bayesian Statistical Science, Alexandria VA, American Statistical Association*, pp. 1–10.

[24] Cox, D. R. (1972): Regression models and life-tables. *Journal of the Royal Statistical Society. Series B (Methodological)* 34:187–220.

[25] Spruance, S. L., Reid, J. E., Grace, M., and Samore, M. (2004): Hazard ratio in clinical trials. *Antimicrobial Agents and Chemotherapy* 48:2787–2792.

[26] Keene, O. N. (2002): Alternatives to the hazard ratio in summarizing efficacy in time-to-event studies: An example from influenza studies. *Statistics in Medicine* 21:3687–3900.

Chapter 15

Cure Rate Models with Applications to Melanoma and Prostate Cancer Data

Ming-Hui Chen and Sungduk Kim

Contents

15.1 Introduction

For modeling censored time-to-event or survival data, the Cox proportional hazards model (PHM) [1,2] is most popular among the practitioners. However, the Cox PHM may not be appropriate for certain survival data such as those from the population, in which a significant proportion of patients are cured. Due to the recent medical advance, a significant proportion of patients are cured from various types of cancers such as breast cancer, head and neck cancer, melanoma, and prostate cancer. Thus, survival data in particular from cancer clinical trials often have a cure fraction. A cure rate model is particularly suitable for modeling these types of survival data as in the cure rate model, we assume that a certain fraction of the population is cured and the corresponding hazard is zero. There has been a vast literature on the cure rate models, including Berkson and Gage [3], Farewell [4,5], Halpern and Brown [6,7], Meeker [8], Kuk and Chen [9], Laska and Meisner [10], Yamaguchi [11], Yakovlev et al. [12], Yakovlev [13], Meeker and LuValle [14], Taylor [15], Asselain et al. [16], Fine [17], Chen et al. [18], Sy and Taylor [19], Peng and Dear [20], Broet et al. [21], Chen and Ibrahim [22,23], Ibrahim et al. [24], Tsodikov [25,26], Chen et al. [27, 28, 29], Ibrahim et al. [30], Yin and Ibrahim [31,32], Chi and Ibrahim [33], Kim et al. [34], and Cooner et al. [35]. Berkson and Gage [3] first introduced the mixture cure rate model. An extensive discussion of frequentist methods of inference for the mixture cure rate model is given in Maller and Zhou [36]. Bayesian formulation of the cure rate model is discussed in Ibrahim et al. ([37], Chapter 5). Tsodikov et al. [38] gave an excellent review on estimating cure rates from both frequentist and Bayesian perspectives.

In this chapter, we primarily focus on the cure-rate models with applications to melanoma and prostate cancer data. Melanoma is the most serious type of cancer of the skin. About 62,000 new cases are diagnosed in the United States each year, and there are about 8000 melanoma deaths. When caught early, melanomas can be easily treated by surgically removing the cancerous patch of skin. Prostate cancer forms in tissues of the prostate (a gland in the male reproductive system found below the bladder and in front of the rectum). Prostate cancer usually occurs in older men. About 186,320 new cases are diagnosed in the United States each year and there are about 28,000 deaths from prostate cancer. When cancer is detected before it spreads beyond the region of the prostate, it can be cured (completely eradicated for the remaining life of the patient) in many patients using treatment techniques that are widely available in the United States today. Although prostate cancer is the second leading cause of cancer death in men. Only 1 man in 34 will die of prostate cancer. As melanoma and prostate cancer can be cured, the cure rate model may be more suitable than the Cox PHM for modeling survival data from melanoma or prostate cancer clinical trials. In this chapter, we consider two such data sets, one from the E1673 trial conducted by Eastern Cooperative Oncology Group (ECOG) and another from a retrospective cohort study of 353 men treated with conventional-dose external beam radiation therapy (RT) at St. Anne's Hospital in Fall River, MA to examine whether the cure rate models fit these data better than the Cox PHM.

The rest of this chapter is organized as follows. A detailed description of the data is given in Section 15.2. Section 15.3 presents the development of cure rate models. The analysis of the data is carried out in detail in Section 15.4. We conclude this chapter with a brief discussion in Section 15.5.

15.2   Data

In this section, we provide a detailed description of two data sets used for the analysis in this chapter.

15.2.1   Melanoma Data

We consider the E1673 data from a melanoma clinical trial conducted by the ECOG. The E1673 trial was conducted by the ECOG to investigate the adjuvant effect of bacillus Calmette-Guerin (BCG) on resected American Joint Committee on Cancer (AJCC) Stage I–III melanoma between 1974 and 1978. Here, we consider a

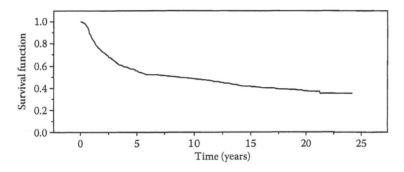

FIGURE 15.1: The Kaplan–Meier plot of overall survival for the E1673 data.

subset of the data published in Agarwala et al. [39] and also analyzed in Kim et al. [34]. This subset consists of $n = 650$ patients. The response variable (y) is overall survival, which is defined as the time from randomization until death or the last follow-up, whichever came first. The three covariates considered include age in years (x_1), gender (1 = male, 2 = female) (x_2), and performance status (PS) (0 = fully active, 1 = other) (x_3). The maximum follow-up in this subset was 24.208 years. The median survival time was 8.80 years. The median age was 48 years. There were 375 and 275 male and female patients, respectively, and 561 patients had fully active performance status. A detailed summary of the data can also be found in Ibrahim et al. ([37], Chapter 5). A Kaplan–Meier plot for overall survival is shown in Figure 15.1.

15.2.2 Prostate Cancer Data

We consider a subset of data published in D'Amico et al. [40]. The subset data consists of 353 men who were treated with RT for localized prostate cancer at St. Anne's Hospital in Fall River, MA, a Harvard Medical School affiliate, from January 1, 1989 to December 1, 2002. The primary endpoint is the time to prostate-specific antigen (PSA) recurrence or to the last follow-up, whichever came first. There were 155 patients who had PSA recurrence after RT. We consider five prognostic factors: age at the time of initial RT, natural logarithm of prostate specific antigen (logpsa) prior to RT, biopsy Gleason score, the 1992 AJCC clinical tumor category, and PSA velocity during the year prior to diagnosis. The covariates age and logpsa are continuous. We dichotomize biopsy Gleason score as G7 and G8H, where (GS7, GS8H) takes values (0, 0), (1, 0), and (0, 1) corresponding to a biopsy Gleason score of 6 or less, 7, and 8 to 10, respectively. Similarly, we dichotomize the clinical tumor category as T23, which takes the values 0 and 1, where 0 denotes the clinical tumor category T1 and 1 indicates the clinical tumor category T2 or T3. In addition, we dichotomize PSA velocity as a binary covariate Vel2, which is defined as Vel2 = 1 if PSA velocity > 2 and 0 otherwise. For this subset data, the maximum follow-up was 10.97 years and the median PSA recurrence time was 4.54 years. The means and the standard deviations (SDs) were 71.80 and 5.65 for age and

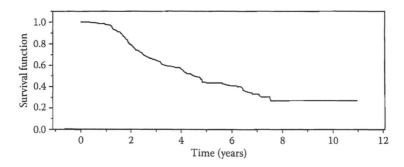

FIGURE 15.2: The Kaplan–Meier plot of PSA recurrence for the prostate cancer data.

11.15 and 11.74 for PSA, respectively. The numbers of patients who had biopsy Gleason score 6 or less, 7 or 8 to 10 were 189, 136, and 28, respectively. 155 patients had AJCC clinical tumor category T1, and 198 patients had AJCC clinical tumor category T2 or T3. There were 146 patients who had PSA velocity greater than 2. Let x_1, x_2, x_3, x_4, x_5, and x_6 denote age, logpsa, (G7, G8H), T23, and Vel2. A Kaplan–Meier plot for PSA recurrence is shown in Figure 15.2.

15.3   Cure Rate Models

Let y_i denote the observed survival time, let ν_i be the censoring indicator that equals 1 if y_i is a failure time and 0 if it is right censored for the ith subject. Also, let x_i denote a k-dimensional vector of covariates for the ith subject, which may include an intercept.

Suppose that a certain fraction π of the population are "cured," and the remaining $1 - \pi$ are not cured. Berkson and Gage [3] assume that the survival function for the population, $S(y_i)$, takes the form

$$S(y_i) = \pi_i + (1 - \pi_i)S^*(y_i), \tag{15.1}$$

where $S^*(y_i)$ denotes the survivor function for the noncured group in the population. Let Y_i denote the survival time for the ith subject. The model (Equation 15.1) essentially assume that

$$Y_i = \begin{cases} \infty & \text{with probability } \pi_i, \\ <\infty & \text{with probability } 1 - \pi_i. \end{cases}$$

For the "noncured" patient, the model (Equation 15.1) further assume $Y_i \sim S^*(y)$. Thus, under the Berkson and Gage model, there is a positive probability mass at ∞, which implies that Y_i does not have any finite moments. Ibrahim et al. [37] refer to the model defined by Equation 15.1 as the standard cure rate model. The standard cure rate model has been extensively discussed in the statistical literature. One way to incorporate covariates in Equation 15.1 is to relate the cure fraction π to the covariates via a standard binomial regression

$$\pi_i = G(x_i'\boldsymbol{\beta}), \tag{15.2}$$

where
  G is a continuous cumulative distribution function and
  $\boldsymbol{\beta}$ is a k-dimensional vector of regression coefficients.

Chen et al. [18] show that if we take an improper uniform prior for $\boldsymbol{\beta}$ (i.e., $\pi(\boldsymbol{\beta}) \propto 1$), the standard cure rate regression model (CRM) defined by Equations 15.1 and 15.2 yields improper posterior distributions for any G. This is a crucial drawback of model (Equation 15.1) since it implies that Bayesian inference with it essentially requires a proper prior for $\boldsymbol{\beta}$.

Yakovlev et al. [12], Yakovlev and Tsodikov [41], and Chen et al. [18] discuss a different type of cure rate model derived from a biological motivation, which is quite different from the standard cure rate model. This alternative cure rate model is derived as follows. Let N_i denote the number of metastatic-competent tumor cells and assume that the N_i's are independent Poisson random variables with mean θ_i. Suppose further that W_{ij} denotes the random time for the jth carcinogenic cell to produce a detectable cancer mass (incubation time for the jth carcinogenic cell) for the ith subject. We assume that the variables W_{ij}, $i = 1, 2, \ldots$, are independent and distributed with a common distribution function $F(y)$, and are independent of N_i. The survival time is defined by the random variable

$$Y_i = \min \{W_{ij}, 0 \leq j \leq N_i\},$$

where $P(W_{i0} = \infty) = 1$. After some algebra, it can be shown that the survival function for the ith subject is given by

$$S_p(y_i) = P(Y_i \geq y_i) = \exp\{-\theta_i F(y_i)\}. \tag{15.3}$$

Using Equation 15.3, the cure rate is given by $S_p(\infty) = \exp(-\theta_i)$, which is also equal to $P(N_i = 0)$. Under this formulation, the "density" corresponding to Equation 15.3 is given by

$$f_p(y_i) = \theta_i f(y_i) \exp\{-\theta_i F(y_i)\},$$

where $f(y_i) = dF(y_i)/dy_i$, and the corresponding hazard function is given by $h_p(y_i) = \theta_i f(y_i)$. Thus, the cure rate model (Equation 15.3) yields an attractive form for the hazard. That is, $h_p(y_i)$ is multiplicative in θ_i and $f(y_i)$ and thus has the proportional hazards structure, with the covariates modeled through θ_i. This form of the hazard is more appealing than the one from the standard cure rate model in Equation 15.1, which does not have the proportional hazards structure if π_i is modeled as a function of covariates. The proportional hazards property is computationally attractive, as Markov chain Monte Carlo (MCMC) methods are relatively easy to implement.

In addition, Chen et al. [18] establish a mathematical connection between Equations 15.1 and 15.3. Specifically, Equation 15.3 can be rewritten as

$$S_p(y_i) = \exp(-\theta_i) + \{1 - \exp(-\theta_i)\}S^*(y_i), \qquad (15.4)$$

where

$$S^*(y_i) = P(Y_i > y_i|N_i \geq 1) = \frac{\exp\{-\theta_i F(y_i)\} - \exp(-\theta_i)}{1 - \exp(-\theta_i)}.$$

Thus, letting $\pi_i = \exp(-\theta_i)$ in Equation 15.4, Equation 15.3 reduces to Equation 15.1. To build a regression model, Chen et al. [18] introduce covariates through θ_i via the standard log-linear model:

$$\theta_i \equiv \theta(x_i' \beta) = \exp(x_i' \beta). \qquad (15.5)$$

Then the joint distribution for (Y_i, N_i) is given by

$$f_p(y_i, N_i|x_i, \beta) = N_i f(y_i)S(y_i)^{N_i-1} \frac{\exp(N_i x_i' \beta)}{N_i!} \exp\{-\exp(x_i' \beta)\} \qquad (15.6)$$

and the resulting survival function is given by

$$S_p(y_i|x_i, \beta) = \exp\{-\exp(x_i' \beta)F(y_i)\}. \qquad (15.7)$$

Unlike the standard CRM defined by Equations 15.1 and 15.2, Chen et al. [18] show that under some mild conditions, the alternative CRM defined by Equations 15.3 and 15.5 yields a proper posterior when an improper uniform prior is assumed for β and $F(.)$ corresponds to a Weibull distribution.

Chen et al. [27] extend a Weibull distribution considered in Chen et al. [18] to a piecewise exponential model for $F(.)$. Let $h(y) = f(y)/(1 - F(y))$, which is the hazard function corresponding to F. The piecewise exponential model for $h(y)$ is constructed as follows. We first partition the time axis into J intervals: $(s_0, s_1]$, $(s_1, s_2], \ldots, (s_{J-1}, s_J]$, where $s_0 = 0 < s_1 < s_2 < \cdots < s_J$. In practice, it is sufficient to choose s_J to be greater than the largest follow-up time. We then assume a constant hazard λ_j over the jth interval $I_j = (s_{j-1}, s_j]$. That is,

$$h(y) = \lambda_j, \quad \text{for } y \in I_j \qquad (15.8)$$

for $j = 1, 2, \ldots, J$. We see that the piecewise exponential model depends on the number (J) of intervals and the choice of the s_j. As discussed in Chen et al. [27], without any prior information, the condition for the λ_j to be estimable is that at least one event occurs in each chosen interval $(s_{j-1}, s_j]$. This condition can be relaxed by putting a correlated or smooth hazard function prior on $h(y)$. Using Equation 15.8, the cumulative distribution function (cdf), denoted by $F(y|\lambda)$, is given by

$$F(y|\lambda) = 1 - \exp\left\{-\lambda_j(y - s_{j-1}) - \sum_{g=1}^{j-1} \lambda_g(s_g - s_{g-1})\right\}, \qquad (15.9)$$

for $s_{j-1} < y \le s_j$, where $\lambda = (\lambda_1, \ldots, \lambda_J)$. We note that when $J = 1$, $F(y|\lambda)$ reduces to the parametric exponential model. Let $D = (n, y, X, \nu)$ denote the observed data, where $y = (y_1, \ldots, y_n)'$, $\nu = (\nu_1, \ldots, \nu_n)'$, and X is the $n \times p$ matrix of covariates with ith row x_i'. Let $D_{\text{comp}} = (n, y, X, \nu, N)$ denote the "complete data," where $N = (N_1, N_2, \ldots, N_n)$. Then, the complete data likelihood for the piecewise exponential CRM defined by Equations 15.3 and 15.8 can be written as

$$\begin{aligned}
L(\beta, \lambda|D_{\text{comp}}) = {}& \prod_{i=1}^{n} \prod_{j=1}^{J} \exp\left\{-(N_i - \nu_i)\delta_{ij}\left[\lambda_j(y_i - s_{j-1}) + \sum_{g=1}^{j-1} \lambda_g(s_g - s_{g-1})\right]\right\} \\
& \times \prod_{i=1}^{n} \prod_{j=1}^{J} (N_i\lambda_j)^{\delta_{ij}\nu_i} \exp\left\{-\nu_i\delta_{ij}\left[\lambda_j(y_i - s_{j-1}) + \sum_{g=1}^{j-1} \lambda_g(s_g - s_{g-1})\right]\right\} \\
& \times \exp\left\{\sum_{i=1}^{n}[N_ix_i'\beta - \log(N_i!) - \exp(x_i'\beta)]\right\},
\end{aligned}$$

where $\delta_{ij} = 1$ if the ith subject failed or was censored in the jth interval I_j, and 0 otherwise. Again, since N is not observed, the observed data likelihood, $L(\beta, \lambda|D)$ is obtained by summing out N from Equation 15.10 as follows

$$L(\beta, \lambda|D) = \prod_{i=1}^{n} \exp\left\{\nu_i\left(x_i'\beta - B_i + \sum_{j=1}^{J} \delta_{ij}\log\lambda_j\right) - \exp\{x_i'\beta\}(1 - \exp\{-B_i\})\right\},$$

$$(15.10)$$

where $B_i = \sum_{j=1}^{J} \delta_{ij}\log\left[\lambda_j(y_i - s_{j-1}) + \sum_{g=1}^{j-1} \lambda_g(s_g - s_{g-1})\right]$.

Ibrahim et al. [24] introduce a smoothing parameter in the prior for λ_j in Equation 15.8, denoted κ, such that the model converges to a parametric model in the right tail of the survival curve as $j \to \infty$. Let $F_0(y|\lambda_0)$ denote the parametric survival model we wish to choose for the right tail of the survival curve, and let $H_0(y)$ denote the corresponding cumulative baseline hazard function. Ibrahim et al. [24] assume that the λ_j's are independent a priori, each having a gamma prior distribution with mean

$$\mu_j = E(\lambda_j|\lambda_0) = \frac{H_0(s_j) - H_0(s_{j-1})}{s_j - s_{j-1}}, \qquad (15.11)$$

and variance

$$\sigma_j^2 = \text{Var}(\lambda_j | \boldsymbol{\lambda}_0, \kappa) = \mu_j \kappa^j, \tag{15.12}$$

where $0 < \kappa < 1$ is a smoothing parameter that controls the degree of parametricity in the right tail. It is easy to see that as $\kappa \to 0$, $\sigma_j^2 \to 0$, which implies that small values of κ imply a more parametric model in the right tail. In addition, as $j \to \infty$, $\sigma_j^2 \to 0$, implying that the degree of parametricity is increased at a rate governed by κ as the number of intervals increases. This property implies that as $j \to \infty$, the survival distribution in the right tail becomes more parametric regardless of any fixed value of κ. The incorporation of κ into the model makes the posterior estimation of the λ_j's much more stable for large j, in which there are fewer subjects at risk. In Ibrahim et al. [24], an exponential distribution and a Weibull distribution are considered for $F_0(.|\boldsymbol{\lambda}_0)$. When $F_0(.|\boldsymbol{\lambda}_0)$ is an exponential distribution, namely, $F_0(y|\boldsymbol{\lambda}_0) = 1 - \exp(-\lambda_0 y)$, $\mu_j = \lambda_0$, and $\sigma_j^2 = \lambda_0 \kappa^j$. If $F_0(.|\boldsymbol{\lambda}_0)$ is a Weibull distribution, i.e., $F_0(y|\boldsymbol{\lambda}_0) = 1 - \exp(-\gamma_0 y^{\alpha_0})$, $\boldsymbol{\lambda}_0 = (\alpha_0, \gamma_0)'$, $\mu_j = \gamma_0(s_j^{\alpha_0} - s_{j-1}^{\alpha_0})/(s_j - s_{j-1})$ and $\sigma_j^2 = \gamma_0(s_j^{\alpha_0} - s_{j-1}^{\alpha_0})/s_j - s_{j-1}\kappa^j$.

In the Cox-type regression model framework, McKeague and Tighiouart [42] model the log-baseline hazard, $(\log \lambda_1, \log \lambda_2, \ldots, \log \lambda_J)$, as a Gaussian Markov random field conditional on the jump times s_j's. In McKeague and Tighiouart [42], the endpoints $\log \lambda_1$ and $\log \lambda_J$ are considered as neighbors due to the neighbor structure of the Gaussian Markov random field, which may not be desirable due to the nature of survival data. Because for the survival data with a cure fraction, there are typically more events and more patients at risk early on and less events and few patients at risk at the later time, there is a need to borrow strength in estimating $\log \lambda_j$ from neighboring $\log \lambda_{j'}$'s in the tail than in the beginning part of the survival curve, which implies that the correlation of $\log \lambda_{j-1}$ and $\log \lambda_j$ should be larger as j increases. To introduce such correlation structure, Kim et al. [34] propose a class of dynamic models for the log-baseline hazard, $\log \lambda_j$, based on the martingale-type process prior. Their dynamic models are constructed as follows. We let $\xi_j = \log(\lambda_j)$, $j = 1, 2, \ldots, J$, and assume that

$$\xi_j - \mu_j = c_j(\xi_{j-1} - \mu_{j-1}) + w_j, \quad w_j \sim N(0, b_j W), \tag{15.13}$$

where

$$b_j = e^{-\alpha \max\{0, \log s_j\}}, \quad c_j = \frac{r}{1 + b_j},$$

r $(0 < r < 1)$ and α are known constants, and
μ_j is the expected value of ξ_j.

The log hazard function for the first interval is based on Gaussian priors, with mean μ_1 and variance $b_1 W$. That is, $\xi_1 \sim N(\mu_1, b_1 W)$. Write ξ_j as follows:

$$\xi_j = \mu_j + \sum_{l=1}^{j} \left\{ \prod_{k=l+1}^{j} c_k \right\} w_l. \tag{15.14}$$

Note that in Equation 15.14, we assume $\prod_{k=j+1}^{j} c_k = 1$. Let $F_0(y|\lambda_0)$ denote the cdf of a parametric survival model and let $H_0(y)$ denote the corresponding cumulative baseline hazard function. We take the μ_j of the expected value of ξ_j to be

$$\mu_j = E(\xi_j|\lambda_0) = \log\left[\frac{H_0(s_j) - H_0(s_{j-1})}{s_j - s_{j-1}}\right].$$

It is easy to show that the variance of ξ_j is given by $\text{Var}(\xi_j|W) = \sum_{l=1}^{j} \{\prod_{k=l+1}^{j} c_k^2\} b_l W$.

In Equation 15.13, b_j is a decreasing function of j and α, and c_j is an increasing function of j and α. Both b_j and c_j depend on j through s_j. The parameters α and r play an important role in the dynamic CRM. Specifically, α is a smoothing parameter that controls the degree of parametricity in the right tail, and r is a correlation parameter, which introduces the correlation between ξ_j and ξ_{j-1}. We see that as $\alpha \to \infty$, $\text{Var}(\xi_j|W) \to 0$, so that small values of $\text{Var}(\xi_j|W)$ imply a more parametric model in the right tail. This property also implies that as $\alpha \to \infty$, the survival distribution in the right tail becomes more parametric. We also see that when $\alpha \to 0$, $c_j \to r/2$, when $\alpha \to \infty$, $c_j \to r$, and when $r \to 0$, ξ_j and ξ_{j-1} are independent. This is a novel construction of the semiparametric model that forces a high degree of parametricity and a large amount of correlation with large α and r. The incorporation of α and r into the model makes the posterior estimation of the ξ_j's much more stable in the tail of the survival curve, in which there are fewer subjects at risk.

As the estimation of the cure rate parameters, θ_i's, may be affected by α, r, J, and $F_0(\cdot|\lambda_0)$, in practice, the analysis should be carried out for several values of these parameters, to examine the sensitivity of the posterior estimates to various choices of these parameters. In the analysis of melanoma and prostate cancer data, we assume a Weibull density for $F_0(\cdot|\lambda_0)$, so that

$$f_0(y|\lambda_0) = \alpha_0 y^{\alpha_0 - 1} \exp\{\gamma_0 - y_0^{\alpha} \exp(\gamma_0)\},$$

where $\lambda_0 = (\alpha_0, \gamma_0)'$. Furthermore, the correlated nature of the dynamic models also allows us to assume J to be random. To this end, we assume that the jump times $s_1, s_2, \ldots$ form a time-homogeneous Poisson process. With random J and s_j, the number and positions of the jump times need not be fixed in advance. However, a random choice of J will lead to a posterior distribution with varying dimensions. In this regard, the posterior computation can be carried out via the reversible jump algorithm (see [42,43]).

To carry out Bayesian inference of the dynamic CRM defined by Equations 15.10 and 15.13, we need to specify a joint prior distribution for $(\beta, \xi, W, \lambda_0, J)$. For fixed J and s_j, $j = 1, \ldots, J$, the joint prior of $(\beta, \xi, W, \lambda_0)$ is taken as

$$\pi(\beta, \xi, W, \lambda_0) = \pi(\beta)\pi(\xi|W, \lambda_0)\pi(W)\pi(\lambda_0)$$

$$\propto \pi(\beta)\left[\prod_{j=2}^{J} \pi(\xi_j|\xi_{j-1}, W, \lambda_0)\right]\pi(\xi_1|W, \lambda_0)\pi(W)\pi(\lambda_0).$$

We assume a vague prior for $\boldsymbol{\beta}$. Thus $\boldsymbol{\beta}$ is assumed to follow a p-dimensional normal distribution $N_p(0, \sigma_\beta^2 I)$, where σ_β^2 is chosen to be large, for example, $\sigma_\beta^2 = 10^3$. As noted earlier, we assume that the prior distribution of ξ_1 is the normal distribution with mean μ_1 and variance $b_1 W$, and $\pi(\xi_j | \xi_{j-1}, W, \lambda_0)$ is normal with mean $\mu_j + c_j(\xi_{j-1} - \mu_{j-1})$ and variance $b_j W$, for $j = 2, 3, \ldots, J$. We specify an inverse gamma prior W, which is given by

$$W \sim IG(a_W, b_W),$$

which is the inverse gamma distribution with shape parameter a_W and scale parameter b_W. In Section 15.4, we take $a_W = 1.1$ and $b_W = 1$. For F_0, we take

$$\pi(\lambda_0) = \pi(\alpha_0 | \zeta_{\alpha_0}, \tau_{\alpha_0}) \pi(\gamma_0),$$

where

$$\pi(\alpha_0 | \zeta_{\alpha_0}, \tau_{\alpha_0}) \propto \alpha_0^{\zeta_{\alpha_0} - 1} \exp(-\tau_{\alpha_0} \alpha_0),$$

ζ_{α_0} and τ_{α_0} are specified hyperparameters and γ_0 is assumed to follow the normal distribution with mean zero and a large variance (10^3). In Section 15.4, we use $\zeta_{\alpha_0} = 1$ and $\tau_{\alpha_0} = 0.01$. When J and s_j, $j = 1, 2, \ldots, J$, are random variables, the time-homogeneous Poisson process assumption on the jump times implies that $J \sim \text{Poisson}(as_{\max})$, where $s_{\max}$ is the maximum observed survival time. In Section 15.4.1, the number of jump times, J, is assumed to follow a Poisson distribution with mean 20 and truncated in the interval 1 to 60. This automatically specifies a to be $20/s_{\max}$. In Section 15.4.2, the Poisson distribution with mean 10 and truncated in the interval 1 to 40 is assumed for J. Given J, the martingale specification implies that

$$\xi | W \sim N_J(\mu, WC^{-1}),$$

where the $J \times J$ matrix C has all elements zero except for $a_{11} = ((1/b_1) + (c_2^2/b_2))$ $a_{jj} = \frac{1}{b_j} + \frac{c_{j+1}^2}{b_{j+1}}$, $j = 2, 3, \ldots, J-1$ and $c_{JJ} = \frac{1}{b_J}$ and $c_{j,j+1} = -(c_j/b_{j+1})$, $j = 1, 2, \ldots, J-1$ and $c_{j+1,j} = -(c_{j-1}/b_j)$, $j = 2, 3, \ldots, J-1$.

In Section 15.4, we examine whether the dynamic CRM defined by Equations 15.10 and 15.13 fits the E1673 data and the prostate cancer data better than the Cox PHM with a piecewise exponential baseline hazard function given by Equation 15.8. Note that under the Cox PHM, the likelihood function of $(\boldsymbol{\beta}, \lambda)$ is given by

$$L(\boldsymbol{\beta}, \lambda | D) = \prod_{i=1}^{n} \prod_{j=1}^{J} \left\{ \lambda_j \exp(x_i' \boldsymbol{\beta}) \right\}^{\delta_{ij} \nu_i}$$

$$\times \exp\left[-\delta_{ij} \left\{ \lambda_j(y_i - s_{j-1}) + \sum_{g=1}^{j-1} \lambda_g(s_g - s_{g-1}) \right\} \exp(x_i' \boldsymbol{\beta}) \right]$$

$$= \prod_{i=1}^{n} \left(\prod_{j=1}^{J} \lambda_j^{\nu_i \delta_{ij}} \right) \exp\{\nu_i x_i' \boldsymbol{\beta}\} \exp\{-B_i^* \exp(x_i' \boldsymbol{\beta})\}, \qquad (15.15)$$

where $B_i^* = \sum_{j=1}^{J} \delta_{ij} \{ \lambda_j (y_i - s_{j-1}) + \sum_{g=1}^{j-1} \lambda_g (s_g - s_{g-1}) \}$. We also note that in Equation 15.15, x_i does not include an intercept, and otherwise the intercept is confounded with the λ_j under the Cox model. To carry out Bayesian inference, we assume that the λ_j's are independent a priori, each having a gamma prior distribution $G(a_\lambda, b_\lambda)$. In Section 15.4, we take $a_\lambda = 1.1$ and $b_\lambda = 0.001$. We also assume that the λ_j's are independent of β and $\beta \sim N(0, 1000)$ in Section 15.4 a priori.

15.4   Data Analysis

In this section, we carry out a detailed data analysis of the E1673 melanoma data as well as the prostate cancer data discussed in Section 15.2. To assess the goodness of fit of the dynamic CRM and Cox PHM, we use the logarithm of pseudomarginal likelihood (LPML) given in Ibrahim et al. ([37], Chapter 6). LPML is a well-established Bayesian model comparison criterion based on the conditional predictive ordinate (CPO) statistics, which is particularly suitable for the cure rate models. Let $D^{(-i)}$ denote the data with the ith observation deleted. The CPO statistic for the ith subject is the marginal posterior predictive density of y_i when $\nu_i = 1$ or the marginal posterior predictive probability of the censored event $\{ Y_i \geq y_i \}$ when $\nu_i = 0$. For the dynamic CRM defined by Equations 15.10 and 15.13, the CPO statistic for the ith subject is computed as

$$
\mathrm{CPO}_i = E\left[\exp\left\{ \nu_i \left(x_i' \beta - B_i + \sum_{j=1}^{J} \delta_{ij} \log \lambda_j \right) \right. \right.
$$
$$
\left. \left. - \exp\{ x_i' \beta \} (1 - \exp\{ -B_i \}) \right\} \Big| D^{(-i)} \right],
\tag{15.16}
$$

where B_i is defined in Equation 15.10, and the expectation is taken with respect to the posterior distribution of the model parameters given the data $D^{(-i)}$. Similarly, for the Cox PHM in Equation 15.15, the CPO statistic is given by

$$
\mathrm{CPO}_i = E\left[\left(\prod_{j=1}^{J} \lambda_j^{\nu_i \delta_{ij}} \right) \exp\{ \nu_i x_i' \beta \} \exp\left\{ -B_i^* \exp(x_i' \beta) \right\} \Big| D^{(-i)} \right],
\tag{15.17}
$$

where B_i^* is defined in Equation 15.15 and the expectation is taken with respect to the posterior distribution of the model parameters given the data $D^{(-i)}$. Then, the LPML measure is defined as

$$
\mathrm{LPML} = \sum_{i=1}^{n} \log(\mathrm{CPO}_i).
$$

The larger the LPML measure, the better the fit of a given model. An efficient Monte Carlo (MC) estimate of LPML has been developed and the detailed development can be found in Ibrahim et al. ([37], Chapter 6). In both data analyses, we standardized all covariates. The standard Gibbs sampling algorithm is used to sample from the posterior distribution under the Cox PHM. For the dynamic CRM, we use the MCMC sampling algorithm developed in Kim et al. [34]. The detailed description of these sampling algorithms is omitted for brevity. In all the computations, 50,000 Gibbs samples for fixed J and 100,000 iterations for random J were used to compute all posterior estimates, including posterior means, posterior SDs, 95% highest posterior density (HPD) intervals and LPMLs, using a burn-in of 2000 sample for fixed J and 20,000 samples for random J. The convergence of the Gibbs sampler was checked using several diagnostic procedures as recommended by Cowles and Carlin [44]. All HPD intervals were computed using a MC method developed by Chen and Shao [45]. The computer codes were written in FORTRAN 95 using IMSL subroutines with double precision accuracy.

15.4.1 Analysis of the E1673 Melanoma Data

For the E1673 data discussed in Section 15.2.1, we use the LPML measure to assess the goodness of fit of Cox PHM for different choices of J and the dynamic CRM for different choices of α, r, and J. Table 15.1 shows the LPMLs for various choices of α, r, and J. From Table 15.1, we see that among all models with fixed J, the best PHM is the one with $J=30$, which has LPML $=-1335.72$, and the best CRM model is the one with $\alpha=0.5$, $r=0.95$, and $J=30$, which has LPML $=-1333.94$. Thus, the best fixed J CRM fits the data better than the PHM. We also observe that among those with fixed J, the LPML measure appears to be concave in J for both PHM and CRM. Among all models considered in Table 15.1, the best model is the CRM with $\alpha=0.1$, $r=0.5$, and random J, which has LPML $=-1329.65$. We note that under this CRM model with random J, the mode of the posterior distribution of J shown in Figure 15.3 is roughly around $J=30$. This result is intuitively appealing because a random J provides an additional source of correlations among the log λ_j's.

TABLE 15.1: LPMLs for the E1673 data with various choices of α, r, and J.

			J				
Model	α	r	**10**	**20**	**30**	**40**	**Random**
PHM			−1340.45	−1336.93	−1335.72	−1346.05	
CRM		0.0	−1342.33	−1338.71	−1335.99	−1343.34	−1343.31
	0.1	0.5	−1342.23	−1338.28	−1335.07	−1341.35	−1329.65
		0.95	−1342.05	−1337.96	−1334.47	−1339.58	−1333.08
		0.0	−1343.34	−1338.30	−1335.74	−1342.70	−1335.92
	0.5	0.5	−1342.06	−1337.71	−1334.67	−1340.24	−1331.49
		0.95	−1341.84	−1337.51	−1333.94	−1338.86	−1347.57
		0.0	−1342.11	−1338.48	−1336.44	−1343.37	−1341.11
	1.0	0.5	−1341.61	−1337.78	−1335.08	−1340.57	−1337.49
		0.95	−1341.66	−1337.58	−1334.79	−1339.41	−1343.88

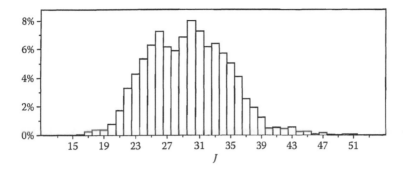

FIGURE 15.3: The posterior distribution of J when J is random, $\alpha = 0.1$ and $r = 0.5$ for the E1673 data.

TABLE 15.2: Posterior estimates under the best PHM for the E1673 data.

Parameter	Posterior Mean	Posterior SD	95% HPD Interval
β_1 (age)	0.180	0.048	(0.083, 0.273)
β_2 (gender)	−0.500	0.102	(−0.700, −0.300)
β_3 (PS)	0.171	0.144	(−0.113, 0.450)

TABLE 15.3: Posterior estimates under the best fixed J CRM for the E1673 data.

Parameter	Posterior Mean	Posterior SD	95% HPD Interval
β_0 (intercept)	0.136	0.081	(−0.021, 0.299)
β_1 (age)	0.188	0.050	(0.091, 0.285)
β_2 (gender)	−0.377	0.104	(−0.586, −0.177)
β_3 (PS)	0.246	0.146	(−0.041, 0.533)
α_0	0.940	0.119	(0.702, 1.172)
γ_0	−1.743	0.303	(−2.362, −1.161)
W	0.545	0.213	(0.216, 0.956)

The posterior estimates of the model parameters under the best PHM model with $J = 30$, the best CRM model with fixed J ($\alpha = 0.5$, $r = 0.95$, and $J = 30$) and the best CRM model with random J ($\alpha = 0.1$ and $r = 0.5$) are reported in Tables 15.2 through 15.4. From these tables, we see that (1) the posterior estimates of the regression coefficients under the PHM are comparable to those under the CRM's in the sense that the HPD intervals for age and gender do not include 0 and the HPD interval for PS contains 0 under each of these three models; and (2) the posterior estimates of the regression coefficients with fixed J are quite similar to those with random J under CRMs. We also examined those posterior estimates under other choices of α, r, and J. We found that the results are quite

TABLE 15.4:   Posterior estimates under the best random J CRM for the E1673 data.

Parameter	Posterior Mean	Posterior SD	95% HPD Interval
β_0 (intercept)	0.140	0.081	$(-0.016,\ \ 0.300)$
β_1 (age)	0.188	0.049	$(0.092,\ \ 0.285)$
β_2 (gender)	-0.379	0.105	$(-0.581,\ -0.168)$
β_3 (PS)	0.246	0.145	$(-0.047,\ \ 0.519)$
α_0	0.888	0.132	$(0.623,\ \ 1.138)$
γ_0	-1.536	0.317	$(-2.156,\ -0.915)$
W	0.566	0.224	$(0.222,\ \ 1.017)$

robust. As age and gender are significant at the 5% significance level under all three models, these two prognostic factors are potentially important for predicting survival in melanoma.

The estimated baseline hazard functions of $h(y)$ in Equation 15.8 with fixed and random J's are displayed in Figure 15.4. As expected, the estimated hazard functions are more nonparametric at the earlier time and more parametric at the tail of the survival curve. Moreover, a more smooth hazard function is obtained under the model with a random J, which is a desirable result as the number and location of jump times can change randomly under the model with a random J.

Figure 15.5 shows the boxplots of the estimated cure rates under the best CRM model with fixed J ($\alpha = 0.5$, $r = 0.95$, and $J = 30$) and the best CRM model with random J ($\alpha = 0.1$ and $r = 0.5$) for all 650 patients. From Figure 15.4, we see that these two boxplots are very similar. The first quartiles, medians, and third quartiles of the estimated cure rates are 0.285, 0.359, and 0.436 under the best fixed J CRM and 0.280, 0.354, and 0.432 under the best random J CRM. These results imply that there are a substantial proportion of patients cured from melanoma cancer.

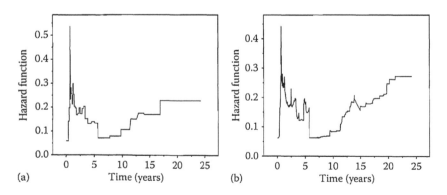

FIGURE 15.4:   Estimated hazard functions for $\alpha = 0.5$, $r = 0.95$, and $J = 30$ (a) and for $\alpha = 0.1$, $r = 0.5$, and random J (b) for the E1673 data.

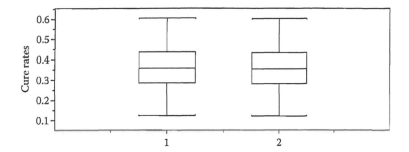

FIGURE 15.5: The boxplots of estimated cure rates under the best fixed J CRM ("1") and the best random J CRM ("2") for the E1673 data.

15.4.2 Analysis of the Prostate Cancer Data

For the prostate cancer data discussed in Section 15.2.2, we again use the LPML measure to assess the goodness of fit of Cox PHM for different choices of J and the dynamic CRM for different choices of α, r, and J. Table 15.5 shows the LPMLs for various choices of α, r, and J. From Table 15.5, we see that among all models with fixed J, the best PHM is the one with $J = 10$, which has LPML $= -400.27$, and the best CRM model is the one with $\alpha = 0.1$, $r = 0.5$, and $J = 20$, which has LPML $= -398.35$. Thus, the best fixed J CRM fits the data better than the PHM. Similarly to the E1673 data, we again see that among those with fixed J, the LPML measure appears to be concave in J for both PHM and CRM. Among all models considered in Table 15.5, the best model is the CRM with $\alpha = 0.1$, $r = 0.0$, and random J, which has LPML $= -395.75$. Figure 15.6 shows that the mode of the posterior distribution of J when $\alpha = 0.1$ and $r = 0.0$ is roughly around $J = 20$. This may partially explain why a better fit is achieved by the models with $J = 20$ when J is fixed.

TABLE 15.5: LPML's for the prostate cancer data with various choices of α, r, and J.

Model	α	r	5	10	15	20	25	30	Random
PHM			−405.42	−400.27	−400.48	−400.84	−403.41	−405.33	
CRM		0.0	−406.97	−402.78	−399.38	−398.45	−399.80	−401.98	−395.75
	0.1	0.5	−407.04	−402.41	−399.07	−398.35	−399.45	−401.03	−396.87
		0.95	−407.07	−402.18	−398.94	−398.38	−399.28	−401.07	−396.52
		0.0	−407.05	−402.58	−399.80	−398.58	−398.58	−401.48	−396.97
	0.5	0.5	−407.03	−402.24	−398.80	−398.55	−398.55	−401.39	−396.84
		0.95	−407.12	−401.90	−398.65	−398.63	−399.02	−401.58	−397.00
		0.0	−406.99	−402.44	−399.36	−399.16	−399.39	−402.12	−397.63
	1.0	0.5	−412.19	−402.60	−398.70	−398.95	−399.16	−402.19	−398.85
		0.95	−407.12	−402.62	−398.60	−399.17	−399.13	−404.22	−398.48

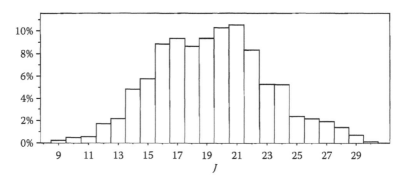

FIGURE 15.6: The posterior distribution of J when J is random, $\alpha = 0.1$ and $r = 0.0$ for the prostate cancer data.

The posterior estimates of the model parameters under the best PHM model with $J = 10$, the best CRM model with fixed J ($\alpha = 0.1$, $r = 0.5$, and $J = 20$) and the best CRM model with random J ($\alpha = 0.1$ and $r = 0.0$) are reported in Tables 15.6 through 15.8. From these tables, we see that under the CRMs, the posterior estimates of the regression coefficients with fixed J are quite similar to those with random J. Also, the posterior estimates of the regression coefficients under the PHM are comparable to those under the CRMs. Specifically, in Tables 15.6 through 15.8, the HPD intervals only for logpsa and GS8H do not include 0, which indicate that logpsa and GS8H are potentially important prognostic factors for predicting PSA recurrence.

The estimated baseline hazard functions of $h(y)$ in Equation 15.8 with fixed and random J's are displayed in Figure 15.7. As expected, the estimated hazard functions are more nonparametric at the earlier time and more parametric at the tail of the survival curve. Moreover, a more smooth hazard function is obtained under the model with a random J. This is a desirable result as the number and location of jump times can change randomly under the model with a random J.

Figure 15.8 shows the boxplots of the estimated cure rates under the best CRM model with fixed J ($\alpha = 0.1$, $r = 0.5$, and $J = 20$) and the best CRM model with random J ($\alpha = 0.1$ and $r = 0.0$) for all 353 patients. Similarly to the E1673 data, we

TABLE 15.6: Posterior estimates under the best PHM for the prostate cancer data.

Parameter	Posterior Mean	Posterior SD	95% HPD Interval
β_1 (age)	−0.113	0.073	(−0.257, 0.029)
β_2 (logpsa)	0.622	0.092	(0.440, 0.800)
β_3 (GS7)	−0.017	0.086	(−0.188, 0.147)
β_4 (GS8H)	0.147	0.069	(0.012, 0.283)
β_5 (T34)	0.157	0.081	(−0.003, 0.315)
β_6 (Vel2)	0.095	0.095	(−0.091, 0.281)

TABLE 15.7: Posterior estimates under the best fixed J CRM for the prostate cancer data.

Parameter	Posterior Mean	Posterior SD	95% HPD Interval
β_0 (intercept)	0.267	0.146	(−0.010, 0.563)
β_1 (age)	−0.119	0.075	(−0.262, 0.030)
β_2 (logpsa)	0.628	0.096	(0.437, 0.813)
β_3 (GS7)	−0.030	0.089	(−0.208, 0.142)
β_4 (GS8H)	0.154	0.071	(0.014, 0.291)
β_5 (T34)	0.149	0.084	(−0.014, 0.315)
β_6 (Vel2)	0.073	0.098	(−0.117, 0.266)
α_0	2.313	0.335	(1.658, 2.975)
γ_0	−3.613	0.495	(−4.595, −2.632)
W	0.411	0.180	(0.137, 0.762)

TABLE 15.8: Posterior estimates under the best random J CRM for the prostate cancer data.

Parameter	Posterior Mean	Posterior S.D.	95% HPD Interval
β_0 (intercept)	0.295	0.150	(0.006, 0.588)
β_1 (age)	−0.119	0.075	(−0.268, 0.023)
β_2 (logpsa)	0.633	0.097	(0.441, 0.822)
β_3 (GS7)	−0.028	0.088	(−0.203, 0.141)
β_4 (GS8H)	0.153	0.071	(0.014, 0.291)
β_5 (T34)	0.151	0.084	(−0.014, 0.315)
β_6 (Vel2)	0.075	0.099	(−0.121, 0.264)
α_0	2.332	0.371	(1.582, 3.057)
γ_0	−3.601	0.574	(−4.739, −2.456)
W	0.664	0.363	(0.167, 1.364)

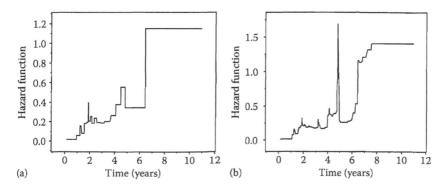

(a)

(b)

FIGURE 15.7: Estimated hazard functions for $\alpha = 0.1$, $r = 0.5$, and $J = 20$ (a) and for $\alpha = 0.1$, $r = 0.0$, and random J (b) for the prostate cancer data.

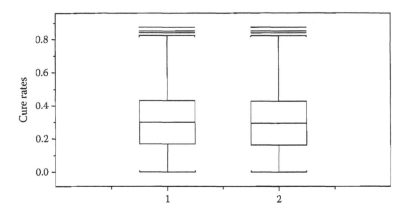

FIGURE 15.8:   The boxplots of estimated cure rates under the best fixed *J* CRM ("1") and the best random *J* CRM ("2") for the prostate cancer data.

see that these two boxplots are very similar. The first quartiles, medians, and third quartiles of the estimated cure rates are 0.168, 0.298, and 0.432 under the best fixed *J* CRM and 0.161, 0.293, and 0.427 under the best random *J* CRM. These results imply that there are a substantial proportion of patients free from PSA recurrence.

15.5   Concluding Remarks

In this chapter, we have provided an overview of the development of the cure rate models. We have also carried out the detailed Bayesian analyses of the E1673 melanoma data and the prostate cancer data. For both data sets, we have demonstrated that the cure rate models fit the data better than the Cox PHM based on the LPML measure.

As discussed in Section 15.3, if a patient is cured, his or her survival time is $Y = \infty$. In practice, $Y = \infty$ is never observed. For a typical survival data set, when $Y = \infty$, we only observe the censored time. In this sense, a cure rate model is not totally identifiable. However, when the follow-up time is longer enough and a patient is free from the disease, he/she is practically "cured." For the data analyzed in this chapter, the E1673 study has had 24 years of follow-up on 650 patients and the prostate cancer study has had nearly 11 years of follow-up on 353 men. This may partially explain why the cure rate models outperform the Cox models in fitting these two data sets.

In this chapter, we use the LPML measure as a model assessment tool. From Equation 15.16 or Equation 15.17, we see that LPML is always well defined as long the posterior predictive density is proper. Thus, LPML is well defined under improper priors, and in addition, it is very computationally stable. Therefore, LPML has a clear advantage over the Bayes factor as a model assessment tool, since it is well-known that the Bayes factor is not well defined with improper priors, and is generally quite sensitive to vague proper priors. In addition, the LPML measure also has clear advantages over other model selection criteria, such as the L measure (see [46–48]). The L measure is a Bayesian criterion requiring finite second moments of the sampling distribution of y_i, whereas the LPML measure does not require existence of any moments. Another useful Bayesian model assessment criterion is the deviance information criterion (DIC) proposed by Spiegelhalter et al. [49]. Similarly to LPML, DIC does not require existence of any moments as well. However, based on our experience and simulation study, the performance of DIC is quite similar to LPML.

Finally, we mention that the smoothing methodology via the martingale-type process prior discussed in Section 15.3 is not only restrict to cure rate models and it can also be useful for other types of models such as Cox-type regression models and frailty models as long as a piecewise hazard function is assumed. Based on our experience, the dynamic CRM is particularly suitable and works the best for survival data with long follow-ups.

References

[1] Cox, D.R. (1972). Regression models and life tables. *Journal of the Royal Statistical Society, Series B, 34*, 187–220.

[2] Cox, D.R. (1975). Partial likelihood. *Biometrika, 62*, 269–276.

[3] Berkson, J. and Gage, R.P. (1952). Survival curve for cancer patients following treatment. *Journal of the American Statistical Association, 47*, 501–515.

[4] Farewell, V.T. (1982). The use of mixture models for the analysis of survival data with long-term survivors. *Biometrics, 38*, 1041–1046.

[5] Farewell, V.T. (1986). Mixture models in survival analysis: Are they worth the risk? *Canadian Journal of Statistics, 14*, 257–262.

[6] Halpern, J. and Brown, B.W. Jr. (1987). Cure rate models: Power of the log rank and generalized Wilcoxon tests. *Statistics in Medicine, 6*, 483–489.

[7] Halpern, J. and Brown, B.W. Jr. (1987). Designing clinical trials with arbitrary specification of survival functions and for the log rank or generalized Wilcoxon test. *Controlled Clinical Trials, 8*, 177–189.

[8] Meeker, W.Q. (1987). Limited failure population life tests: Application to integrated circuit reliability. *Technometrics, 29*, 51–65.

[9] Kuk, A.Y.C. and Chen, C.-H. (1992). A mixture model combining logistic regression with proportional hazards regression. *Biometrika, 79*, 531–541.

[10] Laska, E.M. and Meisner, M.J. (1992). Nonparametric estimation and testing in a cure rate model. *Biometrics, 48*, 1223–1234.

[11] Yamaguchi, K. (1992). Accelerated failure-time regression models with a regression model of surviving fraction: An application to the analysis of "permanent employment" in Japan. *Journal of the American Statistical Association, 87*, 284–292.

[12] Yakovlev, A.Y., Asselain, B., Bardou, V.J., Fourquet, A., Hoang, T., Rochefediere, A., and Tsodikov, A.D. (1993). A simple stochastic model of tumor recurrence and its applications to data on premenopausal breast cancer. In *Biometrie et Analyse de Dormees Spatio-Temporelles*, vol. 12 (Eds. B. Asselain, M. Boniface, C. Duby, C. Lopez, J.P. Masson, and J. Tranchefort). Société Francaise de Biométrie, ENSA Rennes, France, pp. 66–82.

[13] Yakovlev, A.Y. (1994). Letter to the editor. *Statistics in Medicine, 13*, 983–986.

[14] Meeker, W.Q. and LuValle, M.J. (1995). An accelerated life test model based on reliability kinetics. *Technometrics, 37*, 133–146.

[15] Taylor, J.M.G. (1995). Semi-parametric estimation in failure time mixture models. *Biometrics, 51*, 899–907.

[16] Asselain, B., Fourquet, A., Hoang, T., Tsodikov, A.D., and Yakovlev, A.Y. (1996). A Parametric regression model of tumor recurrence: An application to the analysis of clinical data on breast cancer. *Statistics and Probability Letters, 29*, 271–278.

[17] Fine, J.P. (1999). Analysing competing risks data with transformation models. *Journal of the Royal Statistical Society, Series B, 61*, 817–830.

[18] Chen, M.-H., Ibrahim, J.G., and Sinha, D. (1999). A new Bayesian model for survival data with a surviving fraction. *Journal of the American Statistical Association, 94*, 909–919.

[19] Sy, J.P. and Taylor, J.M.G. (2000). Estimation in a proportional hazards cure model. *Biometrics, 56*, 227–336.

[20] Peng, Y. and Dear, K.B.G. (2000). A nonparametric mixture model for cure rate estimation. *Biometrics, 56*, 237–243.

[21] Broet, P., Rycke, Y.D., Tubert-Bitter, P., Lellouch, J., Asselain, B., and Moreau, T. (2001). A semiparametric approach for the two-sample comparison of survival times with long-term survivors. *Biometrics, 57*, 844–852.

[22] Chen, M.-H. and Ibrahim, J.G. (2001). Maximum likelihood methods for cure rate models with missing covariates. *Biometrics, 57*, 43–52.

[23] Chen, M.-H. and Ibrahim, J.G. (2001). Bayesian model comparisons for survival data with a cure fraction. In *Bayesian Methods with Applications to*

Science, Policy and Official Statistics, Office for Official Publications of the European Communities, Luxembourg pp. 81–90.

[24] Ibrahim, J.G., Chen, M.-H., and Sinha, D. (2001). Bayesian semi-parametric models for survival data with a cure fraction. *Biometrics, 57*, 383–388.

[25] Tsodikov, A. (2001). Estimation of survival based on proportional hazards when cure is a possibility. *Mathematical and Computer Modelling, 33*, 1227–1236.

[26] Tsodikov (2002). Semiparametric models of long- and short-term survival: An application to the analysis of breast cancer survival in Utah by age and stage. *Statistics in Medicine, 21*, 895–920.

[27] Chen, M.-H., Harrington, D.P., and Ibrahim, J.G. (2002). Bayesian cure rate models for malignant melanoma: A case-study of Eastern Cooperative Oncology Group trial E1690. *Applied Statistics, 51(2)*, 135–150.

[28] Chen, M.-H., Ibrahim, J.G., and Sinha, D. (2002). Bayesian inference for multivariate survival data with a surviving fraction. *Journal of Multivariate Analysis, 80*, 101–126.

[29] Chen, M.-H., Ibrahim, J.G., and Lipsitz, S.R. (2002). Bayesian methods for missing covariates in cure rate models. *Lifetime Data Analysis, 8*, 117–146.

[30] Ibrahim, J.G., Chen, M.-H., and Sinha, D. (2005). Bayesian approaches to cure rate models. In *Encyclopedia of Biostatistics*, 2nd edn., vol. 1 (Eds. Peter Armitage & Theodore Colton). John Wiley & Sons Ltd., Chichester, pp. 306–313.

[31] Yin, G. and Ibrahim, J.G. (2005). A general class of Bayesian survival models with zero and nonzero cure fractions. *Biometrics, 61*, 403–412.

[32] Yin, G. and Ibrahim, J.G. (2005). Cure rate models: A unified approach. *The Canadian Journal of Statistics, 33*, 559–570.

[33] Chi, Y. and Ibrahim, J.G. (2006). Joint models for multivariate longitudinal and multivariate survival data. *Biometrics, 62*, 432–445.

[34] Kim, S., Chen, M.-H., Dey, D.K., and Gamerman, D. (2007). Bayesian dynamic models for survival data with a cure fraction. *Lifetime Data Analysis, 13*, 17–35.

[35] Cooner, F., Banerjee, S., Carlin, B.P., and Sinha, D. (2007). Flexible cure rate modelling under latent activation schemes. *Journal of the American Statistical Association, 102*, 560–572.

[36] Maller, R. and Zhou, X. (1996). *Survival Analysis with Long-Term Survivors*. Wiley, New York.

[37] Ibrahim, J.G., Chen, M.-H., and Sinha, D. (2001). *Bayesian Survival Analysis*. Springer-Verlag, New York.

[38] Tsodikov, A.D., Ibrahim, J.G., and Yakovlev, A.Y. (2003). Estimating cure rates from survival data: An alternative to two-component mixture models. *Journal of the American Statistical Association, 98,* 1063–1078.

[39] Agarwala, S.S., Neuberg, D., Park, Y., and Kirkwood, J.M. (2004). Mature results of a phase III randomized trial of bacillus Calmette-Guerin (BCG) versus observation and BCG plus dacarbazine versus BCG in the adjuvant therapy of American Joint Committee on Cancer Stage I–III melanoma (E1673): A trial of the Eastern Oncology Group. *Cancer, 100*(8), 1692–1698.

[40] D'Amico, A.V., Renshaw, A.A., Sussman, B., and Chen, M.-H. (2005). Pre-treatment PSA velocity and the risk of death from prostate cancer following external beam radiation therapy. *The Journal of the American Medical Association, 294,* 440–447.

[41] Yakovlev, A.Y. and Tsodikov, A.D. (1996). *Stochastic Models of Tumor Latency and Their Biostatistical Applications.* World Scientific, Singapore.

[42] McKeague, I.W. and Tighiouart, M. (2000). Bayesian estimators for conditional hazard functions. *Biometrics, 56,* 1007–1015.

[43] Green, P.J. (1995). Reversible jump Markov chain Monte Carlo computation and Bayesian model determination. *Biometrika, 82,* 711–732.

[44] Cowles, M.K. and Carlin, B.P. (1996). Markov chain Monte Carlo convergence diagnostics: A comparative review. *Journal of the American Statistical Association, 91,* 883–904.

[45] Chen, M.-H. and Shao, Q.-M. (1999). Monte Carlo estimation of Bayesian credible and HPD intervals. *Journal of Computational and Graphical Statistics, 8,* 69–92.

[46] Chen, M.-H., Dey, D.K., and Ibrahim, J.G. (2004). Bayesian criterion based model assessment for categorical data. *Biometrika, 91,* 45–63.

[47] Gelfand, A.E. and Ghosh, S.K. (1998). Model choice: A minimum posterior predictive loss approach. *Biometrika, 85,* 1–13.

[48] Laud, P.W. and Ibrahim, J.G. (1995). Predictive model selection. *Journal of the Royal Statistical Society, Series B, 57,* 247–262.

[49] Spiegelhalter, D.J., Best, N.G., Carlin, B.P., and van der Linde, A. (2002). Bayesian measures of model complexity and fit (with discussion). *Journal of the Royal Statistical Society, Series B, 64,* 583–639.

Chapter 16

Parametric Likelihoods for Multiple Nonfatal Competing Risks and Death, with Application to Cancer Data

Peter F. Thall and Xuemei Wang

Contents

16.1   Introduction

Statistical analyses of clinical trials involving fatal diseases often focus on overall survival time as the primary outcome. In such settings, typically there are one or more intermediate events that the patient may experience prior to death. Such nonfatal events may be very important in that they characterize morbidity or early treatment effects, and the occurrence of a particular event or the time from the start of treatment to the event may help predict the patient's subsequent survival time [1–5]. Consequently, such intermediate events often are used by physicians for therapeutic decision-making, and many clinical trial designs base their primary treatment evaluation on intermediate event times rather than overall survival time in order to reduce the trial's cost and duration. An example of an important intermediate event in oncology settings where patients have active disease at enrollment is disease progression, which is characterized by a specified amount or type of worsening compared to the patient's baseline disease status. While disease progression increases the patient's risk of death, a technical complication is that each patient may die either with or without disease progression occurring first. A common practice is to use the minimum of the time to progression and the time to death without progression, so-called

371

progression-free survival (PFS) time, as the primary endpoint for treatment evaluation. Similarly, if a trial's entry criteria require that the patient's disease has been brought into remission previously and that the patient is still disease-free, each patient may die either with or without recurrence of disease. In this setting, the minimum of the time to recurrence and the time to death without recurrence, "disease-free survival" (DFS) time, commonly is used as the primary endpoint. Both cases may be described generally in terms of three transition times, $T_1 =$ time from the start of treatment to the intermediate event, $T_2 =$ time from the intermediate event to death, and $T_0 =$ time from the start of treatment to death without the intermediate event occurring, sometimes called regimen-related death. Aside from administrative right censoring or drop-out, overall survival time is actually $T_D = T_0 I(T_0 < T_1) + (T_1 + T_2)I$ $(T_0 > T_1)$, and PFS or DFS is $T_F = \min\{T_0, T_1\}$, where $I(A)$ indicates the event A. The ultimate goal of therapy is to cure the disease, that is, to make T_2 so large that, for a patient with covariates $\mathbf{Z} = (Z_1, \ldots, Z_q)$, the distribution of $[T_2 \mid \mathbf{Z}]$ is close to that of the survival time of an individual with similar covariates but without the disease. Similarly, an ideal treatment would have no regimen-related death, formally, $\Pr(T_0 < T_1) = 0$. A key point is that (T_0, T_1, T_2) are actually potential outcomes, or counterfactuals [6], since either T_0 or (T_1, T_2) but not both are observed for any patient.

There also are many examples in oncology of desirable intermediate events that decrease the risk of death. These include achieving a substantive amount of shrinkage of a solid tumor, achieving complete remission (CR) of acute leukemia, defined in terms of the patient's circulating blast cells, white blood cells, and platelet count all returning to normal levels and, in stem cell transplantation, achieving engraftment of the transplanted cells in the bone marrow, characterized by an absolute neutrophil count achieving a functional level. The issue noted above, that a second-line treatment may be given when an intermediate event occurs, also arises with desirable intermediate events. For example, once frontline treatment of leukemia achieves CR, a second round of "consolidation" treatment to reduce the risk of disease recurrence may be given [7]. Similarly, once a stem cell transplant from a matched donor has engrafted, the patient may receive prophylactic treatment to reduce the risk of graft-versus-host disease.

While the relationships between intermediate events and survival time may seem intuitively obvious, several technical complications arise when analyzing the multivariate event time data that they motivate. In the simplest case with one possible intermediate event motivating potential outcomes (T_0, T_1, T_2), the times to death with or without the antecedent event, specifically $T_1 + T_2$ and T_0, may have very different distributions. Moreover, the time T_1 to the intermediate event and the subsequent survival time T_2 typically are not independent. In more complex settings where two or more different intermediate events are possible, the occurrence of one event may preclude the others, that is, the events may be competing risks. This is the case we consider in this chapter. We describe a multivariate parametric model for the times to the nonfatal events, the residual survival times following the events, and the time to death without any preceding intermediate event. We illustrate the model by fitting it to a data set from patients with acute myelogenous leukemia (AML) or myelodysplastic syndrome (MDS) that includes the times to two intermediate events, one desirable and the other undesirable, as well as overall survival time. The general competing risks model structure, and statistical analyses similar to those presented here, are given in Shen and Thall [8] and Estey et al. [9].

16.2 Data Structure and Probability Models

The following notation generalizes the counterfactual vector (T_0, T_1, T_2) given above in order to accommodate settings where there are $K \geq 2$ possible nonfatal events. Denote the time from the start of treatment to the jth event by $T_{j,1}$, and the subsequent time from the event to death by $T_{j,2}$, with $T_j = (T_{j,1}, T_{j,2})$. Denote $T = \min\{T_{1,1}, \ldots, T_{K,1}\}$ and let T_0 be the time to death without any of the K possible nonfatal events occurring. We assume that the K nonfatal intermediate events are mutually exclusive, that is, at most one can occur, so that these K events and the $K+1$st outcome that the patient dies without any nonfatal event first occurring are competing risks [10,11]. Thus, the patient's overall survival time is $T_D = T_0$ if $T_0 < T$, in which case no nonfatal event occurs, and $T_D = T_{j,1} + T_{j,2}$ if $T_{j,1} = T < T_0$, that is, if nonfatal event j occurs. Since at most one of $T_0, T_1, \ldots, T_K$ can be observed for any patient, and thus any joint distribution or association among them cannot be estimated, we assume that these $K+1$ random quantities are mutually independent. To account for right-censoring at time C, we define $\delta_j = I(T_{j,1} = T < \min\{T_0, C\})$, the indicator that the jth nonfatal event occurs, and $\delta_0 = I(T_D < C)$, the indicator that the time of death is observed.

For $j = 1, \ldots, K$ and $r = 1, 2$, let $f_{j,r}$, $F_{j,r}$, and $\overline{F}_{j,r} = 1 - F_{j,r}$ denote the marginal pdf, cdf, and survivor function of $T_{j,r}$, with f_0, F_0, and $\overline{F}_0$ corresponding to T_0. We will assume that the joint distribution of each pair T_j is characterized by the von Morgenstern distribution [12], which has bivariate cdf

$$F_{j,12}(t_1, t_2) = \Pr(T_{j,1} \leq t_1, T_{j,2} \leq t_2) = F_{j,1}(t_1) F_{j,2}(t_2)\{1 + \alpha \overline{F}_{j,1}(t_1) \overline{F}_{j,2}(t_2)\}, \quad (16.1)$$

for $t_1, t_2 > 0$, where the parameter $\alpha \in [-1, 1]$ characterizes association between $T_{j,1}$ and $T_{j,2}$, with $\alpha = 0$ corresponding to independence. The likelihood for a single patient's event time data thus takes one of the following four possible forms. To reduce notation, denote $T_1 = T_{j,1}$ and $T_2 = T_{j,2}$ if $\delta_j = 1$. If a nonfatal event occurs and the subsequent time of death is observed then the likelihood is

$$\mathcal{L}_1 = \prod_{j=1}^{K} \left[f_{j,12}(T_1, T_2) \overline{F}_0(T_1) \prod_{k \neq j} \overline{F}_{k,1}(T_1) \right]^{\delta_0 \delta_j}. \quad (16.2)$$

If a nonfatal event occurs but the patient is followed for a time C without dying then the likelihood is

$$\mathcal{L}_2 = \prod_{j=1}^{K} \left[\int_{t_2=C-T_1}^{\infty} f_{j,12}(T_1, t_2) dt_2 \overline{F}_0(T_1) \prod_{k \neq j} \overline{F}_{k,1}(T_1) \right]^{(1-\delta_0)\delta_j}. \quad (16.3)$$

If the patient dies without any nonfatal event occurring first then the likelihood is

$$\mathcal{L}_3 = \left[f_0(T_0) \prod_{j=1}^{K} \{ \overline{F}_{j,1}(T_0) \}^{1-\delta_j} \right]^{\delta_0}. \tag{16.4}$$

Finally, if the patient is followed for a time C without any of the $K+1$ events occurring then the likelihood is

$$\mathcal{L}_4 = \left[\overline{F}_0(C) \prod_{j=1}^{K} \{ \overline{F}_{j,1}(C) \}^{1-\delta_j} \right]^{1-\delta_0}. \tag{16.5}$$

The overall likelihood is thus $\mathcal{L} = \prod_{r=1}^{4} \mathcal{L}_r$.

16.3   Leukemia Data

We illustrate the model by fitting it to a data set arising from 1512 patients with AML or MDS treated at M.D. Anderson Cancer Center between 1980 and 1995 [9]. These patients were treated with numerous different chemotherapy combinations, including many different CR induction treatments at the start of therapy (frontline) and many different salvage treatments (second-line). Each patient was enrolled in one of a wide variety of phase II clinical trials, or was treated outside any particular trial protocol. While treatment evaluation typically is the primary focus of a statistical analysis of this type of data, and accounting for trial effects also is an important issue, in order to focus on the event time structure that is the topic of this chapter we will ignore both treatments and trial effects. Arguably, this is not a serious omission here, since the long-term survival of these AML/MDS patients was less than 20%. Unfortunately, there has been very little improvement in survival for AML/MDS patients achieved with any chemotherapeutic regimen in the intervening years, and patient characteristics observed at the time of diagnosis remain by far the strongest predictors of overall survival time.

16.4   Standard Analyses of the Leukemia Data

We begin our analyses of this data set by fitting the two regression models that are used most commonly to assess potential predictive variables in therapy of leukemia and other cancers. As covariates, both in these standard analyses and when fitting the more elaborate competing risks model described in Section 16.2, we will use the following variables measured at baseline, before the start of therapy. "Good PS" indicates a Zubrod performance status of 0, 1, or 2. "AHD" indicates the presence of an antecedent hematologic disorder prior to the diagnosis of AML or MDS. Patients were divided into three categories for the type of cytogenetic abnormality in their leukemic blood cells. "Good Cyto" indicates an inversion of the 16th chromosome, "Poor Cyto" indicates that pieces of the fifth or seventh chromosome were missing, and an intermediate cytogenetic group was comprised of patients with all other types of cytogenetics. In the model fits, the intermediate cytogenetic group was used as the baseline for comparison. We omit patient age since, although older age is strongly predictive of worse outcome in these patients, age and PS have a strong positive association, hence including both as covariates would introduce substantial collinearity into any regression model.

Table 16.1 summarizes a fitted logistic regression model for the probability of CR as a function of the baseline covariates. Since only partial covariate data were available on 23 patients, the fitted model is based on the 1489 patients (98.5%) who had complete covariate data. While the overall CR rate was 946/1512 (62.6%), each of the baseline covariates had a substantive effect on the probability of CR. This is illustrated in Table 16.2 for four selected prognostic subgroups. In fact, the effects of these well-established covariates were much larger than the effects of any available chemotherapeutic treatment regimens for this disease. The Kaplan–Meier

TABLE 16.1: Fitted logistic regression model for the probability of CR as a function of baseline covariates, based on the 1489 patients (98.5%) who had complete data.

Covariate	Est	Odds Ratio	p
Intercept	$1.15_{0.08}$	3.17	—
Poor PS	$-1.60_{0.18}$	0.20	<0.0001
AHD	$-0.77_{0.12}$	0.46	<0.0001
Good Cyto	$1.25_{0.41}$	3.50	0.003
Poor Cyto	$-0.84_{0.15}$	0.43	<0.0001

Note: The standard error of each parameter estimate is given as a subscript.

TABLE 16.2: Illustration of the estimated CR probabilities, with 95% confidence intervals, for selected patient subgroups, under the fitted logistic regression model.

Covariates				
PS	**AHD**	**Cyto**	**Estimated Pr(CR)**	**95% Confidence Interval**
Good	No	Good	0.92	0.83–0.96
Good	No	Poor	0.58	0.51–0.65
Poor	Yes	Good	0.51	0.30–0.71
Poor	Yes	Poor	0.11	0.08–0.16

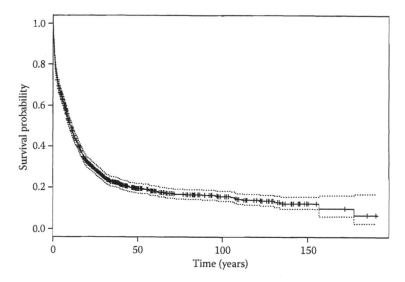

FIGURE 16.1: Plot of the Kaplan–Meier survival time probability estimates, with 95% confidence band, for the 1512 AML/MDS patients.

estimate [13] of the overall survival time distribution of these patients is given in Figure 16.1, and Table 16.3 summarizes a fitted Cox model for overall survival time as a function of the baseline covariates [14], again based on the 1489 patients with complete covariate data. All of the covariates are strongly predictive of survival time. Moreover, if CR is added to the model as a predictor, it has p-value < 0.0001 and an estimated relative risk of 0.16. This quantifies the well-known fact that achieving a CR in these patients greatly reduces the risk of death. However, because CR is an outcome and not a baseline covariate, and moreover many AML/MDS patients die during induction chemotherapy, including the indicator of CR as a covariate in a Cox model is somewhat misleading.

TABLE 16.3: Fitted Cox proportional hazards model for overall survival time as a function of baseline covariates, based on the 1489 patients (98.5%) who had complete data.

Covariate	Est	Relative Risk	p
Poor PS	$1.13_{0.08}$	3.10	<0.0001
AHD	$0.42_{0.06}$	1.52	<0.0001
Good Cyto	$-1.03_{0.20}$	0.36	<0.0001
Poor Cyto	$0.65_{0.08}$	1.92	<0.0001

Note: At the time of final follow up, 1130 (74.7%) of the 1512 patients had died, and the median overall survival time was 10.2 months with 95% confidence interval 9.1–11.4 months. The standard error of each parameter estimate is given as a subscript.

16.5 Two Nonfatal Competing Risks and Death

We now continue our analysis of the AML/MDS data by applying the competing risks model. This data set may be considered a prototype example of the general data structure, since in this clinical setting each patient undergoing induction chemotherapy has one of three competing initial events: CR, RESISTANT = disease declared resistant to frontline chemotherapy, or death during the process of attempting to achieve CR. Figure 16.2 provides a schematic summary of the numbers of patients who had the different possible outcomes when one accounts for CR and RESIST-ANT as intermediate events preceding death. As shown in the figure, of the 946 patients who achieved CR, 588 died after CR with a median residual survival time of 18.3 months (95% CI 16.4–21.2). For the 193 patients with disease resistant to induction chemotherapy, 169 subsequently died with a median residual survival time of 3.9 months (95% CI 2.9–4.7). Among the 373 patients who died during induction chemotherapy, the median survival time was 0.69 months (95% CI 0.63–0.79). Thus, on average, patients for whom induction chemotherapy achieved CR lived over a year longer than those with resistant disease, and death during induction occurred in less than 1 month. These simple analyses, like the conventional model-based analyses given above, again seem to show that achieving CR greatly improves the patient's survival time. Together, these analyses strongly support the common practice in leukemia clinical trials of using CR as a surrogate for overall survival time when evaluating the efficacy of chemotherapy regimens for AML/MDS.

The analyses given above are misleading, or at least incomplete, because they ignore the time it took to achieve CR. The following analyses will show that, among

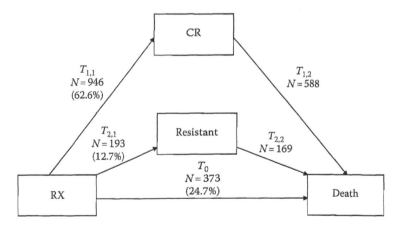

FIGURE 16.2: Schematic of the possible AML/MDS patient outcomes following induction chemotherapy. The three events: CR = {complete remission achieved with induction chemotherapy}, RESISTANT = {patient's disease declared resistant to the induction chemotherapy}, and death without either CR or RESISTANT occurring first are competing risks.

the 946 patients whose induction therapy achieved CR, the time required to do so was critically important. Applying the notation in the general model formulation, and referring to Figure 16.2, $T_{1,1}$ = the time to achieve CR, $T_{1,2}$ = the time from CR to death, $T_{2,1}$ = the time to the patient's disease being declared RESISTANT to the induction chemotherapy, $T_{2,2}$ = the time from RESISTANT to death, T_0 = the time to death without either CR or RESISTANT (death during induction), T = min $\{T_{1,1}, T_{2,1}\}$ = the time to the first nonfatal event, δ_0 is the indicator of death during induction, δ_1 is the indicator that CR was achieved, and δ_2 is the indicator that the patient's disease was resistant.

In the general model formulation given earlier, the marginals may be any distributions that provide a reasonable fit to the transition times in the data at hand. For analysis of the AML/MDS data, we will use the log odds rate distribution for all marginals, since it is very flexible and allows a wide variety of different shapes for the hazard function [15]. The log odds rate distribution is characterized by the survivor function

$$\overline{F}(t \,|\, \mathbf{Z}, \boldsymbol{\beta}, \gamma, \phi, \lambda) = \left[1 + \gamma(t/\lambda)^{\phi} e^{\eta(\mathbf{Z}, \boldsymbol{\beta})}\right]^{-1/\gamma}, \tag{16.6}$$

for $t > 0$. Covariate effects enter through the linear term $\eta(\mathbf{Z}, \boldsymbol{\beta}) = \beta_1 Z_1 + \ldots + \beta_q Z_q$, where $\boldsymbol{\beta} = (\beta_1, \ldots, \beta_q)$ are covariate parameters and $\gamma, \lambda, \phi > 0$ characterize the shape of the hazard function. This includes as special or limiting cases the log logistic distribution when $\gamma = 1$ [16], the Weibull for $\gamma \to 0$, and the Exponential for $\gamma \to 0$ and $\phi = 1$.

In the following, all parameter estimators were obtained by maximum likelihood, and all standard errors were obtained by bootstrapping. The fitted competing risks model is summarized in Table 16.4. A positive value of a covariate parameter estimate corresponds to a smaller value of $\overline{F}(t)$, equivalently, to a smaller value of the event time, on average. Poor PS is strongly predictive of a faster death during induction (smaller T_0), and also a faster death after CR (smaller $T_{1,2}$). An AHD is predictive of a longer time $T_{1,1}$ needed to achieve CR and strongly predictive of a faster death after CR. A result that may seem counterintuitive is that Good Cyto is moderately predictive ($p = 0.07$) of a faster death during induction while Poor Cyto is moderately predictive ($p = 0.05$) of a longer time to death during induction. This may be explained by the common clinical practice of giving more aggressive induction chemotherapy to AML/MDS patients with Good Cyto and less aggressive induction to patients with Poor Cyto, so that the estimated effects on T_0 associated with cytogenetics actually may be due to clinical practice. However, once a patient has achieved CR, Good (Poor) Cyto is strongly predictive of a longer (shorter) subsequent survival time $T_{1,2}$. None of the covariates are predictive of either $T_{2,1}$ or $T_{2,2}$.

The practical utility of using the log odds rate model is shown by the widely varying numerical values of the estimates of ϕ, λ, and γ for the five marginal distributions. The negative value of $\hat{\alpha}$ for the joint distribution of $T_{1,1}$ and $T_{1,2}$ indicates that patients with a longer time to achieve CR had a shorter subsequent survival time. The positive value of $\hat{\alpha}$ for the joint distribution of $T_{2,1}$ and $T_{2,2}$

TABLE 16.4: Fitted competing risks model accounting for covariate effects on each transition time, estimates of the log odds rate model parameters (ϕ, λ, γ) for each marginal transition time distribution, and associations between $(T_{j,1}, T_{j,2})$ for $j=1$ (complete remission) and $j=2$ (resistant disease) in terms of α.

	Death During Induction		Complete Remission				Resistant Disease			
	T_0		$T_{1,1}$		$T_{1,2}$		$T_{2,1}$		$T_{2,2}$	
Covariate	Est	p	Est	p	Est	p	Est	p	Est	p
Poor PS	$0.74_{.18}$	<0.001	$-0.17_{.56}$	0.77	$0.83_{.24}$	0.001	$0.55_{.58}$	0.35	$0.84_{.61}$	0.17
AHD	$-0.12_{.15}$	0.41	$-0.77_{.37}$	0.04	$0.39_{.12}$	0.001	$-0.35_{.35}$	0.32	$0.30_{.25}$	0.23
Good Cyto	$0.49_{.26}$	0.07	$0.58_{1.12}$	0.61	$-0.63_{.25}$	0.01	$1.67_{1.29}$	0.20	$-0.94_{2.35}$	0.69
Poor Cyto	$-0.24_{.12}$	0.05	$-0.24_{.41}$	0.56	$0.58_{.15}$	<0.001	$0.21_{.30}$	0.49	$0.40_{.33}$	0.23
Noncovariate Parameters	T_0		$T_{1,1}$		$T_{1,2}$		$T_{2,1}$		$T_{2,2}$	
$\hat{\phi}$	$1.43_{.09}$		$12.93_{1.32}$		$1.48_{.10}$		$3.27_{.49}$		$1.07_{.15}$	
$\hat{\lambda}$	$0.08_{.01}$		$0.07_{.002}$		$1.23_{.08}$		$0.17_{.02}$		$0.45_{.07}$	
$\hat{\gamma}$	$0.25_{.10}$		$6.12_{.80}$		$0.49_{.09}$		$0.99_{.32}$		$0.31_{.20}$	
$\hat{\alpha}$			$-0.12_{.13}$				$0.54_{.22}$			

Note: The standard error of each parameter estimate is given as a subscript.

indicates that patients for whom the time $T_{2,1}$ to be declared resistant was longer had a longer subsequent survival time $T_{2,2}$. These relationships are illustrated in Figure 16.3, which shows the estimated values of median($T_{1,2} \mid T_{1,1} = t$) as a function of t for patients who achieved CR and, similarly, of median($T_{2,2} \mid T_{2,1} = t$) as a function of t for patients with resistant disease. This figure is extremely revealing since, in terms of the patient's subsequent survival time $T_{1,2}$, it shows that the apparent survival benefit due to CR fell rapidly as the time required to achieve it increased. In fact, patients for whom ≥ 2 months were required to achieve CR died almost as quickly thereafter as patients whose disease was declared resistant to induction chemotherapy. An important implication is that the common practice of using the

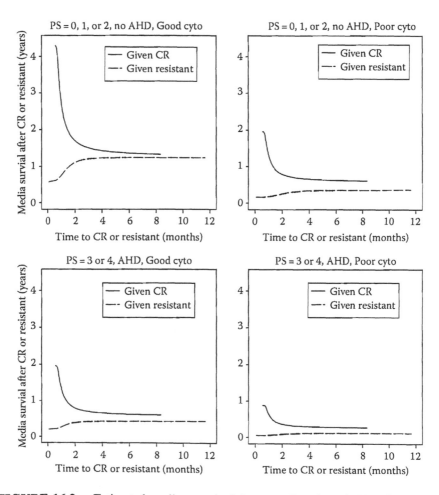

FIGURE 16.3: Estimated median survival time as a function of either time to CR (solid line) or time to the patient's disease being declared resistant (dashed line), based on the fitted parametric competing risks model.

binary indicator of CR as a surrogate for early treatment success in AML/MDS patients receiving chemotherapy is very misleading since, for example, a CR achieved in 2 weeks is of much greater benefit to the patient than a CR achieved in 6 weeks. In any case, a CR requiring 2 months or longer to achieve is of very little benefit.

16.6 Time to First Treatment Failure

The most common approach to complex time-to-event data is to simply use the time to first treatment failure as the outcome. In the simplest case of the data structure considered here, where $K = 1$ and the intermediate event is undesirable, such as PFS or DFS, this is $T_F = \min\{T_0, T_{1,1}\}$. In such settings, there are several common reasons for basing treatment evaluation on T_F:

1. Both analytically and conceptually, the univariate outcome T_F is much easier to deal with than the full counterfactual vector $(T_0, T_{1,1}, T_{1,2})$.

2. When occurrence of the intermediate event increases the risk of death, T_F may be considered the time of treatment failure.

3. T_F may be observed more quickly than T_D because T_F does not involve $T_{1,2}$, and thus a clinical trial may be completed more quickly.

4. Because a second-line, "salvage" treatment typically is given at the time of disease progression or recurrence, the effect of the patient's frontline treatment on overall survival time is confounded with the effect of salvage therapy on $T_{1,2}$. Using T_F avoids this problem.

It is interesting to consider briefly the distribution, under the competing risks model, of the time to first treatment failure in this data set. This is $T_F = \min \{T_{1,1} + T_{1,2}, T_{2,1}, T_0\}$, the minimum of the times to death for a patient who achieved CR, to disease being declared resistant and to death during induction. For each of these three types of failure events, conditional on the event occurring and thus considering the three subgroups of patients separately, median$(T_{1,1} + T_{1,2}) = 19.7$ months (95% CI 17.7–22.5), median$(T_{2,1}) = 2.2$ months (95% CI 2.1–2.5), and median$(T_0) = 0.69$ months (95% CI 0.6–0.8). These competing failures occurred with respective probabilities $\Pr(T_F = T_{1,1} + T_{1,2}) = 0.626$, $\Pr(T_F = T_{2,1}) = 0.127$, and $\Pr(T_F = T_0) = 0.247$. From this viewpoint, the distribution of T_F is a mixture of three very different distributions. The median of T_F based on the entire sample of 1512 patients is 10.2 months with 95% CI 9.1–11.4. This shows that using T_F alone to characterize treatment effect obfuscates what is actually going on, since the distribution of T_F is really a mixture of very small values in the range 0–3 months and much larger values in the range 17–23 months.

16.7   Two-Stage Dynamic Treatment Regimes

We have ignored treatment effects in order to focus on the competing risks model and, in particular, the profound effect of $T_{1,1}$ on $T_{1,2}$. Still, the data structure illustrated in Figure 16.1 raises the issue that a patient's therapy generally consists of more than just the induction regimen. The overall therapeutic process may be regarded as a two-stage *dynamic treatment regime* (DTR) in which a frontline treatment A_0 is given initially and, at the time of CR or RESISTANT, a second-line treatment A_1 is given. Denote the patient's baseline data by L_0 and the data obtained from the start of induction to observing $\min\{T_0, T_{1,1}, T_{2,1}\} = \min\{T_0, T\}$ by L_1. In this setting, a DTR is a sequence of rules for choosing A_0 on the basis of L_0 and, if the patient does not die during induction, choosing A_1 on the basis of the history $\overline{L}_1 = \{L_0, A_0, L_1\}$. In practice, patients who achieve CR are often given consolidation therapy to decrease the chance of disease recurrence [7], while patients who have resistant disease are given salvage in the hope of achieving CR after the frontline treatment has failed. If we denote the set of possible induction chemotherapy combinations by I, the set of possible consolidation treatments by C and the set of possible salvage treatments by S, the DTR may be formalized as a pair of mappings $A_0 : L_0 \rightarrow \mathcal{I}$ and $A_1 : \overline{L}_1 \rightarrow \mathcal{C} \cup \mathcal{S}$, where L_1 for which $T = T_{1,1}$ restricts the range of A_1 to $\mathcal{C}$ and L_1 for which $T = T_{2,1}$ restricts the range of A_1 to $\mathcal{S}$. An analysis of the two-stage DTRs (A_0, A_1) used to treat the patients in the AML/MDS data set would go far beyond the scope of this chapter, however. The interested reader may refer to general developments of DTRs for the analysis of observational data given by Robins [17], Lunceford et al. [18], Murphy et al. [19], Murphy [20], Wahed and Tsiatis [21], Moodie et al. [22], and the references therein.

16.8   Discussion

The class of multivariate parametric models described here is useful primarily because it provides a formal basis for examining the transition times for data where patients are subject to multiple nonfatal competing risks and death. The general approach is to model each transition time marginally using a flexible parametric model and specify bivariate distributions to characterize the associations between each nonfatal event time and subsequent survival time. The particular parametric distributions that we used are not essential to our approach, and other marginal and bivariate distributions may be used, depending on the particular application at hand. For example, an alternative to the von Morgenstern bivariate distribution for each pair $(T_{j,1}, T_{j,2})$ is a frailty model [23,24], which mixes over a random parameter to induce association. This may be formulated in many ways, e.g., by assuming $\Pr[T_{j,1} > t_1, T_{j,2} > t_2] = E[\exp(\xi\{\log S_{j,1}(t_1) + \log S_{j,2}(t_2)\})]$, where the frailty parameter ξ is a nonnegative-valued patient-specific random variable following an assumed distribution that yields a tractable bivariate model. Another approach is to model each $T_{j,1}$ marginally and model each conditional distribution $f(T_{j,2} \mid T_{j,1})$ by using an appropriate function of $T_{j,1}$, such as $\log(T_{j,1})$, as a covariate in the linear term.

An important aspect of our formulation is that we avoid the commonly used Markov assumption that the time to each nonfatal event and subsequent survival time are independent. As shown by Figure 16.3, this was critically important in assessing the relationship between CR and survival time. For one nonfatal event, our formulation generalizes Lagakos [1], who assumed independent exponential distributions for $T_0, T_{1,1}$, and $T_{1,2}$. The Lagakos model is a special case of the semi-Markov process model of Weiss and Zelen [25], and of the bivariate exponential model of Freund [26]. Finkelstein and Schoenfeld [27] presented distribution-free methods for estimating overall survival by assuming that T_0 and $T_{1,1}$ are independent competing risks and using a Cox model with $T_{1,2}$ the outcome variable, either with or without $T_{1,1}$ as a covariate. Andersen [28] applied a multistate model to analyze times to diabetic nephropathy (DN) and death with or without DN in insulin-dependent diabetics, using separate Cox regressions for the transition times to DN, death without DN, and death post-DN. As noted by Andersen, however, this does not provide an overall estimate of survival without assumptions similar to those noted above, namely that the death rates for patients with or without DN are the same. Kalbfleisch and Lawless [29] presented a pseudo-likelihood approach to the general setting of progression from a healthy state to a diseased state or death. Finally, general treatments of multivariate time-to-event data are given in the books by Andersen et al. [30], Hougaard [31], and Klein and Moeschberger [32].

References

[1] S.W. Lagakos, Using auxiliary variables for improved estimates of survival time, *Biometrics* 33, 399–404, 1977.

[2] D.M. Finkelstein and D.A. Schoenfeld, Analyzing survival in the presence of an auxiliary variable, *Statistics in Medicine* 8, 1747–1754, 1994.

[3] T.R. Fleming, R.L. Prentice, M.S. Pepe, and D. Glidden, Surrogate and auxiliary endpoints in clinical trials, with potential applications in cancer and AIDS research, *Statistics in Medicine* 13, 955–968, 1994.

[4] R. Gray, A kernel method for incorporating information on disease progression in the analysis of survival, *Biometrika* 81, 527–534, 1994.

[5] L.D. Epstein and A. Munoz, A bivariate parametric model for survival and intermediate event times, *Statistics in Medicine* 15, 1171–1185, 1996.

[6] P.W. Holland, Statistics and causal inference, *Journal of the American Statistical Association* 96, 1410–1424, 1986.

[7] R.M. Stone, D.T. Berg, S.L. George, R.K. Dodge, P.A. Paciucci, P. Scgulman, E.J. Lee, O.J. Moore, B.L. Powell, and C.A. Schiffer, Granulocyte macrophage colony-stimulating factor after initial chrneotherapy for elderly patients with primary acute myelogenous leukemia. *The New England Journal of Medicine* 332, 1671–1677, 1995.

[8] Y. Shen and P.F. Thall, Parametric likelihoods for multiple non-fatal competing risks and death, *Statistics in Medicine* 17, 999–1016, 1998.

[9] E.H. Estey, Y. Shen, and P.F. Thall, Effect of time to complete remission on subsequent survival and disease-free survival time in AML, RAEB-t, RAEB, *Blood* 95, 72–77, 2000.

[10] M.H. Gail, A review and critique of some models used in competing risk analysis, *Biometrics* 31, 209–222, 1975.

[11] R.L. Prentice, J.D. Kalbfleisch, A.V. Peterson, N. Flournoy, V.T. Farewell, and N.E. Breslow. The analysis of failure time data in the presence of competing risks, *Biometrics* 34, 541–554, 1978.

[12] D. Morgenstern, Einfache beispiele zweidimensionaler verteilungen, *Mittelangsblatt fur Math. Statistik* 8, 234–235, 1956.

[13] E.L. Kaplan and P. Meier, Nonparametric estimator from incomplete observations, *Journal of the American Statistical Association* 53, 457–481, 1958.

[14] D.R. Cox, Regression models and life tables (with discussion), *Journal of the Royal Statistical Society, B* 34, 187–220, 1972.

[15] D.M. Dabrowska and K.A. Doksum, Estimation and testing in a two-sample generalized odds-rate model, *Journal of the American Statistical Association* 83, 744–749, 1988.

[16] S. Bennett, Log-logistic regression models for survival data, *Applied Statistics* 32, 165–171, 1983.

[17] J.M. Robins, A new approach to causal inference in mortality studies with sustained exposure periods—Application to control of the healthy survivor effect, *Mathematical Modeling* 7, 1393–1512, 1986.

[18] S.A. Murphy, M. van der Laan, J.M. Robins, and CPPRG, Marginal mean models for dynamic treatment regimes, *Journal of the American Statistical Association* 96, 1410–1424, 2001.

[19] J.M. Lunceford, M. Davidian, and A.A. Tsiatis, Estimation of the survival distribution of treatment policies in two-stage randomization designs in clinical trials, *Biometrics* 58, 48–57, 2002.

[20] S.A. Murphy, Optimal dynamic treatment regimes (with discussion), *Journal of the Royal Statistical Society, B* 65, 331–366, 2003.

[21] A.S. Wahed and A.A. Tsiatis, Optimal estimator for the survival distribution and related quantities for treatment policies in two-stage randomization designs in clinical trials, *Biometrics* 60, 124–133, 2004.

[22] E.E.M. Moodie, T.S. Richardson, and D.A. Stephens, Demystifying optimal dynamic treatment regimes, *Biometrics* 63, 447–455, 2007.

[23] P. Hougaard, A class of multivariate failure time distributions, *Biometrika* 73, 671–678, 1986.

[24] D. Oakes, Bivariate survival models induced by frailties, *Journal of the American Statistical Association* 84, 487–493, 1989.

[25] G.H. Weiss and M. Zelen, A semi-Markov model for clinical trials, *Journal of Applied Probability* 2, 269–285, 1965.

[26] J.E. Freund, A bivariate extension of the exponential distribution, *Journal of the American Statistical Association* 56, 971–977, 1961.

[27] D.M. Finkelstein and D.A. Schoenfeld, Analyzing survival in the presence of an auxiliary variable, *Statistics in Medicine* 8, 1747–1754, 1994.

[28] P.K. Andersen, Multistate models in survival analysis: A study of nephropathy and mortality in diabetes, *Statistics in Medicine* 88, 661–670, 1988.

[29] J.D. Kalbfleisch and J.F. Lawless, Likelihood analysis of multi-state models for disease incidence and mortality, *Statistics in Medicine* 7, 149–160, 1988.

[30] P.K. Andersen, O. Borgan, R.D. Gill, and N. Keiding, *Statistical Models Based on Counting Processes*, Springer-Verlag, New York, NY, 1993.

[31] P. Hougaard, *Analysis of Multivariate Survival Data,* Springer-Verlag, New York, NY, 2000.

[32] J.P. Klein and M.L. Moeschberger, *Survival Analysis: Techniques for Censored and Truncated Data*, Springer-Verlag, New York, NY, 2003.

Chapter 17

Design, Summarization, Analysis, and Interpretation of Cancer Prevention Trials

Matthew C. Somerville, Jennifer B. Shannon, and Timothy H. Wilson

Contents

17.1   Overview

The focus of this chapter is on issues pertaining to cancer prevention trials. In particular, interest is in large randomized controlled trials with cancer occurrence as the primary endpoint, as these are considered to exhibit rigorous study design [1,2]. It is recognized that many issues discussed here are relevant to a wider group of trials. Additional information regarding such trials can be found in other sources [1,3–10].

Following is a description of relevant considerations in the design, summarization, analysis, and interpretation of cancer prevention trials. Specific aspects of these considerations are illustrated using the reduction by dutasteride of prostate cancer events (REDUCE) prostate cancer (PCa) risk reduction study [11] as an example.

17.2   Design

There are a number of elements that are important in the design of a cancer prevention study. These items include those described in Sections 17.2.1 through 17.2.8.

17.2.1   Interventions

Byar states that the question of which interventions to use is the first issue to address in the design of cancer prevention studies, and notes that these may include supplemental measures that are introduced (such as use of a daily medication) as well as removal of existing factors (such as limiting or abstaining from a certain dietary component) [12]. Chemoprevention is defined as the use of specific natural or synthetic chemical agents to reverse, suppress, or prevent carcinogenic progression to invasive cancer [13]. Use of an intervention regarding foods ingested in a normal diet is not considered to be included in the field of chemoprevention but rather the field of diet and cancer [1]. In addition, an intervention could take the form of other lifestyle modifications. For an intervention to be useful, it should be effective, easy to administer, and have minimal side effects [14]. Candidates may be identified in various ways including results from laboratory research, epidemiological studies, and clinical trials [15]. For a cancer prevention study, a placebo or other active control group should be used as a comparator, unless ethically not feasible [16,17].

17.2.2 Population

A critical factor in the design of cancer prevention trials is determination of the population of interest. This may be influenced by how the intervention(s) of interest are expected to act, as well as by other factors. Three types of cancer prevention have been identified [3]:

- Primary prevention is that of de novo malignancies in a healthy population.

- Secondary prevention is that of progression of premalignant lesions into cancers.

- Tertiary prevention is that of second primary tumors in patients cured of initial cancer or definitively treated for premalignant lesions.

These different prevention types involve different populations which may respond differently to the study interventions. Therefore it is desirable to consider which is most appropriate.

Moreover, it is useful to consider low risk vs. increased-risk populations, since risk will affect study duration, sample size, and power [12,18]. This is the case since study entry and compliance of subjects are affected by perceived risk and, in turn, are important factors in determining the power of statistical tests and the validity of study results [13]. Therefore identifying important risk factors and/or estimating risk is important in identifying the most appropriate study design parameters. This process should be done recognizing the trade-offs between validity and generalizability; that is, although utilizing a higher risk subpopulation may limit generalizability, validity (and cost-effectiveness) may be overriding concerns [19]. Moreover, from a statistical point of view, the basis of inference (randomization vs. model based) has some bearing on this trade-off, since it affects the interpretation of the results (see Section 17.4.1). Finally, interest is focused on risk for progressive versus latent or indolent cancer [20], although it is not always straightforward to classify cancers in such a manner.

An additional need is to establish exclusion criteria. These can address potential safety considerations as well as factors that could affect evaluation of the cancer.

17.2.3 Endpoint Selection

Ideally, a cancer prevention intervention will improve survival [5]. However, although having the advantages of clinical relevance and usually being precisely measurable, this endpoint has drawbacks [21]:

- For many types of cancers, survival studies require large sample sizes and long durations which adversely impact study feasibility.

- Overall survival is an omnibus measure of various effects including those not of direct interest.

- Overall survival may not include other significant outcomes such as quality of life.

Use of cause-specific mortality raises issues regarding how competing risks are handled and how cause of death is determined. Because of these considerations, incidence and prevalence are often used [5,16], and cancer-risk reduction has been accepted by the Food and Drug Administration (FDA) as a measure of clinical benefit [20]. In such cases disease assessment becomes an important issue, with various methods of assessment (such as imaging and biopsy) being used for different types of cancer. For example, in PCa, pathological review of tissue obtained from prostate needle biopsies is the standard approach to determining a diagnosis of PCa. Although recognized as safe, this method is subject to sampling error and grade migration [22].

It should be noted that in the past there has been some controversy regarding the use of the term "prevention" for studies focusing on disease incidence or prevalence. It has been suggested that "risk reduction" may be more appropriate, to acknowledge that such studies may not clearly establish permanent tumor prevention [23–25].

Consistency of endpoint determination is necessary in order to minimize variability from this process and to thereby increase the sensitivity of the trial to detect differences if they exist. Examples of this include the use of central review of imaging results or pathological tissue samples to establish diagnoses. Such review can also facilitate timely and more complete data reporting, and simplify implementation of data quality efforts.

Development of surrogate endpoints is pursued in a desire to utilize resources more efficiently and to enable measurement of precancerous processes [1,26,27]. A surrogate marker is defined as an observable event shown to be a highly significant and predictably accurate correlate of the risk of subsequent malignancy [16]. A useful surrogate is required not only to predict the clinical outcome of interest but also to fully capture the effects of the intervention [28]. As an example, Kelloff describes the use of colon adenomas as a surrogate endpoint for colorectal cancer prevention [29].

An area of prevention research is directed at prevention of infection or the control of chronic infection with specific viruses, parasites, or bacteria that are associated with the development of certain cancers [1]. An example of this is the use of a vaccine to prevent human papilloma virus infection and so also the associated cervical cancer [30].

The selection of a particular endpoint and the corresponding assessment procedures has implications regarding appropriate summary and analysis methods, and the interpretation of results. In particular, it is important to determine whether an endpoint should be considered to be measured on a continuous or categorical scale.

An example of the former would be time-to-death measured in days from randomization over a study period of several years; an example of the latter would be occurrence of PCa diagnosis via needle biopsy conducted at several timepoints during the study.

17.2.4 Duration of Intervention and Follow-Up

The appropriate duration of intervention and follow-up is determined by the mechanism of action as well as by the study population and endpoint, and often is relatively long for prevention studies [12]. Because of this and corresponding potential safety concerns, it is important to plan for appropriate monitoring that may include the use of Data Monitoring Committees (DMCs) [31]. In addition, interim analyses and futility analyses should be considered for subject safety [13] and for wise use of resources.

There are several factors which influence these determinations, including clinical practice, previous studies and information, sample size and powering, as well as regulatory agency input.

17.2.5 Sample Size and Power

In determining sample size, the typical long duration of these studies makes it important to consider associated issues such as compliance and competing risks [5]. Methods to maximize compliance should be considered, such as adopting a run-in period prior to randomization [32]. In addition, the particular risk characteristics of the study population will affect the expected number of events of interest and so should be carefully considered [12]. Other factors include expected rates of cancer in the treatment groups, withdrawal rates, and significance level.

17.2.6 Randomization and Blinding

Various authors have noted the importance of randomization and blinding in the design and conduct of studies. Such methods are useful in avoiding bias [16,33]. Stratification by baseline factors can be utilized to improve precision of estimated rates as well as power to compare rates [34]. In addition, randomization can provide the basis of inference (see Section 17.4.1). Approaches include central randomizations, center-based randomizations, and stratified randomizations. Biased-coin and adaptive methods may be considered, although these are more usually employed in cancer treatment studies. Generally, it is important that rigorous designs be utilized in cancer prevention studies to enable reliable inferences to be made [31].

Consideration of the extent of study blinding should be thorough. For example, although a diagnosis of cancer may be determined in a relatively objective fashion (e.g., via review of imaging or needle biopsy results), assessments of related items such as disease severity and extent could be more susceptible to bias from knowledge of the treatment regimen. In addition, assessment of safety (e.g., adverse events, physical examinations), symptoms, and health outcome questionnaires may be affected by both subject and investigator knowledge of investigational treatment.

17.2.7 Monitoring (DMC)

DMCs are particularly useful in trials of life-threatening diseases or trials of treatments to delay or prevent mortality or serious morbidity [35]. The responsibilities of a DMC include protecting the safety of trial participants, ensuring the credibility of the study, and ensuring the integrity of the data [35]. The responsibilities of the DMC should be spelled out in a charter.

The charter should list all members of the DMC and the roles and responsibilities of each member. The charter should describe the responsibilities of the DMC and the timing and purpose of each meeting.

The DMC should be comprised of members from a variety of areas of expertise [35]. A clinician with relevant experience in the therapeutic area under study must be included. Statisticians are also necessary. Individuals with a financial or other conflict of interest in the study should not serve on the DMC.

In some cases, the DMC may be involved in the review of the trial design and protocol. This involvement allows the DMC members to raise concerns about important scientific issues of the trial while there is time to make changes. The DMC members must be supportive of the trial in order to fulfill their responsibilities [35].

The DMC provides ongoing reviews of the safety and efficacy data collected during a study in order to make recommendations as to whether the study should continue. The DMC may recommend the trial be terminated early for positive or negative results or for safety reasons. It is important that the DMC review both safety and efficacy data in order to evaluate the full benefit-to-risk profile. The DMC typically would receive unblinded summaries of the data [35]. With unblinded summaries, the DMC can more fully evaluate the benefit-to-risk profile. The data provided to the DMC must be as complete and accurate as possible.

There are several statistical considerations that must be addressed. The approach to interpreting the data at each interim timepoint must be addressed. The objectivity of the DMC is enhanced by documenting statistical stopping rules in advance.

The DMC should be the only group with access to the interim data [35]. Maintaining the confidentiality of interim results is critical in order to ensure trial integrity and credibility [35]. Widespread distribution of interim results which are often unreliable can adversely impact the recruitment of the study, the continuation of participants in the trial, the assessments of trial outcomes, as well as influence other ongoing trials with related outcomes.

17.2.8 Examples of Study Design

Table 17.1 shows the design specifications of various cancer prevention trials. These were selected to illustrate relevant characteristics and do not represent an exhaustive list of such trials. These studies show the relatively large sample sizes and long durations that are typical of cancer prevention studies.

TABLE 17.1: Design specifications for selected cancer chemoprevention studies.

Study	Cancer Type	Population	Primary Endpoint/Analysis	Intervention	Duration of Follow-Up	Number of Subjects Randomized
Breast Cancer Prevention Trial [36]	Breast	Women at increased risk of breast cancer, age ≥ 35	Incidence of breast cancer/exact binomial test of difference in rates	Tamoxifen, placebo	4 years (average)	13,388
International Breast Cancer Intervention Study [37]	Breast	Women at increased risk of breast cancer, age between 35 and 70	Incidence of breast cancer/Fishers exact test and odds ratio	Tamoxifen, placebo	4 years (median)	7,152
Study of Tamoxifen and Raloxifene [38]	Breast	Women at increased risk of breast cancer age ≥ 35	Incidence of breast cancer/logrank test and risk ratio	Tamoxifen, raloxifene	4 years (average)	19,747
Alpha-tocopherol, Beta Carotene Lung Cancer Prevention Study [39]	Lung	Male smokers, age between 50 and 69	Incidence of lung cancer/logrank test	2^2 factorial: Alpha-tocoperol, beta-carotene	6 years (median)	29,133
Beta-carotene and Retinol Efficacy Trial [40,41]	Lung	Smokers, former smokers, and workers exposed to asbestos	Incidence of lung cancer/logrank test	Retinol + beta-carotene, placebo	4 years (average)	18,314

(continued)

TABLE 17.1 (continued): Design specifications for selected cancer chemoprevention studies.

Study	Cancer Type	Population	Primary Endpoint/Analysis	Intervention	Duration of Follow-Up	Number of Subjects Randomized
Prostate Cancer Prevention Trial [42,43]	Prostate	Healthy men, age ≥ 55, PSA ≤ 3 ng/mL, normal DRE	Period prevalence of PCa/relative risk reduction, test unknown	Finasteride, placebo	7 years	18,882 (9060 included in analysis)
Selenium and Vitamin E Cancer Prevention Trial [44,45]	Prostate	Healthy men, age > 50, PSA ≤ 4 ng/mL, nonsuspicious DRE	Clinical incidence of PCa/test unknown	2^2 factorial: Selenium, vitamin E	7–12 years	32,400
Reduction by Dutasteride of Prostate Cancer Events Trial [11]	Prostate	Men at increased risk, age between 50 and 75, PSA between 2.5 and 10 ng/mL, negative entry biopsy	Incidence of PCa/Mantel–Cox test and relative risk reduction	Dutasteride, placebo	4 years	8,000
Physician's Health Study I [46]	Various	Healthy U.S. male physicians, age ≥ 40	Total cancer, cardiovascular disease/Cox proportional hazards model and relative risk reduction	2^2 factorial: aspirin, beta-carotene	12 years (average)	22,071

Study		Population	Endpoint/statistical method	Intervention	Duration	N
Physician's Health Study II [47]	Various	Healthy U.S. male physicians, age $\geq$ 55	Total cancer, PCa, and others/Cox proportional hazards model	2^4 factorial: beta-carotene, vitamin E, vitamin C, multivitamin	5 years	15,000
Women's Health Study [48]	Various	Healthy U.S. women, age $\geq$ 45	Total cancer, major cardiovascular event/Cox proportional hazards model and relative risk reduction	2^2 factorial: aspirin, vitamin E	10 years (average)	39,876
Supplementation en Vitamines et Mineraux Antioxydants study [49]	Various	French residents with age between 35 and 60	Total cancer, major cardiovascular event/logrank test	Ascorbic acid + vitamin E + beta carotene + selenium + zinc, placebo	7.5 years (median)	13,017
Linxian vitamin and mineral trial [50]	Various	Linxian, China residents with age between 40 and 69	Mortality, total cancer/Cox proportional hazards model	Half replicate of 2^4 factorial: retinol + zinc, riboflavin + niacin, ascorbic acid + molybdenum, beta carotene + selenium + alpha-tocopherol	5 years	29,584

17.3   Summarization

There are two general approaches to assessment of the event in a time-to-event trial. One is to require an explicit assessment (e.g., a biopsy) at prespecified, scheduled, timepoints; the other is to collect the time to event as a continuous variable without requiring assessments at scheduled timepoints. When the time-to-event is continuous, the summarization of data will be different than when the assessment is categorical (e.g., from a planned biopsy). When scheduled assessments are required, Kaplan–Meier methods must be adapted due to the interval nature of the data collection. Please refer to Table 17.2 for a summary of these approaches.

Two examples from PCa prevention are described to highlight these considerations. The selenium and vitamin E cancer prevention trial (SELECT) was a double-blind, randomized study of selenium and vitamin E on the risk of PCa. The primary endpoint was the incidence of PCa on a recommended routine clinical diagnostic evaluation including yearly digital rectal exam and serum prostate-specific antigen (PSA) measurement. Biopsy was recommended for subjects with a suspicious digital rectal exam and/or elevated PSA [44]. However, biopsies were not required for all subjects during the study. In comparison, the REDUCE study was a double-blind, randomized study of dutasteride on the risk of PCa. The primary endpoint was biopsy proven PCa [11]. The protocol required a biopsy at baseline and at year 2 and year 4; unscheduled biopsies could be performed as needed. Therefore, the SELECT study is an example of the continuous assessment approach since biopsies were not required at specific timepoints whereas the REDUCE study is an example

TABLE 17.2:   Summarization considerations.

	Continuous Assessment Approach	Scheduled Assessment Approach
Summarization of cancer occurrence	Life-table rates Kaplan–Meier estimates	Crude rates Modified crude rates Life table rates
Summarization of cancer treatment effect	Hazard ratio Odds ratio Relative risk	Relative risk Odds ratio
Statistical analysis methods (see Section 17.4)	Logrank test Cox proportional hazards model	Fishers exact test Mantel–Cox test
Handling of withdrawals	Withdrawals are censored at the time of withdrawal	Withdrawals handled several ways via alternative definitions of number at risk
Examples (PCa)	SELECT study [44]	REDUCE study [11]

of the scheduled assessment approach since biopsies were specified to be performed on all subjects at year 2 and year 4.

17.3.1 Withdrawals

If the study design is such that the time-to-event is continuous, then withdrawals can be censored at the time of withdrawal if the status of the event is known at the time of withdrawal or at the last assessment in which the status was known. Subjects who withdraw will contribute to the calculation for the time prior to censoring.

If the study design utilizes the definitive scheduled assessment approach, the summarization of cancer occurrence could be based on crude rates and/or life table rates [51]. The distinction between these methods is in how subjects who withdraw from the study without an endpoint assessment are managed. Subjects who withdraw or for whom no assessment is performed provide incomplete information. In order to demonstrate the robustness of the conclusions, it is of interest to summarize the cancer rates using multiple methods [51].

The crude rate for cancer occurrence is a ratio of the number of subjects with confirmed cancer and the number of subjects who are at risk for cancer. The crude rate would use all eligible subjects as the denominator. Eligible subjects could be defined as all randomized subjects for an intent-to-treat analysis. In this situation, withdrawals are assumed to not have cancer. By treating withdrawals as cancer-free, the crude rate tends to underestimate the true cancer occurrence rate. Standard errors for the crude rates can be calculated by a binomial formula. Crude rates can be calculated for the overall time period of interest as well as for subintervals of interest.

Another possible strategy for summarizing cancer occurrence rates would be a modified crude rate. The modified crude rate is a ratio of the number of subjects with confirmed cancer and the number of subjects with confirmed cancer plus the number of subjects who completed the treatment period and had an assessment indicating no cancer at the end of the study. For practical purposes, a time window could be used around this such that all subjects with an assessment during this time interval would be included.

Additionally, one could define restricted crude rates as the ratio of the number of subjects with confirmed cancer and the number of subjects with an assessment at any time during the study. Subjects who never have an assessment are excluded from the denominator.

Alternatively, life table estimates for the occurrence of cancer can also be cumulatively obtained for the successive time intervals. Subjects contribute information until the time interval of withdrawal.

17.3.2 Other Variables of Interest

It is often important to evaluate the results within various subgroups of interest. Subgroups can be defined using baseline characteristics. For continuous baseline values, subgroups could be defined by dividing the data in tertiles. For categorical baseline values, subgroups can be defined by combining categories as needed. Since cancer prevention trials are often large, these studies lend themselves to subgroup evaluations.

While the primary endpoint of many cancer trials is incidence of cancer, it can also be important to summarize certain characteristics of the cancer, such as severity or extent (see Section 17.5.2).

Summarizing the quality of life of the subjects in each group is also relevant. Improvements in survival rates in the active treatment group would ideally be accompanied by improved quality of life compared to placebo.

As in any clinical study, the safety of the active treatment group(s) is also very important. The benefit of treatment must outweigh the risks. The overall safety of a drug is typically evaluated by summarizing the incidence of adverse events. Summaries of vital signs, ECG measures, and laboratory measures are also important to fully evaluate safety. Persons may be expected to take an active treatment for a long time in order to realize prevention; therefore, understanding long-term safety is also important.

17.4   Analysis

The primary focus of this section is on statistical hypothesis testing and estimation of treatment effect for the primary endpoint of a cancer prevention clinical trial. However, it is acknowledged that analysis of additional study endpoints is also important and may play a key role in the interpretation of the results (see Section 17.5).

17.4.1   Basis for Inference

Design-based and model-based inferences are alternative approaches for interpreting data [52]. The specifics of a particular study (including research question of interest, target population, sampling mechanisms employed, randomization techniques, presence of important covariates, etc.) are relevant in identifying an appropriate approach [53]. The selected approach then will guide the choice of a specific analysis methodology, reflecting important aspects of the study. Design-based inference is that based on random selection or allocation of observational units [52]. Examples of analyses for design-based inference include Fishers exact test and Mantel–Haenszel tests. Advantages include only needing to appeal to randomization for the validity of the inference rather than to assumptions that may be difficult to verify. This approach requires that the analysis reflects the particular randomization actually used for the trial. Model-based inference utilizes assumptions external to the study including postulated probability distributions [52]. Examples of analyses for model-based inference include linear models and the Cox proportional hazards model. Advantages include the relatively straightforward and flexible incorporation of covariates.

17.4.2 Statistical Tests and Estimates of Treatment Effect

The statistical test and estimate of treatment effect should be consistent with the study design and allow for inclusion of the relevant factors. In particular, as noted in Section 17.2, pertinent considerations recognized in the design stage should determine whether a categorical or continuous endpoint is utilized, and how important factors are accommodated (e.g., via stratification, covariate adjustment, etc.). Analysis methods should be selected accordingly. In addition, since prevention trials are typically long in duration, these methods should account for subject withdrawal, as well as competing risks as appropriate. This can be done using various life table methods and censoring approaches.

To provide some specific examples, the studies included in Table 17.1 utilized the following statistical tests:

- Categorical endpoints—difference in binomial proportions, Fishers exact test, and Mantel–Cox test

- Continuous endpoints—logrank test, Cox proportional hazards model

and the following estimates of treatment effect: the odds ratio, the risk ratio, and the difference in binomial proportions. It is recognized that differences may exist between the utility of particular measures of treatment effect from a statistical testing standpoint under the null hypothesis of no effect and those from a clinical interpretational standpoint given that treatment effects have been established [54,55]. Hence it is not necessarily the case that there be a direct correspondence between the test statistic and the measure of treatment effect. Given that a hypothesis test results in rejection of the null hypothesis of no treatment effect, it then may be useful to review various summary statistics in order to get a complete picture regarding the nature of the effect.

Multiplicity can arise in various ways in testing, including analysis of a single endpoint at multiple times, multiple endpoints at a single time, or combinations of these situations. In cancer prevention trials, such cases are not uncommon due to the long duration and large number of subjects typically involved. Interim analyses are an example of multiplicity. This is an issue particularly relevant to DMCs as they may be tasked with reviewing primary efficacy results at multiple times during a clinical trial [56]. Such multiplicity needs to be accounted for in the analysis to ensure that Type I error rates for hypothesis tests are controlled. To accomplish this, the Type I error can be allocated across the tests using various methods including prespecified values and alpha-spending functions [35]. Multiplicity of endpoints at a given time should be dealt with using preplanned methods [57]. For prevention studies there is usually one primary endpoint and one primary analysis; in such cases this form of multiplicity is not a problem.

17.4.3   Number of Studies

FDA discusses the issues concerning the number of clinical studies necessary to establish effectiveness [58]. Typically more than one study is needed to provide independent substantiation of the results. However, in some cases it is possible to rely on a single study, without independent substantiation from another study. Such cases may include effects on mortality, irreversible morbidity, or prevention of a disease with potentially serious outcome. Hence cancer prevention could be included as such a case. Following are characteristics that could contribute to a conclusion that a single study is adequate to support effectiveness:

1. Large multicenter study exhibiting internal consistency of effect

2. Consistency of results across study subsets

3. Multiple studies within a study

4. Multiple endpoints involving different events

5. Statistically very persuasive finding

Analysis approaches should be conducted so as to allow these characteristics to be appropriately and thoroughly investigated.

17.5   Interpretation

17.5.1   Interpretation of Interim Results

Caution must be used when interpreting interim results. The rules for early termination must be described in advance so that the interim results can be interpreted appropriately. Early interim results can be misleading due to the small amount of available data. It is important to recognize that interim analyses require the appropriate strength of inference to control the Type I error rate and to avoid a spurious finding. Additionally, it is important to have appropriately mature data to provide confidence that an early finding is durable. The need for long-term data in cancer prevention studies must be considered when interpreting interim results.

It is also important to limit distribution of the interim results as specified in the DMC charter so that the results are not interpreted out of context. Since early interim analyses can provide very misleading results, confidentiality of the results can be critical to successful completion of the trial following the preplanned termination rules [35]. Widespread prejudgment of early, unreliable efficacy and safety data could adversely impact recruitment into the trial, compliance to the treatment regimens, and complete evaluation of trial outcome measures [35]. The study under consideration may be adversely impacted as well as other ongoing-related trials. The importance of maintaining appropriate confidentiality can be demonstrated by a study of fluorouracil plus levamisole in colon cancer. This study was conducted in 971 subjects with stage III colon cancer. The primary objective was improvement in long-term survival; the rate of disease recurrence was also of key interest. Patient enrollment was completed prior to the first scheduled interim analysis. The interim results indicated that the combined treatment regimen reduced the rate of recurrence of the disease. However, only a small trend for survival improvement was observed and the median follow-up time was short. The DMC recommended to continue the study based on the available data. Several months after the interim review, the DMC decided to share the results with a small group from the FDA and National Cancer Institute in order to facilitate review in the event that the study was stopped after the next interim analysis [35]. Despite the attempt to maintain confidentiality, the interim results were more widely circulated and eventually published in an editorial. The editorial challenged the decision to continue the trial. Although enrollment in this study was already complete, this violation of confidentiality could have impacted subsequent follow-up of the study as well as enrollment into a follow-up study. This example demonstrates the importance of maintaining the confidentiality as planned in the DMC charter such that interim results are not taken out of context.

17.5.2 Efficacy as a Multivariate Response

While the primary objective of the study may be to determine if there is a significant difference in cancer occurrence between the active and placebo treatment groups over a specified time period, an examination of the severity of events is also important. Furthermore, the incidence and severity of side-effects must be considered along with the interpretation of the efficacy results.

For example, in the prostate cancer prevention trial (PCPT), 18,882 males with a PSA ≤ 3.0 ng/mL were randomized to 7 years of treatment with finasteride 5 mg OD or placebo. The primary endpoint was the prevalence of PCa during the study. At the final analysis, PCa had been detected in 803 (18.4%) of the subjects in the finasteride group versus 1147 (24.4%) of the subjects in the placebo group [43]. This represented a 24.8% reduction in the prevalence of PCa over the 7 years [43]. However, tumors of Gleason grade 7–10 (considered high-grade tumors) were more common in the finasteride-treated group. In the finasteride group, 6.4% of the subjects in the final analysis had high-grade tumors compared to 5.1% of the subjects in the placebo group ($p = 0.0005$) [43]. High-grade tumors represented 37.0% of all tumors among finasteride-treated subjects versus 22.2% of all tumors among placebo-treated subjects ($p < 0.001$) [43]. The tendency for more high-grade tumors for finasteride could be due to more placebo subjects having earlier detection of PCa with corresponding earlier study discontinuation. In addition, finasteride-treated subjects reported fewer urinary symptoms and complications but a higher incidence of adverse effects on sexual function [43]. Physicians will use the results of the PCPT trial to counsel men. The reduction in the risk of PCa observed during the study as well as the apparent increase in the risk of high-grade tumors will need to be weighed along with the lower incidence of urinary symptoms and the possibility of negative sexual side-effects [43].

Furthermore, the most appropriate population to be targeted for prevention must be considered. The PCPT study enrolled men from the general population rather than limiting enrollment to men at high risk of PCa [43]. This strategy allowed results to be examined in specific subgroups. However, in the clinical setting, prevention treatments would likely be targeted to men at higher risk of PCa.

The interpretation of the results is also influenced by the overall safety profile of the active treatment. It must be established that the benefits of treatment outweigh the risks.

17.5.3   Compliance and Competing Risks

The potential influence of competing risks must also be considered when interpreting the results from prevention trials. Competing risks such as death due to another cause or morbidity which precludes further participation in the trial lead to missing data. The potential influence of this missing data must be addressed.

Noncompliance to study drug may affect the ability to detect differences by decreasing the difference between treatment and placebo. It is important to examine the nature and extent of noncompliance within treatment groups.

17.5.4   Hierarchy

The primary endpoint and primary analysis must be prespecified in the statistical analysis plan. In addition, the statistical analysis plan should explain which endpoints and analysis are considered secondary. Sensitivity and supportive analyses should be described.

17.5.5   Sensitivity Analyses

In any clinical study, it is important to examine the results in multiple ways. If the same conclusions can be drawn from several different methods of analyzing the data then the results are more convincing. While the crude rate, modified crude rate, and restricted crude rate described previously will all yield different results, it is expected that the overall conclusions would be similar. Important differences between these rates would need to be explored in detail.

17.5.6   Risk Calculators

The identification of the most appropriate population to be treated with an intervention is an important challenge. In practice, an intervention for cancer prevention would likely be targeted to a population at increased risk. In order to most effectively utilize an intervention for cancer prevention it is necessary to determine who would most benefit from treatment. As an example, data from the PCPT trial was used to develop predictive models of PCa [59,60]. The risk of PCa and the risk of high-grade disease were modeled using logistic regression to create risk equations.

These risk equations can be used to individualize assessment of cancer risk and can help translate clinical trial results to clinical practice. When trying to understand risk, the rate of occurrence of cancer, the magnitude of effect, possible interactions, and the overall treatment benefit must be considered.

17.5.7   Interaction

When interpreting the results of a cancer prevention trial, it is important to understand whether any statistical interactions exist. The extent to which an overall treatment effect differs across various subgroups must be explored. It is also important to evaluate the treatment effect across time.

Statistical testing of interactions can be performed using statistical models. In doing so, the reliability of results may depend on certain technical considerations such as numbers of events and numbers of subjects per subgroup, and model goodness of fit.

17.6   Example—the REDUCE Trial

Following is a description of specific approaches to study design, summarization, and analysis utilized in the REDUCE trial. This study is used to illustrate how the various aspects that have been previously described are addressed in a particular application. Specifically, for REDUCE, this application is in PCa risk reduction.

17.6.1   Design

Adverse event data from several Phase III BPH trials indicated a potential effect of dutasteride in reducing PCa incidence; hence it was deemed appropriate to test such an intervention in a definitive clinical trial which came to be known as REDUCE [11]. A placebo control group was used as there was no approved treatment for the prevention of PCa (at the time of the start of the study), and it was considered appropriate to assign subjects to a placebo treatment group for this type of cancer.

Since the goal was PCa risk reduction, the study population was subjects who were at an increased risk of PCa. The subjects included were based upon age, previous suspicion of PCa (negative prostate biopsy prior to enrollment), and serum PSA. An upper age limit was established to target subjects who would be expected to remain in the study for the entire planned duration. A prior negative biopsy was required to eliminate subjects with preexisting detectable disease. Elevated serum PSA is an established marker for PCa.

Subjects with a prostate volume >80 cc at baseline were excluded, in order to adequately sample a prostate using a 10 core biopsy. In addition, men with evidence of high-grade prostatic intraepithelial neoplasia (HGPIN) or atypical small acinar proliferation (ASAP) at the screening biopsy were excluded as these subjects have been identified as having an increased likelihood of developing PCa. Furthermore, subjects with severe BPH symptoms were excluded in order to minimize the number of subjects undergoing benign prostatic hyperlasia (BPA) related surgery (and thus an evaluation of PCa).

Subjects were evaluated at the postbaseline assessments at 2 years and 4 years for PCa using a 10-core transrectal ultrasound-guided biopsy. The location of the 10 cores was standardized. The use of 10 cores was chosen because this reflects a balance between the need to maximize the detection of clinically significant tumors and minimize the over diagnosis of low-grade tumors. Furthermore, all biopsies were to be centrally evaluated. Unscheduled biopsies (between baseline and 2 years or between 2 years and 4 years) were allowed, and subjects who had undergone biopsies within 6 months of the scheduled biopsy did not have to undergo a repeat biopsy.

A 4 year study duration was selected with postbaseline biopsies performed at 2 years and 4 years. For this subject population, it was deemed within clinical practice to have 2 year intervals between prostate biopsies. Furthermore, in the dutasteride phase III BPH studies, the crude incidence rate of PCa (after 27 months) was 50% lower in the dutasteride group than in the placebo group (1.2% vs. 2.5%, $p = 0.002$) [11]. Guidance from regulatory agencies consulted considered 4 years to be an acceptable study duration.

The rate of biopsy detectable PCa was estimated to be 19% in the placebo group after 4 years (12.5% after 2 years), and 15.2% in the dutasteride group after 4 years (10.0% after 2 years). This 20% reduction in the occurrence of PCa was considered to be clinically meaningful. The withdrawal rate for both treatment groups after 4 years was assumed to be 25% based upon projected estimates of mortality, biopsy refusals, and study discontinuations. Since the REDUCE study was planned to be used as a single pivotal study for a regulatory submission, a significance level of 0.01 was identified, with guidance from regulatory agencies. Using sample size formulas for differences in proportions, a two-sided test at the 0.01 significance level, and a 25% withdrawal rate, 4000 subjects per treatment group would provide 90% power to detect a difference between the two treatment groups in terms of the occurrence of PCa. An interim analysis was planned after all subjects had completed the 2 year biopsies. A significance level of 0.001 was determined for this interim analysis also with guidance from regulatory agencies. The power to detect a significant difference between the two treatment groups at this interim analysis using the 0.001 significance level was approximately 50% assuming a 20% risk reduction and was approximately 80% assuming a 25% risk reduction.

Randomization schemes stratified by variables that could affect the occurrence of PCa were considered. These variables included age, race, geographical region, prostate volume, serum total and free PSA, family history of PCa, and number of cores on the screening biopsy. Since there were no clearly dominant factors, it was decided that a center-based randomization (i.e., treatments equally allocated within a study center) without any stratification would be used. Since the sample size for the REDUCE study was large, randomization should insure balance between the treatment groups with regard to the various factors.

Subjects and investigators were blinded with regard to study treatment. An additional consideration in the REDUCE study was with regard to PSA blinding.

TABLE 17.3: REDUCE trial design considerations.

Design Consideration	REDUCE Study
Population	Subjects at increased risk of PCa
Endpoint	Biopsy proven PCa—centrally reviewed
Study control	Placebo-controlled
Blinding	Subject, investigator, and sponsor blinded
Duration	4 years—prostate biopsies at 2 and 4 years
Sample size	8000 subjects (4000 placebo, 4000 dutasteride)
Power	90% (0.01 significance level)
Randomization	Center-based
Interim analyses	Yes—2 years
IDMC	Yes—met every 6 months

PSA is a blood serum laboratory test which is used for determination of PCa. Dutasteride is known to reduce serum PSA by approximately 50%. PSA samples were collected every 6 months in the REDUCE study and were evaluated at a central laboratory. Postbaseline values were reported to the sites as the actual PSA value for subjects randomized to placebo, and reported as the PSA value doubled for subjects randomized to dutasteride (randomly reported as either the actual PSA value multiplied by 2 or the actual PSA value multiplied by 2 plus or minus 0.1 units).

Due to the relatively long time period involved, an independent Data Monitoring Committee (IDMC) was established before the study initiated. The IDMC met every 6 months. All data from the study (which included PCa and safety data) was sent to an independent Statistical Data Center (SDC) approximately one month prior to IDMC meetings. The SDC produced a report of background, efficacy, and safety results (unblinded with regard to randomized treatment group) that was reviewed at the IDMC meetings. Quality control procedures of the results produced by the SDC were established. Results discussed at the IDMC meetings were disclosed only to the members of the IDMC. It was planned that the IDMC would conduct an interim analysis after all subjects had completed 2 year biopsies. A statistically significant treatment effect at the interim analysis (using the 0.001 significance level) was not the sole determining factor for early stopping of the study. The IDMC used the results of this statistical evaluation along with other information regarding the study and prior advice from regulatory agencies to determine whether to stop the study.

Table 17.3 summarizes the major trial design considerations for REDUCE.

17.6.2 Summarization

In the REDUCE study, the primary endpoint is the occurrence of biopsy-detectable PCa after 4 years. Summarization of the occurrence of PCa must be in agreement with the evaluation timepoints, handling of withdrawals, and statistical analysis methods.

The primary population of subjects evaluated in REDUCE was the efficacy population which included subjects randomized to study drug, with a prostate entry biopsy reviewed by the central pathology group revealing no PCa or suspicious tissue and who received at least one dose of study treatment. For the primary analysis, only results from the central pathology group were utilized. Hence, in all respects, the population being evaluated used the intent to treat principle according to the randomized study drug.

Prostate biopsies in REDUCE were scheduled at 2 years and at 4 years. Unscheduled prostate biopsies could occur prior to the 2 year and 4 year evaluations. If an unscheduled prostate biopsy occurred within 6 months prior to the scheduled biopsy, the scheduled biopsy was not mandatory, and therefore for analysis purposes, these unscheduled biopsies were treated as scheduled biopsies.

Several methods for summarization of the occurrence of PCa in REDUCE were prospectively planned. The primary method utilized a crude rate approach (grouping withdrawals with subjects having no PCa), while secondary methods utilized a modified crude rate approach (eliminating withdrawals), and a restricted crude rate approach (utilizing the last postbaseline biopsy information from withdrawals). Differences between the three methods involved subjects included in the risk set. Subjects included in the risk set for the three approaches are illustrated in Table 17.4 below.

TABLE 17.4:   Establishment of crude rate, modified crude rate, and restricted crude rate risk sets in REDUCE.

Rate	Baseline	Month 1–24	Month 25–48	Month 1–48
Crude rate	Negative biopsy	All subjects	Negative biopsy after Month 18 or positive biopsy during Month 25–48	All subjects
Modified crude rate	Negative biopsy	Negative biopsy Month 19–24 or positive biopsy during Month 1–24	Negative biopsy Month 43–48 or positive biopsy during Month 25–48	Negative biopsy Month 43–48 or Positive biopsy during Month 1–48
Restricted crude rate	Negative biopsy	Biopsy during Month 1–24	Biopsy during Month 25–48	Biopsy during Month 1–48

An example of calculating the PCa occurrence rate using the crude rate approach is shown in Table 17.5. Because the REDUCE study was not yet complete at the time of this writing, the results in this example are hypothetical, assuming that the alternative hypothesis of the study was true.

TABLE 17.5: Example of summarization of PCa occurrence using crude rate risk sets.

Time Interval		Placebo	Active
Month 1–24	Number of subjects at risk	4000	4000
	Number of subjects with PCa	500	400
	Proportion of subjects with PCa	500/4000 (12.5%)	400/4000 (10.0%)
	Probability estimate for PCa (standard error)	0.125 (0.005)	0.100 (0.005)
	Mantel–Haenszel statistic (*p*-value)		12.5 (0.0004)
	Mantel–Haenszel relative risk (95% CI)		0.80 (0.71–0.91)
	Relative risk reduction (95% CI)		20% (9% to 29%)
Month 25–48	Number of subjects at risk	3000	3100
	Number of subjects with PCa	260	208
	Proportion of subjects with PCa	260/3000 (8.7%)	208/3100 (6.7%)
	Probability estimate for PCa (standard error)	0.087 (0.005)	0.067 (0.004)
Month 1–48	Number of subjects at risk	4000	4000
	Number of subjects with PCa	760	608
	Proportion of subjects with PCa	760/4000 (19.0%)	608/4000 (15.2%)
	Probability estimate for PCa (standard error)	0.201 (0.007)	0.160 (0.006)
	Mantel–Haenszel statistic (*p*-value)		20.7 (<0.0001)
	Mantel–Haenszel relative risk (95% CI)		0.7911 (0.7149-0.8753)
	Relative risk reduction (95% CI)		20.89% (12.47% to 28.51%)

Note that results in Table 17.5 could be reproduced using the following SAS (version 8) code:

```
data example;
input tx $ time_p pca num_pat;
cards;;
P 1 0 3500
P 1 1 500
A 1 0 3600
A 1 1 400
P 2 0 2740
P 2 1 260
A 2 0 2892
A 2 1 208
;
proc freq data = example;
tables time_p*tx*pca/cmh; weight num_pat;
run;
```

Cumulative probability estimates for PCa for the Month 1–48 time interval were calculated based upon the probability estimates for the Month 1–24 and Month 25–48 time intervals, and the associated cumulative standard error was based on Greenwood's formula [61]. For example, for the placebo treatment group, the cumulative probability estimate for the Month 1–48 time period would be $1 - [(1 - 0.125) \times (1 - 0.087)] = 0.201$.

Similar statistics using the modified crude rate approach and restricted crude rate approach can be calculated as in the crude rate example in Table 17.5. Note that the number of subjects with PCa in each time interval is identical in each approach, with the differences being attributed to the number of subjects at risk. For example, if 25% of the subjects for each treatment group withdrew without either a PCa diagnosis or a biopsy between Month 43–48, the proportion of subjects with PCa for Month 1–48 would be 760/3000 (25.3%) for the placebo group and 608/3000 (20.3%) for the active treatment group using the modified crude rate approach. Similarly, if 20% of the subjects for each treatment group withdrew without either a PCa diagnosis or at least one post baseline biopsy, the proportion of subjects with PCa for Month 1–48 would be 760/3200 (23.8%) for the placebo group and 608/3200 (19.0%) for the active treatment group using the restricted crude rate approach. Note in this example that the relative risk for the Month 1–48 time interval would be similar using either the crude rate, modified crude rate, or restricted crude rate approaches.

17.6.3 Analysis

17.6.3.1 Primary Analysis

The planned primary analysis of the primary endpoint will be done using the Mantel–Cox test (i.e., the life-table extension of the Mantel–Haenszel test) [62] stratified by site cluster and time period using PROC FREQ in SAS.

The rationale for the use of the Mantel–Cox test is that it

- Recognizes the interval censored nature of the primary endpoint

- Corresponds to the protocol-specified biopsy schedule

- Requires no assumptions other than the randomization of subjects to treatment groups

The Mantel–Cox test has been used previously in the analysis of data from a cancer prevention study. Arber indicates such use in the context of the prevention of colorectal adenomatous polyps [63].

For REDUCE, the null hypothesis being tested is that within each investigator site cluster, the distribution of the time to PCa occurrence is the same for the placebo and active treatment groups. A Mantel–Haenszel statistic and corresponding p-value will be computed in order to test this hypothesis.

Relative risk and relative risk reduction will be computed for the Month 1–24 and the Month 1–48 time periods using the Mantel–Haenszel estimate of the relative risk of the active treatment versus placebo. The corresponding confidence intervals will be computed using the Wald method based on the estimated variance of the log of relative risk [64].

Table 17.5 displays the Mantel–Haenszel relative risk for the Month 1–24 and Month 1–48 time periods for the example using the crude rates without stratification for site cluster. The Mantel–Haenszel relative risk for this example was 0.7911 with a 95% confidence interval of 0.7149–0.8753. Therefore, for this example, the null hypothesis of no difference between the two treatment groups was rejected, with the active treatment group having a 20.89% reduction in the risk of PCa compared to the placebo treatment group.

In REDUCE, more than 1000 investigator sites (centers) in 42 countries were utilized and geographical pooling of investigators into 33 investigator site clusters was defined once study enrollment was complete. The investigator site clusters were determined using country as the basis, yielding 150–350 subjects per cluster. These investigator site clusters were defined so that the primary analysis was in harmony with how the randomization (by investigator center) was performed. Countries that contributed a larger number of subjects were divided into several clusters. Since the primary analysis for the time to PCa occurrence was the Mantel–Cox test, at least one event per cluster and time period was needed so that each cluster was informative with regard to treatment differences. For the cluster with the smallest number of subjects (150 subjects) and the time interval with the lowest expected number of PCa events (Month 25–48), a binomial distribution could be used to calculate the probability of at least one PCa event within this cluster and time interval. For the Month 25–48 time interval, assuming 75% of the subjects are evaluated for a cluster of 150 subjects and 7.5% of the subjects with PCa, approximately 8.4 (0.075×112.5) PCa events would be expected with standard deviation of 2.8 PCa events. Hence, at least one PCa event within the smallest investigator cluster and time interval is very likely, as one PCa event is more than 2 standard deviations below the expected number of PCa events. In the event that each cluster and time interval does not contain at least one PCa event, additional pooling of clusters is planned. Furthermore, three geographical regions of investigators were established (Europe, North America, Other) for the analysis of the primary endpoint within subgroups.

Therefore, the planned primary analysis of PCa occurrence in REDUCE consists of 66 (33 clusters × 2 time periods) 2 by 2 tables for the Mantel–Cox test.

Other statistical analyses planned in REDUCE are summarized in Table 17.6.

17.6.3.2   Sensitivity Analysis

Using the crude rate approach, withdrawals from the study (without having been diagnosed with PCa) are managed as not having PCa within the individual time intervals. Other methods for the handling of withdrawals (modified crude and restricted crude rate approaches) were prospectively identified, and similar statistical analyses are planned for these two approaches as in the crude rate approach.

17.6.3.3   Supportive Analysis

Several supportive analyses of the primary endpoint are planned. These analyses were specified in order to evaluate the robustness of the results with regard to the influence of local pathology results and deaths.

The primary analyses will utilize the results from the central pathology group only. For various reasons, some biopsy samples were evaluated by the local pathology group only and the pathology results not verified by the central pathology group. The primary analysis (using the crude rate approach) was planned to be repeated using the results of the central and local pathology group.

Due to age of the target population in REDUCE and the duration of the study, deaths are expected. For these subjects, a PCa diagnosis is likely unknown. The primary analysis (using the crude rate approach) was planned evaluating time to PCa or death with the risk set in Month 25–48 being subjects without PCa or death in Month 1–24.

17.6.3.4   Subgroup Analysis

As in many large clinical trials, there is an interest in evaluating the primary results in various subgroups of interest. Subgroups specified for the REDUCE study included age, race, family history of PCa, baseline prostate volume, baseline PSA, baseline percent-free PSA, baseline PSA density, baseline digital rectal examination result, baseline testosterone level, baseline body mass index, baseline chronic inflammation, number of cores taken at the entry biopsy, and prior use of nonsteroidal anti-inflammatory drugs (NSAIDs), salicylates, selenium, vitamin E, and statins. For each of the subgroups, summaries of PCa occurrence were planned with relative risks and associated confidence intervals calculated within each subgroup. Relative risk within each of the subgroups will be calculated using Mantel–Haenszel estimates. Subgroups results will be displayed as tertiles for the continuous parameters of interest (e.g., baseline prostate volume).

TABLE 17.6: Planned statistical analyses in REDUCE.

Analysis Type	Description	Statistical Test
Primary	Time to PCa occurrence using results of central pathology (crude rate approach)	Mantel–Cox with stratification by investigator site cluster
Sensitivity	Time to PCa occurrence using results of central pathology (modified crude rate approach)	Mantel–Cox with stratification by investigator site cluster
	Time to PCa occurrence using results of central pathology (restricted crude rate approach)	Mantel–Cox with stratification by investigator site cluster
Supportive	Time to PCa occurrence using results of central and local pathology (crude rate approach)	Mantel–Cox with stratification by investigator site cluster
	Time to PCa occurrence using results of central pathology or death (crude rate approach)	Mantel–Cox with stratification by investigator site cluster
Subgroup	Time to PCa occurrence within subgroups using results of central pathology (subgroups based upon baseline characteristics)	Relative risks and confidence intervals using Mantel–Cox with stratification by geographical cluster within subgroup
Severity	Occurrence of high grade PCa using results of central pathology (Gleason grade 7–10)	Fisher's Exact Test
Related variables	Occurrence of other pathological findings using results of central pathology:	
	HGPIN, ASAP	Fisher's exact test
	Treatment Alteration Score	Wilcoxon rank-sum test
	Percent of cores with PCa	Wilcoxon rank-sum test
	Number of cores with PCa	Wilcoxon rank-sum test
	Time to Intervention for PCa	Logrank test
Interactions	Time to PCa occurrence using results of central pathology (treatment by time interval, treatment by investigator site cluster, treatment by subgroup)	Likelihood ratio test (chi-square) from log binomial model
Modeling	Time to PCA occurrence using results of central pathology with effects for baseline parameters	Likelihood ratio statistics from log binomial model

17.6.3.5 Severity Analysis

Gleason grading was performed on the PCa biopsy samples. A higher Gleason score (7–10) was indicative of a more severe PCa. The treatment groups will be compared with regard to the proportion of subjects with a Gleason grade 7–10 PCa using Fisher's exact test.

17.6.3.6 Analysis of Related Variables

As previously noted, entry biopsies of subjects in REDUCE were not to have evidence of HGPIN or ASAP as these conditions have been associated with increased likelihood of PCa. Statistical comparison of the treatment groups in terms of the individual occurrence of HGPIN and ASAP at any postbaseline biopsy will be done using Fisher's exact test.

In addition, the percentage of biopsy cores (average over the total number of cores) with PCa, as well as the number of cores with PCa, and the treatment alteration score (an assessment of the nuclear and architectural changes in the majority of cells) will be statistically evaluated using Wilcoxon's rank-sum test. The time to PCa intervention (surgical and nonsurgical) was also planned to be evaluated using a logrank test.

17.6.3.7 Analysis of Interactions

Evaluations of the treatment effect across time, investigator site clusters, and subgroups are of interest. Statistical testing of treatment interactions for PCa occurrence are planned, using a logarithm binomial model (via PROC GENMOD in SAS).

Using this type of model for the example data in Table 17.5, a relative risk estimate of 0.7913 with a 95% confidence interval of 0.7151–0.8756 would be obtained via a PROC GENMOD model in SAS [66] including class effects for treatment and time interval with a binomial distribution and a log link function (Table 17.7). These results are almost identical to the relative risk results obtained using the Mantel–Cox test in Table 17.5.

Note that results in Table 17.7 could be reproduced using the following SAS (version 8) code:

```
proc genmod data = example descending;
    class time_p tx,
    model pca = time_p tx /
    dist = binomial link = log type3;
    estimate 'treatment difference' tx 1 -1 / exp;
    estimate 'active, time period 1' intercept 1 tx 1 time_p 1 / exp;
    estimate 'placebo, time period 1' intercept 1 tx 0 1 time_p 1 / exp;
    estimate 'active, time period 2' intercept 1 tx 1 time_p 0 1 / exp;
    estimate 'placebo, time period 2' intercept 1 tx 0 1 time_p 0 1 / exp;
    weight num_pat;
run;
```

TABLE 17.7: Log binomial model results via PROC GENMOD in SAS.

Parameter	Estimate	Standard Error	95% Confidence Limits	Chi-Square	Probability > ChiSq
Intercept	−2.4553	0.0500	−2.5533, −2.3574	2411.82	<0.0001
Time period: Month 1–24	0.3807	0.0544	0.2741, 0.4872	49.04	<0.0001
Time period: Month 25–48	0	0			
Treatment: active	−0.2341	0.0516	−0.3353, −0.1329	20.55	<0.0001
Treatment: placebo	0	0			
Relative risk	0.7913	0.0409	0.7151, 0.8756	20.55	<0.0001
Probability PCa—active, Month 1–24	0.0994	0.0043	0.0914, 0.1081		
Probability PCa—placebo, Month 1–24	0.1256	0.0048	0.1165, 0.1355		
Probability PCa—active, Month 25–48	0.0679	0.0036	0.0612, 0.0753		
Probability PCa—placebo, Month 25–48	0.0858	0.0043	0.0778, 0.0947		

An advantage of this model is the ability to be able to provide estimation. For the example in Table 17.7, the probability of PCa in the active treatment group in the Month 1–24 time period was 0.0994 (95% CI of 0.0914–0.1081). In addition, estimation in the presence of other covariates (both categorical and/or continuous) could be performed. Difficulties may be encountered in modeling such as non-convergence or estimates out of range; in these cases alternative approaches such as a logistic model may be useful.

In order to evaluate a treatment by time interval interaction, a treatment by time interval interaction term could be added to the logarithm binomial model, and likelihood ratio statistics computed for Type 3 contrasts. This likelihood ratio (chi-square) statistic is two times the log likelihood for the model including the interaction minus the log likelihood for the model excluding the interaction. For the results in Table 17.7, the log likelihood for the modeling including the treatment by time interval interaction is −4454.4811 and the log likelihood for the model excluding the treatment by time interval interaction is −4454.5259, which yields a chi-square of 0.09 with 1 degree of freedom and a p-value of 0.76. This result can also be obtained directly from the likelihood ratio statistics for the treatment by time interval interaction from the Type 3 analysis in the SAS output. Hence, no significant treatment by time interval interaction was present in this example.

Investigation of treatment by investigator site cluster interaction, and treatment by subgroup interactions could be performed similarly with the log binomial model. In this case the number of PCa events within a cluster and also within a subgroup needs to be considered. At least 5 PCa events per treatment and investigator site cluster combination (for the evaluation of treatment by investigator site cluster interaction) and at least 5 PCa events per treatment and subgroup combination (for the evaluation of treatment by subgroup interaction) is needed [62].

17.6.3.8   Modeling

In order to evaluate the effect of multiple baseline parameters on PCa, a statistical modeling procedure has been planned. This procedure will use the logarithm bino-mial model previously discussed in the analysis of interactions, using the significant subgroups and treatment by subgroup interactions identified, along with treatment, time interval, and geographical cluster, combined into an initial model. Variables other than treatment and time interval which do not obtain significance when combined will be dropped from the model, until the final model is determined which includes treatment, time interval and all other significant variables.

17.6.4   Interpretation

The primary interpretation of any large cancer prevention study such as the REDUCE study should be based upon whether the study achieved statistical significance and clinical relevance with regard to the primary endpoint of the study. Risk reductions and corresponding confidence intervals quantify the level of the treatment effect (e.g., 20.89% risk reduction (95% CI: 12.47%–28.51%) in the hypothetical example in Table 17.5). This risk reduction tends to be the primary message from these clinical trials as the 24.8% reduction in the PCPT study [43].

Additional analyses of the primary endpoint in REDUCE have been planned (and outlined above) to address the effect of withdrawals (sensitivity analyses), and additional local pathology results and deaths (supportive analyses). These analyses will help assess the robustness of the treatment results.

In REDUCE, the interpretation of the results will be affected by the analysis of the severity of the PCas identified (using Gleason grades). In particular, if the active treatment results demonstrate a significant reduction in the occurrence of all PCas, but an increase in the occurrence of high-grade PCas, this could complicate the interpretation as in the PCPT study [43].

Large cancer prevention studies such as REDUCE lend themselves to an evaluation of treatment results across relevant patient subgroups. Consistent treatment results across patient subgroups are desirable. However, identification of parameters affecting the occurrence of cancer, as well as treatment interactions with these parameters, should be evaluated. Risk models or nomograms to estimate probabilities of developing cancer can be developed. For example, risk models to estimate the risk of PCa using the results of the PCPT study were produced using the placebo group [59] and also the active treatment group [60].

Biomarkers of PCa can be evaluated using additional serum collected in the study. The usefulness of these biomarkers in estimating PCa occurrence should be evaluated in conjunction with the significant parameters identified with the risk models or nomograms, to determine if these biomarkers add any predictive value in addition to the parameters already identified.

PSA levels have been used in clinical practice for detection of PCa. Since PSA measurements are collected at 6 month intervals in the REDUCE study, postbaseline changes in PSA in relation to PCa occurrence needs to be carefully evaluated. For example, in the PCPT study, receiver operating characteristic (ROC) curves were developed for PSA for detection of PCa [65].

The interpretation of REDUCE will also be influenced by evaluations other than the occurrence of PCa. Treatment benefits will be investigated for other pathological parameters (e.g., occurrence of ASAP, HGPIN), PCa sequelae (e.g., occurrence of surgical and nonsurgical intervention), BPH-related parameters (e.g., changes in BPH symptoms, occurrence of BPH complications), prostatitis parameters (e.g., changes in prostatitis symptoms), and health outcome parameters (e.g., quality of life).

REDUCE, a large placebo-controlled 4 year study, also allows for a thorough evaluation of safety data, in particular with regard to evaluation of infrequent adverse events. In order for a cancer prevention study to have a positive interpretation (as in any clinical trial study), the benefits of the active treatment must outweigh the risks.

Acknowledgment

The authors would like to thank Professor Gary G. Koch from the Biostatistics Department of the University of North Carolina for his insightful suggestions to this chapter.

References

[1] Lippman SM, Lee JJ, and Sabichi AL. Cancer chemoprevention: Progress and promise. *J Natl Cancer Inst* 90:1514–1528, 1998.

[2] Byers T. What can randomized controlled trials tell us about nutrition and cancer prevention? *CA Cancer J Clin* 49:353–361, 1999.

[3] Tsao AS, Kim ES, and Hong WK. Chemoprevention of cancer. *CA Cancer J Clin* 54:150–180, 2004.

[4] Vogel VG. Breast cancer prevention: A review of current evidence. *CA Cancer J Clin* 50:156–170, 2000.

[5] Tangen CM, Goodman PJ, Crowley JJ, and Thompson IM. Statistical design issues and other practical considerations for conducting phase III prostate cancer prevention trials. *J Urol* 171:S64–S67, 2004.

[6] Lieberman R. Chemoprevention of prostate cancer: Current status and future directions. *Cancer Metastasis Rev* 21:297–309, 2002.

[7] Cohen V and Khuri FR. Chemoprevention of lung cancer. *Curr Opin Pulm Med* 10:279–283, 2004.

[8] Janne PA and Mayer RJ. Chemoprevention of colorectal cancer. *N Engl J Med* 342:1960–1968, 2000.

[9] Hawk ET and Levin B. Colorectal cancer prevention. *J Clin Oncol* 23:378–391, 2005.

[10] Klein EA. Chemoprevention of prostate cancer. *Annu Rev Med* 57:49–63, 2006.

[11] Andriole G et al. Chemoprevention of prostate cancer in men at high risk: Rationale and design of the reduction by dutasteride of prostate cancer events (REDUCE) trial. *J Urol* 172:1314–1317, 2004.

[12] Byar DP. Some statistical considerations for design of cancer prevention trials. *Prev Med* 18:688–699, 1989.

[13] Lippman SM, Benner SE, and Hong WK. Cancer chemoprevention. *J Clin Oncol* 12:851–873, 1994.

[14] Neuget AI, Lebwohl B, and Hershman DL. Cancer chemoprevention: How do we know what works? *J Clin Oncol* 25:1461–1462, 2007.

[15] Greenwald P. Clinical trials in cancer prevention: Current results and perspectives for the future. *J Nutr* 134:3507S–3512S, 2004.

[16] Johnson KA, Beitz J, Justice R, Schmidt W, Andrews P, and DeLap R. Protocol design considerations that relate to demonstrating the safety and effectiveness of chemopreventive agents. *J Cell Biochem Suppl* 27:1–6, 1997.

[17] Lewis JA, Jonsson B, Kreutz G, Sampaio C, and van Zweiten-Boot B. Placebo-controlled trials and the declaration of Helsinki. *Lancet* 359:1337–1340, 2002.

[18] Buring JE and Hennekens CH. Intervention studies. In: *Cancer Epidemiology and Prevention*, ed. by Schottenfeld and Fraumeni, 2nd edn., Oxford University Press, England, pp. 1422–1432, 1996.

[19] Hennekens CH and Buring JE. Validity versus generalizability in clinical trial design and conduct. *J Cardiac Fail* 4:239–241, 1998.

[20] Lee JJ, Lieberman R, Sloan JA, Piantadosi S, and Lippman SM. Design considerations for efficient prostate cancer chemoprevention trials. *Urology* 57:205–212, 2001.

[21] Albertsen PC, Hanley JA, and Murphy-Setzko M. Statistical considerations when assessing outcomes following treatment for prostate cancer. *J Urol* 162:439–444, 1999.

[22] Marks LS, Epstein JI, and Partin AW. The role of prostate needle biopsy in evaluation of chemopreventive agents. *Urology* 57:191–193, 2001.

[23] Fisher B. National surgical adjuvant breast and bowel project breast cancer prevention trial: A reflective commentary. *J Clin Oncol* 17:1632–1639, 1999.

[24] Chlebowski RT. Reducing the risk of breast cancer. *N Engl J Med* 343:191–198, 2000.

[25] Powles TJ. Tamoxifen for the prevention of breast cancer: Contra. *Eur J Cancer* 36:146–147, 2000.

[26] Beitz J. Trial endpoints for drug approval in oncology: Chemoprevention. *Urology* 57:213–215, 2001.

[27] Kelloff GJ, Sigman CC, and Greenwald P. Cancer chemoprevention: Progress and promise. *Eur J Cancer* 35:2031–2038, 1999.

[28] DeGruttola VG, Clax P, DeMets DL, Downing GJ, Ellenberg SS, Friendman L, Gail MH, Prentice R, Wittes J, and Zeger SL. Considerations in the evaluation

of surrogate endpoints in clincial trials: Summary of a National institutes of health workshop. *Control Clin Trials* 22:485–502, 2001.

[29] Kelloff GJ, Schilsky RL, Alberts DS, Day RW, Guyton KZ, Pearce HL, Peck JC, Phillips R, and Sigman CC. Colorectal adenomas: A prototype for the use of surrogate end points in the development of cancer prevention drugs. *Clin Cancer Res* 10:3908–3918, 2004.

[30] Harper DM, Franco EL, Wheeler C, Ferris DG, Jenkins D, Schuind A, Zahaf T, et al. Efficacy of a bivalent L1 virus-like particle vaccine in prevention of infection with human papillomavirus types 16 and 18 in young women: a randomized controlled trial. *Lancet* 364:1757–1765, 2004.

[31] Ellenberg SS. Analytical, practical and regulatory issues in prevention studies. *Stat Med* 23:297–303, 2004.

[32] Kelloff GJ, Johnson JJ, and Crowell JA et al. Approaches to the development and marketing approval of drugs that prevent cancer. *Cancer Epidemiol Biomarkers Prev* 4:1–10, 1995.

[33] Friedman LM, Furberg CD, and DeMets DL. *Fundamentals of Clinical Trials*, Mosby, New York, 1996.

[34] Zelen M. The randomization and stratification of patients to clinical trials. *J Chron Dis* 27:365–375, 1974.

[35] Ellenberg SS, Fleming TR, and DeMets DL. *Data Monitoring Committees in Clinical Trials: A Practical Perspective*, Wiley, New York, 2002.

[36] Fisher B, Costantino JP, Wickerham DL, Redmond CK, Kavanah M, Cronin WM, Vogel V, et al. Tamoxifen for prevention of breast cancer: Report of the National surgical adjuvant breast and bowel project P-1 study. *J Natl Cancer Inst* 90:1371–1388, 1998.

[37] IBIS Investigators. First results from the international breast cancer intervention study (IBIS-I): A randomized prevention trial. *Lancet* 360:817–824, 2002.

[38] Vogel VG, Costantino JP, Wickerham DL, Cronin WM, Cecchini RS, Atkins JN, Bevers TB, et al. Effects of Tamoxifen vs Raloxifene on the risk of developing invasive breast cancer and other disease outcomes. *J Am Med Assoc* 295:2727–2741, 2006.

[39] ATBC Study Group. The effect of vitamin E and beta carotene on the incidence of lung cancer and other cancers in male smokers. *N Engl J Med* 330:1029–1035, 1994.

[40] Thornquist MD and Omenn GS et al. Statistical design and monitoring of the carotene and retinol efficacy trial (CARET). *Control Clin Trials* 14:308–324, 1993.

[41] Omenn GS and Goodman GE et al. Effects of a combination of beta carotene and vitamin A on lung cancer and cardiovascular disease. *N Engl J Med* 334:1150–1155, 1996.

[42] Feigl P, Blumenstein B, and Thompson I et al. Design of the prostate cancer prevention trial (PCPT). *Control Clin Trials* 23:675–685, 1995.

[43] Thompson IM and Goodman PJ et al. The influence of finasteride on the development of prostate cancer. *N Engl J Med* 349:215–224, 2003.

[44] Klein EA, Thompson IM, Lippman SM, Goodman PJ, Albanes D, Taylor PR, and Coltman C. SELECT: The next prostate cancer prevention trial. *J Urol* 166:1311–1315, 2001.

[45] Lippman SM, Goodman PJ, Klein EA et al. Designing the selenium and vitamin E cancer prevention trial (SELECT). *J Natl Cancer Inst* 97:94–102, 2005.

[46] Hennekens CH, Buring JE, Mansom JE et al. Lack of effect of long-term supplementation with beta carotene on the incidence of malignant neoplasms and cardiovascular disease. *N Engl J Med* 334:1145–1149, 1996.

[47] Christen WG, Gaziano JM, and Hennekens CH. Design of physicians' health study II—A randomized trial of beta-carotene, vitamins E and C, and multivitamins, in prevention of cancer, cardiovascular disease, and eye disease, and review of results of completed trials. *Ann Epidemiol* 10:125–134, 2000.

[48] Lee IM, Cook NR, Gaziano JM, Gordon D, Ridker PM, Manson JE, Hennekens CH, and Buring JE. Vitamin E in the primary prevention of cardiovascular disease and cancer. *J Am Med Assoc* 294:56–65, 2005.

[49] Hercberg S, Galan P, Preziosi P et al. The SU.VI.MAX study. *Arch Intern Med* 164:2335–2342, 2004.

[50] Blot WJ, Li JY, Taylor PR et al. Nutrition intervention trials in Linxian, China: supplementation with specific vitamin/mineral combinations, cancer incidence, and disease-specific mortality in the general population. *J Natl Cancer Inst* 85:1483–1492, 1993.

[51] Koch GG, Amara IA, Forster J et al. Statistical issues in the design and analysis of ulcer healing and recurrence studies. *Drug Inform J* 27:805–824, 1993.

[52] Koch GG and Gillings DB. Inference, design based vs model based. In *Encyclopedia of Statistical Sciences*, ed. S. Kotz and N. Johnson, vol. 4, John Wiley and Sons, New York, 1983.

[53] Berger VW. Pros and cons of permutation tests in clinical trials. *Stat Med* 19:1319–1328, 2000.

[54] Walter SD. Choice of effect measure for epidemiological data. *J Clin Epidemiol* 53:931–939, 2000.

[55] Kraemer HC. Reconsidering the odds ratio as a measure of 2 × 2 association in a population. *Stat Med* 23:257–279, 2004.

[56] Whitehead J. On being the statistician on a data and safety monitoring board. *Stat Med* 18:3425–3434, 1999.

[57] Westfall PH, Tobias RD, Rom D, Wolfinger RD, and Hochberg Y. *Multiple Comparisons and Multiple Tests Using the SAS System*, SAS Institute, Carys NC, 1999.

[58] FDA. Guidance for industry: Providing clinical evidence of effectiveness for human drugs and biological products. U.S. Department of Health and Human Services, FDA, CDER, CBER, May 1998.

[59] Thompson IM, Ankerst DP, Chi C, Goodman PJ et al. Assessing prostate cancer risk: Results from the prostate cancer prevention trial. *J Natl Cancer Inst* 98(8):529–534, 2006a.

[60] Thompson IM, Ankerst DP, Chi C, Goodman PJ et al. Prediction of prostate cancer for patients receiving finasteride. *J Clin Oncol* 25(21):3076–3081, 2007.

[61] Collett D. *Modelling Survival Data in Medical Research*, Chapman & Hall, London, 1994.

[62] Stokes ME, Davis CS, and Koch GG. *Categorical Data Analysis Using the SAS System*, SAS Institute, Cary, NC, 2000.

[63] Arber N et al. Celecoxib for the prevention of colorectal adenomatous polyps. *N Engl J Med* 355:885–895, 2006.

[64] Greenland S and Robins JM. Estimation of a common effect parameter from sparse follow-up data. *Biometrics* 41:55–68, 1985.

[65] Thompson IM, Chi C, Ankerst DP, Goodman PJ et al. Effect of finasteride on the sensitivity of PSA for detecting prostate cancer. *J Natl Cancer Inst* 98 (16):1128–1133, 2006.

[66] SAS Institute. SAS online Documentation, Version 8, SAS Institute, Cary NC, 1999.

Chapter 18

LASSO Method in Variable Selection for Right-Censored Time-to-Event Data with Application to Astrocytoma Brain Tumor and Chronic Myelogenous Leukemia

Lili Yu and Dennis Pearl

Contents

18.1 Introduction

We propose models of potential relationships in time-to-event data and we infer whether these associations occur based on the support of the available data. Our inferences are only as good as the models that we use to define these associations of interest.

Cox proportional hazard model [1,2] is the most popular model used in survival analysis due to the computational simplicity of the inference methods and well-established asymptotic properties of the partial likelihood. However, the proportional hazards assumption is not always true since the hazard ratio for real data often converges to 1 as time increases.

421

A linear regression model is often enough to model the relationship between survival time and covariates after suitable transformation [3,4]. Consider a linear model for censored data with n observations:

$$t_i = \beta^T \mathbf{x_i} + \varepsilon_i \qquad (18.1)$$

where
  β is the parameter vector $(\beta_0, \beta_1, \ldots, \beta_p)$
  $\mathbf{x_i}$ is the covariate vector of the ith observation

It is assumed that x_i, that is $\{\varepsilon_i : \varepsilon_i = t_i - \beta^T \mathbf{X}_i\}$ are independent and identically distributed from a distribution F with mean $= 0$ and finite equal variance σ^2. t_i is the failure time of the ith observation. The survival times $\{y_i : y_i = \min(t_i, c_i), i = 1, \ldots, n\}$, together with the indicators $\{\delta_i : \delta_i = I(t_i < c_i)\}$ that indicate whether right-censoring occurs. Assume that given $\mathbf{x_i}$, c_i is independent of t_i, ε_i is independent of $(\mathbf{x_i}, c_i)$, and neither the distribution of $c_i|\mathbf{x_i}$ nor that of $\mathbf{x_i}$ depends on (β, σ^2).

Model (Equation 18.1) is central in survival analysis and is closely related to the linear transformation model [4]. With a monotone transformation h of t_i, Equation 18.1 becomes

$$h(t_i) = \beta^T \mathbf{x_i} + \varepsilon_i \qquad (18.2)$$

When h is known, models (Equations 18.1 and 18.2) are equivalent with time rescaled. Model (Equation 18.2) reduces to the Cox model when ε follows the extreme value distribution; it is the proportional odds model when ε follows the standard logistic distribution.

For our method, we employ the linear model as the candidate model space. Thus, the model selection problem reduces to the issue of variable selection: finding which explanatory variables are statistically significant in predicting the survival time. The optimal model should reflect the trade-off between simplicity and goodness-of-fit.

Many variable selection procedures have been proposed in the literature, however, only a few of them have been generalized to incomplete data and are available for use with survival data. The selection methods that are based on tests such as the subset selection method or the stepwise method are used in survival analysis by assuming the Cox proportional hazard model and are available in many statistical software packages. However, these methods [5] are discrete processes (little change in the data may result in different models). This may increase the prediction error. Selection methods may be based on information theory [6]. For example, the akaike information criterion (AIC) method is constructed to minimize the Kullback–Leibler distance between the distribution of the selected model and the distribution of the true model and is an unbiased estimate of the expectation of the distance. For incomplete data, Shimodaira [7] proposed a natural extension of the AIC called the predictive divergence for incomplete observation (PDIO) model criterion. This criterion is approximately an unbiased estimator of the expectation of the Kullback–Leibler distance. Cavanaugh and Shumway [8] proposed an alternate variant of AIC for incomplete data that is also approximately an unbiased estimator of the expected Kullback–Leibler distance, but it can be evaluated using only complete data tools which are readily available through the expectation maximization (EM) algorithm and the supplemented EM algorithm. However, AIC is intended to minimize the in-sample prediction error [6] defined as the difference between the predicted values and new observations with the same values of the covariates as those in the training data. This in-sample error is quite different from the prediction error of interest in which the covariate realizations for new patients do not necessarily coincide with those in the training set.

Shrinkage methods were introduced to minimize the prediction error needed. Tibshirani [5] developed a model selection technique, least absolute shrinkage and selection operator (LASSO), and extended it for censored data under the proportional hazards model [9]. In this chapter, we further extend it to the proposed model (Equation 18.1)—the linear model for censored data.

To calculate the LASSO criteria, we need to estimate the likelihood and the coefficients in the linear model for censored data. Inference under this model has been extensively investigated because it retains the basic features of linear models, while being able to handle censored observations after suitable transformations. Miller [10] used the weighted least-squares approach with $F(\cdot)$ estimated by the Kaplan–Meier (KM) estimator. Buckley and James [11] introduced modified least-square normal equation by replacing the censored data with its unbiased estimate. Koul et al. [12] suggested using the censored distribution to reweigh the censored data and estimate β without involving iterations. Leurgans [14] described an alternative noniterative method. Schmee and Hahn [15] used an iterated least-squares method that substitutes censored values with the Gaussian estimate. Previous comparisons of these approaches [13,16] found the Buckley and James estimates to be the most reliable. Prentice [17] proposed a class of linear rank statistics for testing the regression coefficients based on the martingale probability of a generalized rank vector with various specified distributions of the error term in the accelerated failure time model. Harrington and Fleming [18] applied a class of rank test procedures for censored survival data. Lai and Ying [19] gave linear rank statistics with censored data for estimating regression parameters. However, the likelihood functions constructed by these methods provide little information about the location of β, leading to an inconsistent estimate of β.

Shen et al. [20] proposed a semiparametric regression technique—using the random-sieve likelihood method which can estimate the distribution $F(\cdot)$ and the coefficients simultaneously. Zhao [4] generalized this technique to include the right-censored data case and proved that these estimates are consistent. In this chapter, we further generalize this work to right-censored data in the constraint regions under the model (Equation 18.1).

This chapter is organized as follows: Section 18.2 gives the detail of calculating the LASSO criterion using a random-sieve likelihood and describes our algorithm including the automatic estimation of the constraint parameter λ; Section 18.3 reports the results of a simulation study and the application of the new method to predicting survival from brain tumors and from leukemia; finally, Section 18.4 contains some discussion.

18.2   Methods

18.2.1   LASSO Procedure Calculated by Random-Sieve Likelihood in the General Linear Model for Censored Data

Consider the right-censored survival data in model (Equation 18.1). The random-sieve likelihood [3] is defined as

$$L_n(\beta, F) = \prod_{\{i \in i: \delta_i = 1\}} p_i \prod_{\{i \in i: \delta_i = 0\}} (1 - F(\varepsilon_i))$$

Subject to the constraint

$$G(\{p_i\}, \beta) = 0$$

where p_i is the probability mass of ε_i and $F(\varepsilon_I^-) = \text{Prob}(\varepsilon < \varepsilon_i)$. $G(\{p_i\}, \beta)$ is specified by the model assumptions, i.e., $E(\varepsilon) = \sum_{i=1}^n \varepsilon_i p_i = 0$ and $E(\varepsilon \mathbf{x_j}) = \sum_{i=1}^n \varepsilon_i x_{ij} p_i = 0$ for $j = 1, \ldots, p$, where $\mathbf{x_j}$ represents the jth covariate.

The parameters p_i and β are estimated simultaneously by maximizing the random-sieve likelihood, which is

$$(\hat{p}_i, \hat{\beta}) = \max_{G(\{p_i\}, \beta)} \prod_{\{i \in i: \delta_i = 1\}} p_i \prod_{\{i \in i: \delta_i = 0\}} (1 - F(\varepsilon_i))$$

The maximum random-sieve likelihood estimates have good properties [4]. For the case without censored data, the estimates of the likelihood are equal to the empirical likelihood and the estimates of coefficients are equivalent to the ordinary least-square estimates. For right-censored data, the estimates of likelihood are equal to the KM estimate if the constraints $G(\cdot, \cdot)$ are not enforced and the estimates for coefficients and the likelihood at the true coefficients are consistent.

Denote the log-random-sieve likelihood by $l(p_i, \beta) = \log L(p_i, \beta)$. In this chapter, we propose to estimate β via the criterion

$$\hat{\beta} = \arg\max \left\{ l(p_i, \beta) - \lambda \sum_{j \neq 0} |\beta_j| \right\}$$

where

$\lambda \geq 0$ is the constraint parameter to be optimized

$l(p_i, \beta) - \lambda \sum_{j \neq 0} |\beta_j|$ is the LASSO value

Under the assumptions of the Cox proportional hazards model, Tibshirani [9] proposed a criterion that maximizes the Cox partial likelihood, subject to a constraint that $\sum_{j \neq 0} |\beta_j| \leq S$. In the comparisons that follow, we call his method the "Cox method" and the new proposed method the "Sieve method."

The Sieve method is a coefficients estimation method using nonparametric likelihood subject to some constraints. The estimates are asymptotically consistent, but it may not perform well for small sample sizes due to the nonparametric property.

However, this property relaxes the assumption on the distribution of the error term like the proportional hazard assumption in the Cox model. Therefore, the Sieve method provides an alternative estimation procedure to Cox method.

18.2.2 Algorithm

In this section, we will describe an algorithm to maximize the LASSO criteria with respect to the pi'^s and β'^s under the constraints $G(\{p_i\}, \beta) = 0$. There is by no means a trivial solution for this high-dimensional optimization problem. Fortunately, we can derive a closed form expression for β for any arbitrary pi'^s, indicating that the parameters that need to be estimated are just the pi'^s. The constraints $G(\{p_i\}, \beta) = 0$ are then rewritten as

$$
\begin{cases}
\sum_{i=1}^{n} p_i = 1 \\[2mm]
\sum_{i=1}^{n} (t_i - \mathbf{x_i}\beta)p_i = 0 \\[2mm]
\sum_{i=1}^{n} x_{i1}(t_i - \mathbf{x_i}\beta)p_i = 0 \\[1mm]
\cdots \\[1mm]
\sum_{i=1}^{n} x_{ik}(t_i - \mathbf{x_i}\beta)p_i = 0
\end{cases}
$$

If the pi'^s are given, the solution of β is $\hat{\beta} = (\mathbf{D'D})^{-1}\mathbf{D'Z}$, where

$$
\mathbf{D} = \left\{ \begin{array}{cccc} \sqrt{p_1} & x_{11}\sqrt{p_1} & \cdots & x_{1k}\sqrt{p_1} \\ \cdots & \cdots & \cdots & \cdots \\ \sqrt{p_n} & x_{n1}\sqrt{p_n} & \cdots & x_{nk}\sqrt{p_n} \end{array} \right\}, \quad \mathbf{Z} = \left\{ \begin{array}{c} \sqrt{p_1}t_1 \\ \cdots \\ \sqrt{p_n}t_n \end{array} \right\}
$$

This is just the least-square estimates based on the new design matrix $\mathbf{D}$ and new dependent variable vector $\mathbf{Z}$ for any fixed pi'^s. Hence, the variance for $\hat{\beta}$ can be calculated as $\text{var}(\hat{\beta}) = (\mathbf{D'D})^{-1}\text{var}(\mathbf{z})$.

For each fixed λ, our algorithm consists of four steps:

1. Initialize $pi'^s = 1/n$.

2. Apply an annealing technique to update the pi'^s. Randomly choose two new pi'^s and assign them to (p^1, p^2). The LASSO value is recalculated for the new (p^1, p^2) and compared with the old LASSO value. The new (p^1, p^2) is accepted if the new LASSO value is larger than the old LASSO value. We also assign a small probability to accept the new (p^1, p^2) when the new LASSO value is a little bit smaller than the old LASSO value.

3. Calculate $\hat{\beta}$ for the new pi'^s.

4. Repeat steps 2 and 3 until the LASSO value converges.

18.2.3 Estimation of the Constraint Parameter λ

To estimate the constraint parameter λ based on the data automatically, we follow Tibshirani's idea [9] to use an approximate generalized cross-validation (GCV) [21] which is defined as

$$\text{GCV}(\lambda) = \frac{1}{N} \frac{-\ell_\lambda(\beta, F)}{N(1 - p(\lambda)/N)^2}$$

where $\ell(\lambda)$ is the log-random-sieve likelihood for the constrained fit with constraint λ; $p(\lambda)$, the number of effective parameters in the constrained fit, is estimated as follows: from the previous result, we have a linear approximation to the LASSO estimates, that is,

$$\tilde{\beta} = (\mathbf{D'D})^{-1}\mathbf{D'Z}$$

In this new setting with design matrix $\mathbf{D}$ and dependent vector $\mathbf{Z}$, we approximate $p(\lambda)$ by

$$p(\lambda) \approx \text{tr}(\mathbf{D(D'D)}^{-1}\mathbf{D}) = \text{number of nonzero parameters}$$

Lemma. The model selected by the Sieve method is consistent.
   Sketch of proof:

1. If n goes to infinity, the denominator will go to N^2. To minimize GCV, we need to select the constraint parameter that can maximize the likelihood. Therefore, constraint parameter is selected to be zero when n goes to infinity.

2. The likelihood and coefficient estimates are consistent using the random-sieve likelihood method [4].

18.3 Application

18.3.1 Simulation

In order to investigate the performance of the Sieve method, here we compare the prediction errors for the Sieve method to those for the Cox method in a variety of settings. The relationship between the linear model in which ε follows the extreme value distribution and the Cox model is as follows:
   From the linear model to the Cox model,

$$t = \mathbf{x}\beta + \varepsilon$$

$$S(t) = p(T \geq t) = p(\mathbf{x}\beta + \varepsilon \geq t)$$
$$= p(\varepsilon \geq t - \mathbf{x}\beta)$$
$$= e^{-e^t e^{-\mathbf{x}\beta}}$$

$$\Lambda(t|x) = -\ln S(t) = -e^t e^{-\mathbf{x}\beta}$$
$$= \Lambda_0(t) e^{-\mathbf{x}\beta}$$

By assuming $\Lambda_0(t) = -e^{e^t}$

Then, $\lambda(t|x) = \lambda_0(t) e^{-\mathbf{x}\beta}$

From the Cox model to the linear model, we can infer the following:

$$\lambda(t|x) = \lambda_0(t) e^{\mathbf{x}\beta}$$
$$\Lambda(t|x) = \Lambda_0(t) e^{\mathbf{x}\beta}$$
$$S(t|x) = e^{-\Lambda(t|x)} = e^{-\Lambda_0(t) e^{\beta \mathbf{x}}}$$

Assume $\Lambda_0(t) = -e^{e^t}$,

$$F(t|x) = 1 - e^{-e^{t+\beta \mathbf{x}}}$$
$$f(t|x) = \frac{dF(t|x)}{dt} = e^{(t+\beta \mathbf{x})-e^{(t-\beta \mathbf{x})}}$$

This belongs to extreme value distribution with mean $(-\beta \mathbf{x} + \gamma)$ where γ is a constant [22]. Then we get

$$E(t|x) = -\beta \mathbf{x} + \gamma$$

And $t = -\mathbf{x}\beta + \varepsilon$ by absorbing γ into β_0.

These model spaces intersect since $\Lambda_0(t)$ is open for Cox model and consider $\Lambda_0(t) = e^t$, the coefficient estimates we get from Cox model correspond to the opposite coefficient in the general linear model.

We simulate 100 datasets for each setting described in Table 18.1 for the linear regression:

$$t = \beta^{\mathrm{T}} \mathbf{X} + \varepsilon$$

The values of the covariates are generated from the multivariate normal distribution with all means $= 0$ and variances $= 1$. The covariates are either independent or any two of them correlated with $\rho = 0.5$.

The error terms are simulated from the normal distribution, the extreme value distribution or bimodal distribution; all with mean 1.77 and variance 1.64. Note that the extreme value distribution satisfies the proportional hazard assumption required by the Cox method. Consequently, it is expected that the Cox method would perform

TABLE 18.1: Simulation settings for the sieve likelihood method under the linear model and the partial likelihood method under the Cox model both using the LASSO criteria.

	Sample	Number of Coefficients	Covariate Association	Censoring Proportion (%)	Error Term Distribution	True Coefficients
1	50	6	Independent	10	Normal	(0,0.6,0.5,0,0.4,0)
2	50	6	Correlated	10	Normal	(0,0.6,0.5,0,0.4,0)
3	50	6	Independent	30	Normal	(0,0.9,0.7,0,0.6,0)
4	50	6	Correlated	30	Normal	(0,0.9,0.7,0,0.6,0)
5	50	6	Independent	10	Extreme	(0,0.6,0.5,0,0.4,0)
6	50	6	Correlated	10	Extreme	(0,0.6,0.5,0,0.4,0)
7	50	6	Independent	30	Extreme	(0,0.9,0.7,0,0.6,0)
8	50	6	Correlated	30	Extreme	(0,0.9,0.7,0,0.6,0)
9	50	6	Independent	10	Bimodal	(0,0.6,0.5,0,0.4,0)
10	50	6	Correlated	10	Bimodal	(0,0.6,0.5,0,0.4,0)
11	50	6	Independent	30	Bimodal	(0,0.9,0.7,0,0.6,0)
12	50	6	Correlated	30	Bimodal	(0,0.9,0.7,0,0.6,0)
13	150	10	Independent	10	Normal	(0,0.6,0.5,0,0,0,0.4,0,0,0)
14	150	10	Correlated	10	Normal	(0,0.6,0.5,0,0,0,0.4,0,0,0)
15	150	10	Independent	30	Normal	(0,0.9,0.7,0,0,0,0.6,0,0,0)
16	150	10	Correlated	30	Normal	(0,0.9,0.7,0,0,0,0.6,0,0,0)
17	150	10	Independent	10	Extreme	(0,0.6,0.5,0,0,0,0.4,0,0,0)
18	150	10	Correlated	10	Extreme	(0,0.6,0.5,0,0,0,0.4,0,0,0)
19	150	10	Independent	30	Extreme	(0,0.9,0.7,0,0,0,0.6,0,0,0)
20	150	10	Correlated	30	Extreme	(0,0.9,0.7,0,0,0,0.6,0,0,0)
21	150	10	Independent	10	Bimodal	(0,0.6,0.5,0,0,0,0.4,0,0,0)
22	150	10	Correlated	10	Bimodal	(0,0.6,0.5,0,0,0,0.4,0,0,0)
23	150	10	Independent	30	Bimodal	(0,0.9,0.7,0,0,0,0.6,0,0,0)
24	150	10	Correlated	30	Bimodal	(0,0.9,0.7,0,0,0,0.6,0,0,0)

Note: There are 24 settings in the simulation study. For the column of covariate association, if the covariates are correlated, the correlation between any two covariates is

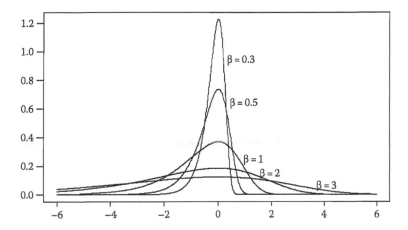

FIGURE 18.1: Family of minimum extreme value distributions.

better than the Sieve method for this case. Extreme value distributions are the limiting distributions for the minimum or the maximum of a very large collection of random observations from the same arbitrary distribution. The general formula for the probability density function of the minimum extreme value distribution is

$$f(x) = \frac{1}{\beta} e^{(x-\mu)/\beta} e^{-e^{(x-\mu)/\beta}}$$

where
  μ is the location parameter
  β is the scale parameter

The density functions for $\mu = 0$ and different β values are shown in Figure 18.1. The general formula for the probability density function of the maximum extreme value distribution is

$$f(x) = \frac{1}{\beta} e^{-((x-\mu)/\beta)} e^{-e^{-((x-\mu)/\beta)}}$$

Similarly, μ is the location parameter and β is the scale parameter. The density functions are symmetric to those for minimum values. We choose the extreme value distribution for the minimum distribution with $\mu = 0$ and $\beta = 1$.

For the bimodal distribution, we generate the random variables from $|x| \sim$ gamma (4,scale $= 0.287$). The three distributions for the simulation study are in Figure 18.2.

The bimodal distribution used here is more different from the extreme value distribution than the normal distribution. Hence, it might be expected that the Cox method will perform worse for the settings with the bimodal distribution.

To calculate the prediction error, 100,000 new noncensored observations are generated for each setting from the true distribution of the failure time t. We then

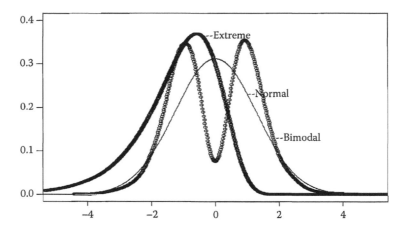

FIGURE 18.2: Simulation distributions for error terms.

calculate the prediction error for each data set. The prediction error for each setting is approximated by the average of the prediction errors across the 100 datasets.

The simulation results are in Table 18.2 while Figures 18.3 and 18.4 show the results for prediction errors for both methods.

For the small sample size ($n = 50$), we can see the expected trend that the Cox method performs better than the Sieve method when there is less censoring and when the error distribution is closer to the extreme value distribution; while the Sieve method will do better as we move farther from the extreme value distribution aligned with the proportional hazards model. Overall, the Sieve method has a smaller prediction error in 6 of 12 settings when $n = 50$ including 5 of the 6 cases with the higher (30%) censoring rate.

For the larger sample size ($n = 150$), the prediction errors of the Sieve method were smaller than those given by the Cox method in 11 of the 12 settings studied. Surprisingly, the Sieve method performs better than the Cox method for the larger sample size even in the settings when the proportional hazards assumption is true. We suspect that the use of partial likelihood and the approximation in the algorithm of the Cox method results in the reduction of the power of the approach.

Although the Sieve method appears to generally outperform the Cox method with respect to prediction error, this comes at the expense of an overall smaller percentage of times it chooses the correct model. However, even by this criterion, the Sieve method does show better performance when the error distribution is far from the proportional hazards model as in the bimodal case for the large sample size.

18.3.2   Application to Astrocytoma Brain Tumor Data Sets

The data analyzed in this study come from the surgical specimens of patients who were diagnosed with astrocytoma brain tumor by a consensus of at least three

TABLE 18.2: Simulation results for the sieve likelihood method under the linear model and the partial likelihood method under the Cox model both using the LASSO criteria.

Setting	Sample	Error Term Distribution	Sieve Method Correct Model %	ase	sdse	Cox Method Correct Model %	ase	sdse
1	50	Normal	7	2.24	0.009	20	2.21	0.010
2	50	Normal	12	2.32	0.009	36	2.18	0.009
3	50	Normal	13	2.20	0.008	43	2.30	0.010
4	50	Normal	20	2.16	0.008	38	2.48	0.011
5	50	Extreme	14	2.52	0.015	18	2.47	0.015
6	50	Extreme	25	2.14	0.012	36	2.39	0.015
7	50	Extreme	22	2.63	0.016	36	2.36	0.015
8	50	Extreme	17	2.06	0.012	40	2.55	0.015
9	50	Bimodal	16	2.16	0.008	14	2.22	0.009
10	50	Bimodal	26	2.26	0.007	38	2.17	0.008
11	50	Bimodal	26	2.15	0.007	51	2.32	0.009
12	50	Bimodal	19	2.10	0.006	48	2.49	0.010
13	150	Normal	33	1.83	0.008	26	1.90	0.008
14	150	Normal	13	1.80	0.008	12	1.93	0.009
15	150	Normal	7	1.87	0.008	9	1.99	0.009
16	150	Normal	0	1.79	0.008	15	2.19	0.010
17	150	Extreme	35	1.78	0.011	17	2.08	0.014
18	150	Extreme	11	1.76	0.011	10	2.11	0.014
19	150	Extreme	0	1.75	0.012	14	2.19	0.015
20	150	Extreme	0	1.78	0.011	20	2.37	0.015
21	150	Bimodal	70	1.84	0.006	36	1.91	0.007
22	150	Bimodal	26	1.82	0.006	14	1.92	0.007
23	150	Bimodal	22	1.90	0.007	16	2.01	0.007
24	150	Bimodal	22	2.07	0.007	16	2.34	0.009

Note: ase, average prediction errors; sdse, standard deviation of the average prediction errors.

neuropathologists in the National Cancer Institute's Glioma Marker Network. Sung et al. [23,24] and Singh et al. [25] have analyzed an overlapping set of data (that also included other gliomas besides astrocytomas) in detail to investigate the relationship of the glycolipid composition of primary brain tumors with the histological diagnosis and with the survival of the patients using Cox regression. Later, the Glioma Marker Network provided an independent set of astrocytoma brain tumor data. The same laboratory (e.g., Comas et al.; Yates et al.) [26] and Oblinger et al. [27] further investigated the relationship between tumor histology or patient prognosis and the pattern of glycolipids and the enzymes involved in their formation (glycosyltrans-ferases) based on this new data set. These two independent datasets include survival times which may be subject to right censoring along with key data on factors that might influence survival—such as age, gender, and tumor grade, as well as

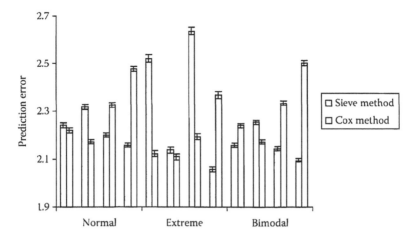

FIGURE 18.3:   Prediction errors for both methods for small sample size.
Note: Normal represents normal error distribution; extreme represents extreme value error distribution; bimodal represents bimodal error distribution.

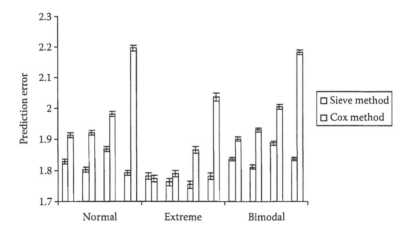

FIGURE 18.4:   Prediction errors for both methods for large sample size. *Note*: Same representation as Figure 18.3.

laboratory measures of the pattern of gangliosides and glycosyltransferases. We combined these two data sets and discarded the nonastrocytic tumors as well as any observations without laboratory values to arrive at 69 observations and among them, 53 are uncensored.

The variables in the dataset are

Y: The natural log of the number of days between the surgery and death (either due to Glioblastoma or other reasons)

δ: 1 if Y is log of time to death; 0 if survival time is censored

Gender: 0 = female; 1 = male

Grade: 0 = grade 1 or 2; 1 = grade 3 or 4

Age at surgery in years

Log(B3G): log of amount of β3 galactosyltransferase

%GM3: The percentage of the total ganglioside content of the tissue that is of the GM3 type
%GD3
%GM2

Log(GD3): log of amount of GD3 synthase
%GM1
%GD1a

Log(GNA): log of amount of GalNac transferase

We combined grades 1 and 2 (nonmalignant astocytomas) and also grades 3 and 4 (malignant astrocytomas) together since few observations are in grade 2 or 3. To examine survival time on a relative, rather than absolute, basis, we take the natural log for the survival time as the response variable.

Checking the proportional hazard assumption of this data set using Schoenfeld residuals, we did not find any strong departures from the assumption either for the model as a whole or for the individual variables (Table 18.3). Only the covariate Log (GD3) shows some evidence of failing to meet the proportional hazards assumption.

We applied both the Sieve and Cox LASSO methods to this data set and the results are shown in Table 18.4. Since the proportional hazards assumption fits reasonably well, it is encouraging that the Sieve method pointed to the same model in this case.

TABLE 18.3: Checking the proportional hazards assumption for the astrocytoma data.

Variable	Rho	Chi-sq	P
Gender	0.16	1.88	0.17
Grade	0.10	0.66	0.42
Age	−0.11	0.92	0.34
Log(B3G)	0.08	0.35	0.55
%GM3	0.02	0.01	0.91
%GD3	0.18	2.06	0.15
%GM2	0.18	1.84	0.18
Log(GD3)	0.29	4.61	0.03
%GM1	0.15	1.42	0.23
%GD1a	−0.02	0.02	0.89
Log(GNA)	0.01	0.00	0.95
Global	NA	12.3	0.34

Note: Rho = the correlation between the transformed survival times and the scaled Schoenfeld residuals. The chi-square statistics and the corresponding two-sided. *P*-values are also provided.

TABLE 18.4:   Variable selection results for the astrocytoma brain tumor data.

Variable	Sieve Method			Cox Method		
	Coefficient	SE	Z-Score	Coefficient	SE	Z-Score
Intercept	7.66	—	0.00	7.68	—	0.00
Gender	0.00	0.1	0.00	0.00	0.01	0.00
Grade	−0.74	0.14	−0.25	−0.81	0.24	−0.27
Age	−0.02	0.13	−0.28	−0.03	0.00	−0.44
Log(B3G)	0.00	0.12	0.00	0.00	0.01	0.00
%GM3	0.00	0.11	0.00	0.00	0.01	0.00
%GD3	0.00	0.15	0.00	0.00	0.01	0.00
%GM2	0.00	0.1	0.00	0.00	0.02	0.00
Log(GD3)	0.00	0.11	0.00	0.00	0.02	0.00
%GM1	0.00	0.14	0.00	0.00	0.02	0.00
%GD1a	0.00	0.13	0.00	0.00	0.00	0.00
Log(GNA)	0.22	0.09	0.09	0.11	0.07	0.04

Both methods select grade, age, and Log(GNA) as the significant variables which concur with results from work of Oblinger et al. [27].

18.3.3   Application to Chronic Myelogenous Leukemia Data Sets

The data in this example are from a study of chronic myelogenous leukemia (CHL) patients transplanted as part of the National Marrow Donor Program. Here, we have taken the subset of patients who experienced T-depleted transplantation and have the laboratory measurements of interest. This includes 283 observations, among them, 200 are uncensored. The variables in the data set are

Y: Survival time in months
δ: 1 if Y is the time to the event of interest; 0 if censored
Disease grades: 1 = grade I; 2 = grade II; 3 = grade III or IV
Donor age category: 0 = less than 40 years; 1 = over 40 years
Donor CMV(Cytomegalovirus) status: 0 = negative; 1 = positive
Disease stage: 0 = early; 1 = advanced
Donor gender: 0 = female; 1 = male

HLA matching overall group: general grouping of HLA matching for HLA-A, -B, -C, -DRB1, and -DQ in both directions:

1 = allele matched at all loci;
2 = single allele mismatch but antigen matched;
3 = single antigen mismatch;
4 = two or more mismatches (any combination of allele and/or antigen mismatches)

HLA matching in graft versus host direction: general grouping of HLA matching for HLA-A, -B, -C, -DRB1, and -DQ in GvH direction:

1 = allele matched at all loci;
2 = single allele mismatch but antigen matched;
3 = single antigen mismatch with no additional allele mismatches;
4 = two or more mismatches (any combination of allele and/or antigen mismatches)

HLA matching in host versus graft direction: general grouping of HLA matching for HLA-A, -B, -C, -DRB1, and -DQ in HvG direction:

1 = allele matched at all loci;
2 = single allele mismatch but antigen matched;
3 = single antigen mismatch with no additional allele mismatches;
4 = two or more mismatches (any combination of allele and/or antigen mismatches)

Log(indxtx): log time interval from diagnosis to transplant (in months)
Age interaction: The interaction between donor age and recipient age
CMV interaction: Interaction between donor cmv and recipient cmv
Gender interaction: Interaction between donor sex and recipient sex
KPS category: Karnofsky performance score. 0 = 10–90; 1 = 90–100
Recipient age category: 0 = under 50 years; 1 = over 50 years
Recipient CMV status: 0 = negative; 1 = positive
Caucasian: 1 = Caucasian; 0 = other
Black: 1 = black; 0 = other
Hispanic: 1 = Hispanic; 0 = other
Recipient gender: 0 = female; 1 = male
TBI conditioning: Indicator for whether total body irradiation (TBI) was used in conditioning regimen. 1 = yes; 0 = no

First, examining the Schoenfeld residuals, we find the variables related to age donor age, recipient age, and the interaction of donor and recipient age—all show significant departure from the proportional hazards assumption (Table 18.5).

Many researchers have investigated the factors that affect the survival time of CML patients after transplantation and HLA matching is typically found to be the most important [28]. Goldman [29] and others have also found that longer time intervals from diagnosis to transplant in CML is associated with increased mortality. Davies et al. [30] found that older age had an adverse effect on survival for unrelated donor bone marrow transplantation. McGlave et al. [31] found that transplant in chronic phase, transplant within 1 year of diagnosis, younger recipient age, and a cytomegalovirus seronegative recipient were all associated with improved disease-free survival. Algara et al. [32] confirmed that lower KPS was related to higher risk of early death. TBI is an important treatment that can affect the survival time for unrelated marrow transplantation. Dini et al. [33] reported that a TBI containing regimen led to higher disease-free survival.

TABLE 18.5:   Checking the proportional hazards assumption for the CML data.

Variable	Rho	Chi-sq	P
Disease grade	0.01	0.01	0.93
Donor age category	0.14	4.84	0.03
Donor CMV status	0.01	0.02	0.90
Disease Stage	−0.01	0.03	0.85
Donor gender	0.03	0.17	0.68
HLA matching overall	−0.06	0.58	0.45
HLA matching gvh	0.00	0.00	0.97
HLA matching hvg	0.06	0.87	0.35
Time from dx to tx	0.01	0.01	0.91
Age interaction	−0.22	9.89	0.00
CMV status interaction	0.01	0.03	0.86
Gender interaction	−0.03	0.20	0.66
KPS	−0.05	0.56	0.45
Recipient age category	0.15	4.79	0.03
Recipient CMV status	−0.03	0.20	0.65
Caucasian(recipient)	0.02	0.11	0.74
Black (recipient)	0.00	0.00	0.95
Hispanic (recipient)	−0.00	0.00	0.99
Recipient gender	0.07	1.03	0.31
TBI conditioning	0.02	0.12	0.73
Global	NA	19.3	0.50

The covariates selected by each method are displayed in Table 18.6. Following the literature, both methods select disease grade, HLA matching, and TBI conditioning as the significant covariates. The Sieve method also selects donor and recipient age, the disease stage, the Karnofsky performance score, and the recipient's gender as significant covariates. Except for the gender of the recipient, these are aligned with covariates seen as important in the literature. The Cox method misses the donor and recipient age as being important, possibly because the association with survival does not appear to satisfy the proportional hazards assumption. The Cox method does identify log(time from diagnosis to transplant) as important while it is missed by the Sieve method. In summary, overall, it seems that the Cox method prefers a more parsimonious model that does not include some variables found to be important in the literature, compared to the Sieve method for this data set.

18.4   Discussion

The LASSO technique for variable selection in the linear model for censored data using the sieve likelihood approach appears to provide a robust alternative to the

TABLE 18.6: Variable selection results for the CML data.

Variable	Sieve Method			Cox Method		
	Coefficient	SE	Z-score	Coefficient	SE	Z-score
Intercept	17.02	—	0	36.26	—	0
Disease grade	−8.85	0.07	−0.12	−0.02	0.01	−0.26
Donor age category	−6.26	0.08	−0.05	0	0	0
Donor CMV status	0	0.09	0	0	0	0
Disease stage	0.38	0.07	0	0	0	0
Donor gender	0	0.11	0	0	0	0
HLA matching overall	0	0.32	0	−0.07	0.02	−1.29
HLA matching GvH	−8.98	0.26	−0.19	0	0	0
HLA matching HvG	0	0.23	0	0	0	0
Time from dx to tx	0	0.08	0	−0.08	0.03	−1.04
Age interaction	0	0.09	0	0	0	0
CMV status interaction	0	0.11	0	0	0	0
Gender interaction	0	0.14	0	0	0	0
KPS	10.43	0.07	0.06	0	0	0
Recipient age category	−14.60	0.09	−0.07	0	0	0
Recipient CMV status	0	0.09	0	0	0	0
Caucasian (recipient)	6.58	0.18	0.04	0	0	0
Blank (recipient)	−18.85	0.15	−0.08	−0.14	0.03	−0.48
Hispanic (recipient)	0	0.14	0	0	0	0
Recipient gender	17.99	0.11	0.14	0	0	0
TBI conditioning	2.1	0.07	0.01	0.27	0.05	0.98

corresponding technique using the partial likelihood under the Cox model, especially for data sets with large sample sizes. In simulations the Sieve method appeared to work well over a variety of error distributions, even in the difficult cases of correlated covariates and a large amount of censoring that have a pronounced deleterious effect on other methods. In applications to real data it appeared to find interpretable models aligned with knowledge in the literature for predicting both brain tumor and chronic myelogenous leukemia prognosis. However, because of its relative computational complexity and nonparametric nature, the Sieve method would not be preferred in situations when the proportional hazards assumption is known to at least approximately hold.

As Tibshirani [9] pointed out, it is important to standardize the covariates in order to penalize them fairly. An appropriate transformation of survival time should also be chosen before applying the Sieve method. Techniques to produce efficient and interpretable plots to address this issue need to be explored in future work.

The Sieve method presented here can be easily extended to other kinds of incomplete data such as interval censoring since the random-sieve likelihood method has been already applied to them [3].

Although the Sieve method can find a model that is consistent theoretically, it is computationally difficult to apply to large sample size data sets with a large number of variables. This is due to the time-consuming nature of finding the maximum over a high-dimensional nonparametric function model space. Further work to speed the program (e.g., taking advantage of theoretical approximations, parallel computing architectures, and faster movement strategies in model space) will thus be the key to increasing its value in practice.

References

[1] Cox D. Regression models and life tables (with discussion). *Journal of the Royal Statistical Society, Series B* 1972; 74: 187–220.

[2] Lee ET and Go OT. Survival analysis in public health research. *Annual Review of Public Health* 1997; 18: 105–134.

[3] Shen XT. Linear regression with current status data. *Journal of the American Statistical Association* 2000; 95(451): 842–852.

[4] Zhao Y. The general linear model for censored data. Department of Statistics, The Ohio State University, Columbus, OH, 2003.

[5] Tibshirani R. Regression shrinkage and selection via the LASSO. *Journal of the Royal Statistical Society Series B-Methodological* 1996; 58(1): 267–288.

[6] Hastie T, Tibshirani R, and Friedman J. *The Elements of Statistical Learning: Data Mining, Inference, and Prediction.* New York: Springer, 2001.

[7] Shimodaira H. A new criterion for selecting models from partially observed data, *Selecting Models from Data: Artificial Intelligence and Statistica IV*, in *Lecture Notes in Statistics*, P Cheeseman and RW Oldford (eds.), pp. 21–29. Springer: Berlin, 1994.

[8] Cavanaugh JE and Shumway RH. An akaike information criterion for model selection in the presence of incomplete data. *Journal of Statistical Planning and Inference* 1998; 67: 45–65.

[9] Tibshirani R. The lasso method for variable selection in the Cox model. *Statistics in Medicine* 1997; 16(4): 385–395.

[10] Miller RG. Least-squares regression with censored data. *Biometrika* 1976; 63 (3): 449–464.

[11] Buckley J and James I. Linear-regression with censored data. *Biometrika* 1979; 66(3): 429–436.

[12] Koul H, Susarla V, and Vanryzin J. Regression-analysis with randomly right-censored data. *Annals of Statistics* 1981; 9(6): 1276–1288.

[13] Miller R and Halpern J. Regression with censored-data. *Biometrika* 1982; 69 (3): 521–531.

[14] Leurgans S. Linear-models, random censoring and synthetic data. *Biometrika* 1987; 74(2): 301–309.

[15] Schmee J and Hahn GJ. Simple method for regression-analysis with censored data. *Technometrics* 1979; 21(4): 417–432.

[16] Heller G and Simonoff JS. A comparison of estimators for regression with a censored response variable. *Biometrika* 1990; 77(3): 515–520.

[17] Prentice RL. Linear rank-tests with right censored data. *Biometrika* 1978; 65(1): 167–179.

[18] Harrington DP and Fleming TR. A class of rank test procedures for censored survival-data. *Biometrika* 1982; 69(3): 553–566.

[19] Lai TZ and Ying Z. Linear rank statistics in regression analysis with censored or truncated data. *Journal of multivariate analysis* 1990; 19: 531–536.

[20] Shen XT, Shi J, and Wong WH. Random sieve likelihood and general regression models. *Journal of the American Statistical Association* 1999; 94(447): 835–846.

[21] Wahba G. Spline bases, regularization, and generalized cross-validation for solving approximation problems with large quantities of noisy data. In *Proceedings of the International Conference on Approximation Theory in Honour of George Lorenz*. Austin, TX: Academic Press, 1980.

[22] Gumbel EJ. *Statistics of Extremes*. New York: Columbia University Press, 1958.

[23] Sung CC, Pearl DK, Coons SW, et al. Gangliosides as diagnostic markers of human astrocytomas and primitive neuroectodermal tumors. *Cancer* 1994; 74 (11): 3010–3022.

[24] Sung CC, Pearl DK, Coons SW, et al. Correlation of ganglioside patterns of primary brain-tumors with survival. *Cancer* 1995; 75(3): 851–859.

[25] Singh LPK, Pearl DK, Franklin TK, et al. Neutral glycolipid composition of primary human brain-tumors. *Molecular and Chemical Neuropathology* 1994; 21(2–3): 241–257.

[26] Comas TC, Tai T, Kimmel D, et al. Immunohistochemical staining for ganglioside gd1b as a diagnostic and prognostic marker for primary human brain tumors. *Neuro-Oncology* 1999; 1(14): 261–267.

[27] Oblinger JL, Pearl DK, Boardman CL, et al. Diagnostic and prognostic value of glycosyl transferase mRNA in glioblastoma multiforme patients. *Neuropathology Applied Neurobiology* 2006; 32(4): 410–418.

[28] Petersdorf EW, Anasetti C, Martin PJ, et al. Limits of HLA mismatching in unrelated hematopoietic cell transplantation. *Blood* 2004; 104(9): 2976–2980.

[29] Goldman JM. Chronic myeloid leukemia. *Current Opinion in Hematology* 1997; 4(4): 277–285.

[30] Davies SM, Shu XO, Blazer BR, et al. Unrelated donor bone marrow transplantation: Influence of HLA A and B incompatibility on outcome. *Blood* 1995; 86(4): 1636–1642.

[31] McGlave PB, Shu XO, Wen WQ, et al. Unrelated donor marrow transplantation for chronic myelogenous leukemia: 9 years' experience of the National marrow donor program. *Blood* 2000; 95(7): 2219–2225.

[32] Algara M, Valls A, Ruiz V, et al. Prognostic factors of early mortality after bone-marrow transplantation in patients with chronic myeloid-leukemia. *Revista Clinica Espanola* 1994; 194(8): 607–612.

[33] Dini G, Lamparelli T, Rondelli R, et al. Unrelated donor marrow transplantation for chronic myelogenous leukaemia. *British Journal of Haematology* 1998; 102(2): 544–552.

Chapter 19

Selecting Optimal Treatments Based on Predictive Factors

Eric C. Polley and Mark J. van der Laan

Contents

19.1   Introduction

With the increasing interest in individualized medicine there is a greater need for robust statistical methods for prediction of optimal treatment based on the patient's characteristics. When evaluating two treatments, one treatment may not be uniformly superior to the other treatment for all patients. A patient characteristic may interact with one of the treatments and change the effect of the treatment on the response. Clinical trials are also collecting more information on the patient. This additional information on the patients combined with the state of the art in model selection allows researchers to build better optimal treatment algorithms.

In this chapter we introduce a methodology for predicting optimal treatment. The methodology is demonstrated first on a simulation and then on a phase III clinical trial in neuro-oncology.

19.2   Predicting Optimal Treatment Based on Baseline Factors

Start with a randomized controlled trial where patients are assigned to one of two treatment arms, $A \in \{0, 1\}$, with $\Pr(A = 1) = \Pi_A$. The main outcome for the trial is defined at a given time point t as $Y = I(T > t)$, where T is the survival time. For example, the main outcome may be the 6 month progression-free rate and T is the progression time. Also collected at the beginning of the trial is a set of baseline covariates W. The baseline covariates may be any combination of continuous and categorical variables. The baseline covariates can be split into prognostic and predictive factors. Prognostic factors are patient characteristics which are associated with the outcome independent of the treatment given, while predictive factors are patient characteristics which interact with the treatment in their association with the outcome. To determine the optimal treatment, a model for how the predictive factors and treatment are related to the outcome needs to be estimated.

The observed data is $O_i = (W_i, A_i, Y_i = I(T_i > t)) \sim P$ for $i = 1, \ldots, n$. For now assume Y is observed for all patients in the trial but this assumption is relaxed in Section 19.3. The optimal treatment given a set of baseline variables is found using the W-specific variable importance parameter:

$$\Psi(W) = E(Y|A = 1, W) - E(Y|A = 0, W) \qquad (19.1)$$

$\Psi(W)$ is the additive risk difference of treatment A for a specific level of the prognostic variables W. The conditional distribution of Y given W is defined as $\{Y|W\} \sim \text{Bernoulli}(\pi_Y)$. The subscript W is assumed on π_Y and left off for clarity of the notation. Adding the treatment variable A into the conditioning statement we define $\{Y|A = 1, W\} \sim \text{Bernoulli}(\pi_{+1})$ and $\{Y|A = 0, W\} \sim \text{Bernoulli}(\pi_{-1})$. Again the subscript W is dropped for clarity but assumed throughout the Chapter. The parameter of interest can be expressed as $\Psi(W) = \pi_{+1} - \pi_{-1}$. For a given value of W, $\Psi(W)$ will fall into one of three intervals with each interval leading to a different treatment decision. The three intervals for $\Psi(W)$ are

1. $\Psi(W) > 0$: indicating a beneficial effect of the intervention $A = 1$

2. $\Psi(W) = 0$: indicating no effect of the intervention A

3. $\Psi(W) < 0$: indicating a harmful effect of the intervention $A = 1$

Knowledge of $\Psi(W)$ directly relates to knowledge of the optimal treatment.

As noted in Ref. [1], the parameter of interest can be expressed as

$$\Psi(W) = E\left(\left(\frac{I(A = 1)}{\Pi_A} - \frac{I(A = 0)}{1 - \Pi_A}\right)Y\Big|W\right) \qquad (19.2)$$

When $\Pi_A = 0.5$, the conditional expectation in Equation 19.2 can be modeled with the regression of $Y(A - (1 - A))$ on W. Let $Z = Y(A - (1 - A))$ and since A and Y are binary variables:

$$Z = \begin{cases} +1 & \text{if } Y = 1 \text{ and } A = 1 \\ 0 & \text{if } Y = 0 \\ -1 & \text{if } Y = 1 \text{ and } A = 0 \end{cases}$$

The observed values of Z follow a multinomial distribution. The parameter $\Psi(W)$ will be high dimensional in most settings and the components of $\Psi(W)$ are effect modifications between W and the treatment A on the response Y. The parameter can be estimated with a model $\Psi(W) = m(W|\beta)$. The functional form of $m(W|\beta)$ can be specified a priori, but since the components of the model represent effect modifications, knowledge of a reasonable model may not be available and we recommend a flexible approach called the super learner (described in Section 19.3) for estimating $\Psi(W)$. In many cases a simple linear model may work well for $m(W|\beta)$, but as the true functional form of $\Psi(W)$ becomes more complex, the super learner gives the researcher flexibility in modeling the optimal treatment function. With the squared error loss function for a specific model $m(W|\beta)$, the parameter estimates are

$$\beta_n = \underset{\beta}{\text{argmin}} \sum_{i=1}^{n} (Z_i - m(W_i|\beta))^2 \tag{19.3}$$

The treatment decision for a new individual with covariates $W = w$ is to treat with $A = 1$ if $m(w|\beta_n) > 0$, otherwise treat with $A = 0$.

A normal super learner model for $m(W|\beta)$ would allow for a flexible relationship between W and Z but these models do not respect the fact that $\Psi(W)$ is bounded between -1 and $+1$. The regression of Z on W does not use the information that the parameter $\Psi(W) = \pi_{+1} - \pi_{-1}$ is bounded between -1 and $+1$. The estimates in Equation 19.3 have a nice interpretation since the model predicts the additive difference in survival probabilities. In proposing an alternative method, we wanted to retain the interpretation of an additive effect measure but incorporate the constrains on the distributions. Starting with the parameter of interest in Equation 19.1 we add a scaling value based on the conditional distribution of Y given W as in

$$\Psi'(W) = \frac{E_P(Y|A = 1, W) - E_P(Y|A = 0, W)}{E_P(Y|W)} = \frac{\pi_{+1} - \pi_{-1}}{\pi_Y} \tag{19.4}$$

Since $\pi_Y = \Pr(Y = 1|W) = \Pr(Z \neq 0|W)$, the new parameter $\Psi'(W) = E(Z|Z \neq 0, W)$. When we restrict the data to the cases with $Z \neq 0$ (i.e., $Y = 1$) the outcome becomes a binary variable and binary regression methods can be implemented. For example, the logistic regression model:

$$\text{logit}(\Pr(Z = 1|Z \neq 0, W)) = m'(W_i|\beta) \tag{19.5}$$

The treatment decision is based on $m'(W_i|\beta_n) > 0$ where β_n is the maximum likelihood estimate for the logistic regression model. With the binary regression setting, we are now incorporating the distribution information in creating the prediction model, but losing information by working on a subset of the data. These trade-offs depend on the probability π_Y and we will evaluate both methods on the trial example below. In Section 19.3 we propose a data-adaptive method for estimating $\Psi(W)$.

19.3   Super Learner

Many methods exist for prediction, but for any given dataset it is not known which method will give the best prediction. A good prediction algorithm should be flexible to the true data generating distribution. One such algorithm is the super learner [2]. The super learner is applied to predict the optimal treatment based on the observed data. The super learner algorithm starts with the researcher selecting a set of candidate prediction algorithms (candidate learners). This list of candidate learners should be selected to cover a wide range of basis functions. The candidate learners are selected prior to analyzing the data; selection of the candidates based on performance on the observed data may introduce bias in the final prediction model. A flow diagram for the super learner algorithm is provided in Figure 19.1. With the candidate learners selected and the data collected, the initial step is to fit all of the candidate learners on the entire dataset and save the predicted values for $\Psi_n(W) = m_j(W|\beta_n)$, where j indexes the candidate learners. The data is then split into V equal sized and mutually exclusive sets as is typically done for cross fivefold validation. Patients in the fifth fold are referred to as the fifth fold validation set, and all patients not in the fifth fold are referred to as the fifth fold training set. For the fifth fold, each candidate learner is fit on the patients in the fifth fold training set and the predicted values for $\Psi(W) = m_j(W|\beta_n)$ for the patients in the fifth fold validation set are saved. This process of training the candidate learners on the out of fold samples and saving the predicted values in the fold is repeated for all V folds. The predictions from all V folds are stacked together in a new data matrix X^v. With the prediction data, regress the observed outcome Z on the columns of X^v,

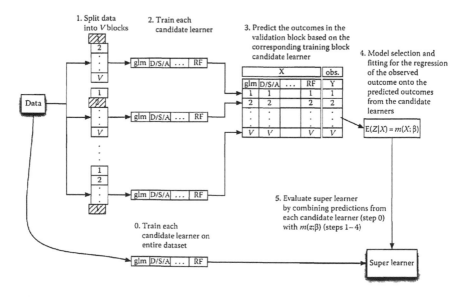

FIGURE 19.1:   Flow diagram for super learner.

which represent the predicted outcomes for each candidate learner. This regression step selects weights for each candidate learner to minimize the cross-validated risk. With the estimates, β_n, from the model $E(Z|X^v) = m(X|\beta)$ the super learner only saves the weights (β_n) and the functional form of the model. The super learner prediction is then based on combining the predictions from each candidate learner on the entire dataset with the weights from the cross-validation step.

19.4   Extensions for Censored Data

In a prospective trial the data may be subject to right censoring. In both methods above, right censoring leads to the outcome Z being missing. The data structure is extended to include an indicator for observing the outcome. Let C be the censoring time (for individuals with an observed outcome we set $C = \infty$). Define $\Delta = I(C > t)$. $\Delta = 1$ when the outcome is observed and $\Delta = 0$ when the outcome is missing. The observed data is the set $(W, A, \Delta, Y \Delta)$. For the first method, we propose using the doubly robust censoring unbiased transformation [3]. The doubly robust censoring unbiased transformation generates a new variable Z^* which is a function of the observed data but has the additional property:

$$E(Z^*|W, \Delta = 1) = E(Z|W)$$

The transformation allows estimation of the parameter $\Psi(W)$ by applying the super learner on the uncensored observations with the transformed variable Z^* as the outcome. The doubly robust censoring unbiased transformation is

$$Z^* = \frac{Z\Delta}{\pi(W)} - \frac{\Delta}{\pi(W)} Q(W) + Q(W) \tag{19.6}$$

where
$$\pi(W) = \Pr(\Delta = 1|W)$$
$$Q(W) = E(Z|W, \Delta = 1)$$

Both $\pi(W)$ and $Q(W)$ need to be estimated from the data. If either $\pi(W)$ or $Q(W)$ is consistently estimated, then the prediction function $E(Z^*|W, \Delta = 1) = m(W|\beta_n)$ is an unbiased estimate for the true parameter $\Psi(W)$. The censoring mechanism $\pi(W)$ can be estimated with a logistic regression model or a binary super learner on the entire dataset. Similarly, $Q(W)$ may be fit with a linear regression model or a super learner, but on the subset of the data with observed values for Z.

For the second method which relies on modeling $E(Z|Z \neq 0, W)$, the main feature was the ability to use the knowledge of the distributions to develop a better model. To retain the binary outcome, the doubly robust censoring unbiased transformation will not work. An alternative method for the right censoring which will retain the binary outcome would be inverse probability of censoring weighting. Inverse probability of censoring weights uses the same $\pi(W)$ as above, but does not incorporate the other nuisance parameter $Q(W)$. When applying the binary super learner for $E(Z|Z \neq 0, W, \Delta = 1)$ the weights $1/\pi(W)$ will be applied for both the candidate learners and the fivefold cross-validation steps. The super learner will minimize the weighted loss function.

19.5   Simulation Example

We first demonstrate the proposed method on a simulation example where the true value of $\Psi(W)$ is known. The baseline variables were all simulated as normally distributed, $W_j \sim N(0, 1), j = 1, \ldots, 10$. The treatment was randomly assigned with $\Pi_A = 0.5$. The true model for the outcome was:

$$\Pr(Y = 1|A, W) = g^{-1}(0.405A - 0.105W_1 + 0.182W_2 + 0.039AW_2$$
$$+ 0.006AW_2W_3 - 0.357AW_4 - 0.020AW_5W_6 - 0.051AW_6) \quad (19.7)$$

where
  $g^{-1}(\cdot)$ is the inverse logit function
  W_j refers to the jth variable in W

The true model was selected to include interactions between the treatment and some of the baseline variables. With knowledge of the true model for the outcome Y, the true value of $\Psi(W)$ is calculated for every individual.

The first method involves the regression of Z on W. We applied the super learner for $m(W|\beta)$. Tenfold cross validation was used for estimating the candidate learner weights in the super learner. The super learner for the first method included five candidate learners. The first candidate was ridge regression [4]. Ridge regression used an internal cross validation to select the penalty parameter. Internal cross validation means the candidate learner performed a fivefold cross-validation procedure within the folds for the super learner. Structurally, when the candidate learner also performs cross validation within the super learner cross validation we have nested cross validation; therefore, we refer to the candidate learner cross validation as internal cross validation. The second candidate was random forests [5]. For the random forest candidate learner, 1000 regression trees were grown. The third candidate was least angle regression [6]. An internal 10-fold cross-validation procedure was used to determine the optimal ratio of the L1 norm of the coefficient vector compared to the L1 norm of the full least squares coefficient vector. The fourth candidate was adaptive regression splines for a continuous outcome [7]. The final candidate was linear regression. Table 19.1 contains reference for the R packages implemented for the candidate learners in the super learner.

The prediction model from the super learner is

$$\Psi_n(W) = -0.01 + 7.24\left(X_n^{\text{ridge}}\right) + 1.16\left(X_n^{\text{rf}}\right) - 0.20\left(X_n^{\text{lars}}\right)$$
$$- 7.07\left(X_n^{\text{lm}}\right) - 0.03\left(X_n^{\text{mars}}\right)$$

TABLE 19.1: R packages for candidate learners.

Method	R Package	Authors
Adaptive regression splines	polspline	Kooperberg
Least angle regression	lars	Efron and Hastie
Penalized logistic	stepPlr	Park and Hastie
Random forests	randomForest	Liaw and Wiener
Ridge regression	MASS	Venables and Ripley

Note: R is available at http://www.r-project.org

where

X_n^j is the predicted value for Z based on the jth candidate learner

$j =$ ridge is the ridge regression model

$j =$ rf is the random forests model

$j =$ lars is the least angle regression model

$j =$ lm is the main effects linear regression model

$j =$ mars is the adaptive regression splines model

The largest weights are for ridge regression and the linear regression model. For example, the estimates for the linear regression model is:

$$X_n^{lm} = 0.06 + 0.02W_1 + 0.01W_2 - 0.03W_3 - 0.07W_4 + 0.01W_5 + 0.05W_6$$
$$- 0.02W_7 - 0.00W_8 - 0.01W_9 - 0.06W_{10}$$

The linear regression model has the largest coefficient on W_4, which is the variable with the strongest effect modification with the treatment in the true model (Equation 19.7). The second largest coefficient is on W_{10} which is a variable unrelated to the outcome. The super learner helps smooth over these errors by having multiple candidate learners. For example, W_{10} has a small coefficient (-0.01) in the ridge regression model. When all the candidates are combined into the final super learner prediction model the spurious effect estimates will often disappear resulting in a better predictor. The third largest coefficient from the linear regression model is on W_6 which is also a strong effect modifier in the true model. To evaluate how the super learner is performing in comparison to the other candidate learners, each candidate learner was also fit as a separate estimate. We looked at two risk values, first the $E(\Psi_n(W) - Z)^2$ which was minimized by each algorithm. For the simulation, the risk $\hat{E}(Z - \Psi(W))^2 = 0.540$ gives a lower bound for the risk $E(\Psi_n(W) - Z)^2$. Since the true $\Psi(W)$ is known in the simulation, the risk $E(\Psi_n(W) - \Psi(W))^2$ was also evaluated. Table 19.2 contains the risk values for the simulation. The super learner achieved the smallest $E(\Psi_n(W) - Z)^2$ and is comparable to MARS and LARS on the risk for the true parameter value $\Psi(W)$.

The super learner for the second method included three candidate learners. The first candidate was adaptive regression splines for polychotomous outcomes [8]. The second candidate was the step-wise penalized logistic regression algorithm [9].

TABLE 19.2: Risk for all candidate learners and the super learner.

	$E(\Psi_n(W) - \Psi(W))^2$	$E(\Psi_n(W) - Z)^2$
Super learner	0.012	0.544
MARS	0.012	0.549
LARS	0.012	0.549
Ridge	0.026	0.558
Linear model	0.028	0.559
Random forests	0.038	0.565

The final candidate was main terms logistic regression. The super learner for the second method is

$$\Psi'_n(W) = -1.20 + 1.43\left(X_n^{\text{poly}}\right) - 0.50\left(X_n^{\text{plr}}\right) + 1.61\left(X_n^{\text{glm}}\right)$$

where
  X_n^j is the predicted value for Z based on the jth candidate learner
  $j = \text{poly}$ is the polyclass adaptive spline model
  $j = \text{plr}$ is the penalized logistic regression model
  $j = \text{glm}$ is the main effects logistic regression model

19.6 Example of Prediction Model on Clinical Trial

A phase III clinical trial was conducted to evaluate a novel treatment for brain metastasis. The study recruited 554 patients with newly diagnosed brain metastasis and the patients were randomized to receive either standard care ($A = 0$) or the novel treatment ($A = 1$). The researchers were interested in determining an optimal treatment to maximize the probability of surviving 6 months from treatment initiation without progression. Of the 554 patients, 246 are censored prior to 6 months. For the 308 patients with an observed 6 month progression time, 130 progressed or died (42.2%). In addition to the treatment and event time data, the researchers collected baseline prognostic and predictive factors on every patient. We apply the super learner to estimate a model for selecting the optimal treatment given a patient's baseline factors. A breakdown of the sample size and treatment allocations available for each method is given in Table 19.3.

19.6.1 Super Learner for Optimal Treatment Decisions

Both methods proposed above were applied to the data. The first method looks for a model of Z on W treating Z as a continuous variable. The second method looks for a model of Z on W conditional on $Z \neq 0$ treating the outcome as binary.

TABLE 19.3: Number of subjects in each treatment arm at enrollment and available for each method.

		A	
	Total	**0**	**1**
Enrolled	554	275	279
Method 1	308	158	150
Method 2	130	67	63

The same super learners from the simulation example above were used here in the trial example. The predicted model for the first method is

$$\Psi_n(W) = -0.01 + 0.02\left(X_n^{\text{ridge}}\right) + 1.21\left(X_n^{\text{rf}}\right) - 0.84\left(X_n^{\text{lars}}\right)$$
$$- 0.28\left(X_n^{\text{lm}}\right) + 0.50\left(X_n^{\text{mars}}\right)$$

where
  X_n^j is the predicted value for Z based on the *j*th candidate learner
  $j = $ ridge is the ridge regression model
  $j = $ rf is the random forests model
  $j = $ lars is the least angle regression model
  $j = $ lm is the main effects linear regression model
  $j = $ mars is the adaptive regression splines model

The coefficient estimates for each candidate learner from the super learner can be interpreted as a weight for each candidate learner in the final prediction model. Random forests has the largest absolute weight. When interpreting the weights, be cautious of the often near collinearity of the columns of X. To evaluate the super learner in comparison to the candidate learners, a 10-fold cross validation of the super learner and each of the candidate learners themselves was used to estimate $E(\Psi_n(W) - Z)^2$. Table 19.4 contains the risk estimates. For the trial example, both the

TABLE 19.4: Tenfold honest cross-validation estimates of $E(\Psi_n(W) - Z)^2$ for the super learner and each of the candidate learners on their own.

Method	Risk
Lars	0.426
Mars	0.426
Super learner	0.445
Ridge regression	0.505
Random forests	0.509
Linear model	0.525

lars algorithm and the mars algorithm outperform the super learner. As observed in the simulation, minimizing the risk $E(\Psi_n(W) - Z)^2$ should directly relate to minimizing the risk $E(\Psi_n(W) - \Psi(W))^2$. These cross-validation estimates may be used to select an optimal final model for the treatment decisions.

The second method evaluates $E(Z|Z \neq 0, W) = m'(W|\beta)$. The estimated super learner model for the second method is

$$\Psi'_n(W) = -0.53 - 0.40(X_n^{\text{poly}}) + 0.55(X_n^{\text{plr}}) + 0.81(X_n^{\text{glm}})$$

where
  X_n^j is the predicted value for Z based on the jth candidate learner
  $j = $ poly is the polyclass adaptive spline model
  $j = $ plr is the penalized logistic regression model
  $j = $ glm is the main effects logistic regression model

To compare the two methods, we created a confidence interval at the mean vector for W. Let $\bar{w}$ be the vector of observed means for the baseline variables using all observations in the trial. Confidence intervals were created based on 1000 bootstrap

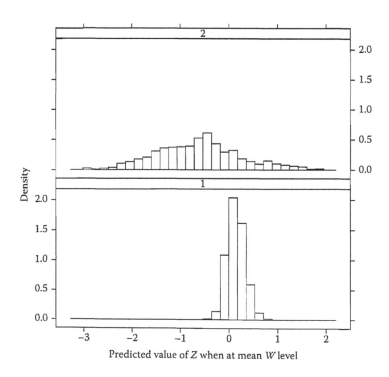

FIGURE 19.2: Histograms from 1000 bootstrap samples for $\Psi'(W = \bar{w})$ and $\Psi(W = \bar{w})$. The number in the title bar refers to the method used.

samples of the entire super learner. The 95% confidence interval for $m(\bar{w}|\beta)$ based on the first method is $(-0.20, 0.52)$. The 95% for $m(\bar{w}|\beta)$ based on the second method is $(-2.23, 1.23)$. Although the second method is able to use the distributional information, the penalty for the smaller sample size is great (308 patients for the first method down to 130 patients for the second method). As can be seen in Figure 19.2, the second method has a wide confidence interval compared to the first method.

19.7   Variable Importance Measure

An additional feature of having a good prediction model is better variable importance measures. The variables in $E(Z|W)$ are effect modifications and when applying the targeted maximum likelihood estimation (tMLE) variable importance measure [10] the results will be causal effect modification importance measures. The targeted maximum likelihood effect modification variable importance allows the researcher to focus on each variable in W individually while adjust for the other variables in W. An initial variable importance estimate is based on an univariate regression, $Z^* = \beta_{0j} + \beta_{1j}W_j$, $j = 1, \ldots, p$ where p is the number of baseline covariates in W. The top five baseline variables based on the ranks of the univariate p-values is presented in Table 19.5. The top unadjusted effect modification variable is an indicator of whether the patients lives in the United States or Europe, followed

TABLE 19.5:   Top five effect modifiers based on univariate regression, LARS, and super learner with targeted maximum likelihood. The standard error was based on a bootstrap with 1000 samples.

Method	Baseline Variable	Effect	p-Value
Univariate regression	United States versus Europe	−0.222	0.007
	RPA class 2	−0.229	0.017
	Primary tumor control	0.165	0.052
	Extracranial mets	−0.133	0.069
	Age > 65 years	−0.157	0.075
LARS	United States versus Europe	−0.124	0.350
	Primary tumor control	0.080	0.405
	Age > 65 years	−0.050	0.412
	Extracranial mets	−0.028	0.413
	Squamous cell	0.034	0.419
tMLE	Mets Dx > 6 Mo	0.864	<0.001
	Squamous cell	1.012	<0.001
	Adeno carcinoma	0.129	0.007
	Extracranial mets	−0.102	0.022
	Caucasian	0.172	0.035

by an indicator for the patients being in RPA class 2, an indicator for the primary tumor being controlled, an indicator for extracranial metastasis, and finally an indicator for the patient's age greater than 65 years. The top five baseline variables from the LARS procedure are similar to those from the univariate regression with the exception of Squamous cell indicator replacing the RPA class 2 indicator. For the tMLE variable importance, the effect of W_j on Z is adjusted by all other covariates in W. Let $W_{(-j)}$ be all covariates in W excluding the jth variable. The targeted maximum likelihood variable importance measure as outlined in Ref. [11] was then applied using the predictions from the super learner as the initial estimate of $E(Z|W)$. The targeted effect modification parameter is then:

$$\psi_j = E(E(Z|W_j = 1, W_{(-j)}) - E(Z|W_j = 0, W_{(-j)})), \quad j = 1, \ldots, p \qquad (19.8)$$

The top five baseline variables are presented in Table 19.5. The effect estimates from the tMLE procedure can be considered causal effect modifiers. Only extracranial mets appears in both the adjusted and unadjusted top five list, although Squamous cell indicator does appear in both the LARS procedure and the tMLE procedure. The top variable (Mets Dx > 6 Mo) is an indicator for the metastasis diagnosis occurring greater than 6 months after previous cancer. The tMLE list contains two indicators for histology of the tumor cells (Squamous and Adeno carcinoma) suggesting that some tumor types my respond better to the treatment compared to others. Comparing the variable importance lists, the indicator for the patient being in the United States compared to Europe is on top of the list for the univariate regression and the LARS model, but absent from the tMLE list. There is no biological evidence for geographical location to interact with the treatment in this trial. The variable importance based on targeted maximum likelihood is able to appropriately adjust for the confounding on the other variables in W and remove the United States versus Europe indicator from the list of top variables. The variable importance list from the tMLE has a better interpretation and is informative as to which patient characteristics have a causal interaction with the treatment.

19.8   Discussion

Two methods were proposed for predicting the optimal treatment based on baseline factors. The first method involves modeling Z on W disregarding the knowledge that $E(Z|W)$ is bounded between -1 and $+1$. The second method incorporates the bounds, but does so at a cost in sample size by modeling $E(Z|Z \neq 0, W)$. The second method predicts a scaled version of the parameter of interest, and so is still valid for making treatment decisions. In the simulation and trial example presented here, the loss of sample size in the second method greatly increased the variability of the final prediction. But both the simulation and trial example had a high fraction of patients with $Z = 0$ (equivalently, $Y = 0$). The second method may outperform the first method in settings where $\Pr(Y=0)$ is very small. For the examples presented here, no problems were observed with the first method not respecting the bounds on $E(Z|W)$.

In the trial example, the super learner did perform better than the main terms linear regression based on the estimate of the risk $E(\Psi_n(W) - Z)^2$. Even though the super learner has shown to have excellent performance across a range of simulations [2,12] and in various of our data analyses in breast cancer research, there is a risk that the super learner will result in a slight over-fit. In the data analysis we observed that the super learner was ranked third, but competitive with the top two candidate learners, LARS and MARS. We have also proposed an extension to the super learner outlined here to adaptively select the number of candidates [13] so that the weaker candidates are not selected, which we believe will protect the super learner against possible over-fitting, but this was not implemented in the current data analysis yet.

We observed that the difference in sample size between the two methods may make the second method unusable in this example, but the two methods also differed in the treatment of right censoring. The first method incorporated the doubly robust censoring unbiased transformation while the second method used the inverse probability of censoring weights. If the model for $Q(W)$ was correctly specified, but the model for the censoring mechanism was not consistently estimating $\pi(W)$, the doubly robust estimator would still be unbiased but the inverse probability of censoring weighted method will be biased. Alternatively, if $\pi(W)$ was correctly specified, but $Q(W)$ was inconsistent, then both methods will be unbiased. The doubly robust transformation gives the researcher two chances to correct the nuisance parameters, while the inverse weighting method relies solely on the model for $\pi(W)$. When there is uncertainty regarding the model for the censoring mechanism, the doubly robust transformation is preferred.

The methods presented above are not limited to randomized clinical trials. Optimal treatment prediction models could also be estimated from observational or registry datasets. As long as the variables needed to estimate $\Pr(A = 1|W))$ are collected in the study the above methods easily extend to the non randomized setting. Registry datasets are often larger than randomized trials and therefore have more power to detect the interaction effects necessary for predict optimal treatments.

References

[1] M. J. van der Laan. Statistical inference for variable importance. *The International Journal of Biostatistics*, 2(2), 2006.

[2] M. J. van der Laan, E. C. Polley, and A. E. Hubbard. Super learner. *Statistical Applications in Genetics and Molecular Biology*, 6(25), 2007.

[3] D. Rubin and M. J. van der Laan. Doubly robust censoring unbiased transformations. Technical report 208, Division of Biostatistics, University of California, Berkeley, CA, 2006.

[4] A. E. Hoerl and R. W. Kennard. Ridge regression: Biased estimation for nonorthogonal problems. *Technometrics*, 12(3):55–67, 1970.

[5] L. Breiman. Random forests. *Machine Learning*, 45:5–32, 2001.

[6] B. Efron, T. Hastie, I. Johnstone, and R. Tibshirani. Least angle regression. *Annals of Statistics*, 32(2):407–499, 2004.

[7] J. H. Friedman. Multivariate adaptive regression splines. *Annals of Statistics*, 19(1):1–141, 1991.

[8] C. Kooperberg, S. Bose, and C. J. Stone. Polychotomous regression. *Journal of the American Statistical Association*, 92:117–127, 1997.

[9] M. Y. Park and T. Hastie. l_1-regularization path algorithm for generalized linear models. *Journal of the Royal Statistical Society, Series B*, 69(4):659–677, 2007.

[10] M. J. van der Laan and D. Rubin. Targeted maximum likelihood learning. *International Journal of Biostatistics*, 2(11), 2006.

[11] O. Bembom, M. L. Petersen, S. Rhee, W. J. Fessel, S. E. Sinisi, R. W. Shafer, and M. J. van der Laan. Biomarker discovery using targeted maximum likelihood estimation: Application to the treatment of antiretroviral resistant HIV infection. Technical report 221, Division of Biostatistics, University of California, Berkeley, CA, 2007.

[12] S. E. Sinisi, E. C. Polley, M. L. Petersen, S. Y. Rhee, and M. J. van der Laan. Super learning: An application to the prediction of HIV-1 drug resistance. *Statistical Applications in Genetics and Molecular Biology*, 6(7), 2007.

[13] E. C. Polley and M. J. van der Laan. Adaptive selection of the functional form for the super learner, in preparation, 2009.

Chapter 20

Application of Time-to-Event Methods in the Assessment of Safety in Clinical Trials

Kelly L. Moore and Mark J. van der Laan

Contents

20.1   Introduction

Safety analysis in randomized controlled trials (RCTs) involves estimation of the treatment effect on the numerous adverse events (AEs) that are collected in the study. RCTs are typically designed and powered for efficacy rather than safety. Even when assessment of AEs is a major objective of study, the trial size is generally not increased to improve likelihood of detecting AEs [1]. As a result, power is an important concern in the analysis of the effect of treatment on AEs in RCTs [2].

Typically in an RCT, crude incidences of each AE are reported at some fixed end point such as the end of study [3–5]. These crude estimates often ignore missing observations that frequently occur in RCTs due to early patient withdrawals [6]. A review of published RCTs in major medical journals found that the censored data are often inadequately accounted for in their statistical analyses [7]. A crude estimator that ignores censoring can be highly biased when the proportion of dropouts differs between treatment groups (see Ref. [3] for examples).

The crude incidence is an important consideration in the evaluation of safety for very rare, severe, or unexpected AEs. Such AEs require clinical evaluation for each case and are not the focus of this chapter. Instead, we focus on those AEs that are routinely collected in RCTs and most often are not associated with a prespecified hypothesis. These AEs are typically reported as an observed rate with a confidence interval or p-value.

Patient reporting of AEs occurrence usually occurs at many intervals throughout the study often collected at follow-up interviews rather than only at a single fixed end point. As such, time-to-event methods that exploit these data structures may provide further insight into the safety profile of the drug. The importance of considering estimators of AE rates that account for time due to differential lengths of exposure and follow-up is discussed in Ref. [8]. Furthermore, in most RCTs in oncology, most if not all patients suffer from some AEs [9] and thus investigators may be interested in the probability of the occurrence of a given AE by a certain time rather than simply the incidence. Time-to-event analysis techniques may be more sensitive than crude estimates in that they readily handle missing observations that frequently occur in RCT due to early patient withdrawals. For example, in Ref. [10] AEs from the Beta-Blocker Heart Attack Trial were analyzed by comparing distributions of the time to the first AE in the two treatment arms. The results of this analysis were contrasted to the cross-sectional crude percentage analysis and were found to be more sensitive in detecting a difference by taking into account the withdrawals. A vast amount of literature exists for time-to-event analysis but these methods are often not applied to the analysis of AEs in RCTs. A general review of survival analysis methods in RCTs (without a particular focus on AEs) is provided in Ref. [11].

In this chapter, we focus on the estimation of treatment-specific survival at a fixed end point for right-censored survival outcomes using targeted maximum likelihood estimation [12]. Survival is estimated based on a hazard fit and thus the time-dependent nature of the data are exploited. There are two main goals of the methodology presented in this chapter over unadjusted crude proportions and

Kaplan–Meier estimators. The first is to provide an estimator that exploits covariates to improve efficiency in the estimation of treatment-specific survival at fixed end points. The second is to provide a consistent estimator in the presence of informative censoring.

20.2 Motivation and Outline

Consider the estimation of the effect of treatment on a particular AE at some fixed end point in the study. From estimation theory [13], it is known that the nonparametric maximum likelihood estimator (MLE) is the efficient estimator of the effect of interest. In most RCTs, data are collected on baseline (pretreatment) covariates in addition to the treatment and the AEs of interest. The unadjusted or crude estimator is defined as the difference in proportions of the AEs between treatment groups. This estimator ignores the covariates and is thus not equivalent to the full MLE. It follows that application of the unadjusted estimator can lead to a loss in estimation efficiency (precision) in practice.

Conflicting results in initial applications of covariate adjustment in RCTs for estimating the treatment effect for fixed end-point efficacy studies were found. For continuous outcomes using linear models for adjustment demonstrated gains in precision over the unadjusted estimate [14]. However, adjustment using logistic models for binary outcomes was shown to actually reduce precision and inflate point estimates [15,16].

This apparent contradiction was resolved through the application of estimation function methodology [17,18] and targeted maximum likelihood estimation [19]. In these references consistent estimators that do not require parametric modeling assumptions were provided and shown to be more efficient than the unadjusted estimator, even with binary outcomes. It just so happens that the coefficient for the treatment variable in a linear regression that contains no interactions with treatment coincides with the efficient estimating function estimator and thus the targeted MLE. This fortunate property does not hold for the logistic regression setting, i.e., the exponentiated coefficient for treatment from the logistic regression model does not equal the unadjusted odds ratio. This conditional estimator does not correspond to the marginal estimator in general and in particular not in the binary case. The efficient estimate of the marginal (i.e., unconditional) effect obtained from the conditional regression is the weighted average of the conditional effect of treatment on the outcome given covariates according to the distribution of the covariates.

With this principle of developing covariate adjusted estimators that do not require parametric modeling assumptions for consistency in mind, in this chapter, we provide a method for covariate adjustment in RCT for the estimation of treatment-specific survival at a fixed end point for right-censored survival outcomes. Thereby we can estimate a comparison of survival between treatment groups at a fixed end point that is some function of the two treatment-specific survival estimates.

Examples of such parameters are provided in Section 20.4 such as the marginal additive difference in survival at a fixed end point. Under no or uninformative censoring, the estimator provided in this chapter does not require any additional parametric modeling assumptions. Under informative censoring, the estimator is consistent under consistent estimation of the censoring mechanism or the conditional hazard for survival.

It is important to note that the conditional hazard on which the estimate is based is not meant to infer information about subgroup (conditional) effects of treatment. By averaging over the covariates that have terms in the hazard model, we obtain a marginal or unconditional estimate. The methodology presented in this chapter can be extended to the estimation of subgroup-specific effects however we focus only on marginal (unconditional) treatment effects on survival at fixed end point(s).

We also note that the methodology can be extended to provide a competitor test to the ubiquitous logrank test. Methods have been proposed for covariate adjustment to improve power over the logrank test [20–22]. These are tests for an average effect of treatment over time. Our efficiency results are not in comparison to these methods but rather to the treatment-specific Kaplan–Meier estimate at that fixed end point.

In itself treatment-specific survival at a fixed end point, and thereby the effect of treatment on survival at that end point can provide useful information about the given AE of interest. This is a very common measure to report, however, most of the currently applied estimation approaches ignore covariates and censoring and do not usually exploit the time-dependent nature of the data [3,4,5,6].

We present our method of covariate adjustment under the framework of targeted maximum likelihood estimation originally introduced in Ref. [12]. Specifically, this chapter is outlined as follows. We first begin with a brief introduction to targeted maximum likelihood estimation in Section 20.3. We then outline the data, model, and parameter(s) of interest in Section 20.4. The application of targeted maximum likelihood estimation to our parameter of interest with its statistical properties and inference are presented in Section 20.5. In Section 20.6, we present a simulation study to demonstrate the efficiency gains of the proposed method over the current methods in an RCT under no censoring and uninformative censoring. Furthermore, under informative censoring we demonstrate the bias that arises with the standard estimator in contrast to the consistency of our proposed estimator. The targeted MLE requires estimation of an initial conditional hazard. Methods for fitting this initial hazard as well as the censoring mechanism are provided in Section 20.7. In Section 20.8, we outline the inverse weighting assumption for the censoring mechanism. Alternative estimators and their properties are briefly outlined in Section 20.9. AE data are multivariate in nature in that many AEs are collected and analyzed in any given RCT. In Section 20.10, we outline the multiple testing issues involved in the analysis of such data. Section 20.11 provides extensions to the methodology including time-dependent covariates, and postmarket safety analysis. Finally, we conclude with a discussion in Section 20.12.

20.3 Introduction to Targeted Maximum Likelihood Estimation

Traditional maximum likelihood estimation aims for a trade-off between bias and variance for the whole density of the observed data O, whereas investigators are typically interested in a specific parameter of the density of O, rather than the whole density itself. In this section, we discuss the algorithm generally, for technical details about this estimation approach we refer the reader to its seminal article [12].

Define a model $\mathcal{M}$ which is a collection of probability distributions of $O{\sim}p_0$ and let $\hat{p}$ be an initial estimator of p_0. We are interested in a particular parameter of the data, $\psi_0 = \psi(p_0)$. To estimate this parameter, the targeted maximum likelihood algorithm's goal is to find a density $\hat{p}* \in \mathcal{M}$ that solves the efficient influence curve estimating equation for the parameter of interest that results in a bias reduction in comparison to the maximum likelihood estimate $\psi(\hat{p})$ but also to find $\hat{p}*$ that increases the log-likelihood relative to $\hat{p}$.

To estimate this $\hat{p}*$, the algorithm finds a fluctuation of the initial $\hat{p}$ that results in a maximum change in ψ by constructing a path denoted by $\hat{p}(\varepsilon)$ through $\hat{p}$ where ε is a free parameter. The score of this path at $\varepsilon = 0$ equals the efficient influence curve. The optimal fluctuation is obtained by maximizing the likelihood of the data over ε and applying this fluctuation to $\hat{p}$ to obtain $\hat{p}^1$. This is the first step of the targeted maximum likelihood algorithm and the process is iterated until the fluctuation is essentially zero. The final step of the algorithm gives the targeted maximum likelihood estimate $\hat{p}*$ which solves the efficient influence curve estimating equation and thus the resulting substitution estimator $\psi(\hat{p}*)$ inherits the desirable properties of the estimating function based methodology, namely local efficiency and double robustness [13]. It is also completely based on the maximum likelihood principle, resulting in robust finite sample behavior.

Targeted MLEs not only share the optimal properties with estimating equation estimators, but they also overcome some of their drawbacks. Estimating equation methodology requires that the efficient influence curve can be represented as an estimating function in terms of a parameter of interest and nuisance parameters which is not required by the targeted maximum likelihood algorithm since it simply solves the efficient influence curve estimating equation in p itself. Estimating equation estimators require external estimation of the nuisance parameters, while in the targeted maximum likelihood estimation procedure the estimator of the parameter of interest and the nuisance parameters are compatible with a single density estimator. Finally, estimating equation methodology lacks a criterion for selecting among candidate solutions in situations where multiple solutions in the parameter of interest exist, where the targeted maximum likelihood estimation approach can use the likelihood criterion to select among the targeted MLEs indexed by initial density estimators.

20.4   Data, Model, and Parameter of Interest

We assume that in the study protocol, each patient is monitored at K equally spaced clinical visits. At each visit, M AEs are evaluated as having occurred or not occurred. We focus on the first occurrence of the AE and thus let T represent the first visit when the AE reported as occurring and thus can take values $\{1, \ldots, K\}$. The censoring time C is the first visit when the subject is no longer enrolled in the study. Let $A \in \{0, 1\}$ represent the treatment assignment at baseline and W represents a vector of baseline covariates. The observed data are given by $O = (\tilde{T}, \Delta, A, W) \sim p_0$ where $\tilde{T} = \min(T, C)$, $\Delta = I(T \leq C)$ is the indicator that that subject was not censored and p_0 denotes the density of O. The conditional hazard is given by $\lambda_0(\cdot | A, W)$ and the corresponding conditional survival is given by $S_0(\cdot | A, W)$. We present the methodology for estimation of the treatment effect for a single AE out of the M total AE collected. This procedure would be repeated for each of the M AE. For multiplicity considerations see Section 20.10.

Let T_1 represent a patient's time to the occurrence of an AE had the possibly contrary to fact been assigned to the treatment group and let T_0 likewise represent the time to the occurrence of the AE had the patient been assigned to the control group.

Let $\mathcal{M}$ be the class of all densities of O with respect to an appropriate dominating measure where $\mathcal{M}$ is nonparametric up to possible smoothness conditions. Let our parameter of interest be represented by $\Psi(p_0)$. Specifically, we aim to estimate the following treatment-specific parameters,

$$P_0 \to \Psi_1(p_0)(t_k) = \Pr(T_1 > t_k) = E_0(S_0(t_k | A = 1, W)), \qquad (20.1)$$

and

$$P_0 \to \Psi_0(p_0)(t_k) = \Pr(T_0 > t_k) = E_0(S_0(t_k | A = 0, W)), \qquad (20.2)$$

where the subscript for Ψ denotes the treatment group, either 0 or 1. In order to estimate the effect of treatment A on survival T we can thereby estimate a parameter that is some combination of $\Pr(T_1 > t_k)$ and $\Pr(T_0 > t_k)$. Examples include the marginal log hazard of survival, the marginal additive difference in the probability of survival, and the marginal log relative risk of survival at a fixed time t_k given, respectively, by

$$P_0 \to \Psi_{\mathrm{HZ}}(p_0)(t_k) = \log\left(\frac{\log(\Pr(T_1 > t_k))}{\log(\Pr(T_0 > t_k))}\right), \qquad (20.3)$$

$$P_0 \to \Psi_{\mathrm{AD}}(p_0)(t_k) = \Pr(T_1 > t_k) - \Pr(T_0 > t_k), \qquad (20.4)$$

and

$$P_0 \to \Psi_{\mathrm{RR}}(p_0)(t_k) = \log\left(\frac{\Pr(T_1 > t_k)}{\Pr(T_0 > t_k)}\right). \qquad (20.5)$$

We note that if one averaged $\Psi_{\mathrm{HZ}}(p_0)(t_k)$ over t, this would correspond with the Cox proportional hazards parameter and thus the parameter tested by the logrank test. However, we focus only on the t_k-specific parameter in this chapter.

20.5 Targeted Maximum Likelihood Estimation of Marginal Treatment-Specific Survival at a Fixed End Point

Consider an initial fit $\hat{p}^0$ of the density of the observed data O identified by a hazard fit $\hat{\lambda}^0(t|A, W)$, the distribution of A identified by $\hat{g}^0(1|W)$ and $\hat{g}^0(0|W) = 1 - \hat{g}^0(1|W)$, the censoring mechanism $\hat{G}^0(t|A, W)$ and the marginal distribution of W being the empirical probability distribution of $W_1, \ldots, W_n$. In an RCT, treatment is randomized and $\hat{g}^0(1|W) = \frac{1}{n}\sum_{i=1}^{n} A_i$.

Let the survival time be discrete and let the initial hazard fit $\hat{\lambda}(t|A, W)$ be given by a logistic regression model,

$$\mathrm{logit}(\hat{\lambda}(t|A, W)) = \hat{\alpha}(t) + m(A, W|\hat{\beta}),$$

where m is some function of A and W. The targeted maximum likelihood estimation algorithm updates this initial fit by adding to it the term $\varepsilon h(t, A, W)$, i.e.,

$$\mathrm{logit}(\hat{\lambda}(\varepsilon)(t|A, W)) = \hat{\alpha}(t) + m(A, W|\hat{\beta}) + \varepsilon h(t, A, W). \qquad (20.6)$$

The algorithm selects $h(t, A, W)$ such the score for this hazard model at $\varepsilon = 0$ is equal to the projection of the efficient influence curve on scores generated by the parameter $\lambda(t|A, W))$ in the nonparametric model for the observed data assuming only coarsening at random (CAR).

The general formula for this covariate $h(t, A, W)$ for updating an initial hazard fit was provided in Ref. [23] and is given by

$$h(t, A, W) = \frac{D^{\mathrm{FULL}}(A, W, t|\hat{p}) - E_{\hat{p}}[D^{\mathrm{FULL}}(A, W, T|\hat{p})|A, W, T > t)]}{\bar{G}(t_-|A, W)}, \qquad (20.7)$$

where D^{FULL} is the efficient influence curve of the parameter of interest in the model in which there is no right censoring. This is also the optimal estimating function in this model. This full data estimating function for $\Psi_1(p_0)$ (t_k) provided in Equation 20.1 is given by

$$D_1^{\mathrm{FULL}}(T, A, W|p)(t_k)$$
$$= [I(T > t_k) - S(t_k|A, W)]\frac{I(A = 1)}{g(1|W)} + S(t_k|1, W) - \psi_1(p), \qquad (20.8)$$

and for $\Psi_0(p_0)$ (t_k) provided in Equation 20.2 it is given by

$$D_0^{\mathrm{FULL}}(T, A, W|p)(t_k)$$

$$= [I(T > t_k) - S(t_k|A, W)]\frac{I(A = 0)}{g(0|W)} + S(t_k|0, W) - \psi_0(p). \qquad (20.9)$$

To obtain the specific covariates for targeting the parameters $\Psi_1(p_0)$ and $\Psi_0(p_0)$, the full data estimating functions provided in Equations 20.8 and 20.9 at $t = t_k$ are substituted into Equation 20.7. Evaluating these substitutions gives the covariates,

$$h_1(t, A, W) = -\frac{I(A = 1)}{g(1)\bar{G}(t_-|A, W)} \frac{S(t_k|A, W)}{S(t|A, W)} I(t \le t_k), \qquad (20.10)$$

and

$$h_0(t, A, W) = -\frac{I(A = 0)}{g(0)\bar{G}(t_-|A, W)} \frac{S(t_k|A, W)}{S(t|A, W)} I(t \le t_k), \qquad (20.11)$$

for the treatment-specific parameters $\Psi_1(p_0)(t_k)$ and $\Psi_0(p_0)(t_k)$, respectively.

Finding $\hat{\varepsilon}$ in the updated hazard provided in Equation 20.6 to maximize the likelihood of the observed data can be done in practice by fitting a logistic regression in the covariates $m(A, W|\hat{\beta})$ and $h(t, A, W)$. The coefficient for $m(A, W|\hat{\beta})$ is fixed at 1 and the intercept is set to 0 and thus the whole regression is not refit, rather only ε is estimated. These steps for evaluating $\hat{\varepsilon}$ correspond with a single iteration of the targeted maximum likelihood algorithm. In the second iteration, the updated $\hat{\lambda}^1(t|A, W)$ now plays the role of the initial fit and the covariate $h(t, A, W)$ is then reevaluated with the updated $\hat{S}^1(t|A, W)$ based on $\hat{\lambda}^1(t|A, W)$. In the third iteration, $\hat{\lambda}^2(t|A, W)$ is fit and the procedure is iterated until $\hat{\varepsilon}$ is essentially zero. The final hazard fit at the last iteration of the algorithm is denoted by $\hat{\lambda}^*(t|A, W)$ with the corresponding survival fit given by $\hat{S}^*(t|A, W)$.

As we are estimating two treatment-specific parameters, we could either carry out the iterative updating procedure for each parameter separately or update the hazard fit simultaneously. To update the fit simultaneously, both covariates are added to the initial fit, i.e.,

$$\mathrm{logit}(\hat{\lambda}(\varepsilon)(t|A, W)) = \hat{\alpha}(t) + m(A, W|\hat{\beta}) + \varepsilon_1 h_1(t, A, W) + \varepsilon_2 h_0(t, A, W).$$

The iterative procedure is applied by now estimating two coefficients in each iteration as described above until both ε_1 and ε_2 are essentially zero.

Finally, the targeted maximum likelihood estimates of the probability of surviving past time t_k for subjects in treatment arms 1 and 0 given by $\Psi_1(p_0)(t_k)$ and $\Psi_0(p_0)(t_k)$ are computed by

$$\hat{\psi}_1^*(t_k) = \frac{1}{n} \sum_{i=1}^{n} \hat{S}^*(t_k|1, W_i),$$

and

$$\hat{\psi}_0^*(t_k) = \frac{1}{n} \sum_{i=1}^{n} \hat{S}^*(t_k|0, W_i).$$

20.5.1   Rationale for Updating Only Initial Hazard

The initial fit $\hat{p}^0$ of p_0 is identified by $\hat{\lambda}^0(t|A, W)$, $\hat{g}^0(A|W)$, $\hat{G}^0(t|A, W)$, and the marginal distribution of W. However, the algorithm only updates $\hat{\lambda}^0(t|A, W)$. Assuming CAR the density of the observed data p factorizes into the marginal distribution of W given by p_W, the treatment mechanism $g(A|W)$, the conditional probability of censoring up to time t given by $\bar{G}(t|A, W)$, and the product over time of the conditional hazard at $T=t$ given by $\lambda(t|A, W)$. This factorization implies the orthogonal decomposition of functions of O in the Hilbert space $L^2(p)$. We can thus apply this decomposition to the efficient influence curve $D(O|p)$. As shown in Ref. [13] $D(O|p)$ is orthogonal to the tangent space T_{CAR} (p) of the censoring and treatment mechanisms. Thus, the components corresponding with $g(A|W)$ and $\bar{G}(t|A, W)$ are zero. This leaves the nonzero components p_W and $\lambda(t|A, W)$. We choose the initial empirical distribution for W to estimate p_W which is the nonparametric maximum likelihood estimate for p_W and is therefore not updated. Thus, the only element that does require updating is $\hat{\lambda}^0(t|A, W)$.

The efficient influence curve for $\Psi_1(p_0)(t_k)$ can be represented as

$$D_1(p_0) = \sum_{t<=t_k} h_1(g_0, G_0, S_0)(t, A, W)[I(\tilde{T} = t, \Delta = 1) - I(\tilde{T} >= t)$$

$$\lambda_0(t|A = 1, W)] + S_0(t_k|A = 1, W) - \Psi_1(p_0)(t_k), \tag{20.12}$$

where $S_0(t_k|A=1, W)$ is a transformation of $\lambda_0(t|A=1, W)$. This representation demonstrates the orthogonal decomposition described above. The empirical mean of the second component of $D_1(p_0)$ given by $S_0(t_k|A=1, W) - E_0 S_0(t_k|A=1, W)$ is always solved by using empirical distribution to estimate the marginal distribution of W. Thus, the targeted MLE solves this second component. The first component, the covariate times the residuals, is solved by performing the iterative targeted maximum likelihood algorithm with logistic regression fit of the discrete hazard $\lambda_0(t|A, W)$. We note that similarly, the efficient influence curve for $\Psi_0(p_0)(t_k)$ can be represented as

$$D_0(p_0) = \sum_{t<=t_k} h_0(g_0, G_0, S_0)(t|A, W)[I(\tilde{T} = t, \Delta = 1) - I(\tilde{T} >= t)$$

$$\lambda_0(t|A = 0, W)] + S_0(t_k|A = 0, W) - \Psi_0(p_0)(t_k) \tag{20.13}$$

20.5.2   Statistical Properties

The targeted maximum likelihood estimate $\hat{p}^* \in \mathcal{M}$ of p_0 solves the efficient influence curve which is the optimal estimating equation for the parameter of interest. It can be shown that $E_0 D_1(p_0) = E_0 D_1(S, g, G) = 0$ if either $S = S(\cdot|A, W)$ (and thus $\lambda(\cdot|A, W)$) is consistently estimated or $g_0(A|W)$ and $\bar{G}_0(\cdot|A, W)$ are consistently estimated. When the treatment is assigned completely at random as in an RCT, the treatment mechanism is known and $g(A|W) = g(A)$. Thus consistency of $\hat{\psi}_1^*(t_k)$ in an RCT relies on only consistent estimation of $\bar{G}_0(\cdot|A, W)$ or $S(\cdot|A, W)$. When there is no censoring or censoring is missing completely at random (MCAR), $\hat{\psi}_1^*(t_k)$ is consistent even when the estimator $\hat{S}(\cdot|A, W)$ of $S(\cdot|A, W)$ is inconsistent (e.g., if it relies on a misspecified model). One is hence not concerned with estimation bias with this method in an RCT. Under informative or missing at random (MAR) censoring, if $\bar{G}_0(\cdot|A, W)$ is consistently estimated then $\hat{\psi}_1^*(t_k)$ is consistent even if $\hat{S}(\cdot|A, W)$ is misspecified. If both are correctly specified then $\hat{\psi}_1^*(t_k)$ is efficient. These same statistical properties also hold for $\hat{\psi}_0^*(t_k)$.

20.5.3   Inference

Let $\hat{p}^*$ represent the targeted maximum likelihood estimate of p_0. One can construct a Wald-type 0.95 confidence interval for $\hat{\psi}_1^*(t_k)$ based on the estimate of the efficient influence curve $D_1(\hat{p}^*)(O)$ where $D_1(p)$ is given by Equation 20.12. The asymptotic variance of $\sqrt{n}(\hat{\psi}_1^*(t_k) - \Psi_1(p_0)(t_k))$ can be estimated with

$$\hat{\sigma}^2 = \frac{1}{n} \sum_{i=1}^{n} D_1^2(\hat{p}^*)(O_i).$$

The corresponding asymptotically conservative Wald-type 0.95 confidence interval is defined as $\hat{\psi}_1^*(t_k) \pm 1.96 \frac{\hat{\sigma}}{\sqrt{n}}$. The null hypothesis $H_0 : \Psi_1(p_0)(t_k) = 0$ can be tested with the test statistic

$$T_n = \frac{\hat{\psi}_1^*(t_k)}{\frac{\hat{\sigma}}{\sqrt{n}}},$$

whose asymptotic distribution is $N(0, 1)$ under the null hypothesis. Similarly, confidence intervals and test statistics for $\Psi_0(p_0)(t_k)$ can be computed based on the estimate of the efficient influence curve $D_0(\hat{p}^*)(O)$ where $D_0(p)$ is given by Equation 20.13.

If our parameter of interest is some function of the treatment-specific survival estimates we can apply the δ-method to obtain the estimate of its influence curve. Specifically, the estimated influence curve for the log hazard of survival, additive difference in survival, and relative risk of survival at t_k provided in Equations 20.3, through 20.5 are, respectively, given by

1. $\Psi_{HZ}(p_0)(t_k) : \frac{1}{\hat{\psi}_1^*(t_k) \log(\hat{\psi}_1^*(t_k))} D_1(\hat{p}^*)(O) - \frac{1}{\hat{\psi}_0^*(t_k) \log(\hat{\psi}_0^*(t_k))} D_1(\hat{p}^*)(O)$

2. $\Psi_{AD}(p_0)(t_k) : D_1(\hat{p}^*)(O) - D_1(\hat{p}^*)(O)$

3. $\Psi_{RR}(p_0)(t_k) : -\frac{1}{1-\hat{\psi}_1^*(t_k)} D_1(\hat{p}^*)(O) + \frac{1}{1-\hat{\psi}_0^*(t_k)} D_1(\hat{p}^*)(O)$

We can again compute confidence intervals and test statistics for these parameters using the estimated influence curve to estimate the asymptotic variance.

As an alternative to the influence curve-based estimates of the asymptotic variance, one can obtain valid inference using the bootstrap procedure.

The inference provided in this section is for the estimates of the treatment effect for a single AE. For multiplicity adjustments for the analysis of a set of AE see Section 20.10.

20.6   Simulation Study

The targeted maximum likelihood estimation procedure was applied to simulated data to illustrate the estimator's potential gains in efficiency. The conditions under which the greatest gains can be achieved over the standard unadjusted estimator were explored in addition to the estimators' performance in the presence of informative censoring.

20.6.1   Simulation Protocol

We simulated 1000 replicates of sample size 300 from the following data generating distribution where time is discrete and takes values $t_k \in \{1, \ldots, 10\}$:

- $\Pr(A = 1) = \Pr(A = 0) = 0.5$

- $W \sim U(0.2, 1.2)$

- $\lambda(t|A, W) = \frac{I(t_k < 10)I(Y(t_k - 1) = 0)}{1 + \exp(-(-3 - A + \beta_w W^2))} + I(t_k = 10)$

- $\lambda_C(t|A, W) = \frac{I(\Delta(t_k - 1) = 0)}{1 + \exp(-(-\gamma_0 - \gamma_1 A - \gamma_2 W))}$

where
$\lambda(t|A, W)$ is the hazard for survival
$\lambda_C(t|A, W)$ is the hazard for censoring

Two different data generating hazards for survival were applied corresponding with two values for β_W. These two values were set to $\beta_W \in \{1, 3\}$ corresponding with correlations between W and failure time of -0.22 and -0.63, respectively. We refer to the simulated data with $\beta_W = 1$ as the weak covariate setting and $\beta_W = 3$ as the strong covariate setting.

Three different types of censoring were simulated, no censoring, MCAR, and MAR. Each type of censoring was applied to the weak and strong covariate settings for a total of six simulation scenarios. For both the weak and strong covariate settings, the MCAR an MAR censoring mechanisms were set such that approximately 33% of the observations were censored. The censoring was generated

TABLE 20.1:   Summary of simulation settings.

Scenario	Censoring	γ	Corr W and T	β_W
1	No censoring	NA	−0.22 (Weak)	1
2	MCAR	(−2.7,0,0)	−0.22 (Weak)	1
3	MAR	(−1.65,0.5,−2)	−0.22 (Weak)	1
4	No censoring	NA	−0.65 (Strong)	3
5	MCAR	(−2,0,0)	−0.65 (Strong)	3
6	MAR	(−1.15,0.5,−2)	−0.65 (Strong)	3

Note: "Corr" is correlation, $\gamma = (\gamma_0, \gamma_1, \gamma_2)$ are the coefficients for the hazard for censoring, and β_W is the coefficient for W in the hazard for survival.

to ensure that $\bar{G}(t|A, W) > 0$ (see Section 20.8 for details of this assumption). If censoring and failure time were tied, the subject was considered uncensored. For a summary of the simulation settings and the specific parameter values, see Table 20.1.

The difference in treatment-specific survival probabilities given by $\psi(t_k) = E_0(S_0(t_k|A = 1, \ W) - S_0(t_k|A = 0, \ W))$ was estimated at each time point $t_k = 1$ through 9. The unadjusted estimator is defined as the difference in the treatment-specific Kaplan–Meier estimators at t_k. The targeted MLE was applied using two different initial hazard fits. The first initial hazard was correctly specified. The second initial hazard was misspecified by including A and W as main terms and an interaction term between A and W. For both initial hazard fits, only time points 1 through 9 were included in the fit as the AE had occurred for all subjects by time point 10 and thus the hazard was one at $t_k = 10$. In the MCAR censoring setting, the censoring mechanism was estimated using Kaplan–Meier. In the MAR censoring setting, the censoring mechanism was correctly specified. The update of the initial hazard was performed by adding to it the two covariates h_1 and h_0 provided in Equations 20.10 and 20.11, respectively. The corresponding coefficients ε_1 and ε_2 were simultaneously estimated by fixing the offset from the initial fit and setting the intercept to 0. The procedure was iterated until ε_1 and ε_2 were sufficiently close to 0.

The estimators were compared using a relative efficiency measure based on the mean squared error (MSE) computed as the MSE of the unadjusted estimates divided by the MSE of the targeted maximum likelihood estimates. Thus, a value greater than 1 indicates a gain in efficiency of the covariate adjusted targeted MLE over the unadjusted estimator.

In addition to these six simulation scenarios, to explore the relationship between relative efficiency and the correlation between the covariate and failure time, we generated data by varying β_W in the data generating distribution above for six values, $\beta_W \in \{0.5, 1, 1.5, 2, 2.5, 3\}$ corresponding with correlations between W and failure time of $\{−0.10, −0.22, −0.36, −0.46, −0.56, −0.63\}$ under no censoring. The parameter $\psi(5)$ was estimated based on 1000 sampled datasets with sample size $n = 300$.

20.6.2   Simulation Results and Discussion

20.6.2.1   Strong Covariate Setting

In the no censoring and MCAR censoring scenarios, the bias should be approximately 0. Thus, the relative MSE is essentially comparing the variance of the unadjusted and targeted maximum likelihood estimates. Any gain in the MSE can therefore be attributed to a reduction in variance due to the covariate adjustment. In this strong covariate setting, exploiting this covariate by applying the targeted MLE should provide a gain precision due to a reduction in the residuals. In the informative censoring setting (MAR), in addition to the expected gain in efficiency we expect a reduction in bias of the targeted MLE with the correctly specified treatment mechanism over the unadjusted estimator. The informative censoring is accounted for through the covariates h_1 and h_0 that are inverse weighted by the subjects' conditional probability of being observed at time t given their observed history.

Figure 20.1 provides the relative MSE results for $\hat{\psi}(t_k)$ for $t_k \in \{1, \ldots 9\}$ for the strong covariate setting with $\beta_W = 3$. Based on these results, we observe that indeed the expected gain in efficiency is achieved. The minimum observed relative MSE was 1.25 for $t_k = 1$ in the MAR censoring setting with a misspecified initial hazard fit. A maximum relative MSE of 1.9 is observed under the no censoring setting with the correctly specified initial hazard at $t_k = 3$. The approximate overall average relative MSE was 1.6. Consistently across all time points and censoring scenarios, the targeted MLE is outperforming the unadjusted estimator.

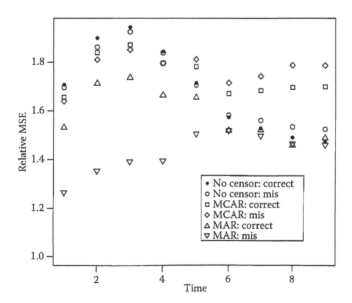

FIGURE 20.1:   Relative MSE: strong covariate setting ($\beta_W = 3$).

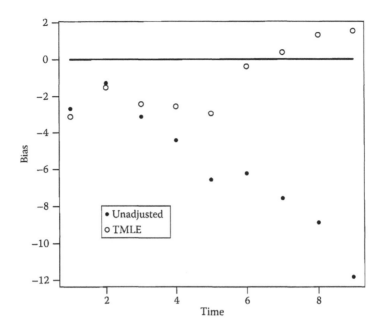

FIGURE 20.2:   Bias: strong covariate setting ($\beta_W = 3$) with informative censoring.

Figure 20.2 provides the bias as a percent of the truth for the two estimators under the MAR censoring setting with the correctly specified initial hazard. Clearly as t_k increases, the bias of the unadjusted estimates increases whereas the targeted maximum likelihood estimates is relatively close to 0 in comparison. Thus, the targeted maximum likelihood approach can not only provide gains in efficiency through covariate adjustment, but can also account for informative censoring as well.

20.6.2.2   Weak Covariate Setting

In this weak covariate setting, again in the no censoring and MCAR censoring scenarios, the bias should essentially be 0. However, we expect a lesser gain in efficiency if any as compared to the strong covariate setting since the covariate in this setting is not as useful for hazard prediction. We do again expect a bias reduction in the MAR censoring setting for the targeted MLE over the unadjusted estimator.

Figure 20.3 provides the relative MSE results for the weak correlation simulation with $\beta_W = 1$. As expected, the relative MSEs are all close to 1 indicating that only small efficiency gains are achieved when only weak covariates are present in the data. However, as the gains are small, they are also achieved across all time points as in the strong covariate setting. Regardless of the correlation between the covariate and failure time, in the informative censoring scenario the targeted maximum likelihood estimate is consistent under consistent estimation of the censoring mechanism as evidenced in the plot of the %bias in Figure 20.4.

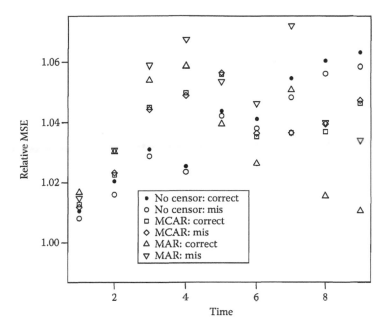

FIGURE 20.3:   Relative MSE: weak covariate setting ($\beta_W = 1$).

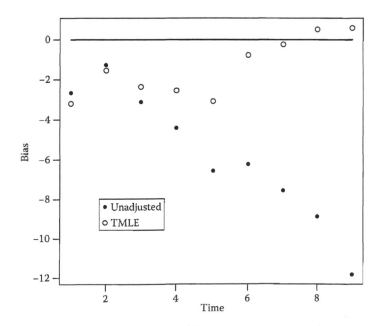

FIGURE 20.4:   Bias: weak covariate setting ($\beta_W = 1$) with informative censoring.

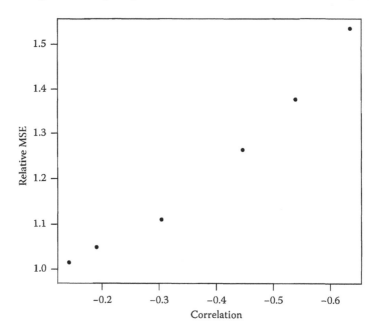

FIGURE 20.5:   Efficiency gain and correlation between covariate and failure time.

20.6.2.3   Relationship between Correlation of Covariate(s) and Failure Time with Efficiency Gain

As the correlation between W and failure time increases we expect to observe increasing gains in efficiency. Selecting an arbitrarily selected time point $t_k = 5$ for ease of presentation, Figure 20.5 clearly demonstrates that as the correlation between W and failure time increases so does the relative MSE. In fact, for this particular data generating distribution, at time $t_k = 5$ the relationship is nearly linear. These results reflect similar findings in RCT with fixed-end point studies where relations between R^2 and efficiency gain have been demonstrated [14,19]. This relationship indicates that if indeed the particular dataset contains covariates that are predictive of the failure time of the AE of interest, one can achieve gains in precision and thus power by using the targeted MLE.

20.7   Fitting Initial Hazard and Censoring Mechanism

Despite these potential gains in efficiency as demonstrated by theory and simulation results, there has been concern with covariate adjustment in RCTs with respect to investigators selecting covariates to obtain favorable inference. We conjecture that such cheating can be avoided if one uses an *a priori* specified algorithm for model selection. When the model selection procedure is specified in an analysis protocol, the analysis is protected from investigators guiding causal inferences based on selection of favorable covariates and their functional forms in a parametric model. In safety analysis, if investigator (sponsor) bias does indeed exist, it would be reasonable to assume that it would lean toward the treatment having no effect on the AEs and thus the concerns are the reverse from efficacy analysis. The investigator bias would tend toward the less efficient unadjusted estimator. The analysis of AEs is often exploratory in nature and the results are meant to flag potential AEs of concern which may reduce the motivation for dishonest inference using covariate adjustment. Regardless of the covariate selection strategy, it should be explicitly outlined to avoid any such concerns.

There are a number of model selection algorithms that can be applied to data-adaptively select the initial hazard fit. One such approach is the D/S/A algorithm [24] that searches through a large space of functional forms using deletion, substitution, and addition moves. One can apply this algorithm to the pooled data (over time) to fit the initial hazard. One can also fit hazards using the hazard regression (HARE) algorithm developed by Kopperberg et al. [25], which uses piecewise linear regression splines and adaptively selects the covariates and knots. As another alternative, one could also include all covariates that have a strong univariate association with failure time in a hazard fit as main terms in addition to the treatment variable. Since one is often investigating many AEs, a fast algorithm such as the latter may be an appropriate alternative for computational efficiency.

We also note that if weights are required as they are for the inverse probability of censoring weighted (IPCW) reduced data targeted MLEs as outlined in Section 20.11.1, the D/S/A algorithm can be run with the corresponding weights.

In addition to the hazard for survival, the hazard for censoring must also be estimated. One of the algorithms discussed above can also be applied to estimate the censoring mechanism. We note that the application of the targeted MLE to a set of M AEs requires M hazard fits whereas only one fit for censoring is required. Thus, the censoring mechanism is estimated once and for all and is used in the analysis of each of the M AEs.

20.8 Inverse Weighting Assumption

The targeted MLE, as well as other inverse weighted estimators (see Section 20.9) for the parameters presented in this chapter, relies on the assumption that each subject has a positive probability of being observed (i.e., not censored) at time t, which can be expressed by

$$\bar{G}(t_-|A, W) > 0, \quad t = t_k.$$

This identifiability assumption has been addressed as an important assumption for right-censored data [26]. In Ref. [27] it was demonstrated that practical violations of this assumption can result in severely variable and biased estimates.

One is alerted of such violations by observing very small probabilities of remaining uncensored based on the estimated censoring mechanism, i.e., there are patients with a probability of censoring of almost 1 given their observed past.

20.9   Alternative Estimators

Prior to the introduction of targeted maximum likelihood estimation, there were two main approaches to estimating the treatment-specific survival at a fixed end point t_k: maximum likelihood estimation and estimating function estimation. In the maximum likelihood approach, one obtains an estimate $\hat{p}$ for p identified by perhaps a Cox proportional hazards model for continuous survival or logistic regression for discrete survival. The parameter of interest is then evaluated via substitution, i.e., $\hat{\psi} = \psi(\hat{p})$. These maximum likelihood substitution estimators involve estimating some hazard fit using an *a priori* specified model or a model selection algorithm that is concerned with performing well with respect to the whole density rather than the actual parameter of interest, e.g., the difference in treatment-specific survival at a specific time t_k. These type of estimators often have poor performance and can be heavily biased whenever the estimated hazard is inconsistent [28]. Furthermore, inference for such MLEs that rely on parametric models are overly optimistic and thus their corresponding p-values are particularly unreliable. This is in contrast to the inference for the targeted MLEs which respects that no *a priori* models are required.

An alternative to the likelihood-based approach is the extensively studied estimating function-based approach. Recall that the full data estimating functions provided in Equations 20.8 and 20.9 are estimating functions that could be applied to estimate the treatment-specific survival at time t_k if we had access to the full data, i.e., the uncensored survival time. The full data estimating function can be mapped into an estimating function based on the observed data using the IPCW method. The IPCW estimators based on the IPCW estimating function denoted by $D^{\text{IPCW}}(T, A, W | \psi_1, g, G)$ have been shown to be consistent and asymptotically linear if the censoring mechanism G can be well approximated [13,29]. While the IPCW estimators have advantages such as simple implementation, they are not optimal in terms of robustness and efficiency. Their consistency relies on correct estimation of the censoring mechanism whereas MLEs rely on correct estimation of the full likelihood of the data.

The efficient influence curve can be obtained by subtracting from the IPCW estimation function the IPCW projection onto the tangent space T_{CAR} of scores of the nuisance parameter G [13]. The efficient influence curve is the optimal estimating function in terms of efficiency and robustness and the corresponding solution to this equation is the so-called double robust IPCW (DR-IPCW) estimator. The "double" robust properties of this estimator are equivalent to those of the targeted MLE as the targeted MLE solves the efficient influence curve estimating equation, see Section 20.5.2. Despite the advantageous properties of such efficient estimating function-based estimators, maximum likelihood-based estimators are much more common in practice.

The more recently introduced targeted maximum likelihood estimation methodology that was applied in this chapter can be viewed as a fusion between the likelihood and estimating function-based methods. A notable advantage of the targeted MLEs is their relative ease of implementation in comparison to estimating equations which are often difficult to solve.

20.10 Multiple Testing Considerations

An important consideration in safety analysis is multiple testing in that often as many as hundreds of AEs are collected. The ICH guidelines indicate that it is recommended to adjust for multiplicity when hypothesis tests are applied [30]. However, the ICH guidelines do not provide any specific methods for adjustment. The need for adjustment is demonstrated by the following example outlined in Ref. [31]. In this study, out of 92 safety comparisons the investigators found a single significant result according to unadjusted *p*-values. A larger hypothesis driven study for this AE that had no known clinical explanation was carried out and did not result in any significant findings. Such false positive results for testing the effect of treatment on a series of AEs based on unadjusted *p*-values can cause undue concern for approval/labeling and can affect postmarketing commitments. On the other hand, over adjusting could also result in missing potentially relevant AEs. Thus appropriate adjustment requires some balance between no adjustment and a highly stringent procedure such as Bonferroni.

Many advances have been made in the area of multiple testing over the Bonferroni-type methods including resampling-based methods to control the family-wise error rate (FWER), for example see Ref. [32] and the Benjamini–Hochberg method for controlling the false discovery rate (FDR) [33]. With FWER approaches, one is concerned with controlling the probability of erroneously rejecting one or more of the true null hypotheses, whereas the FDR approach controls the expected proportion of erroneous rejections among all rejections. The resampling-based FWER method makes use of the correlation of test statistics which can provide a gain in power over assuming independence. However, the Benjamini–Hochberg FDR approach has been shown to perform well with correlated test statistics as well [34]. The selection of the appropriate adjustment depends on whether or not a more conservative approach is reasonable. In safety analysis, one certainly does not want to miss flagging an important AE and thus might lean toward an FDR approach.

FDR methods have been proposed specifically in the analysis of AEs in Ref. [35]. Their method involves a two-step procedure that groups AEs by body system and performs an FDR adjustment both within and across the body system. Presumably this method attempts to account for the dependency of the AEs by grouping in this manner. Thus, the multiple testing considerations and the dependency of the test statistics in safety analysis has indeed received some attention in literature.

The multiple testing adjustment procedure to be applied in the safety analysis should be provided in the study protocol to avoid potential for dishonest inference.

In addition, the unadjusted p-values should continue to be reported with the adjusted p-values so all AEs can be evaluated to assess their potential clinical relevance.

20.11 Extensions

20.11.1 Time-Dependent Covariates

It is not unlikely that many time-dependent measurements are collected at each follow-up visit in addition to the many AEs and efficacy outcome measurements. Such time-dependent covariates are often predictive of censoring. The efficiency and robustness results presented in this chapter have been based on data structures with baseline covariates only. The targeted maximum likelihood estimation procedure for data structures with time-dependent covariates is more complex as demonstrated in Ref. [36]. To overcome this issue and avoid modeling the full likelihood, van der Laan [36] introduced IPCW reduced data targeted MLEs. We provide only an informal description of this procedure here, for details we refer readers to the formal presentation provided in Ref. [36].

In this framework, the targeted maximum likelihood estimation procedure is carried out for a reduced data structure X^r, which in this case is the data structure that only includes baseline covariates. The IPCW reduced data procedure differs from the procedure where X^r is the full data in that the log-likelihoods are weighted by a time-dependent stabilizing weight given by

$$sw(t) = \frac{I(C > t)\bar{G}^r(t|X^r)}{\bar{G}(t|X)}.$$

This stabilizing weight is based on $\bar{G}^r(t|X^r)$ which is the censoring mechanism based on the reduced data structure that includes baseline covariates only and $\bar{G}(t|X)$ which is the censoring mechanism based on the complete data structure that includes time-dependent covariates.

In practice, in the estimation of the parameter $\psi(t_k) = E_0(S_0(t_k|A = 1, W) - S_0(t_k|A = 0, W))$, one must apply these weights anytime maximum likelihood estimation is performed. Thus, the IPCW reduced data targeted maximum likelihood estimation procedure differs from the standard targeted maximum likelihood procedure provided in Section 20.5 in that each time the conditional hazard is fit it is weighted by $sw(t)$. These weights are time-specific and thus each subject receives a different weight at each point in time. The initial hazard estimate $\hat{\lambda}^0(t|A, W)$ is weighted by $sw(t)$. The algorithm then updates $\hat{\lambda}^0(t|A, W)$ by adding the time-dependent covariates $h_1(t, A, W)$ and $h_0(t, A, W)$ and estimating their corresponding coefficients ε_1 and ε_2. In the IPCW reduced data targeted maximum likelihood estimation procedure one includes the weights $sw(t)$ in estimation of ε_1 and ε_2. These weights are applied in each iteration of the algorithm to obtain the final fit

$\hat{\lambda}^*(t|A, W)$ that is achieved when $\hat{\varepsilon}_1$ and $\hat{\varepsilon}_2$ are sufficiently close to 0. Thus, the estimation can again be achieved using standard software with the only additional requirement of weighting each of the regressions by these time-dependent weights.

Estimation of these time-dependent weights requires estimation of $\bar{G}^r(t|X)$ and $\bar{G}(t|X)$. Model selection algorithms that can be applied to estimate $\bar{G}^r(t|X)$ were described in Section 20.7. Similarly, the censoring mechanism $\bar{G}(t|X)$ can be estimated using a Cox proportional hazards model with time-dependent covariates for continuous censoring times or logistic regression model with time-dependent covariates for discrete censoring times. Model selection algorithms such as those described in Section 20.7 can also be applied by including these time-dependent covariates as candidates.

Let $\hat{\psi}^r(t_k)$ represent the IPCW reduced data targeted MLE of $\psi(t_k)$. By applying this IPCW weighting in the reduced data targeted maximum likelihood estimation procedure a particular type of double robustness is obtained. If there are no time-dependent covariates that are predictive of censoring time, then the ratio of estimated survival probabilities of censoring in the above weight $sw(t)$ is 1. In this case, if $\bar{G}(t|X)$ is consistently estimated or $\lambda(\cdot|A, W)$ is consistently estimated then $\hat{\psi}^r(t_k)$ is consistent; if both are consistent then it is even more efficient than the estimator that was based on the reduced data structure. If there are indeed time-dependent covariates that are predictive of censoring time, and $\bar{G}(t|A, W)$ is well approximated then $\hat{\psi}^r(t_k)$ is consistent and the desired bias reduction is achieved.

20.11.2 Postmarket Data

As RCTs are powered for efficacy, it is often the case that many AEs are either not observed at all during the premarket phase or so few are observed that statistically conclusive results are often exceptions [2]. In an RCT of a rotavirus vaccine in which the AE of intussusception among vaccine recipients compared to controls was not found to be statistically significant. After the vaccine was approved and had been widely used, an association between this AE and the vaccine was found and it was pulled off the market. A subsequent analysis demonstrated that to obtain power of 50% to detect a difference as small as the actual observed Phase III incidence of the AE, a sample size of approximately 90,000 would be required (six times the actual sample size) [37]. Due to the high cost and complications involved in running an RCT, such large sample sizes are not feasible.

It is not only the rarity of many AEs that causes issues in detection during RCT, but also the fact that RCT may have restrictive inclusion criteria whereas the drug is likely applied to a less restrictive population in postmarket. Furthermore, the follow-up time in the premarket phase may not be long enough to detect delayed AEs. For a discussion regarding the difficulties in "proving" safety of a compound in general see Ref. [38]. Postmarket monitoring is therefore an important aspect of safety analysis.

There are a number of types of postmarket data (for a thorough description of the various types of postmarket data see Ref. [39]) including spontaneous AE reporting systems (e.g., "MedWatch"). These data can be useful for detecting potentially new or unexpected adverse drug reactions that require further analysis; however, they often suffer from under-reporting by as much as a factor of 20 [40].

In this section, we focus on observational postmarket studies or pharmacoepidemiological studies. Since patients in these type of studies are not randomized to a drug versus placebo (or competitor), confounding is typically present. Of particular concern is the fact that sicker patients are often selected to receive one particular drug versus another. There exists a vast amount of literature for controlling for confounding in epidemiological studies. Popular methods in pharmacoepidemiology include propensity score (PS) methods and regression-based approaches. However, consistency with these methods rely on correct specification of the PS or the regression model used. Furthermore, it is not clear how informative censoring is accounted for with these methods. The targeted MLEs are double robust and are thus more advantageous than these commonly applied alternative approaches.

Before we proceed with discussion of estimation of causal effects with observational data, we first outline the data and assumptions. Suppose we observe n independent and identically distributed copies of $O = (\tilde{T}, \Delta, A, W) \sim p_0$ as defined in Section 20.4. Causal effects are based on a hypothetical full data structure $X = (T_{1,1}, T_{1,0}, T_{0,1}, T_{0,0}, W)$ which is a collection of action-specific survival times where this action is comprised of treatment and censoring. Note that we are only interested in the counterfactuals under this joint action-mechanism that consists of both censoring and treatment mechanisms where censoring equals 0, i.e., $T_{1,0}$ and $T_{0,0}$. In other words, we aim to investigate what would have happened under each treatment had censoring not occurred.

The consistency assumption states that the observed data consist of the counterfactual outcome corresponding with the joint action actually observed. The CAR assumption implies that the joint action is conditionally independent of the full data X given the observed data. We denote the conditional probability distribution of treatment A by $g_0(a|X) \equiv P(A = a|X)$. In observational studies, CAR implies $g_0(A|X) = g_0(A|W)$, in contrast to RCT in which treatment is assigned completely at random and $g_0(A|X) = g_0(A)$.

We aim to estimate $\psi(t_k) = E_0(S_0(t_k|A = 1, W) - S_0(t_k|A = 0, W)) = \Pr(T_{1,0} > t_k) - \Pr(T_{0,0} > t_k)$. Even under no censoring or MCAR, we can no longer rely on the unadjusted treatment-specific Kaplan–Meier estimates being unbiased due to confounding of treatment.

Under the assumptions above, the targeted MLE for $\psi(t_k)$ is double robust and locally efficient. Thus, the targeted maximum likelihood estimation procedure described in this chapter is theoretically optimal in terms of robustness and efficiency. In our presentation, we assumed that treatment was assigned at random. In observational studies, in addition to estimating $\lambda(\cdot|A, W)$ and possibly $\bar{G}(\cdot|A, W)$ (when censoring is present), observational studies require estimation of the treatment mechanism $g(A|W)$ as well. It has been demonstrated that when censoring is MCAR in an RCT, the targeted maximum likelihood estimate $\hat{\psi}^*(t_k)$ is consistent under misspecification of $\lambda(\cdot|A, W)$ since $g(A|W)$ is always correctly specified. However, even under MCAR, in observational studies, consistency of $\hat{\psi}^*(t_k)$ relies on consistent estimation of $\lambda(\cdot|A, W)$ or $g(A|W)$ and is efficient if both are consistently estimated [12]. When censoring is MAR, then consistency of $\hat{\psi}^*(t_k)$ also relies on consistent estimation of the joint missingness $g(A|W)$ and $\bar{G}(\cdot|A, W)$ or $\lambda(\cdot|A, W)$.

We also note that the targeted MLEs as well as the commonly applied PS methods rely on the experimental treatment assignment (ETA) assumption. Under this assumption, each patient must have a positive probability of receiving each treatment. The inverse weighted PS estimator is known to suffer severely from violations of this assumption in practice [26,27,41]. This poor performance is evident with inverse weighting, however, we note that all other PS methods rely on this assumption as well, but are not as sensitive to practical violations. This assumption is essentially about information in the data and violations of it indicate that for certain strata of the data, a given treatment level is never or rarely experienced. When the ETA is violated estimation methods rely on extrapolation.

If it is the case that a given treatment level is very rare or nonexistent for given strata of the population, an investigator may want to reconsider the original research question of interest. To this end [42] developed causal effect models for realistic intervention rules. These models allow estimation of the effect of realistic interventions, that is only intervening on patients for whom the intervention is reasonably "possible" where "possible" is defined by $g(A|W)$ greater than some value, e.g., 0.05. We note that targeted maximum likelihood estimation can be applied to estimate parameters from such models. For applications of such models see Ref. [43].

The ETA assumption and development of realistic causal models are simply examples of some of the many considerations that arise with observational data as compared to RCT data. However, despite the many issues, the rich field of causal inference provides promising methods for safety analysis in postmarket data. As it is not possible to observe all AEs in the premarket phase, postmarket safety analysis is an important and emerging area of research.

20.12 Discussion

Safety analysis is an important aspect in new drug approvals and has become increasingly evident with the recent cases of drugs withdrawn from the market (e.g., Vioxx). Increasing estimation efficiency is one area that can help overcome the issue that RCT are not powered for safety. Using covariate information is a promising approach to help detect AEs that may have remained undetected with the standard crude analysis. Furthermore, time-to-event methods for AE analysis may be more appropriate particularly in studies where the AEs often occur for all patients, such as oncology studies. Exploiting the time-dependent nature can further provide more efficient estimates for the effect of treatment on AEs occurrence.

In this chapter, we provided a method for covariate adjustment in RCT for estimating the effect of treatment on the AEs failing to occur by a fixed end point. The method does not require any parametric modeling assumptions under MCAR censoring and thus is robust to misspecification of the hazard fit. The methods advantages were twofold. The first is the potential efficiency gains over the unadjusted estimator. The second is that the targeted MLE accounts for informative censoring through inverse weighting of the covariate(s) that is added to an initial hazard fit. The standard unadjusted estimator is biased in the informative censoring setting.

The estimator has a relatively straightforward implementation. Given an initial hazard fit either logistic for discrete failure times or Cox proportional hazards for continuous survival times, one updates this fit by iteratively adding a time-dependent covariate(s).

The simulation study demonstrated the potential gains in efficiency that can be achieved in addition to the relation of the correlation between the covariate(s) and failure time and efficiency gains. When no predictive covariates were present the relative efficiency was approximately 1 indicating that one is protected from actually losing precision from applying this method even when the covariates provide little information about failure time. The simulations also demonstrated the reduction in bias in the informative censoring setting.

Considerations for balancing the potential for false positives and the danger of missing possibly significant AEs are an important aspect of safety analysis. The strategies from the rich field of multiple testing briefly discussed in this chapter can exploit the correlation of the AE outcomes and thus provide the most powerful tests.

While this chapter focused on estimation of treatment-specific survival at a specific end point an overall average effect of treatment over time may be of interest. The targeted maximum likelihood estimation procedure described in this chapter can be extended to estimate this effect to provide a competitor to the ubiquitous logrank test. Future work includes providing a method for exploiting covariate information using the targeted maximum likelihood estimation procedure to improve power over the logrank test.

References

[1] Friedman LM, Furberg CD, and DeMets DL. *Fundamentals of Clincal Trials*, 3rd edn. Springer-Verlag, New York, 1998

[2] Peace KE. Design, monitoring and analysis issues relative to adverse events. *Drug Information Journal* 1987; 21:21–28.

[3] Gait JE, Smith S, and Brown SL. Evaluation of safety data from controlled clinical trials: the clinical principles explained. *Drug Information Journal* 2000; 34:273–287.

[4] Guttner A, Kubler J, and Pigeot I. Multivariate time-to-event analysis of multiple adverse events of drugs in integrated analysis. *Statistics in Medicine* 2007; 26:1518–1531.

[5] Liu GF, Wang J, Liu K, and Snavely DB. Confidence intervals for an exposure adjusted incidence rate difference with applications to clincial trials. *Statistics in Medicine* 2006; 25:1275–1286.

[6] Menjoge SS. On estimation of frequency data with censored observations. *Pharmaceutical Statistics* 2003; 2(3):191–197.

[7] Wood AM, White IR, and Thompson SG. Are missing outcome data adequately handled? A review of published randomized controlled trials in major medical journals. *Clinical Trials* 2004; 1:368–376.

[8] O'Neill RT. The assessment of safety. In *Biopharmaceutical Statistics for Drug Development*, Chapter 13 Peace KE (eds.). Marcel Dekker, New York, 1988.

[9] Nishikawa M, Tango T, and Ogawa M. Non-parametric inference of adverse events under informative censoring. *Statistics in Medicine* 2006; 25:3981–4003.

[10] Davis BR, Furberg CD, and Williams CB. Survival analysis of adverse effects data in the beta-blocker heart attack trial. *Clinical Pharmacology Theraphy* 1987; 41:611–15.

[11] Fleming TR. Survival analysis in clinical trials: Past developments and future directions. *Biometrics* 2000; 56(4):971–983.

[12] van der Laan MJ and Rubin D. Targeted maximum likelihood learning. *The International Journal of Biostatistics* 2006; 2(1), Article 11.

[13] van der Laan MJ and Robins JM. *Unified Methods for Censored Longitudinal Data and Causality*. Springer, New York, 2002.

[14] Pocock SJ, Assmann SE, Enos LE, and Kasten LE. Subgroup analysis, covariate adjustment and baseline comparisons in clinical trial reporting: current practice and problems. *Statistics in Medicine* 2002; 21:2917–2930.

[15] Hernández AV, Steyerberg EW, and Habbema JDF. Covariate adjustment in randomized controlled trials with dichotomous outcomes increases statistical power and reduces sample size requirements. *Journal of Clinical Epidemiology* 2004; 57(5):454–460.

[16] Robinson LD and Jewell NP. Some surprising results about covariate adjustment in logistic regression models. *International Statistical Review* 1991; 59:227–240.

[17] Tsiatis AA, Davidian M, Zhang M, and Lu X. Covariate adjustment for two-sample treatment comparisons in randomized clinical trials: A principled yet flexible approach. *Statistics in Medicine* 2007; 27(23): 4658–4677.

[18] Zhang M, Tsiatis AA, and Davidian M. Improving efficiency of inferences in randomized clinical trials using auxiliary covariates. *Biometrics* 2008; 64(3): 707–715.

[19] Moore KL and van der Laan MJ. Covariate adjustment in randomized trials with binary outcomes: Targeted maximum likelihood estimation. *Statistics in Medicine* 2009; 28(1):39–64.

[20] Hernández AV, Eijkemans MJC, and Steyerberg EW. Randomized controlled trials with time-to-event outcomes: How much does prespecified covariate adjustment increase power? *Annals of Epidemiology* 2006; 16(1):41–48.

[21] Li A. Covariate adjustment for non-parametric tests for censored survival data. *Statistics in Medicine* 2001; 20:1843–1853.

[22] Tsiatis AA, Rosner GL, and Tritchler DL. Group sequential tests with censored survival data and adjusting for covariates. *Biometrika* 1985; 72:365–373.

[23] van der Laan MJ and Rubin D. A note on targeted maximum likelihood and right censored data. Technical Report 226, Division of Biostatistics, University of California, Berkeley, CA, 2007.

[24] Sinisi S and van der Laan MJ. The deletion/substitution/addition algorithm in loss function based estimation: Applications in genomics. *Statistical Applications in Genetics and Molecular Biology* 2004; 3(1), Article 18.

[25] Kooperberg C, Stone CJ, and Truong YK. Hazard regression. *Journal of the American Statistical Association* 1995; 90:78–94.

[26] Robins JM and Rotniztky A. Recovery of information and adjustment for dependent censoring using sorrogate markers. In *AIDS Methodology—Methodological Issues*, Jewell N, Dietz K, and Farewell W (eds.). Birkhauser, Boston, 1992.

[27] Neugebauer R and van der Laan MJ. Why prefer double robust estimators in causal inference? *Journal of Statistical Planning and Inference* 2005; 129:405–426.

[28] Robins JM and Ritov Y. Toward a curse of dimensionality appropriate (CODA) asymptotic theory for semi-parametric models. *Statistics in Medicine* 1997; 16:285–319.

[29] Robins JM and Rotnitzky A. Inverse probability weighted estimation in survival analysis. *Encyclopedia of Biostatistics*, 2nd edn., Armitage P and Colton T (eds.). Wiley, New York, 2005.

[30] ICH E3. Structure and content of clinical study reports. *Federal Register* 1996; 61:37320–37343.

[31] Kaplan KJ, Rusche SA, Lakkis HD, Bottenfield G, Guerra FA, Guerrero J, Keyserling H, Felicione E, Hesley TM, and Boslego JW. Post-licensure comparative study of unusual high-pitched crying and prolonged crying following COMVAX2 and placebo versus PedvaxHIB2 and RECOMBIVAX2 in healthy infants. *Vaccine* 2002; 21:18187.

[32] van der Laan MJ, Dudoit S, and Pollard KS. Augmentation procedures for control of the generalized family-wise error rate and tail probabilities for the

proportion of false positives. *Statistical Applications in Genetics and Molecular Biology* 2004; 3(1): Article 15.

[33] Benjamini, Y and Hochberg T. Controlling the false discovery rate: A practical and powerful approach to multiple testing. *Journal of the Royal Statistical Society, Series B.* 1995; 85:289–300.

[34] Benjamini Y, Hochberg Y, and Kling Y. False discovery rate control in multiple hypotheses testing using dependent test statistics. Research Paper 97-1, Department of Statistics and Operations Research, Tel Aviv University, Tel Aviv, Israel, 1997.

[35] Mehrotra DV and Heyse JF. Use of the false discovery rate for evaluating clinical safety data. *Statistical Methods in Medical Research* 2004; 13:227–238.

[36] van der Laan MJ. The construction and analysis of adaptive group sequential designs 232. U.C. Berkeley Division of Biostatistics Working Paper Series, 2008.

[37] Jacobson RM, Adedunni A, Pankratzc VS, and Poland GA. Adverse events and vaccination-the lack of power and predictability of infrequent events in pre-licensure study. *Vaccine* 2001; 19:2428–2433.

[38] Bross ID. Why proof of safety is much more difficult than proof of hazard. *Biometrics* 1985; 41(3):785–793.

[39] Glasser SP, Salas M, and Delzell E. Importance and challenges of studying marketed drugs: What is a phase IV study? Common clinical research designs, registries, and self-reporting systems. *Journal of Clinical Pharmacology* 2007; 47:1074–1086.

[40] Edlavitch SA. Adverse drug event reporting. Improving the low U.S. reporting rates. *Archives of Internal Medicine* 1988; 148:1499–1503.

[41] Wang Y, Petersen ML, Bangsberg D, and van der Laan MJ. Diagnosing bias in the inverse-probability-of-treatment-weighted estimator resulting from violation of experimental treatment assignment. Technical Report 211, U.C. Berkeley Division of Biostatistics Working Paper Series, 2006.

[42] van der Laan MJ and Petersen ML. Causal effect models for realistic individualized treatment and intention to treat rules. *The International Journal of Biostatistics* 2007; 3(1): Article 3.

[43] Bembom O and van der Laan MJ. Analyzing sequentially randomized trials based on causal effect models for realistic individualized treatment rules. Technical Report 216, Division of Biostatistics, University of California, Berkeley, CA, 2007.

Chapter 21

Design and Analysis of Chronic Carcinogenicity Studies of Pharmaceuticals in Rodents*

Mohammad Atiar Rahman and Karl K. Lin

Contents

---

* The views expressed in this chapter are those of the authors and not necessarily those of the Food and Drug Administration.

21.1 Introduction

The incidence of cancer was so frightening that in 1971 President Richard Nixon declared a war against cancer. An enormous amount of resources has been directed toward the fight against cancer. However, the battle against this leading killer disease has not been very successful. Continued human suffering due to this disease has prompted the demand for strategies to effectively identify human carcinogens. In the development of new drugs, the assessment of the carcinogenic potential of chemical compounds in humans is a fundamental step. The risk assessment of the carcinogenic potential of a new drug usually begins with experiments in animals. The law requires the sponsor of a new drug to conduct short- and long-term carcinogenicity studies in animals to assess the carcinogenic effect of the drug compounds. There are different applications of these short- and long-term animal carcinogenicity studies in the determination of the carcinogenic potential of chemical compounds. The first is to use the results merely for screening the unsafe chemical compounds. The second is to conduct risk assessments of chemicals in humans. This process involves the extrapolation of results from animals to humans and from high to low doses. The third is to verify specific scientific hypotheses about the mechanisms of carcinogenesis.

Various federal government agencies in the United States play important roles in the national effort to reduce the threat of cancer. Two of the most important agencies in this effort are the U.S. Environmental Protection Agency (EPA) and the U.S. Food and Drug Administration (FDA). The EPA is responsible for protecting Americans from environmental cancer-causing agents. The FDA is responsible for ensuring the safety of human drugs, animal drugs, medical devices, and food additives. The evaluation of the carcinogenic effect of medical products is one of FDA's most important responsibilities. These two agencies regularly review and evaluate carcinogenicity studies conducted by various sponsors mostly in different rodent species. Other U.S. government agencies involved in the review and evaluation of animal oncology experiments include the National Toxicological Program (NTP), the National Cancer Institute (NCI), and the National Center for Toxicological Research (NCTR). The International Agency for Research on Cancer, a branch of the World Health Organization (WHO), also monitors animal carcinogenicity data from different sources.

The Pharmacology and Toxicology (Pharm/Tox) Team at the Office of Biostatistics (OB) of the Center for Drug Evaluation and Research (CDER) in the FDA is responsible for the statistical review and evaluation of carcinogenicity studies of pharmaceuticals included in investigational new drug (IND) and new drug application (NDA) submissions. The statistical review and evaluation of pharmacology and toxicology studies is an important and integral part of the FDA approval process for new drugs. In a regular carcinogenicity study review the FDA statisticians review and evaluate the appropriateness of designs of experiments, methods of statistical analysis of data, and methods of interpreting the study results. In addition to reviewing the reports submitted by the drug sponsor, statisticians in the CDER/FDA also perform analyses of their own using the tumor data submitted by the sponsors to verify the sponsor's results and to answer questions that are not addressed by the sponsor. The designs, methods of statistical analysis of data, and interpretation of results recommended in the 2001 FDA draft document titled *Guidance for Industry; Statistical Aspects of the Design, Analysis, and Interpretation of Chronic Rodent Carcinogenicity Studies of Pharmaceuticals* are generally followed by CDER/FDA statisticians in their reviews of regular 2 year studies for IND and NDA submissions. This FDA draft guidance for industry document includes methods of analyzing data from carcinogenicity studies using regular rodents but does not cover the designs and methods of data analysis and interpretation of study results for short-term studies using special mice, known as transgenic mice. The CDER/FDA statisticians have been using methods developed both within the FDA and outside the FDA in their statistical reviews of this type of carcinogenicity study for new drugs.

The purpose of this chapter is to provide an update, with detailed discussions on the topics presented in the FDA guidance for industry document and in chapters on the same subject in various editions of other books by the second author, and to present some new designs and methods of data analysis and interpretation of results currently used by FDA/CDER statisticians in the review of carcinogenicity studies using transgenic mice that were not included in publications mentioned here.

21.2 Experimental Designs and Collection of Data

Theoretically, animal carcinogenicity studies may be conducted using any species of animals, for example, dog, monkey, guinea pig, and other small rodents. However, for logistical convenience, long-term carcinogenicity studies of pharmaceuticals are usually conducted in small rodents. As a regulatory requirement for the development of a new drug, animal carcinogenicity studies are conducted in two sexes of rats and mice (a total of four experiments) for the majority of those animals' normal life spans of approximately 2 years. Each of these experiments generally includes four treatment groups, namely, control, low-, medium-, and high-dose groups. There are various routes of administration of a drug to test animals, for example, oral through dietary mix, oral by gavage, cutaneous or subcutaneous injection, dermal on skin surface and so on. All animals alive at the end of 2 years are terminally sacrificed. Organs/tissues of all animals, whether these animals die during the study or are terminally sacrificed, are microscopically examined for neoplastic (tumors) and nonneoplastic lesions.

Because of the high cost and long time necessary to conduct a 2 year carcinogenicity study and the increased insight into the mechanisms of carcinogenicity provided by the advances in molecular biology, currently there are two alternative designs available for carcinogenicity studies of new drugs. The International Conference on Harmonization (ICH) has recommended the use of either two 2 year studies in regular rats and mice or alternatively one 2 year study in regular rats along with one short- or medium-term study in transgenic mice, which provides rapid observation of carcinogenic endpoints. The main strains of transgenic mice include p53+/−, Tg.AC, Tg rasH2, and XPA+/−. Studies with Tg rasH2, p53+/−, and XPA+/− generally include a positive control group (treated with a known carcinogen, for example, p-cresidine, benzene, or 12-O-Tetradecanolyphorbol-13-acetate (TPA)) in addition to the regular three or four treatment groups (negative control, low, medium, and high). The group size is generally 25–30 animals per sex/treatment group. The duration is about 26 weeks. As in the long-term studies, organs/tissues of all animals of experiments with p53+/−, Tg rasH2, and XPA+/− animals that die during the study or are terminally sacrificed are microscopically examined for neoplastic and nonneoplastic lesions. In Tg.AC transgenic mouse studies, only weekly incidence rates and weekly counts of skin papillomas are collected for the evaluation of the drug effects.

The statistical issues in the design of carcinogenicity studies include randomization, sample size selection, dose selection, confounding factors, and so on. In a well-designed experiment, animals are assigned to the treatment groups following a well-defined randomization scheme to ensure that there is no selection bias. If needed, stratification may be applied to balance some physical characteristics (e.g., body weight). A formal calculation of sample size depends on the required power of the proposed statistical tests. However, considering some practical limitations (e.g., expenses on the conduct of experiments with large numbers of animals, concerns about cruelty to animals) the sizes of the treatment groups are generally limited to 50–70 animals per group per sex. Although traditionally treatment groups are of equal size, in certain situations, unequal allocations may be preferred.

Doses used in a chronic carcinogenicity study are based on results of a series of short-term (2 weeks to 3 months) dose-ranging studies. There are various criteria for actual dose selection for animal studies. However, the general accepted criterion is that the testing should be carried out at doses that well exceed a typical human exposure to ensure reasonable challenge of carcinogenic activities. Because limited numbers of animals per sex/group are used in a study, and small numbers of those animals develop tumors, it is important that animals be tested at high multiples of the human therapeutic dose to ensure reasonable levels of power of statistical tests to detect the true carcinogenic effects of the tested chemical compound. Although not generally a statistical issue, dose selection is particularly critical in the design of a carcinogenicity study. The ICH guidance entitled *SIC Dose Selection for Carcinogenicity Studies of Pharmaceuticals* is an internationally accepted guidance for dose selection for carcinogenicity studies. The guidance allows for approaches to high-dose selection based on toxicity endpoints, pharmacokinetic endpoints (multiple of maximum human exposure), pharmacodynamic endpoints, and maximal feasible dose. Based on toxicity endpoints, Sontag et al. [1] presented a general criterion for selection of high dose in a study based on toxicity endpoints. They recommended that the highest dose employed should be the maximum tolerated dose (MTD) which was defined as "The highest dose of the test agent during the chronic study that can be predicted not to alter the animals' normal longevity from effects other than carcinogenicity." Demonstration of a toxic effect in the carcinogenicity study, without compromising survivability or physiological homeostasis, ensures that the animals are sufficiently challenged and provides confidence in the reliability of a negative outcome.

Factors recommended in establishing other doses in a study include all information about linearity of pharmacokinetics, saturation of metabolic pathway, anticipated human exposure levels, pharmacodynamics in the test species, potential for threshold effects in the test species, and the unpredictability of the progression of toxicity observed in short-term rodent studies. It has been recommended that the medium dose be about 50% of MTD and the low dose be between 20% and 30% of MTD (Portier and Hoel 1983) [2]. There has been some criticism of this recommendation by various experts and practitioners. Some details of this criticism are included in appropriate sections of this chapter.

The CDER/FDA statisticians play very limited supportive roles in the determination of the appropriateness of the dose selection. Currently, the CDER carcinogenicity assessment committee (CAC), consisting of senior pharm/tox reviewers, is solely responsible for reviewing and approving of protocols of carcinogenicity studies. The committee reviews study dose levels proposed by the sponsor. The committee either approves the proposed doses or recommends a separate set of doses deemed to be more appropriate by the committee members. Sponsors are strongly encouraged to submit their study protocols to the Agency for the CAC to review before conducting the studies.

There are other nonstatistical issues in animal carcinogenicity studies, for example, appropriateness of species and strain of animals chosen, choice of route of administration, diet, caging, interim or early sacrifice, study duration, and so on, that require careful consideration and attention. A specific strain of animals may be more susceptible to the development of a particular tumor than other strains. The route of administration determines appropriate delivery of drug into the animal body. The position of the cage in the laboratory may sometimes produce unwanted results, for example, the effect of fluorescent lights on animals constantly within their close proximity may increase the incidences of cataracts and retinopathy. It is recommended that the cages be rotated within the test facilities to limit such extraneous effects.

The physical and clinical conditions of animals and their mortality and morbidity need to be regularly observed and recorded. The animals should be palpated and otherwise observed on a regular basis for the presence of any masses or unusual growth. All organs of all animals that died during the study or were terminally sacrificed at the end of the study should be appropriately preserved and microscopically examined by a designated pathologist, in a blinded fashion, for the presence of neoplastic lesions (tumors). For the accuracy of the microscopic findings, a repeat examination may also be performed by a second pathologist.

Data of neoplastic and nonneoplastic lesions, mortality, body weight, food consumption, and so on, are collected from a study. The analysis of the tumor data is the most important part of an FDA statistical review and evaluation of a carcinogenicity study. Sponsors are asked by the FDA to submit the tumor data in an electronic form and in accordance with a format set up by the Agency for the statistical review. The FDA data format includes variables and values, as presented in Table 21.1.

TABLE 21.1:   Variables and possible variable values included in the FDA data format.

Variable	Possible Variable Values
Study number	
Animal number	
Species	
Sex	
Dose group	
Death sacrifice time	
Death sacrifice status	Natural death or moribund sacrificed
	Terminally sacrificed
	Planned interim sacrifice
	Accidental death
Animal examined	No tissues were examined
	At least one tissue was examined
Tumor code	
Tumor name	
Organ code	
Organ name	
Tumor detection time	
Tumor malignancy status	Malignant
	Benign
	Undetermined
Animals' cause of death	Tumor caused the death
	Tumor did not cause the death
	Undetermined
Whether or not a particular organ was ever examined	Organ/tissue was examined and was usable
	Organ/tissue was examined but not usable (e.g., autolyzed tissue)
	Organ/tissue was not examined

21.3   Analysis Endpoints

As mentioned earlier, in a typical carcinogenicity experiment, data of food consumption, bodyweight, organ weight, mortality, and histopathology are regularly observed and recorded. In general, the data of neoplastic lesions (tumor) are used to evaluate the carcinogenicity potential of the related compound, and the data of mortality, body weight, organ weight, and food consumption are used in evaluating the validity of the study.

Typical statistical analyses of 2 year carcinogenicity data primarily include tests for dose–response relationship (also known as positive trends) among the increasing doses in mortality and tumor incidence rates. Tumor data are analyzed by organ/tumor combination for each species/sex. Additionally, the analyses also include pairwise comparisons of mortality and tumor incidence rates between individual treated groups with the control. There are two major concerns in analyzing tumor data, namely, adjustment for mortality differences due to drug toxicity and adjustment for multiple testing due to the large number of dose–response tests and pairwise comparisons for different organ/tumor combinations. The details of the statistical methods for analyzing mortality and tumor incidence data, methods for adjusting mortality differences, and methods for multiple testing are given in related sections of this chapter.

21.4   Sample Tumor Count Data

A typical summary of tumor count data of a tumor type and organ combination (tumor/organ) in an experiment with $r+1$ numbers of dose groups (one control and r treated groups) is given in Table 21.2, where x_i denotes the ith dose level, N_i, the total number of animals assigned to the ith dose group, n_i, the number of tumor-bearing animals in the ith dose group, and $N_i - n_i$, the number of animals without developing the particular tumor (nontumor-bearing animals) in the ith dose group. This notation is used consistently throughout this chapter.

TABLE 21.2:   Summary table for tumor count data.

Treatment Group	0	1	...	i	...	r	Total
Dose	x_0	x_1	...	x_i	...	x_r	
NTBA	n_0	n_1	...	n_i	...	n_r	n
NNTBA	$N_0 - n_0$	$N_1 - n_1$	...	$N_i - n_i$	...	$N_r - n_r$	$N - n$
Total	N_0	N_1	...	N_i	...	N_r	N
Proportion at risk $P_i = N_i/N$	$P_0 = N_0/N$	$P_1 = N_1/N$		$P_i = N_i/N$		$P_r = N_r/N$	1
Proportion of TBA	$p_0 = n_0/N_0$	$p_1 = n_1/N_1$		$p_i = n_i/N_i$		$p_r = n_r/N_r$	$p_0 = n/N$

Note: NTBA, number of tumor-bearing animals; NNTBA, number of nontumor-bearing animals.

21.5   Tumor Classification

As mentioned previously, it is important to adjust the differences in mortality among treatment groups for both trend tests and pairwise comparisons of tumor incidences. Two examples in Section 21.6 demonstrate that results of analyses of tumor data based solely on overall incidence rates without adjusting for differences among treatment groups can be misleading.

There are methods proposed to adjust the difference in mortality in trend tests and pairwise comparisons of tumor incidence. The Peto method [2] and the poly-k method have been used by the CDER/FDA statisticians in their review of carcinogenicity studies of new drugs. The Peto methods require the cause-of-death information of animals (whether the tumor was the cause of death or not) in the adjustment for mortality difference, whereas the poly-3 method does not require such information. The requirement of the cause-of-death information of animals for the adjustment of mortality difference in Peto methods is a controversial issue in the analysis of carcinogenicity study data. There have been arguments among animal pathologists on the accuracy of providing real cause-of-death information of animals. Since pathologists discover most of the tumors on an animal in the microscopic examination after it dies of different causes, it is difficult for them to trace back when the tumors developed and to determine which tumors caused the animal's death and which did not.

In Peto methods, tumors are classified mainly in two different ways, that is, by the context of the observations and by their malignancy status. A tumor that is detectable before the animal dies, mainly by palpation or visual inspection, is known as a tumor observed in a "mortality-independent context," whereas a tumor that can be detected only after the animal dies, mainly by microscopic examination, is known as observed in a "mortality-dependent context." Based on the malignancy status, a tumor that does not directly or indirectly cause the animal's death is known as an incidental tumor, whereas a tumor that is either a direct or an indirect cause of death of the animal is known as a "fatal tumor." Tumors are also classified as "rare" and "common" tumors, based on their spontaneous background incidence rates. A tumor is defined as rare if its published spontaneous tumor rate is less than 1%, whereas it is defined as common if its published spontaneous tumor rate is equal to or more than 1%.

21.6   Statistical Analysis Methods

21.6.1   Statistical Analysis of Mortality Data

Intercurrent mortality refers to all deaths unrelated to the development of the particular type or class of tumors to be analyzed for evidence of carcinogenicity. Older rodents have a higher chance of developing tumors than younger ones. Consequently, if animals of a treatment group die earlier, they may not have enough life span and time of exposure to the study compound to develop late occurring tumors. If there is a significant difference in the survival patterns of animals among treatment groups, the usual statistical comparisons may be biased. Therefore, it is essential to identify and statistically adjust the possible differences in intercurrent mortality among treatment groups to reduce biases caused by this difference to make the statistical tests meaningful. Peto et al. [2] commented that "the effects of differences in longevity on numbers of tumor-bearing animals can be very substantial, and so, whether or not they appear to be, they should routinely be corrected for when presenting experimental results." Bancroft [3] suggested that if we treat the test for heterogeneity in survival distributions or dose–response relationship in mortality as a preliminary test of significance, then a level of significance larger than 0.05 should be used. A very large level of significance used in the preliminary tests in turn means that the survival-adjusted methods should always be used in the subsequent analyses of tumor data. The following examples clearly demonstrate this important point.

Example 21.1 [Peto et al.]

Consider an experiment consisting of one control group and one treated group of 100 animals each of a strain of mice. A very toxic but not tumorigenic new drug was administered to the animals in the diet for 2 years. Assume that the spontaneous incidental tumor rates for both groups are 30% at 15 months and 80% at 18 months of age and that the mortality rates at 15 months for the control and the treated groups are 20% and 60%, respectively, due to the toxicity of the drug. The results of the experiment are summarized in Table 21.3.

TABLE 21.3:   Tumor incidence and death rates at months 15 and 18.

	Control			Treated		
	T	$D\%$	$T\%$	T	$D\%$	$T\%$
15 months	6	20	30	18	60	30
18 months	64	80	80	32	40	80
Total	70	100	70	50	100	50

Note: T, number of incidental tumors found at necropsy; D%, percentage of deaths; T%, percentage of incidental tumors found at necropsy.

If one looks only at the overall tumor incidence rates of the control and the treated groups (70% and 50%, respectively) without considering the significantly higher early deaths in the treated group caused by the toxicity of this new drug, he/she will misleadingly conclude that there is a significant ($p = 0.002$, one-tailed) negative dose–response relationship for this tumor type (i.e., the new drug prevents tumor occurrences). However, the one-tailed p-value is 0.5 when the survival-adjusted method is used.

Example 21.2

In a slightly different variation of the above data, Gart et al. [4] showed the following results. Assume that the design used in this experiment is the same as the one used in the previous example. However, assume that the treated group has much higher early mortality than the control (20% versus 90%) before 15 months. Also, assume that the tumor prevalence rates for the control and treated groups are 5% and 20%, respectively, before 15 months of age and 30% and 70%, respectively, after 15 months of age. The results of this experiment are summarized in Table 21.4.

TABLE 21.4:   Tumor incidence and death rates before and after 15 months.

	Control			Treated		
	T	*D%*	*T%*	*T*	*D*	*T%*
Before 15 months	1	20	5	18	90	20
After 15 months	24	80	30	7	10	70
Total	25	100	25	25	100	25

Note: *T*, number of incidental tumors found at necropsy; *D%*, percentage of deaths; *T%*, percentage of incidental tumors found at necropsy.

It should be noted that the age-specific tumor incidence rates are significantly higher in the treated group than those in the control group. The survival-adjusted method yielded a one-tailed *p*-value of 0.003. This shows a clear tumorigenic effect of the new drug. However, the overall tumor incidence rates are 25% for the two groups. Without considering the significantly higher early mortality in the treated group, one will conclude that the positive dose–response relationship is not significant.

The above examples show that to meaningfully analyze the tumorigenicity data, it is important to analyze the mortality data to detect any significant difference in them among treatment groups. However, the methods of mortality-adjusted analysis of tumor data are nonunique and may be controversial sometimes. If no statistically significant difference in mortality is found, a survival-unadjusted analysis is often conducted because of its simplicity of implementation and interpretation.

The statistical analyses of mortality data include calculations of descriptive statistics, for example, percentage of survivals and death by dose group in different subintervals of the entire study period, visual presentation of mortality pattern (e.g., the graph of the Kaplan–Meier product limit estimation, etc.), and the formal tests that include tests for dose–response relationship, homogeneity among dose groups, and pairwise comparisons between treatment groups, especially control and treated groups.

To test for dose–response relationship and for homogeneity, the parametric method given in the articles of Tarone [5], Cox [6], Thomas et al. [7], and Gart et al. [4] and the nonparametric method of generalized Wilcoxon or Kruskal–Wallis tests [7–9] are widely used. Pairwise comparisons can also be performed using all these methods along with other methods, for example, the log-rank test [2], the chi-square test described in Snedecor and Cochran [10], and Fisher's exact test. Besides these methods, there are a host of other methods available for analyzing mortality data.

The following are typical summary tables (Tables 21.5 and 21.6) and a graphical (Figure 21.1) representation of the analysis of mortality data from carcinogenicity experiments.

TABLE 21.5: Intercurrent mortality rate in male mice.

Week	Control No. of Death	Control Cum. %	Low No. of Death	Low Cum. %	Medium No. of Death	Medium Cum. %	High No. of Death	High Cum. %
0–52			1	1.8	2	3.6		
3–78	10	18.2	3	5.5	8	16.4	6	14.5
79–91	10	36.4	2	9.1	5	25.5	6	25.5
92–104	12	58.2	14	34.5	11	45.5	7	38.2
Term. Sac.	23	41.8	36	65.5	30	54.5	34	61.8

TABLE 21.6: Intercurrent mortality comparison in male rats.

Method	Test	Statistic	*P*-Value
Cox	Dose response	1.1963	0.2741
	Homogeneity	8.9134	0.0305
Kruskal–Wallis	Dose response	0.8660	0.3521
	Homogeneity	9.6772	0.0215

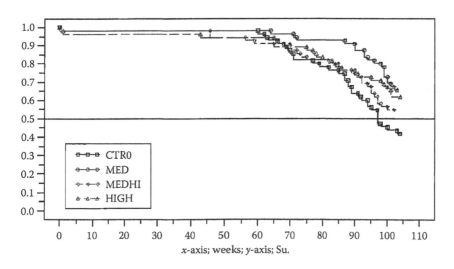

FIGURE 21.1: Kaplan–Meier survival curve for male rats.

21.6.2 Statistical Analysis of Tumor Data

As was true for survival data, the statistical analysis of tumor data consists of a descriptive part and an analytic part. The descriptive part mainly includes the calculation of frequencies of different observed tumor types in different treatment groups. These frequencies or rates are presented in tabular form. Generally, there is no visual representation in tumor data analysis. However, if needed Kaplan–Meier type graphs may be plotted for time to first tumor. The formal statistical analysis of tumor data includes an analysis of dose–response relationship as well as pairwise comparisons of treated groups, especially control and treated groups.

To test for dose–response relationship, the logistic regression [11–14], the Cochran–Armitage trend test [15,16], the method suggested by Peto et al. [2], and the Poly-K method suggested by Bailer and Portier [17] and Bieler and Williams [18] are widely used. Pairwise comparisons can also be performed using all the methods described here, along with other methods, for example, the Fisher's exact test.

The subsequent subsections contain detailed discussions of some widely used tests methods for trend and pairwise comparisons in tumor incidence rates. They are (1) logistic regression, (2) Cochran–Armitage regression test, (3) Armitage analysis of variance (ANOVA) test, (4) Peto method, and (5) Poly-K method.

21.6.2.1   Logistic Regression

This method of tumor data analysis is discussed in the article by Thomas et al. [7] and Dinse and Lagakos [13]. Let Y be the indicator of occurrence of a tumor, with value 1 if the tumor occurred and 0 if the tumor did not occur on an animal. Y will have one value for each animal (multiple occurrences of the same tumor on the same animal do not matter). Assume that Y values in dose group i have a binomial distribution with parameter P_i, which is modeled by a logistic density in terms of dose levels and other covariates. Formally, let x_i denote the ith dose level and t_{ij}, the survival time of the jth animal in the ith dose group. Then, P_i is modeled as

$$P_i = E(Y_i) = \left(e^{\alpha+\beta x_i}\right) / \left[1 + \left(e^{\alpha+\beta x_i}\right)\right]$$

without the adjustment of intercurrent mortality difference and as

$$P_i = E(Y_i) = \left[e^{\alpha+\beta x_i + F(t_{ij})}\right] / \left\{1 + \left[e^{\alpha+\beta x_i + F(t_{ij})}\right]\right\}$$

with the adjustment of intercurrent mortality difference. Where α and β are unknown parameters, $E(Y_i)$ is the expected value of Y_i of animal i, and $F(t_{ij})$ is a polynomial in survival time, that is,

$$F(t_{ij}) = c_1 t_{ij} + c_1 t_{ij}^2 + \cdots + c_p t_{ij}^p$$

The null hypothesis is that there is no dose–response relationship, against an alternative of positive dose response. In notation $H_0 : \beta = 0$ against $H_0 : \beta < 0$ (the direction of β is always in the opposite sense).

Let $\hat{\beta}$ be an unbiased estimate of β and $V(\hat{\beta})$, the variance of $\hat{\beta}$. A test statistic, Z, for dose response is then defined as

$$Z = \hat{\beta} / [V(\hat{\beta})]^{1/2}$$

Z is approximately distributed as standard normal and is used to test for the positive dose–response relationship in a specific incidental tumor. For survival-adjusted logistic regression models, there is an issue of defining $F(t_{ij})$. The functional form of $F(t_{ij})$ has to be specified in the logistic regression model to indicate the effect of survival time on tumor prevalence rate. However, there is no unique way of determining the functional form. Different functional forms of $F(t_i)$ could yield different results. Estimations of α and β are not straightforward.

As defined in Table 21.2, $n_0, n_1, \ldots, n_i, n_r$ are $r+1$ observations of tumor occurrence with probability $p_0, p_1, \ldots, p_i, \ldots, p_{r+1}$ the $r+1$ treatment groups. The associated binomial density for the ith dose group is

$$B(n_i, p_i) = \binom{N_i}{n_i} p_i^{n_i}(1-p_i)^{N_i-n_i} = \binom{N_i}{n_i}\left(\frac{e^{\alpha+\beta x_i}}{1+e^{\alpha+\beta x_i}}\right)^{n_i}\left(\frac{1}{1+e^{\alpha+\beta x_i}}\right)^{N_i-n_i}$$

$$= \binom{N_i}{n_i}\left(\frac{e^{\alpha n_i + \beta n_i x_i}}{(1+e^{\alpha+\beta x_i})^{N_i}}\right).$$

The likelihood function is

$$L = K\Pi\binom{N_i}{n_i}\left(\frac{e^{\alpha n_i + \beta n_i x_i}}{(1+e^{\alpha+\beta x_i})^{N_i}}\right) = K\frac{\exp(\alpha n + \beta \sum n_i x_i)}{\Pi\{1+\exp(\alpha+\beta x_i)\}^{N_i}}.$$

The log likelihood is

$$\log(L) = \log K + \alpha n + \beta \sum n_i x_i - \sum N_i \log\{1+\exp(\alpha+\beta x_i)\}.$$

Taking the derivatives and setting them to 0 we have

$$\frac{d\log(L)}{d\alpha} = n - \sum N_i \frac{\exp(\alpha+\beta x_i)}{1+\exp(\alpha+\beta x_i)} = 0 \tag{21.1}$$

and

$$\frac{d\log(L)}{d\beta} = \sum n_i x_i + \sum N_i x_i \frac{\exp(\alpha+\beta x_i)}{1+\exp(\alpha+\beta x_i)} = 0 \tag{21.2}$$

Clearly, Equations 21.1 and 21.2 are nonlinear in α and β, and there is no closed-form solution for them. Some iterative optimization methods are often applied to solve these sets of equations.

Example 21.3

Consider the incidence rates of interstitial cell tumor in testis in the carcinogenicity dataset given in Appendix 21.B, summarized in Table 21.7.

TABLE 21.7: Incidence of interstitial cell tumor in testis in male rats.

Treatment Group	Control	Low	Medium	High	Total
Dose level (mg)	0	100	300	1000	
NTBA	5	1	0	7	13
NNTBA	50	54	55	48	207
Total (N_i)	55	55	55	55	220
Proportion at risk $P_i = N_i/N$	0.250	0.250	0.250	0.250	1.000

Note: NTBA, number of tumor-bearing animals, NNTBA, number of nontumor-bearing animals, $N = \Sigma N_i$.

Using the SAS proc logistic with actual dose levels, we have $\hat{\beta} = 0.0012$ and $SE(\hat{\beta}) = 0.000666$. This gives $z = 1.8018$ and $p = 0.0358$.

From the above likelihood function, Thomas et al. pointed out that n and $\Sigma n_i x_i$ is a minimal set of sufficient statistics. Therefore, an optimal test of H_0 can be based on $\Sigma n_i x_i$ using the conditional distribution of number of tumor-bearing animals in treated groups with observed total number of events n fixed. This is the r-dimensional hypergeometric distribution:

$$f(n_0, n_1, \ldots, n_r \mid n; N_0, N_1, \ldots, N_r) = \frac{\prod_{i=1}^{r} \binom{N_i}{n_i}}{\binom{N}{n}}$$

The tail probability is $p = \sum_R f(n_0, n_1, \ldots, n_r \mid n; N_0, N_1, \ldots, N_r)$, where R is the set of $r+1$ fold partitions $\{Z\}$ of n such that $\Sigma_i Z x_i \geq \Sigma n_i x_i$ (the observed value). When $r = 1$, the test is equivalent to the Fisher exact test. The corresponding asymptotic test statistic for positive dose–response relationship is

$$z = \frac{\sum n_i x_i - n \sum N_i x_i / N}{[V(\sum x_i n_i \mid n; \beta = 0)]^{1/2}},$$

where

$$V\left(\sum x_i n_i \mid n; \beta = 0\right) = \frac{n(N-n)}{N(N-1)} \left(\sum N_i x_i^2 - \frac{(\sum N_i x_i)^2}{N}\right).$$

Example 21.4

Consider the incidence rates of interstitial cell tumor in testis with tumor incidence rates shown in Table 21.7. We have $n = 13$, $N = 220$, $\Sigma n_i x_i = 7100$, $\Sigma N_i x_i = 77,000$, and $\Sigma N_i x_i^2 = 60,500,000$. Therefore, $V(\Sigma n_i x_i) = 1,873,869.86$, $z = 1.86282$, and $p = 0.031244$.

21.6.2.2   Cochran–Armitage Regression Test

Armitage [15] proposed the following regression test procedure for frequency data in groups following some natural order. An implicit assumption of this test procedure is that all animals are at equal risk of getting the tumor over the duration of the study. For an illustration of this method consider similar data used to discuss the logistic regression method (given in Table 21.2), where $r + 1$ doses of a drug are applied to observe the occurrence of events, for example, occurrence of tumors. Let Y denote a response variable that takes the value of 1 if the event happens and 0 if the event does not happen, and let x_i denote the dose level for the ith dose group. As defined earlier, the proportion of successes in the ith group is $P_i = n_i/N_i$, and the overall proportion is

$P = n/N = \bar{Y}$. Also, let $\bar{x} = \sum N_i x_i / N$. Suppose there is a linear dose–response relationship between Y and x that is modeled by $E(Y) = a + bx$.

The least-square estimate $\hat{b}$ of b is

$$\hat{b} = \frac{\sum N_i (x_i - \bar{x}) Y_i}{\sum N_i (x_i - \bar{x})^2}.$$

Since Y can take values 0 and 1 only, we have

$$\hat{b} = \frac{\sum n_i (x_i - \bar{x})}{\sum N_i (x_i - \bar{x})^2} = \frac{\sum N_i p_i (x_i - \bar{x})}{\sum N_i (x_i - \bar{x})^2} = \frac{\sum n_i x_i - P \sum N_i x_i}{\sum N_i x_i^2 - \frac{\left(\sum N_i x_i\right)^2}{N}}.$$

The variance $V(\hat{b})$ of $\hat{b}$ is

$$V(\hat{b}) = \frac{\sigma^2}{\sum N_i (x_i - \bar{x})^2} = \frac{P(1 - P)}{\sum N_i (x_i - \bar{x})^2}.$$

With these notations, the statistic

$$\chi_0^2 = \frac{\hat{b}^2}{V(\hat{b})} = \frac{\left\{ \sum n_i x_i - P \sum N_i x_i \right\}^2}{P(1 - P)\left\{ \sum n_i x_i - \left(\sum N_i x_i\right)/N \right\}}$$

$$= \frac{\left\{ \sum n_i x_i - n/N \sum N_i x_i \right\}^2}{\frac{n(N - n)}{N^2} \left\{ \sum N_i x_i^2 - \left(\sum N_i x_i\right)^2 / N \right\}} \tag{21.3}$$

has a χ^2 distribution with 1 degree of freedom.

Alternatively, the square root of this statistic

$$z = \sqrt{\chi^2} = \frac{\left\{ \sum n_i x_i - (n/N) \sum N_i x_i \right\}}{\sqrt{\frac{n(N - n)}{N^2} \left\{ \sum N_i x_i^2 - \left(\sum N_i x_i\right)^2 / N \right\}}} \tag{21.4}$$

has approximately the standard normal distribution. This z statistic may be used to test a two-sided dose–response relationship test (positive or negative dose–response relationship). It may be noted that this statistic is the same as that suggested by Thomas, except for a slight difference in the calculation of variance of $\sum x_i n_i$.

Example 21.5

Consider the data of interstitial cell tumor in testis with tumor incidence rates shown in Table 21.7. We have $n = 13$, $N = 220$, $\sum n_i x_i = 7100$, $\sum N_i x_i = 77{,}000$, and $\sum N_i x_i^2 = 60{,}500{,}000$. Therefore, $V(\sum n_i x_i) = 1{,}865{,}352.27$, $z = 1.86707$, and $p = 0.030946$.

21.6.2.3   Armitage Analysis of Variance Test

Armitage [15] also proposed the following ANOVA test for frequency data in groups. He applied a one-way analysis of the variance model with Y as the dependent variable and the dose levels (x) as the classification factor. He first partitioned the total sum of squares (TSS) into treatment sum of squares (TrSS) and error sum of squares (ESS). He then further partitioned the TrSS into the sum of the squares due to the linear regression (LSS), that is, the part of variation explained by the linear model and the sum of squares due to departure from linearity (DLSS). That is,

$$\sum N_i(Y_i - P)^2 = \sum N_i(Y_i - P_i)^2 + \sum N_i(P_i - P)^2$$

$$\sum N_i(Y_i - P)^2 = \sum N_i(Y_i - P_i)^2 + \sum N_i(P_i - \hat{y}_i)^2 + \sum N_I(\hat{y}_i - P)^2$$

or

$$\text{TSS} = \text{ESS} + \text{LSS} + \text{DLSS}.$$

In Armitage notation, total $= S_3 + S_2 + S_1$. His proposed ANOVA table is as follows (Table 21.8):

TABLE 21.8:   ANOVA for Armitage model.

Source of Variation	Degrees of Freedom	Sum of Squares
Treatment	r	$S_1 + S_2$
Linear regression (linearity)	1	S_1
Departure from linearity	$r - 1$	S_2
Error	$N - r - 1$	S_3
Total	$N - 1$	$S_1 + S_2 + S_3$

Note: N, total number of animals; $r+1$, number of treatment groups (including the control).

where, total $= S_1 + S_2 + S_3 = \sum N_i(Y_i - P)^2 = \sum N_i Y_i^2 - 2P \sum N_i Y_i - P^2 \sum N_i$.

Since Y_i can take values 0 and 1 only, and there are nY_i's with values 1 and $P = n/N$, we have

$$S_1 + S_2 + S_3 = n - 2Pn - P^2N = n - \frac{n^2}{N} = n\left(1 - \frac{n}{N}\right).$$

The sum of squares due to treatment is

$$S_1 + S_2 = \sum N_i(P_i - P)^2 = \sum \frac{n_i^2}{N_i} - \frac{n^2}{N},$$

and the sum of squares due to linear regression is

$$S_1 = \sum N_i(\hat{y}_i - P)^2 = \hat{b}^2 \sum N_i(x_i - \bar{x})^2.$$

Putting

$$\hat{b} = \frac{\sum n_i x_i - P \sum N_i x_i}{\sum N_i x_i^2 - \frac{\left(\sum N_i x_i\right)^2}{N}},$$

we have

$$S_1 = \frac{\left(\sum n_i x_i - P \sum N_i x_i\right)^2}{\sum N_i x_i^2 - \frac{\left(\sum N_i x_i\right)^2}{N}}.$$

The sum of squares due to departure from linearity, S_2, and the sum of squares due to error, S_3, can be obtained by subtraction.

Since the dependent variable Y assumes only values 0 and 1, the test statistic for the linear contrast in regular ANOVA needs to be modified. Armitage suggested the use of the alternative statistic $\chi^2_{LR} = \frac{S_1}{(S_1+S_2+S_3)/N}$, which is distributed approximately as χ^2 with 1 degree of freedom under the null hypothesis of no positive dose–response relationship. It should be noted that $\frac{S_1}{(S_1+S_2+S_3)/N} = \frac{\hat{b}^2}{V(\hat{b})}$ defined above in Equation 21.3. Using the same denominator, we can define the test statistic for the test for departure from linearity as $\chi^2_{DL} = \frac{S_2}{(S_1+S_2+S_3)/N}$. The ANOVA results can be used to test for linear dose–response relationship as well as for departure from linearity.

The Cochran–Armitage regression test and the Armitage ANOVA tests are survival-unadjusted. The results from the unadjusted methods are reasonably unbiased if the differences in intercurrent mortality among the treatment groups are not significant. For experiments experiencing significant differences in intercurrent mortality, the Cochran–Armitage trend test procedures can be modified to adjust the effect of the survival differences. Two different modifications can be made. The first modification is to use the survival time as a covariate and perform the analysis of covariance. The second modification is to include the survival time as a linear term or quadratic term or both in the regression analysis as other independent variables in addition to the score variable X.

The computations in the modified Cochran–Armitage regression method are much simpler than those in the logistic regression method. However, they may not satisfy the condition of constant variance in regression analysis. The modified Cochran–Armitage regression method also has a shortcoming similar to that of the logistic regression method. That is, there is no unique way to determine the functional relationship between survival time and tumor incidence.

Example 21.6

Consider again the data of interstitial cell tumor in testis with tumor incidence rates shown in Table 21.7. The ANOVA table is as follows (Table 21.9):

TABLE 21.9: ANOVA for Armitage model.

Source of Variation	Degrees of Freedom	Sum of Squares	χ^2-Value	Z-Value	P-Value Using Z-Values
Treatment	3	0.5955			
Linear regression (linearity)	1	0.1938	3.4859	1.8671	0.0309
Departure from linearity	2	0.4016	7.22384	2.6877	0.00036
Error	216	11.6364			
Total	219	12.2318			

The ANOVA results show a highly significant departure from linearity.

21.6.2.4 Peto Method

As mentioned before, if there are significant differences in mortality among treatment groups, an analysis without appropriate adjustment for the mortality differences may yield a misleading result. Therefore, methods capable of appropriately adjusting mortality difference are preferred. Peto et al. [2] suggested such a method, popularly known as the Peto method. This method corrects the intercurrent mortality differences among treatment groups for a positive dose–response relationships test. Operationally, this method partitions the entire study period into a set of nonoverlapping intervals plus interim sacrifices and terminal sacrifice time points or periods. Animals are stratified by their survival times into those intervals. Data are then analyzed separately in each interval using the Cochran–Armitage test, and the results of individual intervals are then combined using the Mantel–Haenszel [19] procedure to get an overall result. The Mantel–Haenszel procedure states that if $z_0, z_1, \ldots, z_r$ are $r+1$ independent normal variates with means $E(z_0), E(z_1), \ldots, E(z_r)$, and variances $V(z_0), V(z_1), \ldots, V(z_r)$, then $z = z_0 + z_1 + \cdots + z_r$ has a normal distribution with mean $E(z) = \Sigma E(z_i)$ and variance $V(z) = \Sigma V(z_i)$.

Commonly, the Peto method uses a normal approximation for the test for positive dose–response relationship in tumor prevalence rates. The accuracy of the normal approximation depends on the numbers of tumor-bearing animals in each group in each interval, the number of intervals used in the partition, and the mortality patterns. However, it is known that the approximation will not be stable and reliable when the numbers of tumor-bearing animals across treatment groups are small. The *p*-values based on asymptotic normal approximation are underestimated. In this situation, an exact permutation test is used to test the positive dose–response relationship in tumor prevalence rates. In this section we discuss the Peto analysis using the normal approximation. We will discuss the exact analysis separately in a later section.

The choice of positions, number, and width of these intervals depends on the type of context of observation of tumors (incidental, fatal, or mortality-independent). Although Peto et al. [2] proposed the general guidance for partitioning the experimental period into intervals, there is no unique way to do the partition. Test results could be different when different sets of intervals are used. Dinse and Haseman [12] applied 10 different sets of intervals to the same tumor dataset and got 10 different p-values ranging from 0.001 to 0.261.

It is recommended in Peto et al. [2] that the intervals should be chosen in such a way that they "are not so short that the prevalence of incidental tumors in the autopsies they contain is not stable, nor yet so large that the real prevalence in the first half of one interval could differ markedly from the real prevalence in the second half." In particular for predetermined intervals, we have to make sure that none of the intervals ends up with zero number of tumor-bearing animals. The consequence of a poor choice of intervals may sometimes be catastrophic. The following artificial example of a two-group comparison by permutation test (an equivalence to the Fisher exact test) will illustrate the point. The same serious problem of a poor choice of intervals exists in Peto trend tests and pairwise comparisons in incidence rate based on asymptotic approximation.

Example 21.7

Suppose we have two treatment groups, namely, control and treated groups, with 50 animals each. Also, suppose the treated group showed 14 animals with a particular tumor compared with none in the control group. A pairwise comparison using the permutation test shows a highly significant ($p = 0.00002$) increase in tumor incidence in the treated group compared with the control. This result seems to be justified for this pattern of tumor occurrences.

	Treatment Groups		
	Control	Treated	
Table A	0/50	14/50	$p = 0.00002$

Now suppose we have three preselected intervals to stratify the animals for their mortality difference and this stratification gives us the following tumor incidences in different intervals. A pairwise comparison using the age-adjusted permutation test produces a p-value of 0.700, not significant. This result seems unjustified for this pattern of tumor occurrences.

		Treatment Groups		
		Control	Treated	
Table B	Interval 1	0/0	12/13	$p = 0.700$
	Interval 2	0/4	2/21	
	Interval 3	0/46	0/16	
	Total	0/50	14/50	

Clearly, a bad selection of interval positions is responsible for this result. In this analysis the analysis process of permutation test ignored the complete row with the 0/0 element in any cell. The permutation test also ignored the complete row with no tumor-bearing animals in any treatment group. For these kinds of situations, the permutation test practically throws away data and calculates the p-value based on data from the remaining animals. In this example the test procedure ignored the data in intervals 1 and 3 and calculated the p-value using the data from interval 2 only, that is, as follows.

		Treatment Groups		
		Control	Treated	
Table C	Interval 2	0/4	2/21	$p = 0.700$

Because of the earlier-mentioned problems and the lack of uniqueness of partitioning the experiment period, some regression-type methods have been proposed as alternatives for analyzing tumor data from animal carcinogenicity experiments. The logistic regression involving survival time as a continuous regression variable [11–14], the Cochran–Armitage trend test methods involving survival time as a continuous regression variable [15,16], and the Poly-K methods are three examples of those proposed alternatives. These methods do not need to partition the experimental period into intervals. Another advantage of these methods is that other variables that have effects on the prevalence rates, such as body weight and cage location, can also be incorporated into the model as covariates.

The ad hoc runs procedure, also described in Peto et al. [2], may be used to correct the problem caused by using a preselected set of partitioned intervals. This procedure determines different sets of intervals for different tumors based on the times of death of animals and the incidence rates of individual tumors. The disadvantages of using this procedure in the analysis of tumor data are that it increases the false-positive rate and that it involves more computations.

In addition to the problems caused by the choice of partition of study period, there are other difficulties in the use of the Peto method. As mentioned previously, The Peto test requires the cause-of-death information to adjust for differences in mortality among treatment groups. The death-rate method, the onset-rate method, and the prevalence method (defined and discussed in later sections) are selected for survival-adjusted tests for trend and pairwise difference in the Peto method for fatal tumors, mortality-independent tumors, and incidental tumors, respectively. It is a controversy whether pathologists can specify the cause-of-death information accurately. There are consequences of yielding wrong results if inaccurate cause-of-death information is used.

The test statistic Z suggested by Peto et al. may be described as follows. Consider the following dataset, in which the animals have been stratified by their survival time into m nonoverlapping strata as follows:

Interval	Treatment Group	0	1	...	i	...	r	Total
1	Dose	x_0	x_1	...	x_i	...	x_r	
	NTBA	n_{01}	n_{11}	...	n_{i1}	...	n_{r1}	n_1
	NNTBA	$N_{01}-n_{01}$	$N_{11}-n_{11}$	...	$N_{i1}-n_{i1}$	...	$N_{r1}-n_{r1}$	N_1-n_1
	Total	N_{01}	N_{11}	...	N_{i1}	...	N_{r1}	N_1
	Proportion at risk $P_{i1}=N_{i1}/N_1$	P_{01}	P_{11}	...	P_{i1}	...	P_{r1}	1

Interval	Treatment Group	0	1	...	i	...	r	Total
k	Dose	x_0	x_1	...	x_i	...	x_r	
	NTBA	n_{0k}	n_{1k}	...	n_{ik}	...	n_{rk}	n_k
	NNTBA	$N_{0k}-n_{0k}$	$N_{1k}-n_{1k}$	...	$N_{ik}-n_{ik}$	...	$N_{rk}-n_{rk}$	N_k-n_k
	Total	N_{0k}	N_{1k}	...	N_{ik}	...	N_{rk}	N_k
	Proportion at risk $P_{ik}=N_{ik}/N_k$	P_{0k}	P_{1k}	...	P_{ik}	...	P_{rk}	1

Interval	Treatment Group	0	1	...	i	...	r	Total
m	Dose	x_0	x_1	...	x_i	...	x_r	
	NTBA	n_{0m}	n_{1m}	...	n_{im}	...	n_{rm}	n_m
	NNTBA	$N_{0m}-n_{0m}$	$N_{1m}-n_{1m}$	...	$N_{im}-n_{im}$	...	$N_{rm}-n_{rm}$	N_m-n_m
	Total	N_{0m}	N_{1m}	...	N_{im}	...	N_{rm}	N_m
	Proportion at risk $P_{im}=N_{im}/N_m$	P_{0m}	P_{1m}	...	P_{im}	...	P_{rm}	1

Note: NTBA, number of tumor-bearing animals; NNTBA, number of nontumor-bearing animals.

For the kth table the Cochran–Armitage test statistic is

$$z_k = \frac{\sum n_{ik}x_i - (n_k/N_k)\sum N_{ik}x_i}{\sqrt{\dfrac{n_k(N_k-n_k)}{N_k^2}\left\{\sum N_{ik}x_i^2 - \left(\sum N_{ik}x_i\right)^2\Big/N_k\right\}}} = \frac{T_k}{\sqrt{V(T_k)}}.$$

Defining $T = \sum T_k$ and $V = \sum V(T_k)$, results in the Mantel–Haenszel statistic

$$Z = \frac{T}{\sqrt{V}} = \frac{\sum\{\sum n_{ik}x_i - (n_k/N_k)\sum N_{ik}x_i\}}{\sqrt{\sum \dfrac{n_k(N_k-n_k)}{N_k^2}\left\{\sum N_{ik}x_i^2 - \left(\sum N_{ik}x_i\right)^2\Big/N_k\right\}}}, \tag{21.5}$$

which has a standard normal distribution and is the test statistic for the overall dose–response relationship test.

Following the work by Cox [6], an alternative expression of this statistic is given by Peto et al. as follows: For the kth table and the ith dose group, let the observed number of success be $O_{ik}=n_{ik}$ and the expected number of success, $E_{ik}=n_k * P_{ik}$. The covariance of tumor frequencies in the ith and jth dose groups $E\{(n_{ik}-E_{ik})(n_{jk}-E_{ik})\}$ is

$$V_{ijk} = \frac{n_k(N_k-n_k)}{N_k-1}P_{ik}(\delta_{ij}-P_{jk}),$$

where $\delta_{ij} = 1$ if $i = j$ and 0 otherwise. Summing over the intervals defines the total observed number of successes for the ith dose group, $O_i = \sum_k n_{ik}$, and total expected number of successes, $E_i = \sum_k E_{ik}$, with $E(O_i - E_i) = 0$ and covariance $V_{ij} = E\{(O_i - E_i)(O_j - E_j)\} = \sum_k V_{ijk}$.

Also, we define $T = \sum x_i(O_i - E_i)$, then $E(T) = 0$, and $V(T) = \sum\sum x_i x_j V_{ij}$. With these notations $Z = T/\sqrt{V(T)}$ is approximately normally distributed and is the test statistic suggested by Peto et al. Because

$$\sum T_j = \sum x_i(O_i - E_i) = \sum x_i\left(n_i - \sum n_k \frac{N_{ik}}{N_k}\right) = \sum\left(x_i \sum n_{ik} - x_i \sum n_k \frac{N_{ik}}{N_k}\right),$$

the numerator of Peto statistic is the same as that of Cochran–Armitage. The relation between the denominators (variances) of the two statistics may be observed as follows:
The variance from the Peto formula is

$$V = \sum_i \sum_j x_i x_j V_{ij} = \sum_i \sum_j x_i x_j \sum_k V_{ijk} = \sum_i \sum_j x_i x_j \sum_k \frac{n_k(N_k - n_k)}{N_k - 1} \frac{N_{ik}}{N_k}\left(\delta_{ij} - \frac{N_{jk}}{N_k}\right)$$

$$= \sum_k \sum_i x_i^2 \frac{n_k(N_k - n_k)}{N_k - 1} \frac{N_{ik}}{N_k}\left(1 - \frac{N_{jk}}{N_k}\right)$$

$$+ \sum_k \sum_{i \neq j} x_i x_j \frac{n_k(N_k - n_k)}{N_k - 1} \frac{N_{ik}}{N_k}\left(-\frac{N_{jk}}{N_k}\right)$$

$$= \sum_k \frac{n_k(N_k - n_k)}{N_k(N_k - 1)}\left\{\sum_i x_i^2 \frac{(N_k - N_{ik})N_{ik}}{N_k} - \sum_{i \neq j} x_i x_j \frac{N_{ik}N_{jk}}{N_k}\right\}. \qquad (21.6)$$

The variance from the Cochran–Armitage formula is

$$V = \sum_k \frac{n_k(N_k - n_k)}{N_k^2}\left\{\sum_i N_{ik}x_i^2 - \frac{1}{N_k}\left(\sum_i N_{ik}x_i\right)^2\right\}$$

$$= \sum_k \frac{n_k(N_k - n_k)}{N_k^2}\left\{\sum_i N_{ik}x_i^2 - \frac{1}{N_k}\left(\sum_i N_{ik}x_i\right)\left(\sum_j N_{jk}x_j\right)\right\}$$

$$= \sum_k \frac{n_k(N_k - n_k)}{N_k^2}\left\{\sum_i N_{ik}x_i^2 - \frac{1}{N_k}\left(\sum_i N_{ik}^2 x_i^2 - \sum_{i \neq j} N_{ik}N_{jk}x_i x_j\right)\right\}$$

$$= \sum_k \frac{n_k(N_k - n_k)}{N_k^2}\left\{\sum_i N_{ik}x_i^2\left(\frac{N_k - N_{ik}}{N_k}\right) - \frac{1}{N_k}\left(\sum_{i \neq j} N_{ik}N_{jk}x_i x_j\right)\right\}$$

$$\approx \sum_k \frac{n_k(N_k - n_k)}{N_k(N_k - 1)}\left\{\sum_i x_i^2 \frac{(N_k - N_{ik})N_{ik}}{N_k} - \left(\sum_{i \neq j} x_i x_j \frac{N_{ik}N_{jk}}{N_k}\right)\right\}. \qquad (21.7)$$

Equations 21.6 and 21.7 show that the variance calculated using the Peto formula is slightly larger.

The Peto analysis is conducted for all tumor types. However, the choice of intervals and animals at risk in each interval differs from tumor type to tumor type.

The methods used are also named differently for different tumor types. For example, the death-rate method, the onset-rate method, and the prevalence method are used to analyze data of tumors observed in fatal, mortality-independent, and incidental contexts of observation, respectively. In the same paper, Peto et al. demonstrate the possible biases resulting from misclassifications of incidental tumors as fatal tumors or fatal tumors as incidental tumors.

In the following subsections we discuss the Peto method of analysis for incidental, fatal, and mortality-independent tumors separately.

21.6.2.4.1 Incidental Tumors (Prevalence Method) In analyzing data of incidental tumors, the study period is first divided into a reasonable number of intervals. This selection of number and position of intervals can be predetermined or can be determined by the tumor data, using the ad hoc runs procedure.

For the estimation of the proportion of tumor-bearing animals in each time interval for each treatment group, the observed number of tumor-bearing animals is compared (numerator) with the number of animals that died in the interval (denominator). Data are analyzed for the dose–response relationship using the Z statistic pooled over all selected intervals. This procedure of analyzing incidental tumor data is known as the "prevalence method." The null hypothesis is that there is no dose–response relationship.

Example 21.8

Consider the data of interstitial cell tumor in testis. To adjust the mortality difference let us divide the entire study period into three intervals I_1, I_2, and I_3 with the following outcomes (Table 21.10):

TABLE 21.10: Incidence of interstitial cell tumor in testis in male rats by intervals.

Interval	Dose Group	Control	Low	Medium	High	Total
I_1	Dose level (mg)	0	100	300	1000	
	NTBA	0	0	0	1	1
	NNTBA	10	2	5	5	22
	Total	10	2	5	6	23
	Proportion at risk $P_{i1} = N_{i1}/N_1$	0.434	0.087	0.217	0.261	1.00
I_2	Dose level (mg)	0	100	300	1000	
	NTBA	1	1	0	0	2
	NNTBA	11	13	11	7	42
	Total	12	14	11	7	44
	Proportion at risk $P_{i2} = N_{i2}/N_2$	0.286	0.583	0.250	0159	1.00
I_3	Dose level (mg)	0	100	300	1000	
	NTBA	4	0	0	6	10
	NNBA	19	36	30	28	113
	Total	23	36	30	34	123
	Proportion $P_{i3} = n_{i3}/N_{i3}$	0.187	0.293	0.243	0.276	1.00

Note: NTBA, number of tumor-bearing animals; NNTBA, number of nontumor-bearing animals.

Using the Cochran–Armitage formula we have

	Statistic	
Interval	T	$V(T)$
I_1	665.22	161,867.35
I_2	−431.82	217,760.61
I_3	2211.38	1,449,381.71
Total	2444.78	1,829,009.67

and $z = \frac{2{,}444.78}{\sqrt{1{,}829{,}009.67}} = 1.80772$ and $p = 0.035325$.

Using Peto's formula produces Table 21.11:

TABLE 21.11: Observed and expected tumor incidences along with their estimated variance covariances.

Interval	Dose1	Dose2	P1	δ-P2	Observed	Expected	Total Observed	vijk
I1	0	0	.435	.565	0	0.435	5	0.246
		100	.435	−.09	0	0.087	1	−0.038
		300	.435	−.22	0	0.217	0	−0.095
		1000	.435	−.26	1	0.261	7	−0.113
	100	0	.087	−.43	0	0.435	5	−0.038
		100	.087	.913	0	0.087	1	0.079
		300	.087	−.22	0	0.217	0	−0.019
		1000	.087	−.26	1	0.261	7	−0.023
	300	0	.217	−.43	0	0.435	5	−0.095
		100	.217	−.09	0	0.087	1	−0.019
		300	.217	.783	0	0.217	0	0.170
		1000	.217	−.26	1	0.261	7	−0.057
	1000	0	.261	−.43	0	0.435	5	−0.113
		100	.261	−.09	0	0.087	1	−0.023
		300	.261	−.22	0	0.217	0	−0.057
		1000	.261	.739	1	0.261	7	0.193
I2	0	0	.273	.727	1	0.545	5	0.387
		100	.273	−.32	1	0.636	1	−0.170
		300	.273	−.25	0	0.5	0	−0.133
		1000	.273	−.16	0	0.318	7	−0.085
	100	0	.318	−.27	1	0.545	5	−0.170
		100	.318	.682	1	0.636	1	0.424
		300	.318	−.25	0	0.5	0	−0.155
		1000	.318	−.16	0	0.318	7	−0.099
	300	0	.250	−.27	1	0.545	5	−0.133
		100	.250	−.32	1	0.636	1	−0.155
		300	.250	.750	0	0.5	0	0.366
		1000	.250	−.16	0	0.318	7	−0.078
	1000	0	.159	−.27	1	0.545	5	−0.085
		100	.159	−.32	1	0.636	1	−0.099
		300	.159	−.25	0	0.5	0	−0.078
		1000	.159	.841	0	0.318	7	0.261

TABLE 21.11 (continued): Observed and expected tumor incidences along with their estimated variance covariances.

Interval	Dose1	Dose2	P1	δ-P2	Observed	Expected	Total Observed	vijk
I3	0	0	.187	.813	4	1.87	5	1.408
		100	.187	−.29	0	2.927	1	−0.507
		300	.187	−.24	0	2.439	0	−0.422
		1000	.187	−.28	6	2.764	7	−0.479
	100	0	.293	−.19	4	1.87	5	−0.507
		100	.293	.707	0	2.927	1	1.917
		300	.293	−.24	0	2.439	0	−0.661
		1000	.293	−.28	6	2.764	7	−0.749
	300	0	.244	−.19	4	1.87	5	−0.422
		100	.244	−.29	0	2.927	1	−0.661
		300	.244	.756	0	2.439	0	1.708
		1000	.244	−.28	6	2.764	7	−0.624
	1000	0	.276	−.19	4	1.87	5	−0.479
		100	.276	−.29	0	2.927	1	−0.749
		300	.276	−.24	0	2.439	0	−0.624
		1000	.276	.724	6	2.764	7	1.853

Summing over intervals (k) we have the following (Table 21.12):

TABLE 21.12: Calculated values V_{IJ} and $d_i d_j v_{ij}$.

Dose1	Dose2	Vij	didjvij
0	0	2.041	0.00
	100	−0.714	0.00
	300	−0.650	0.00
	1000	−0.677	0.00
100	0	−0.714	0.00
	100	2.421	24206.66
	300	−0.835	−25064.81
	1000	−0.871	−87092.84
300	0	−0.650	0.00
	100	−0.835	−25064.81
	300	2.245	202005.78
	1000	−0.759	−227661.60
1000	0	−0.677	0.00
	100	−0.871	−87092.84
	300	−0.759	−227661.60
	1000	2.307	2306737.71

The calculated T, V, Z statistics and the p-values are as follows (Table 21.13):

TABLE 21.13: Calculated T, V, Z statistics and p-values.

T	V	z	P-Value
2444.78	1853311.66	1.7958323	0.03626

21.6.2.4.2   Fatal Tumors (Death-Rate Method)   For fatal tumor data analysis, a separate time interval is selected for each distinct tumor-onset time point. One implicit assumption is made for the analysis of fatal tumor that animals die instantaneously or in a very short time after the onset of tumor. Therefore, in this analysis the tumor-onset time and the time of death are supposed to be the same. Operationally, when an animal dies from a fatal tumor, the time of death is used for the time of onset. Suppose $t_1 < t_2 < \cdots < t_m$ are the time points when one or more animals died due to a fatal tumor. The collection of these m time points is used to form the total number of intervals to analyze the fatal tumor. For the estimation of the proportion of tumor-bearing animals at each time point for each treatment group, the observed number of tumor-bearing animals at time point t_i is compared (numerator) with the number of animals alive at time point t_i (denominator). The analysis then follows similarly as was described for the incidental tumor. That is, analyze data separately for each incidence time point using the Cochran–Armitage test and then combine the results using the Mantel–Haenszel procedure. This procedure of analyzing fatal tumor data is known as the "death-rate method." The null hypothesis is that there is no dose–response relationship.

21.6.2.4.3   Tumors Observed as Both Incidental and Fatal (Mixed Method)   When a tumor is observed in an incidental context for a set of animals and is observed in a fatal context for the remaining animals, data should be analyzed separately by the prevalence methods for the first set of animals and by the death-rate method for the remaining animals. Results from the different methods are then combined by the Mantel–Haenszel procedure.

21.6.2.4.4   Tumors Observed in Mortality-Independent Context (Onset-Rate Method)   For the analysis of tumors observed in a mortality-independent context, Peto et al. suggested a method similar to the death-rate method. This method uses the time of detection of the tumor instead of time of death to form the number of intervals. With this modification, the numerator for the estimation of the proportion of tumor-bearing animals at time t_i is the number of animals detected with tumor at t_i, and the denominator is the number of animals alive at the detection time. This method is known as the onset-rate method.

One important question is whether one should test dose–response relationship with respect to dose or based on an ordinal scale (rank of the used dose level). Peto et al. [2] made the following recommendation:

> If two or more dose levels are studied, statistical tests for positive trend with respect to the actual dose-levels tested will usually be more sensitive than the standard alternative statistical methods would be to any real carcinogenic effects that may exist (p. 338).

Therefore, use of the actual dose level for dose–response relationship tests is recommended.

21.6.2.4.5   Exact Peto Test   As mentioned in previous subsections, the prevalence and the death-rate methods described in Peto et al. [2] use a normal approximation in the test for the positive dose–response relationship in tumor incidence rates. Mortality patterns, the numbers of intervals used in the partition of the study period, and the numbers and patterns of tumor occurrence in each individual interval have effects on the accuracy of the normal approximation. It is particularly true that when the number of tumor-bearing animals across all treatment groups is "small," the normal approximation is unreliable and tends mostly to underestimate the exact p-values [20]. Under this situation, the use of an exact permutation trend test is suggested [4] to test for a dose–response relationship in tumor incidence rates. The exact dose–response relationship test is a generalization of the Fisher exact test to a sequence of $2X(r+1)$ tables for experiment with r dose groups and one control group, which is derived by conditioning on the fixed row and column marginal totals of each of the $2X(r+1)$ tables. As pointed out earlier under the assumption of fixed row and column totals, $n_{0k}, n_{1k}, \ldots, n_{rk}$ have a hypergeometric distribution.

Consider the following data from the kth time interval of a Peto analysis, with fixed row and column totals (Table 21.14).

TABLE 21.14: Summary data in the kth time interval I_k.

Treatment Group	0	1	i	$\ldots$	r	Total
Dose	x_0	x_1	x_i		x_r	
NTBA	n_{0k}	n_{1k}	n_{ik}		n_{rk}	n_k
NNTBA	$N_{0k} - n_{0k}$	$N_{1k} - n_{1k}$	$N_{ik} - n_{ik}$		$N_{rk} - n_{rk}$	$N_k - n_k$
Total	N_{0k}	N_{1k}	N_{ik}		N_{rk}	N_k

Note: NTBA, number of tumor-bearing animals; NNTBA, number of nontumor-bearing animals.

Consider the Cochran–Armitage z statistic

$$z = \frac{\left\{ \sum n_i x_i - n/N \sum N_i x_i \right\}}{\sqrt{n(N-n)/N^2 \left\{ N_i x_i^2 - \left(\sum N_i x_i \right)^2 / N \right\}}}$$

or the alternative expression of Peto test statistic

$$Z = \frac{\sum x_i n_i - \dfrac{n}{N} \sum x_i N_i}{\sqrt{\sum x_i^2 \dfrac{N_i}{N} \left(1 - \dfrac{N_i}{N}\right)}}.$$

Since the row totals, column totals, and dose levels are all fixed, the only random variable in these expressions is $y = \sum n_i x_i$.

Because of this reasoning and also from Thomas et al.'s argument of sufficient statistics, it is possible to construct a conditional test procedure based on $y = \sum n_i x_i$. The tail distribution is defined as the probability that y will be greater than the observed $y = y_0$ among all possible permutations of n_{ik} values in the kth table satisfying the fixed value of row and column totals. That is, cumulating the probabilities of possible tables that are more extreme than the observed table in terms of y $[P(Y \geq y_{\text{obs}})]$. For an exact test the table probabilities are calculated using the hypergeometric distribution, for example, the probability of the kth table defined above is given by

$$P(Y_k = y_k) = \frac{\binom{N_{0k}}{n_{0k}}\binom{N_{1k}}{n_{1k}} \cdots \binom{N_{ik}}{n_{rk}}}{\binom{N_k}{n_{.k}}}.$$

If we have a total of K tables, then y_k is calculated from the kth table and the overall test statistic is defined as $y = \sum y_k$, and if we assume that they are all independent, then the overall probability involving all tables is calculated by multiplying probabilities from all individual tables; that is,

$$P(Y = y) = P(Y_0 = y_0, Y_1 = y_1, \ldots, Y_k = y_k)$$
$$= P(Y_0 = y_0) \times P(Y_1 = y_1) \times \cdots \times P(Y_K = y_K).$$

The overall probability that Y is greater than the observed y (y_{obs}) is calculated as

$$p\text{-value} = P(Y >= y_{\text{obs}}) = \sum_R [P(Y_1 = y_1) \ldots P(Y_k = y_K)],$$

where R is the region such that $y \geq y_{\text{obs}}$ (right-hand tail). Statistical significance is declared if this right-hand tail p-value is extreme (i.e., smaller than the test level α).

Example 21.9

Consider an experiment with three treatment groups (control, low, and high) with dose levels $D_0 = 0$, $D_1 = 1$, and $D_2 = 2$, respectively. Suppose the study period is partitioned into two intervals I_1 and I_2. Consider a tumor type (classified as incidental) with the following data (Table 21.15).

TABLE 21.15: Tumor count table.

Time Interval	Animals	Dose Levels 0	1	2	Total
I_1	n_1	0	1	2	3
	N_1	10	12	16	38
I_2	n_2	0	1	1	2
	N_2	40	38	34	112

Note: n_i, observer number of tumor-bearing animals in the ith interval; N_i, number of animals at risk (examined) in the ith interval.

The observed tables formed from the two intervals are as follows:

Observed Table O_1 from I_1					Observed Table O_2 from I_2				
	Dose Levels					Dose Levels			
	0	1	2	Total		0	1	2	Total
n_1	0	1	2	3	n_2	0	1	1	2
$N_1 - n_1$	10	11	14	35	$N_2 - n_2$	40	37	33	110
N_1	10	12	16	38	N_2	40	38	34	112

The y value for observed Table O_1 is $y_1 = 0 \times 0 + 1 \times 1 + 2 \times 2 = 5$, the y value for the observed Table O_2 is $y_2 = 0 \times 0 + 1 \times 1 + 2 \times 1 = 3$, and the overall y value $y = 5 + 3 = 8$. The probability of observed Table O_1 is

$$P(Y_1 = 5) = \frac{\binom{10}{0}\binom{12}{1}\binom{16}{2}}{\binom{38}{3}} = \frac{(12 \times 16 \times 15)/2}{(38 \times 37 \times 36)/3 \times 2} = 0.17070,$$

and the probability of observed Table O_2 is

$$P(Y_1 = 32) = \frac{\binom{40}{0}\binom{38}{1}\binom{34}{1}}{\binom{112}{2}} = \frac{(38 \times 34)/2}{(112 \times 111)/2} = 0.20785.$$

For all possible outcomes of this experiment, satisfying the observed marginal total, all configurations of observed Table O_1 associate with all configurations of observed Table O_2. This will produce $10 \times 6 = 60$ possible configurations with values $y = y1 + y2$ and probability $p(y) = p(y1) \ast p(y2)$. All possible values of y with their corresponding probabilities, in ascending order of y, are given in Table 21.16.

TABLE 21.16: All possible configurations of tumor occurrences with corresponding y- and p-values (presented in ascending order of y values).

Config Number	Interval 1					Interval 2					Overall	
	G1	G2	G3	y1	P1	G1	G2	G3	y2	P2	$y=y1+y2$	$p=p1\ast p2$
1	3	0	0	0	.014	2	0	0	0	.125	0	.002
2	3	0	0	0	.014	1	1	0	1	.245	1	.003
3	2	1	0	1	.064	2	0	0	0	.125	1	.008
4	3	0	0	0	.014	0	2	0	2	.113	2	.002
5	3	0	0	0	.014	1	0	1	2	.219	2	.003
6	2	1	0	1	.064	1	1	0	1	.245	2	.016
7	2	0	1	2	.085	2	0	0	0	.125	2	.011
8	1	2	0	2	.078	2	0	0	0	.125	2	.010
9	3	0	0	0	.014	0	1	1	3	.208	3	.003

(continued)

TABLE 21.16 (continued): All possible configurations of tumor occurrences with corresponding *y*- and *p*-values (presented in ascending order of *y* values).

Config	Interval 1					Interval 2					Overall	
Number	G1	G2	G3	y1	P1	G1	G2	G3	y2	P2	y=y1+y2	p=p1*p2
10	0	3	0	3	.026	2	0	0	0	.125	3	.003
11	2	1	0	1	.064	0	2	0	2	.113	3	.007
12	2	1	0	1	.064	1	0	1	2	.219	3	.014
13	2	0	1	2	.085	1	1	0	1	.245	3	.021
14	1	2	0	2	.078	1	1	0	1	.245	3	.019
15	1	1	1	3	.228	2	0	0	0	.125	3	.029
16	3	0	0	0	.014	0	0	2	4	.090	4	.001
17	0	3	0	3	.026	1	1	0	1	.245	4	.006
18	0	2	1	4	.125	2	0	0	0	.125	4	.016
19	2	1	0	1	.064	0	1	1	3	.208	4	.013
20	2	0	1	2	.085	0	2	0	2	.113	4	.010
21	2	0	1	2	.085	1	0	1	2	.219	4	.019
22	1	2	0	2	.078	0	2	0	2	.113	4	.009
23	1	2	0	2	.078	1	0	1	2	.219	4	.017
24	1	0	2	4	.142	2	0	0	0	.125	4	.018
25	1	1	1	3	.228	1	1	0	1	.245	4	.056
26	0	3	0	3	.026	0	2	0	2	.113	5	.003
27	0	3	0	3	.026	1	0	1	2	.219	5	.006
28	0	2	1	4	.125	1	1	0	1	.245	5	.031
29	0	1	2	5	.171	2	0	0	0	.125	5	.021
30	2	1	0	1	.064	0	0	2	4	.090	5	.006
31	2	0	1	2	.085	0	1	1	3	.208	5	.018
32	1	2	0	2	.078	0	1	1	3	.208	5	.016
33	1	0	2	4	.142	1	1	0	1	.245	5	.035
34	1	1	1	3	.228	0	2	0	2	.113	5	.026
35	1	1	1	3	.228	1	0	1	2	.219	5	.050
36	0	3	0	3	.026	0	1	1	3	.208	6	.005
37	0	0	3	6	.066	2	0	0	0	.125	6	.008
38	0	2	1	4	.125	0	2	0	2	.113	6	.014
39	0	2	1	4	.125	1	0	1	2	.219	6	.027
40	0	1	2	5	.171	1	1	0	1	.245	6	.042
41	2	0	1	2	.085	0	0	2	4	.090	6	.008
42	1	2	0	2	.078	0	0	2	4	.090	6	.007
43	1	0	2	4	.142	0	2	0	2	.113	6	.016
44	1	0	2	4	.142	1	0	1	2	.219	6	.031
45	1	1	1	3	.228	0	1	1	3	.208	6	.047
46	0	3	0	3	.026	0	0	2	4	.090	7	.002
47	0	0	3	6	.066	1	1	0	1	.245	7	.016
48	0	2	1	4	.125	0	1	1	3	.208	7	.026
49	0	1	2	5	.171	0	2	0	2	.113	7	.019
50	0	1	2	5	.171	1	0	1	2	.219	7	.037
51	1	0	2	4	.142	0	1	1	3	.208	7	.030
52	1	1	1	3	.228	0	0	2	4	.090	7	.021
53	0	0	3	6	.066	0	2	0	2	.113	8	.008
54	0	0	3	6	.066	1	0	1	2	.219	8	.015
55	0	2	1	4	.125	0	0	2	4	.090	8	.011
56	0	1	2	5	.171	0	1	1	3	.208	8	.035
57	1	0	2	4	.142	0	0	2	4	.090	8	.013
58	0	0	3	6	.066	0	1	1	3	.208	9	.014
59	0	1	2	5	.171	0	0	2	4	.090	9	.015
60	0	0	3	6	.066	0	0	2	4	.090	10	.006

The right-hand tail probability of the distribution of y from the observed $y = 8$ is $p = 0.0075 + 0.0145 + 0.0113 + 0.0355 + 0.0128 + 0.0138 + 0.0154 + 0.0060 = 0.11684$ (the sum of all p-values in the above table corresponding to a y value greater than or equal to 8). For the purpose of comparison it may be noted that the normal approximated p-value for the dataset in the above example is 0.0697. Also for the purpose of comparison, the exact p-value for the dose–response relationship for the data given in Table 21.10 is $p = 0.0453$ (calculated using the StatXact software).

When a tumor type is observed in a fatal context, or when it is observed in a fatal context in some animals and in an incidental context in other animals, the appropriate method is to combine each analysis by a pooled Z statistic, as described in Section 21.6.2.4.3. A parallel exact method may be constructed when the total number of fatal and incidental tumors is small. Tumor count tables are formed corresponding to each context of observation, that is, with the appropriate denominator, and the exact p-values are computed based on the combined collection of tables from both contexts. For example, suppose that in the time interval I_1, all tumors were observed in an incidental context, whereas in the time interval I_2, tumor from one animal was observed in fatal contexts along with a few other tumors from other animals that were obtained in an incidental context. Then there will be three observed tumor count tables for this tumor type—two tables for the incidental context in I_1 and I_2 and a new one, I_3, for the tumor observed in the fatal context corresponding to its date of death. The exact p-value is now computed using these three observed tables according to the method described in the previous subsection. However, this procedure has some technical problems. In a given interval of a partition of the study period, if a tumor is classified as an incidental tumor for some animals and as a fatal one for the remaining animals, then, as mentioned earlier, the prevalence method and the death-rate method are applied to the incidental and fatal parts of the data, respectively. Under this situation, the denominators of the incidence rates of the incidental part of the tumor change in each of the possible permutations of the tumor-bearing animals. For example, consider the following situation where in a single interval one fatal and six incidental tumors were observed. The two tables present results of two permutations of the observed tumor incidence.

Permutation 1

Tumor Type	Dose Groups			
	Control	Low	Medium	High
Fatal	0/45	0/42	1/42	0/42
Incidental	3/10	0/12	2/12	1/15

Permutation 2

Tumor Type	Dose Groups			
	Control	Low	Medium	High
Fatal	1/45	0/42	0/42	0/42
Incidental	3/10	0/12	2/12	1/15

The denominators for the incidental tumors in Permutation 2 table are incorrect. The correct table for Permutation 2 is

Permutation 2 (Corrected)

Tumor Type	Dose Groups			
	Control	Low	Medium	High
Fatal	1/45	0/42	0/42	0/42
Incidental	3/**9**	0/12	2/**13**	1/15

The p-value obtained from tables without this adjustment of the denominators will not be correct.

Some available software for the calculation of exact p-values for the Peto test perform only the permutations of tumor-bearing animals for the numerators, ignoring the need to change the denominators in the permutations. Therefore, in using software for the calculation of p-values for Peto test, we should verify that they construct correct permuted tables.

21.6.2.5   Poly-K Test

As mentioned earlier in great detail, Peto et al. based their analysis method on two factors, namely, context of observation (or cause-of-death information) and choices of number and position of partitioning time intervals. Because of these and other limitations in the Peto analysis method, some alternative methods have been proposed for analyzing carcinogenicity study data. The methods that were discussed earlier, such as the logistic regression method, are possible alternatives. Another widely used alternative is the Poly-K method. In the following section, we discuss this method in detail.

The Poly-K test was suggested by Bailer and Portier [17]. This test is a natural extension of the Cochran–Armitage test. As mentioned before, an implicit assumption of the Cochran–Armitage test procedure is that all animals are at equal risk of developing the tumor over the duration of the study. However, because some tumors may have long latency periods and some treatment compounds may be moderately to seriously toxic, they can significantly shorten the survival time of animals. Animals with shorter life spans may have a reduced risk of tumor onset, especially in the medium- and high-dose groups, if the drug is toxic. The Poly-K method suggests correcting this problem by modifying the number of animals at risk N_i to reflect the compensation due to early death. Operationally, this method considers less than a whole animal for animals dying early without tumor. Unlike the Peto test, this test does not need any arbitrary partitioning of the study period or the cause-of-death information. This test adjusts the proportion of tumor-bearing animals by applying an appropriate polynomial weight to the surviving period of each animal. The proportion of tumor-bearing animals is calculated as

$$p_i^* = x_i/N_i^*, \quad x_i = \sum x_{ij}, \quad N_i^* = \sum w_{ij}.$$

The weight w_{ij} is defined as
$w_{ij} = (t_{ij}/t_{max})^k$ for animals dying before the end of the study without the tumor
and
$= 1$ otherwise

where
t_{ij} = the survival time of the jth animal in the ith dose group
t_{max} = the maximum survival time (length of the study)

The exponent k of the risk weight corresponds to the shape of the tumor-onset distribution. For carcinogenicity data analysis $K = 3$ is most widely used. As Bailer and Portier mentioned, this weighting scheme, resulting from the observation of the large amount of tumor data from previous studies, shows that many tumors seem to appear at the rate of a third- to fifth-order polynomial in time. These modified proportions are then analyzed using the Cochran–Armitage test. However, since N^* is a random variable (not fixed as required by the Cochran–Armitage test), the calculation of the variance of the test statistic needs to be modified. Bieler and Williams [18] suggested an estimate of this variance, using the delta method and the weighted least-squares technique.

Example 21.10
For the above dataset, the incidence table with the adjusted N values (N^*) is given in Table 21.17.

TABLE 21.17: Incidence of interstitial cell tumor and adjusted N in testis in male rats.

Treatment Group	Control	Low	Medium	High	Total
Dose level (mg)	0	100	300	1000	
NTBA	5	1	0	7	13
NNTBA	36	49	44	39	168
N_i^* = Adjusted N_i	41	50	44	46	181 (N)
Proportion at risk $P_i = N_i/N$	0.227	0.276	0.243	0.254	1.000

Note: NTBA, number of tumor-bearing animals; NNTBA, number of nontumor-bearing animals; $N = \Sigma N_i$

The dose–response relationship p-value $= 0.03386$.

21.6.2.5.1   Exact Poly-K   An exact version of the Poly-K test can be derived by a simple modification of the method discussed for the exact version of the Peto test. Consider the following outcome of a tumor type:

Treatment Group	0	1	...	i	...	R	Total
Dose	x_0	x_1	...	x_i	...	x_r	
NTBA	n_0	n_1	...	n_i	...	n_r	N
NNTBA	$N_0 - n_0$	$N_1 - n_1$	...	$N_i - n_i$	...	$N_r - n_r$	$N - n$
Total	N_0	N_1	...	N_i	...	N_r	N

Note: NTBA, number of tumor-bearing animals; NNTBA, number of nontumor-bearing animals.

We can use the suggested weight w_{ij} for the Poly-K procedure and calculate the corresponding $N_i^* s$. We now have a new table as shown below:

Treatment Group	0	1	...	i	...	r	Total
Dose	x_0	x_1	...	x_i	...	x_r	
NTBA	n_0	n_1	...	n_i	...	n_r	N
NNTBA	$N_0^* - n_0$	$N_1^* - n_1$	...	$N_i^* - n_i$	...	$N_r^* - n_r$	$N^* - n$
Total	N_0^*	N_1^*	...	N_i^*	...	N_r^*	N^*

Note: NTBA, number of tumor-bearing animals; NNTBA, number of nontumor-bearing animals.

The exact Poly-K test can now be conducted on the data in the new adjusted table. Note that because the exact test is based on hypergeometric distribution, N_i needs to be an integer; however, N_i^* is not necessarily an integer. Therefore, for operational purpose a rounding of N_i^* to the nearest integer is necessary.

Example 21.11

The dose–response relationship p-value for the data given in Table 21.17 is $p = 0.0427$ (calculated using the StatXact software).

21.6.2.6   Comparison of Exact and Approximate Methods

As mentioned before, the use of exact p-values has been suggested when the total number of tumor-bearing animals across all treatment groups is small. However, the magnitude of this "smallness" is not well studied. Mantel [21] suggested the use of the exact procedure whenever the total tumor frequency is 5 or less. However, a simulation study by Ali [20], imitating an actual study of a new drug development, showed that in a four-group experiment with 50 animals in each, the normal approximated p-value may severely underestimate the exact p-value even when the total number of tumor-bearing animals is as large as 10. In Ali's simulation, survival data for the four groups were generated under the proportional hazard assumption with a baseline Weibull model for tumor generation. The tumor-bearing animals were distributed in one of the four survival time intervals: 0–50, 51–80, 81–104, and the terminal sacrifice depending on the survival length of the animals.

An inherent feature of the exact method is that p-values are computed from the conditional null distribution, which is discrete. Depending on the extent of this discreteness, the exact method will result in a conservative test in the sense that its actual significance level will usually be smaller than the nominal level. When performing multiple tests of significance in an experiment designed to test an "overall experimentwise" hypothesis, the extent of this conservativeness may play an important role in determining the experimentwise Type-I error rate (also referred to as the false-positive rate). The topic of the effect of multiple testing is further discussed in a later section. Under such circumstances, it is useful to gain knowledge of the actual significance levels of the individual tests.

In a typical animal carcinogenicity study, four parallel experiments (two species each with two sexes) are run. In each experiment, a combination of 20 or more organs/tissues with several neoplastic lesions is tested for a positive linear trend in tumor rates across the treatment groups. Thus, the number of tests performed per experiment could be as high as 60 (or even higher). Out of these observed tumor types, it is usually the case that a large number of tumor types are observed in only a few animals (relatively rare). Hence, the number of exact trend tests performed will also be large. Thus, the experimentwise false-positive rates depend heavily on the actual significance levels of the individual exact tests. In addition to the issue of false-positive rates, the question of "false-negative" rates also arises in a parallel context.

Some knowledge about the Type-I and Type-II error rates of an exact trend test compared to those of approximate tests can be found in the results of a simulation study by Ali [22]. In this study, the actual significance levels and the power of the exact trend test were compared with those of three approximate tests for some special cases of small numbers of total tumor-bearing animals across all treatment groups. Data for the simulation were generated under various Weibull models for survival time and time to tumor, and tests were computed using four different score sets for the treatment groups. For details of the results of this study readers are referred to the article cited earlier. Here we will state only the main results comparing the exact test and its normal approximation version reported in the paper.

The actual significance levels attained (as estimated by 10,000 simulated experiments) were compared to the nominal 5% and 1% levels. Five Weibull models, each with three score sets resulting in 15 simulation conditions, are considered. The average number of tumor-bearing animals among these 15 conditions ranged from 2.5 to 7.9. The significance levels attained of the exact test ranged from 0.82% to 1.7% when 5% was used as the nominal level and from 0.08% to 0.32% when 1% was used. Hence it is clear that the exact test was always very conservative in rejecting the null hypothesis of "no positive dose response" when the tumor prevalence rates across treatment groups were equal. On the other hand, the significance levels attained by the normal approximated test ranged from 3.01% to 8.36%, corresponding to a nominal level of 5%, and from 0.31% to 2.09% when the nominal level was 1%. The normal approximation was very unstable in the sense that the significance levels fluctuated above and below the nominal level.

Ali [22] also performed power comparisons between the two tests. The power was computed under various Weibull alternatives for tumor prevalence functions. The average number of tumor-bearing animals ranged from 4.4 to 9.5. The power of the exact test corresponding to a 5% nominal level ranged from 2.14% to 15.09% and between 0.35% and 4.46% when the nominal level was 1%. Thus, in the case of very low total tumor rates, it is almost impossible for the exact test to detect increasing tumor prevalence across the treatment groups. In the case of the normal approximation test, the power ranged from 6.2% to 33%, corresponding to a 5% nominal level and between 1% and 12.8% when the nominal level was 1%. Hence, although the normal approximation improved the power, it was not high enough to make a real difference.

21.6.2.7   Use of Historical Control

The concurrent control group is always the most relevant and important comparator in testing drug-related increases in tumor rates. However, the outcome of an experiment is often impaired due to background noise unrelated to the treatment. Therefore, if used appropriately, historical control data can be valuable in the final interpretation of the study results.

The incorporation of stable historical control data would serve to (a) increase the power of hypothesis testing [23], particularly when the group size is small; (b) decrease the false-positive rate; (c) carry out hypothesis testing meaningfully when the occurrence of response is rare; and (d) validate the judgment that the observed significance is a realization of Type-I errors. There are other important uses of historical control data. The data can be used as a quality control mechanism for a carcinogenicity experiment by assessing the reasonableness of the spontaneous tumor rates in the concurrent control group. These data are also useful in classifying tumors as rare or common. A statistically significant increase in a rare tumor is unlikely as a chance occurrence, so it is critical to decide whether a tumor is rare or not. Rare tumors are generally tested with less-stringent statistical decision rules. For common tumors, in cases of marginally significant trends or differences, historical control data can help investigators determine whether the findings are real or false positives. Historical control data can also help investigators determine whether nonsignificant findings in rare tumors are true-negative or false-negative results due to the lack of power in the statistical tests used.

For an appropriate interpretation, it is extremely important that the historical control data chosen be from studies comparable to the current study. The choice and availability of such historical control are challenging. Large differences between studies can result from differences in nomenclature, pathologist's judgment in reading slides, the specific animal strain used, and laboratory conditions.

21.6.2.7.1   Informal Use of Historical Control Data   The informal method frequently used by researchers is to compare the incidence rates of the treated groups of a tumor type in the current study with the range of its occurrence in the historical control data. The range of historical control data is simply defined as incidence rates between the maximum and the minimum of the historical control rates. This definition of range does not consider the shape of the distribution of the rates. The above informal method of using historical control data in the interpretation of statistical test results is not very satisfactory because the ranges of historical control rates are usually too wide. This problem becomes especially serious in the situation in which the historical control rates of the tumor in most studies are clustered together but a few other studies have rates far away from the cluster. Some analytic methods suggested by Louis [24], Blyth [25], Vollset [26], Jovanovic and Viana [27], and Jovanovic and Levy [28] for the construction of the upper confidence intervals for binomial proportions are more stable and should replace the historical range calculated using this informal method.

21.6.2.7.2 Formal Use of Historical Data Consider a study with $r+1$ treated groups (one control and r treated groups) with doses $x_0 = 0 < \cdots < x_i < \cdots < x_r$ and $N_0, \ldots, N_i, \ldots, N_r$ number of animals, respectively. Suppose the number of animals in these groups that developed a particular tumor are $n_0, \ldots, n_i, \ldots, n_r$. Also, suppose for a given historical control with N number of animals, n number of animals develop the tumor. Assume that the number of tumor-bearing animals follows a binomial distribution with parameter p:

$$f(x) = \binom{N}{n} p^n (1-p)^{N-n} \quad \text{for } n = 0, 1, \ldots, N,$$

where p is the true spontaneous rate of the tumor. In the published literature, a beta distribution is proposed to model the spontaneous tumor rate p that may vary from experiment to experiment. Therefore,

$$B(p|\alpha, \beta) = \frac{\Gamma(\alpha+\beta)}{\Gamma(\alpha)\Gamma(\beta)} p^{\alpha-1}(1-p)^{\beta-1}, \quad \text{for } 0 \le p \le 1,$$

with mean $= \alpha/(\alpha+\beta)$ and variance $= (\alpha\beta)/\{(\alpha+\beta)^2(\alpha+\beta+1)\}$. The unknown parameters α and β can be estimated by statistical methods, for example, the method of moments or the method of maximum likelihood. It is well known that the beta distribution is flexible and can fit many data. A visual representation of the shapes of the family of beta distributions $B(z|\alpha, \beta)$ is presented in Figure 21.2:

Finally, p is assumed to be $p(a) = e^a/\{1+e^a\}$. Therefore,

$$f(x) = \binom{N}{n}\left[\frac{e^a}{(1+e^a)}\right]^n\left[1 - \frac{e^a}{(1+e^a)}\right]^{N-n} = \binom{N}{n}\frac{e^a}{(1+e^a)^N}, \quad \text{for } x = 0, 1, \ldots, n$$

and the beta distribution has the form

$$B(a) = \frac{\Gamma(\alpha+\beta)}{\Gamma(\alpha)\Gamma(\beta)}\left[\frac{e^a}{1+e^a}\right]^{\alpha-1}\left[1 - \frac{e^a}{1+e^a}\right]^{\beta-1} = \frac{\Gamma(\alpha+\beta)}{\Gamma(\alpha)\Gamma(\beta)}\frac{e^{a(\alpha-1)}}{[1+e^a]^{\alpha+\beta-2}}.$$

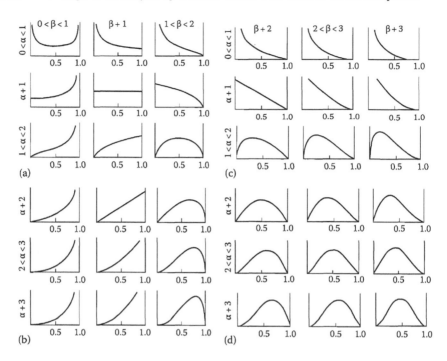

FIGURE 21.2: Family of beta distributions $Be(\alpha, \beta)$. (From Lee, P.M., *Bayesian Statistics: An Introduction*, 2nd edn., Arnold, London, 1997. With permission.)

For a given experiment, the probability of a tumor corresponding to dose x_i is modeled by a logistic model as $p_i = \frac{e^{a+bx_i}}{1+e^{a+bx_i}}$.

If x_0 is the total number of tumor-bearing animals out of a total number of N_0 animals in the combined historical controls, then the conditional likelihood function of x_0 for given a will be

$$L(x_0|a) = \binom{N_0}{n_0} \frac{e^{an_0}}{[1+e^a]^{N_0}} \prod_{i=1}^{r} \binom{n_i}{x_i} \frac{e^{(a+bx_i)n_i}}{[1+e^{a+bx_i}]^{N_i}}.$$

The full likelihood is

$$L(x_0, x_i, a) = L(b|a).B(a) = K(n, x, \alpha, \beta) \frac{e^{a(n_0+\alpha-1)}}{[1+e^a]^{N_0+\alpha+\beta-2}} \prod_{i=1}^{r} \frac{e^{(a+bx_i)n_i}}{[1+e^{a+bx_i}]^{N_i}}.$$

The positive trend in tumor incidence with the incorporation of historical control data is updated from the Cochran–Armitage test to the following statistic (compared to Equation 21.3):

$$\chi^2 = S^2/V,$$

where

$$S = \Sigma n_i x_i - \hat{p} \Sigma N_i d_i,$$

$$V = \hat{p}\hat{q} \left[\sum N_i x_i^2 - \left(\sum N_i x_i \right)^2 \Big/ N \right], \quad N = N + \hat{\alpha} + \hat{\beta},$$

and

$$\hat{p} = (n + \hat{\alpha})/n \quad \text{and} \quad \hat{q} = 1 - \hat{p}, \; N = \Sigma N_i, \quad \text{and} \quad n = \Sigma n_i.$$

The statistic χ^2 is distributed asymptotically as a chi-square with 1 degree of freedom.

Example 21.12 (A Case Study)

Tumor incidence rates of hemangiosarcoma and hemangioma in male rats from a rat carcinogenicity study (Table 21.18) of a drug are now analyzed taking into account historical information (Table 21.19).

The Cochran–Armitage dose–response relationship test in total hemangiosarcoma and hemangioma combined incidence is significant (asymptotic $p = 0.0011$).

The historical control incidence rates of hemangiosarcoma and hemangioma combined of the RITA historical control data of the thirty studies is $48/1677 = 0.02862$. The standard deviation of the historical control rate is 0.031957 (standard error $= 0.005835$). The parameters α and β of the beta distribution are estimated by the method of moments. We have the mean $= \alpha/(\alpha + \beta) = 0.0097$ and variance $= (\alpha\beta)/\{(\alpha + \beta)^2(\alpha + \beta + 1)\} = 0.0003$. The solution to the system of equations is $\alpha = 0.31$ and $\beta = 31.26$. Incorporating the estimated values of α and β using these historical control data into the Cochran–Armitage test statistic, we get $\chi^2 = 8.085$ for hemangiosarcoma and hemangioma combined. The p-value of the test is about 0.004463.

TABLE 21.18: Case studies: Tumor incidence rates of hemangiosarcoma and hemangioma of male rats in the rat carcinogenicity study of drug XXXX.

	Males (mg/kg/day)				
	0	**0**	**1.5**	**5**	**15**
Spleen					
B-hemangioma	0/50	0/50	0/50	0/50	0/50
M-hemangiosarcoma	0/50	0/50	0/50	0/50	2/50
Kidney					
M-hemangiosarcoma	1/50	0/50	0/50	0/50	1/50
Skin and adnexa					
N-hemangiosarcoma	0/50	0/50	0/50	0/50	1/50
Total hemangioma plus hemangiosarcoma[a]	1/50	0/50	0/50	0/50	4/50

[a] To calculate the total hemangioma plus hemangiosarcoma, an animal was counted only once if it developed more than one of these tumors in one or more of these organs.

TABLE 21.19: Thirteen sample Registry of Industrial Toxicology Animal (RITA) historical control data of 30 studies of hemangiosarcoma and hemangioma of male rats.

Male Rats

Study #	Total Examined	Kidneys Hemangioma	Liver Hemangioma	Liver Hemangiosarcoma	Lymph Node Mesenteric Hemangioma	Lymph Node Mesenteric Hemangiosarcoma	Skin/Subcutaneous Tissue Hemangioma	Skin/Subcutaneous Tissue Hemangiosarcoma	Spleen Hemangioma	Spleen Hemangiosarcoma
1	69	0	0	0	0	0	0	1	0	0
10	50	0	0	0	3	0	0	0	0	0
14	50	0	0	0	0	0	0	0	0	0
15	50	0	0	0	0	0	0	0	0	0
16	70	0	0	0	2	0	0	0	0	0
18	70	0	0	0	5	1	1	0	2	0
19	69	0	0	0	0	1	0	0	1	0
—	—	—	—	—	—	—	—	—	—	—
—	—	—	—	—	—	—	—	—	—	—
—	—	—	—	—	—	—	—	—	—	—
100	50	0	0	0	0	0	0	0	0	1
101	55	0	0	0	1	0	0	0	0	0
102	55	0	0	0	1	0	0	0	0	0
106	60	0	0	1	0	0	0	0	0	0
111	60	0	0	0	1	0	0	0	1	1
125	50	0	0	0	1	1	0	0	0	3
Total	1677	2	1	1	23	4	1	5	5	6

The above method is illustrated in Tarone's article in 1982. A limitation of Tarone's method (and other available formal methods of using historical control data) is that it applies only to lifetime incidence tests. In practice, it is well known that time-adjusted tests are needed because of possible toxic effects of the test compound that can cause differences in mortality among treatment groups. Ibrahim and Ryan [30] developed a method to incorporate historical control information into time-adjusted tests for trend. They first divided the time axis into s disjoint intervals $\{[0, \gamma_1), [\gamma_1, \gamma_2), \ldots, [\gamma_{s-2}, \gamma_{s-1}), [\gamma_{s-1}, \infty)\}$ and used a multinomial distribution to model the tumor incidence in each time interval. They then used a Dirichlet distribution to characterize prior information on the tumor rates in various intervals. From the resulting Dirichlet-multinomial distribution on the observed tumor counts, they derived a score test for trend, which generalized the test suggested by Tarone. The test statistic is $\chi^2 = S^2/V$, where $S = \frac{d}{db} \log L(b)|_{b=0}$ and $V = -\frac{d^2}{db^2} \log L(b)|_{b=0}$. A closed form for S is given as

$$S = \sum_{k=1}^{s-1} \sum_{i=0}^{r} di(x_{ik} - \hat{p}_k m_{ik}), \quad \text{where } \hat{p}_k = E(\theta_{0k}|D) = \frac{\gamma_k + \sum_{i=0}^{r} x_{ik}}{\gamma_k + \nu_k + \sum_{i=0}^{r} m_{ik}},$$

$$V = \sum_{k=1}^{s-1} \hat{p}\hat{q}\left(\frac{\hat{m}_k}{1+\hat{m}_k}\right)\left[\sum_{i=0}^{r} d_i^2 m_{ik} - \left(\sum_{i=1}^{r} d_i m_{ik}\right)^2 \Big/ \hat{m}_k\right],$$

with $\hat{m} = \gamma_k + \nu_k + \sum_{i=0}^{r} m_{ik}$, and $\hat{q} = 1 - \hat{p}_k$.

A drawback of the Ibrahim and Ryan method is that it does not take care of the variation due to the estimation of parameter τ (the vector of parameters of the beta priors on the θ_{0k}'s), which needs to be estimated from the log likelihood function $l_{i>_i}(\tau)$ based on the historical control data. Sun in 1999 developed a new test that includes this term. He showed that this could greatly affect the analysis results. The suggested statistic is

$$T^*(\hat{\alpha}) = S^*(\hat{\alpha})/V^*(\hat{\alpha}),$$

where

$$S^*(\hat{\alpha}) = S(b = 0; \hat{\alpha}) = S(b = 0; \alpha_0) + \frac{1}{n^{1/2}} A^t(\alpha_0)\left[n^{1/2}(\hat{\alpha} - \alpha_0)\right],$$

$$V^*(\hat{\alpha}) = V(b = 0; \hat{\alpha}) + A^t(\hat{\alpha})B^{-1}(\hat{\alpha})A(\hat{\alpha}), \quad \text{with } A(\alpha) = \partial S(b = 0; \alpha)/\partial\alpha,$$

$$B(\alpha) = -\partial W(\alpha)/\partial\alpha,$$

and

$$W(\hat{\alpha}) = W(\alpha_0) - \frac{1}{n^{1/2}} B(\alpha_0)\lfloor n^{1/2}(\hat{\alpha} - \alpha_0)\rfloor.$$

Asymptotically $T^*(\hat{\alpha})$ has a chi-square distribution with 1 degree of freedom.

Example 21.13

The following example is taken from an article by Tarone [31]. The data used in the example were taken from a Carcinogenesis Bioassay of the NCI. The example is to test if there is a significant positive dose–response relationship in the incidence of lung tumors in female F344 rats in the Bioassay of nitrilotriacetic acid [32]. The data are summarized in the following table. Since the dose levels were equally spaced, the doses are presented as 0, 1, and 2 (Table 21.20).

TABLE 21.20:   Summary of lung-tumor incidence in female F433 rats in the bioassay of nitrilotriacetic acid.

Dose level:	0	1	2	Total
Animals with tumor	0	3	7	10
Sample size	15	49	46	110
Percent of animals with tumor	0	6	15	9

The Cochran–Armitage test statistic yields $\chi^2_{CA} = 4.04$ with an associated p-value of 0.044. This result is a marginally statistically significant dose–response relationship at the 5% level. The historical control lung-tumor rates from 70 experiments with female F344 rats are given in Table 21.21.

TABLE 21.21:   Control lung-tumor rates (Y_i/M_i) from 70 experiments with female F344 rats.

Y_i/M_i	Frequency	Y_i/M_i	Frequency	Y_i/M_i	Frequency
0/50	3	0/19	6	1/23	2
0/49	3	0/18	4	1/20	14
0/47	2	0/10	1	1/19	1
0/25	2	1/53	1	1/18	1
0/24	2	1/50	2	2/20	6
0/22	1	1/49	2	2/19	1
0/20	14	1/47	1	2/18	1

The pooled historical control rate based on the examination of lungs from 1805 rats is $40/1805 = 0.022$. The maximum likelihood estimates for the beta-binomial parameters are $\hat{\alpha} = 11.52$ and $\hat{\beta} = 501.93$. Thus $\hat{p} = 0.035$, $\hat{n} = 623.45$, and $\chi^2_T = 21.96$, and the associated P-value is $p < 10^{-5}$. This example shows that the incorporation of historical control information can provide evidence of a highly statistically significant dose–response relationship associated with the administration of nitrilotriacetic acid. For analysis using the Ibrahim and Ryan method, we need to divide the entire study period into a few intervals and know the tumor incidence information in each of the chosen intervals. However, such information is not available in the data. Therefore, the only possibility is to use two intervals, namely, the start of the study to before the termination and the termination period. However, as mentioned earlier the method given by Ibrahim and Ryan for $s = 2$

gives the same result as Cochran–Armitage. Therefore, using $s = 2$ the Ibrahim and Ryan test statistics $\chi_{IR}^2 = 21.96$ with associated P-value is $p < 10^{-5}$. Lastly, the test statistic using the method given by Sun using $s = 2$ is $\chi_S^2 = 3.26$ with a P-value of 0.07, showing that the dose–response relationship is not statistically significant.

21.6.2.8 Multiplicity Issue

As stated, the analysis is performed by tumor/organ combination. There are usually 2 species, 2 sexes, and 20 or more tumors/organs examined per experiment. A total of 80 or more simultaneous tests are performed. Therefore, this is a high-dimensional multiplicity problem. This large number of multiple tests increases the overall false-positive rate or family wise error rate (FWER), defined as the probability of making at least one false-positive detection out of all tests. The magnitude of the overall false-positive rate grows dramatically with the increase in number of tests. This may lead to many missed findings and make the test procedure practically useless. Hence, the problem of multiplicity is severe. It is, therefore, important to adjust the effect of multiple testing in the statistical analysis of tumor data. It should be noted that the multiplicity issue is more serious for common tumors than rare tumors. A statistically significant trend test or a pairwise comparison in incidence of a rare tumor is less likely to be a false-positive finding. Therefore, the need to adjust for the effect of multiple testing is less for rare tumors than for common tumors. Operationally, we want to control the overall false positive defined as the probability of rejecting at least one true hypothesis, over the four experiments. There are many available methods for this purpose, for example, methods suggested by Bonferroni and Hochberg, the false discovery rate, methods based on bootstrap/resampling procedures, and methods based on Bayesian approaches. However, as mentioned already, carcinogenicity data analysis is a high-dimensional problem. Methods such as Bonferroni, Hochberg, and many other proposed ones are suitable for low-dimensional problems, that is, a small number of multiple testing adjustments. Not many suitable methods are available for the adjustment for multiple testing in high-dimensional problems. A few suggested approaches for the analysis of carcinogenicity study data are using the weighted FWER-controlling method; allowing a specific number (U say) of false-positive errors; controlling the false discovery rate; and applying an ad hoc method. Brief descriptions of these methods follow.

21.6.2.8.1 Weighted FWER-Controlling Method This method is useful when some hypotheses are more important than others. More weight for a hypothesis leads to higher power. The weighting may be based on biological importance. In the simplest weighting multiple testing procedure, assign weight w_i to hypothesis H_i such that each $w_i \geq 0$ and $\Sigma w_i = 1$. Reject H_i if $p_i \leq w_i \alpha$ [33].

Another approach similar to the above method is as follows: Let $q_i = p_i / w_i$ and $q_{(1)} \leq q_{(2)} \leq \cdots \leq q_{(m)}$ be their ordered values. Let $S_j = \{i_j, \ldots, i_m\}$ for $j = 1, \ldots, m$ and $H_{(j)}^w$ be the hypothesis corresponding to $q_{(j)}$. Reject $H_{(i)}^w$ if $q_{(i)} \leq \alpha / \Sigma_{h \in s_i} w_h$ for all $i = 1, \ldots, j$. When all weights are equal the method reduces to an ordinary step-down Holm method.

21.6.2.8.2   Allowing a Specific Number (*U*) of False-Positive Errors   Failing to control for the effect of multiplicities will make statistical tests too anticonservative, whereas strict controlling for the effect might make the tests too stringent. An intermediate and more acceptable criterion may be to allow a few acceptable numbers of false positives. For example, allowing an arbitrary $\alpha = 0.001$ for testing $m = 10,000$ hypotheses will allow $0.001*10,000 = 10$ false positives. The method works for an average number of rejected hypotheses.

To adjust with exactly U number of false positives, set the first U smallest number of observed p-values $(p_{(1)} \leq p_{(2)} \leq \cdots \leq p_{(u)})$ to be zero. For other tests, the adjusted p-value for the kth test is given by the permutation test. First, permute the level of the comparators (animals). Then let $(p_{(1)}^* \leq p_{(2)}^* \leq \cdots \leq p_{(m)}^*)$ be the ordered unadjusted p-values from a permutation. The adjusted p-value for the kth test (not in the set whose p-values have already been set to zero) is set by the permutation test, that is,

$$\text{Adj } p(k) = \frac{1 + \text{of random permutations where } p^*(u+1) \leq p(k)}{1 + \text{of random permutations}}.$$

Lehmann and Romano [34] proposed testing each hypothesis at $\alpha' = U^*\alpha/m$, where U is the number of false-positive errors in a total of m number of tests.

21.6.2.8.3   False Discovery Rate   There are two types of control: controlling the average false discovery rate to be less than a specified value and controlling the false discovery rate to be less than a specified value with high confidence:

Controlling the average number of false discovery rate: Let the ordered unadjusted p-values be denoted as $p(1) \leq p(2) \leq \cdots \leq p(m)$. To keep the average false discovery rate less than γ, one identifies all tests that are statistically significant with indices $1, 2, \ldots, D$, where D is the largest index satisfying $p(D)^*m/D < \gamma$.

Keeping the false discovery rate less than γ with high confidence: Let $|[x]|$ denote the greatest integer less than or equal to x. For k with $|[k\gamma]| > |[(k-1)\gamma]|$ set the adjusted p-value of test k to be 0. For other values of k, the adjusted p-value is set by the permutation test method, that is,

$$\text{Adj } p(k) = \frac{1 + \text{of random permutations where } p^*(|[k\gamma]|+1) \leq p(k)}{1 + \text{of random permutations}}.$$

21.6.2.8.4   Ad Hoc Methods   There are ad hoc methods developed specially for carcinogenicity data analysis by Haseman [35] and Lin and Rahman [36] based on the method of allowing a specific number of false-positive errors discussed earlier. To keep an overall false-positive error around 10% in a regular 2-year-two-species-two-sex study, Haseman recommends the use of the significance levels of 0.05 and 0.01 for the pairwise comparisons of control with treated groups for a rare tumor and a common tumor, respectively. For dose–response relationship test, Lin and Rahman recommend the use of $\alpha = 0.025$ and $\alpha = 0.005$ for a rare and a common tumor.

A rare tumor type is defined as a tumor with less than 1% background rate. Lin and Rahman showed through some empirical and simulation studies with 20 organ/tumor types in each sex/species with various background rates that the use of their recommended levels of significance on dose–response relationship tests in Peto test resulted in an overall false-positive rate of about 10%. In their simulation they assumed that the tumors occurred independently of each other. This assumption is reasonable since there is very little evidence showing correlations among tumor types. An empirical study also showed similar results. A spontaneous tumor rate data of Crt:CDBR rats and Crt:CD-1(ICR) BR mice were compiled in the Division of Biometrics using information provided by the Charles River Company. In their empirical study Lin and Rahman used prevalence rates from this dataset. Results of a separate similar simulation study by the same authors showed that the false-positive rates using the Peto method and the Poly-3 method are very close. Because of this closeness in false-positive error between the two different methods, it was concluded that for 2 year regular rodent carcinogenicity studies the use of Lin and Rahman method for the adjustment of multiple testing in Poly-3 test will also keep the overall false-positive rate at an acceptable rate.

21.7 Carcinogenicity Studies Using Transgenic Mice

The long time and the high cost needed to conduct regular rat and mouse carcinogenicity studies and the increased insight into the mechanisms of carcinogenicity due to the advances made in molecular biology have led to alternative approaches that can be performed more quickly than the traditional ones for the assessment of carcinogenicity. An approach for this purpose is the use of biologically altered mice, popularly known as transgenic mice. These biologically altered mice provide rapid observation of carcinogenic endpoints. It is argued that some genetically altered mice are better animal surrogates for human cancer, because they carry some specifically activated oncogenes that are known to function in human cancers. The ICH has developed a document entitled "Guidance on testing for carcinogenicity of pharmaceuticals," *Federal Register*, vol. 63, pp. 8983–8986, 1998. The guidance outlines experimental approaches to the evaluation of carcinogenic potential that may obviate the necessity for the routine use of two long-term rodent carcinogenicity studies for the new drug approval process. This would allow drug sponsors either to conduct two long-term carcinogenicity studies in regular rats and mice or to use the alternative approach of conducting one long-term carcinogenicity study in rats together with a short- or medium-term study in transgenic mice.

Studies using transgenic mice have become the most important alternative to carcinogenicity testing among the short or medium rodent test systems recommended in the ICH guideline. Many new studies of known carcinogens and noncarcinogens from previous 2 year bioassays using transgenic rodents have been carried out by the NTP and by the International Life Science Institute (ILSI) to evaluate the specificity and sensitivity of the alternative test system. Different strains of transgenic mice (models) have been proposed and used in the alternative system of testing carcinogenicity of pharmaceutical and environmental chemical compounds. The following are the main strains (models) proposed and used in the studies mentioned previously: (a) p53+/− transgenic mice (with knockout of one of the two alleles of the tumor suppression gene p53), (b) Tg.AC transgenic mice (with genetically initiated skin to induce epidermal papillomas in response to dermal or oral exposure to chemical agents and act as a reporter phenotype of the activities of the tested chemicals), (c) TgrasH2 transgenic mice (with 5–6 copies of the stable human c-Ha-ras gene. They were first developed and patented in Japan), and (d) XPA−/− repair deficient mice (developed in Europe).

The standard study protocol described here has been used in these studies.

1. Study duration: 26 weeks

2. A positive control group in addition to the regular three or four treatment groups (negative control, low, medium, and high)

3. A total of 15–30 animals per sex/treatment group

4. Tissues/organs from all animals of studies with p53+/−, TgrasH2, and XPA−/− repair deficient mice, which died or were terminally sacrificed, are microscopically examined for neoplastic and nonneoplastic lesions

5. For studies using Tg.AC transgenic mice, incidence rates and numbers of only skin papillomas are observed over time

In studies using p53+/−, TgrasH2, and XPA−/− repair deficient mice, tumor data and methods of analysis are similar to those of 2 year studies. Interpretation of results may be different due to smaller group size and fewer tumor types developed on the tested animals.

Methods for analyzing the numbers of skin papillomas in studies using Tg.AC transgenic mice are somewhat different from those for studies using other types of transgenic mice. Incidence rates of skin papillomas (proportions of animals with the tumor) are analyzed by the same methods in regular 2 year studies. However, numbers of skin papillomas data can be analyzed by Mann–Whitney and Jonckhere tests for pairwise difference and positive trend, respectively.

A more recently developed method [37] uses data that include the number and time points of all papilloma development in one analysis. This method decomposes the carcinogenic effects into two components, namely, (1) the dose–response relationship in papilloma latency time and (2) the dose–response relationship in papilloma multiplicity after the appearance of the first papilloma. The following model was fitted:

$$E(Y_{ij}) = \exp\{\beta_1 + (b_1 + \gamma_1)t_{ij}d_i\} \quad \text{if } M_{ij} = 0$$
$$= \exp\{\beta_1 + \gamma_1 d\}_i \quad \text{if } M_{ij} > 0,$$

where

d_i is the dose level for ith mouse

T is the duration of the study

$t_{ij} = j/T$ is the fraction of time that the ith mouse stayed in the study

M_{ij} is the maximum number of papillomas burden observed for the ith mouse prior to week j

$Y_{ij} = (M_{ij} - M_{ij-1})$ is the increase in the maximum papilloma burden observed for the ith mouse between week $j - 1$ and j

Y_{ij} is assumed to follow a Poisson sampling distribution with mean specified via this model. The interpretations of the parameters are as follows:

b_1 = mouse-specific susceptibility variable

β_1 and β_2 = intercepts related to the rate of appearance of spontaneous papillomas

γ_1 and γ_2 = slopes associated with the dose–response relationships in papilloma latency time (that is, time of developing the first papilloma) and in papilloma multiplicity after the appearance of the first papilloma.

The hypotheses of interest are H_{01}: $\gamma_1 = \gamma_2 = 0$, H_{02}: $\gamma_1 = 0$, and H_{03}: $\gamma_2 = 0$, corresponding to incidence, latency, and multiplicity of papillomas. If H_{01} is not rejected, it can be concluded that there is no evidence of a dose response in papilloma incidences. However, if H_{01} is rejected, then it will be of interest to know whether the trend is due to a shortening of the latency time or an increment in papilloma multiplicity. If H_{02} is rejected, then it can be concluded that there is a significant decrease in papilloma latency with increasing dose. If H_{03} is rejected, then it can be concluded that there is a significant increase in papilloma multiplicity with increasing dose.

The following are comments on the analysis of data from carcinogenicity studies using transgenic mice:

1. Since the endpoints of studies using TgrasH2, P53, or XPA$-/-$ transgenic mice are the same as those in the traditional 2 year studies, for the data analysis, the exact and the asymptotic tests for dose–response relationship analysis and tests for difference in tumor incidences between treatment groups for the traditional 2 year study can be applied.

2. Since only 15–30 animals per sex/group are used (most recent studies used 25–30 animals), the power of the trend and pairwise comparison tests should be evaluated.

3. For carcinogenicity studies using TG.AC transgenic mice, the exact and asymptotic trend tests and pairwise comparison tests in tumor incidence can also be applied to the papilloma incidence rate data. For number of papillomas data, the proposed nonparametric procedures of Dunson et al., Jonckheere's test for trend, and the Mann–Whitney test for pairwise comparison are reasonable.

4. Since the number of papillomas in an animal can be counted only up to a prespecified number, 32, there will exist a large number of observations with papilloma counts of 32. The large number of tied observations could be a problem in applying the nonparametric procedures.

5. Since skin papilloma is the only tumor type test, the adjustment for multiplicity is no longer an issue. However, there are suggestions that the examination of only skin papilloma may not be sufficient in detecting a carcinogen in studies using TG.AC transgenic mice.

Example 21.14

A study was designed to assess the carcinogenic potential of a topically applied compound using Tg.AC mice. Two separate experiments, one in males and one in females, were conducted. In each of these two experiments there were three treated groups along with a positive control group and a vehicle control group. The treated groups received 125, 250, and 500 mg/kg of the test drug per day. The positive control group received 1.25 μg TPA three times per week and the vehicle control received methanol. One hundred Tg.AC mice of each gender were randomly allocated to the control and treated groups of equal size of 20 animals.

The Dunson model was fitted to analyze the data of skin papillomas observed in male mice. Table 21.22 contains the estimate of the parameters. The parameters were estimated using a SAS PROC MIXED program originally written by Dunson et al.

TABLE 21.22:   MLE estimators of the parameters for male mice using PROC NLMIXED.

Parameter	Estimate	Standard Error	DF	t-Value	P-Value	Alpha	Lower CL	Upper CL
beta1	−6.8438	1.1787	79	−5.81	<0.0001	0.05	−9.1900	−4.4976
beta2	−10.0021	105.06	79	−0.10	0.9244	0.05	−219.11	199.10
gamma1	−7.3770	15.6458	79	−0.47	0.6386	0.05	−38.5192	23.7651
gamma2	−0.00094	167.19	79	−0.00	1.0000	0.05	−332.78	332.78
sd	29.1658	79.8247	79	0.37	0.7158	0.05	−129.72	188.05

The above results do not show any statistically significant dose responses in papilloma latency time or in papilloma multiplicity after the appearance of the first papilloma.

21.8   Interpretation of Study Results

The evaluation of the results of long-term animal carcinogenicity experiments of a new drug is a complex process. The final interpretation of the study results involves issues that require statistical as well as biomedical judgments. The statistical issues include the validity of the design of the experiment, the appropriateness of the statistical data analysis methods, adjustment for multiple testing, and the use of comparable historical data in the final interpretation of the results. There is a vast amount of statistical literature regarding these issues. In the evaluation of the validity of experimental designs, we need to check if randomization of animals in treatment groups was conducted appropriately; an inappropriate allocation may produce bias in the results. For this reason it is necessary to determine whether a sufficient number of animals were used in an experiment to ensure reasonable power in the statistical tests used. Typically, a group size of about 50 per sex is recommended. If interim sacrifices are planned, the initial number of animals should be increased by the number of animals scheduled for the interim sacrifices. In general, the dose levels are selected based on the results of early phase single-dose, short-term subchronic toxicity studies and in consultation with related experts and government agencies. In negative studies (i.e., studies in which no significant positive dose–response relationships or drug-related increases in tumor incidence rates were found), it is important to evaluate if there were sufficient animals living long enough to get an adequate exposure to the chemical for risk of late developing tumors. In addition, for negative studies, it is important to evaluate whether the high dose used was high enough and close enough to the MTD or appropriate by other endpoint criteria, to present a reasonable tumor challenge to the tested animals.

The adequacy of the number of animals surviving, the length of exposure, and the appropriate dose strength depend on species and strains of animals used, routes of administration, and a few other factors. A general rule proposed by Haseman [38] is that a 50% survival rate in any group between weeks 80 and 90 of a 2 year study is considered a sufficient number and an adequate exposure. However, the percentage can be lower or higher if the number of animals used in each treatment or sex group is larger or smaller than 50, so that there will be between 20 and 30 animals still alive during these weeks. Also in another article Chu et al. [39] suggested that "to be considered adequate, an experiment that has not shown a chemical to be carcinogenic should have groups of animals with greater than 50% survival at one-year."

Regarding the question of adequate dose levels, it is generally accepted that the high dose should be close to the MTD. In the study by Chu et al. [39], the following criteria are mentioned for dose adequacy. A high dose is considered as close to MTD if any of the criteria is met.

1. A dose is considered adequate if there is a detectable loss in weight gain of up to 10% in a dosed group relative to the controls.

2. The administered dose is also considered an MTD if dosed animals exhibit clinical signs or severe histopathologic toxic effects attributed to the chemical.

3. In addition, doses are considered adequate if the dosed animals show a slight increased mortality compared to the controls.

The appropriateness of the high dose is always an important and complicated issue. Information about body weight gain, mortality, and clinical signs and histo-pathologic toxic effects are used to resolve this issue. Other information, such as pharmacokinetic and metabolic data, is also often considered in the evaluation of the appropriateness of doses used.

Because of the inherent limitations, such as small number of animals used, low tumor incidence rates, and biological variation, a carcinogenic drug may not be detected (i.e., a false-negative error occurs). Also because of a large number of statistical tests performed on the data (usually 2 species, 2 sexes, 20–30 tissues examined, and 4 dose levels), there is a great probability that statistically significant positive dose–response relationships in some tumor types are purely due to the chance of variation alone (i.e., a false-positive error occurs). Controlling the above two types of error to acceptable levels is the central element in the interpretation of study results. Again, the control of the two types of error involves both statistical and nonstatistical issues, which require statistical as well as biological judgments. It is important that an overall evaluation of the tumorigenic potential of a drug should be made based on knowledge of statistical significance of positive dose–response relationship and information of biological relevance. The controls of the two types of error are also related to statistical procedures.

The overall false-positive error in animal tumorigenicity studies caused by the effect of multiple tests of statistical significance can be controlled by reducing the number of variables evaluated. This can be achieved by combining certain tumor types based on the biological knowledge of tumor origination. McConnell et al. [40] proposed the following guidelines for combining tumors: (a) Tumors of the same histomorphogenic type with substantial evidence of progression from benign to malignant stage; (b) tumors, such as hyperplasia and benign tumors, in which the criteria for differentiating them become unclear; (c) tumors in other organs/tissues but of the same histomorphogenic type; and (d) tumors of different morphologic classification but with comparable histomorphogenesis.

There are statistical methods proposed for controlling the overall false-positive error rates, as described in Section 21.6.2.8. Appropriate use of these methods will help in keeping the overall false-positive rate at its desired level.

The false-negative error issue in animal carcinogenicity studies, although equally important, has not received as much attention as the false-positive error issue has. This may be in part due to two reasons. First, this issue is less familiar to people. Statistically, the theory of false-negative error is more complicated than that of the false-positive error. The false-negative error is a function of the alternative hypotheses one is interested in testing. The statistical distributions used in the evaluation of false-negative errors are complicated and involve noncentrality parameters. Second, because of the cost involved in developing a new drug, the drug sponsors pay more attention to false-positive errors than to false-negative errors.

As mentioned at the beginning of this section, the large false-negative error committed in animal carcinogenicity study is caused by the inherent limitations of the small numbers of animals used and the low incidence rates in the majority of tumors examined. Due to the above limitations, the power of statistical tests for a positive dose–response relationship will be small. That is, the false-negative errors are expected to be large. A study by Ali [22] shows that under the conditions he simulated assuming tumor incidence rates following Weibull models, the powers of the exact permutation trend test, the Peto prevalence test for trend, and some modified forms of Peto prevalence test are no more than 0.25. That is, the false-negative errors are greater than 0.75. If the above simulation results reflect the general magnitudes of the power of statistical trend tests, then the false-negative error issue should cause concerns to investigators and be weighted at least equally with the false-positive error issue in the overall evaluation of results of an animal carcinogenicity study.

Table 21.23 contains some of Haseman's [41] calculations of tumor rates needed to be induced in the treated group to achieve certain levels of power in the Fisher's exact test at 0.05 and 0.01 levels of significance under various assumed spontaneous rates in the control group (assuming 50 animals in the treated group and in the control).

TABLE 21.23: Tumor rates (%) needed to be induced in the treated group to achieve levels of power of 0.50 and 0.90.

Spontaneous Tumor	$\alpha = 0.05$		$\alpha = 0.01$	
Rate in Control (%)	Power = 0.5	Power = 0.9	Power = 0.5	Power = 0.9
0.1%	9.5%	15.8%	13.5%	20.5%
1.0	11.0	18.4	15.1	23.4
3.0	14.0	22.9	18.9	29.0
5.0	17.0	27.0	22.5	33.3
10.0	24.2	35.7	30.2	41.9
20.0	36.8	49.0	43.2	56.0
30.0	48.1	61.1	54.8	67.0

Statistically, there are at least three ways to increase the power of tests to ensure that the overall false-negative errors are not excessive. The most obvious way is to increase group sizes. However, the increase in power probably will not be significant unless the group size is drastically increased, say, from 50 to 250 animals per group. This approach of increasing power may not be financially or logistically feasible.

The second way to ensure adequate power in statistical tests of positive dose–response relationship in tumor rates is to treat animals with dose levels that are high enough to induce tumors. However, the determination of an MTD dose is a controversial and complicated issue. Information about clinical signs, histopathologic toxic effects, body weight gain and mortality, as well as pharmacokinetic and metabolic data is needed for the evaluation of MTD. Haseman used results of some NTP studies to emphasize the importance of using dose levels that provide adequate tumor challenge to the treated animals. He found that half of the carcinogens tested in those studies would be judged as noncarcinogens if half of the MTDs were used as the highest dose. Under the current four-group design in which a medium group was added as a cushion for cases where the high dose used may be over the MTD, it is feasible to take a greater risk of using the highest possible dose level to ensure adequate power in statistical tests.

The third way to increase power in statistical tests is to assume a larger overall false-positive error. One may have to be willing to assume an overall false-positive error in the 15%–20% range to balance out the low power of statistical tests.

Statistical books tell us that the false-positive error and the false-negative error are two opposite forces.

If one wants to control one of the two types of error to a small magnitude, then he or she has to pay the price for committing the other type of error with a large magnitude other than increasing the sample size). In the general case, a statistical test is performed at a prespecified level of false-positive error, usually at 0.05, and a decision rule is derived to maximize the power (or to minimize the false-negative error) of the test under the alternative hypothesis tested. However, because of the intertwining and conflicting relationship between the two types of error, the magnitudes of the false-positive error and false-negative error have to be determined by the cost-risk (or cost-risk-benefit factor in new drug evaluation). For drug products, such as cancer and AIDS drugs, intended for treating terminally ill patients, one may take a greater risk (false-negative error) by taking a smaller overall false-positive error. This will be especially true when there is no alternative approved drug available in the market. On the other hand, for drug products for treating common cold symptoms, which will be used by a larger population with other available approved alternative drugs, one can be more cautious about the overall false-negative error. To ensure that the false-negative error is not excessive, one may have to assume a larger overall false-positive error. It is true that limited resources shall not be wasted by rejecting an effective drug that costs hundreds of millions of dollars to develop. However, for the protection of the health of the public, it is also equally important that drugs with carcinogenic potential should not be misinterpreted as safe and allowed to enter the market.

In the FDA, to make sure that the committed false-negative error is not excessive, the FDA statistical reviewers collaborate with the reviewing pharmacologists, pathologists, and medical officers to evaluate the adequacy of the gross and histological examination of both control and treated groups, the adequacy of dose selection, and the durations of experiments in relation to the normal life span of the tested animals.

Although concurrent control groups are the most relevant controls in testing drug-related increases in tumors in a study, there are situations in which historical control data from previously comparable studies can be useful for the overall evaluation of the results of the study. One of the situations is when the comparable historical control information is used to define rare tumors, which have less effect on overall false-positive error, and therefore, can be tested at higher levels of significance. The other situation where the historical control may be useful is when checking whether a marginally significant finding is really drug-related or purely due to chance of variation. The third situation is to use historical control data to determine whether a study was conducted properly. In the first situation, a tumor is defined as rare if it was so classified by reviewing pharmacologists and pathologists or if the background spontaneous incidence rate is less than 1%. In the second situation, the incidence rates of the treated groups are compared with the incidence rates of the historical control data. The significant finding will not be considered biologically meaningful if the incidence rates of the treated groups are within the ranges of historical control incidence rates. In the third situation, a question about the quality of the study will be raised if incidence rates of tumors of the control group(s) of the study are not consistent with those in the comparable historical control data. Haseman [41] alerted

"However, before historical control data can be used in a formal testing framework, a number of issues must first be considered." The issues include the nomenclature conventions and diagnostic criteria used by pathologists, conducting laboratories, study durations, strains and species of animals used, and time (calendar year) a study was conducted. It is important that the historical control data be comparable with the concurrent control data. The comparability in general includes identical nomenclature conventions and diagnostic criteria, same species/strain/sex, same source of supplier, same testing laboratory, comparable survival and age at termination, comparable time frame of studies (within 5 years), and comparable food consumption and body weight gain.

21.9 Practice of Statistical Review and Evaluation Generally Followed in the FDA

The FDA receives a huge number of animal carcinogenicity studies submitted by drug sponsors as a part of drug safety evaluation of INDs or NDAs. These studies generally include two 104 week long-term studies in rats and mice or one 104 week long-term study in rats and one short- or medium-term study in transgenic mice. In the long-term studies, usually there will be three treated groups, known as low-, medium-, and high-dose groups and one positive control. However, often there are submissions with different designs, for example, submissions with two identical controls or with one positive and one negative control, and submissions with more than three treated groups. Statisticians in the Divisions of Biometrics, CDER, FDA, are responsible for statistical reviews of the results of these animal carcinogenicity experiments.

These reviewers are neither involved in extrapolating animal carcinogenicity study findings beyond the ranges of doses studied nor to species other than those studied, nor are they involved in the investigation of mechanisms of carcinogenesis. They perform a quantitative assessment of the risk of a drug for each species and sex of rodent. The reviewing pharmacologists and medical officers apply their knowledge of mammalian similarities and interspecies differences to extrapolate qualitatively from rodent to human beings.

Before analyzing the tumor data, the FDA statisticians routinely analyze the intercurrent mortality data to see if the survival distributions of the treatment groups are significantly different and if there exist significant dose–response relationships. For regular review of the long-term studies, the survival distributions of animals in all treatment groups are estimated by the Kaplan–Meier product limit method. The homogeneity and dose–response relationship of survival distributions are tested using the Cox test [6] and the Generalized Wilcoxon test [9].

The primary statistical procedure in detecting the carcinogenic potential of a new drug is to test whether there are statistically significant positive dose–response relationships in tumor incidence rates induced by the new drug. Additional analyses include pairwise comparisons of treated groups with concurrent control for drug-induced increased tumor incidence. The phrase "positive dose–response relationship" refers to the increasing linear component of the effect of treatment but not necessarily to a strictly increasing tumor rate as the dose increases. For a dose–response relationship test as well as pairwise comparisons, generally the methods outlined by Peto et al. or alternatively the Poly-K method are used. Since the sponsor generally classifies the tumor types as "cause of death" and "not a cause of death," following Peto et al. [2], the reviewers apply the "death-rate method" and the "prevalence method" for these two categories of tumors, respectively, to test the dose–response relationship. For tumor types occurring in both categories, a combined test of "death-rate method" and the "prevalence method" is performed. For the calculation of p-values, the exact permutation method is used. The actual dose levels of treatment groups are used as the weight for the dose–response test. The time intervals used are 0–52, 53–78, 79–91, 92–104 weeks, and terminal sacrifice.

For the use of the Poly-K test one critical point is the choice of the appropriate value of k. For the long-term 104 week standard rat and mouse studies, a value of $k = 3$ is suggested in the literature. Hence, the FDA reviewers use $k = 3$ for the analysis of tumor data. If there are two identical control groups and there is no significant difference in survival rates between them, in their analysis of tumor data FDA statisticians combine the two control groups to form a single control group (combined control). Such combining of controls increases the power of the tests and reduces the dimension of the multiple testing. On the other hand, if the two controls are identical with statistically significantly different survival patterns or the two controls are not identical, two separate analyses are done using each control once.

In addition to tumor data analysis, the FDA statisticians routinely perform evaluations of the validity of the study in case the study turns out to be negative. The evaluation includes the investigation whether enough animals were exposed for a sustained amount of time to the risk of developing tumors, especially the late developing tumors, and the investigation whether the dose levels were high enough to pose a reasonable tumor challenge to the animals.

For the adjustment for the multiple dose–response relationship testing, the ad hoc method proposed by Lin and Rahman [36] is used. This method recommends the use of a significance level of $\alpha = 0.025$ for rare tumors and $\alpha = 0.005$ for common tumors for a submission with two studies and a significance level of $\alpha = 0.05$ for rare tumors and $\alpha = 0.01$ for common tumors for a submission with one study to keep the false-positive rate at the nominal level of approximately 10%. A rare tumor is defined as one for which the published spontaneous tumor rate is less than 1%. Adjustment for multiple pairwise comparisons is done using the criterion proposed by Haseman [35], which recommends the use of a significance level $\alpha = 0.05$ for rare tumors and $\alpha = 0.01$ for common tumors, also to keep the false-positive rate at the nominal level of approximately 10%. Comparable historical control data, when available and reliable, are also used to assist in classifying common and rare tumors and in deciding whether significant findings are biologically relevant.

21.10   Presentation of Results and Data to FDA

To facilitate statistical reviews, sponsors should present study results and summary data in such a way that that the FDA statistical reviewers are able to verify the sponsors' findings, evaluate the validity of the study, and reanalyze the data, if necessary, in order to explore alternatives or to gain greater insight into the relationships between various events of the studies. In the sponsor's report, in addition to the volumes containing study data of individual animals, a statistical analysis section should be included containing summary statistics of the study data, results of statistical analyses of the data, results and findings, and main conclusions of the study. In the statistical analysis section, the sponsor should include descriptions of the statistical procedures used and pertinent literature references. The descriptions of statistical methodology and references are particularly important if the sponsor decides to use designs and methods of analysis and interpretation other than those recommended in the FDA 2001 guidance for industry document. Tables 21.15 through 21.17 in the FDA 2001 guidance for industry document are examples of formats for presenting summaries and results of analyses of survival and tumor data.

For FDA statistical reviewers to perform statistical analyses to verify the sponsor's results, and to answer questions that are not addressed by the sponsor, the sponsor is asked to submit the electronic tumor datasets in appropriate formats with the NDA or IND submission. For 2 year studies as well as transgenic mouse studies using all except the TgAC mouse models, the sponsor is requested to recreate the tumor data in conformance to the electronic format specified in the Agency's April 2006 guidance document entitled *Guidance for Industry: Providing Regulatory Submissions in Electronic Format—Human Pharmaceutical Applications and Related Submissions Using the eCTD Specifications*. The guidance document can be found at http://www.fda.gov/cder/regulatory/ersr/ectd.htm under the title of this guidance document.

In Section III.D.3 of the guidance document, the Agency gives a general description of the data formats for the pharmacology and toxicology datasets and refers readers to the associated document *Study Data Specifications* for more information about the format specifications of the data submission. This associated document can also be found at the previously mentioned FDA Web site under the title of this document (or directly at http://www.fda.gov/cder/regulatory/ersr/Studydata.pdf). At this time, the sponsor is expected to submit the tumor dataset in the format described on page 7 (Appendix 1) of the associated document. The table containing the format for tumor data in the document is presented in Appendix 21.A. A sample tumor dataset using this format is given in Appendix 21.B.

For studies using TgAC transgenic mice, the sponsor is requested to recreate the weekly count data of skin papillomas of individual animals as a SAS dataset in the format presented in Appendix 21.C. Numbers of skin papillomas developed on the site of application (SOA) and other sites of the body (nonsites of application [NSOA]) should be listed separately. A period (.) should be used for the count of each of the weeks after death if an animal died before the end of the study.

21.11   Concluding Remarks

In designing an animal carcinogenicity experiment, randomization methods should be used in allocating animals to treatment groups to avoid possible biases caused by animal selection. A sufficient number of animals should be used in an experiment to ensure reasonable power in subsequent statistical tests. In negative studies where analysis results show no significant positive dose–response relationships in tumor incidence rates, a further evaluation of the validity of the experimental designs should be performed to see if there are sufficient numbers of animals living long enough to get adequate exposure to the drug compounds and to be at risk of forming tumors and if the doses used are high enough and sufficiently close to the MTD to present a reasonable tumor challenge to the tested animals.

The intercurrent mortality data should be evaluated to see if the survival distributions of the treatment groups are similar (homogeneity). If a difference is detected, it is of interest to see whether there is a dose–response relationship in mortality. Since the effects of differences in intercurrent mortality on number of tumor-bearing animals can be substantial, in case of a significant difference in survival among treatment groups, survival-adjusted methods should be used in the dose–response relationships analysis as well as in pairwise comparisons to test increased tumorigenicity in treated groups compared to the concurrent control.

When the number of tumor occurrences across treatment groups is small, the test results of asymptotically normal approximations are not stable and reliable. Under this circumstance, exact permutation methods should be used for dose–response relationships as well as pairwise comparisons.

Controlling the overall false-positive error and the overall false-negative error to acceptable levels is the central element in the interpretation of study results. The control of the two types of error involves both statistical and nonstatistical issues. Appropriate statistical methodology should be used to control the effects of multiple testing. It is important that an overall evaluation of the carcinogenic potential of a drug be based on knowledge of statistical significance and the biological relevance.

Sponsors of new drugs should present their data in the FDA data submission format, outlined in the FDA guidance for carcinogenicity data submission, to facilitate the FDA's statistical reviewer in verifying the sponsors' calculations, to validate their statistical methods, and to trace back the sponsors' conclusions through their summaries and necessary additional analyses. The sponsors should make the raw data in an appropriate format and easily accessible to the statistical reviewers. The sponsor is expected to consult the appropriate FDA guidelines and guidance for detailed information regarding data and report submission.

When relevant and reliable historical data are available, formal or informal use of them may improve the power of the tests as well as the interpretation of the study results. The informal method of using historical control data in the interpretation of results of a carcinogenicity study is not very satisfactory because the ranges of historical control rates are usually too wide. This problem becomes especially serious in the situation in which the historical control rates of the tumor in most studies used are clustered together but only a few other studies with rates far away from the cluster. The formal statistical procedure works well in situations in which historical data from a large number of studies with relatively large control groups are available to provide reliable estimations of the parameters of the assumed prior distributions.

Acknowledgments

The authors express their thanks to Dr. Karl Peace for giving the opportunity to contribute to this very important book. The authors are grateful to the director of the Division of Biometrics-6, Dr. Stella Machado, deputy director Dr. Yi Tsong, and other colleagues for their continuous support of this work. The authors express special thanks to Dr. Steven Thomas and his wife Patricia Lynn Carter Thomson for taking the time and for their patience in reading and editing the earlier manuscripts. Finally, Mohammad Rahman personally thanks Dr. Mohammad Huque, director, Division of Biometrics-3, for his encouragement to continue research and academic activities in the drug development statistical area.

References

[1] Sontag, J.M., Page, N.P., and Safiotti, U. (1976): *Guidelines for Carcinogen Bioassay in small Rodents, DHHS Publication (NIH) 76–801*. National Cancer Institute, Bethesda, MD.

[2] Peto, R. et al. (1980): Guidelines for simple, sensitive significance tests for carcinogenic effects in long-term animal experiments. In *Long-term and Short-term Screening Assays for Carcinogens: A Critical Appraisal*, World Health Organization, Geneva; Portier, C. and Hoel, D.G. (1983): Optimal design of the chronic animal bioassay. *Journal of Toxicology and Environmental Health* 12: 1–19.

[3] Bancroft, T.A. (1964): Analysis and inference for incompletely specified models involving the use of preliminary test(s) of significance. *Biometrics* 20: 427–442.

[4] Gart, J.J., Krewski, D., Lee, P.N., Tarone, R.E., and Wahrendorf, J. (1986): *Statistical Methods in Cancer Research, Volume III—The Design and Analysis of Long-Term Animal Experiments*. International Agency for Research on Cancer, World Health Organization, Geneva.

[5] Tarone, R.E. (1975): Tests for trend in life table analysis. *Biometrika* 62: 679–682.

[6] Cox, D.R. (1972): Regression models and life tables (with discussion). *Journal of Royal Statistical Society, Series B* 34: 187–220.

[7] Thomas, D.G., Breslow, N., and Gart, J.J. (1977): Trend and homogeneity analyses of proportions and life table data. *Computer and Biomedical Research* 10: 373–381.

[8] Breslow, N. (1970): A generalized Kruskal-Wallis test for comparing K samples subject to unequal patterns of censorship. *Biometrics* 57: 579–594.

[9] Gehan, E.A. (1965): A generalized Wilcoxon test for comparing K samples subject to unequal patterns of censorship. *Biometrika* 52: 203–223.

[10] Snedecor, G.W. and Cochran, W.G. (1971): *Statistical Methods*, 6th edn. Iowa State University Press, Ames, IA.

[11] Dinse, G.E. (1985): Testing for trend in tumor prevalence rates: I. Nonlethal tumors. *Biometrics* 41: 751–770.

[12] Dinse, G.E. and Haseman, J.K. (1986): Logistic regression analysis of incidental-tumor data from animal carcinogenicity experiments. *Fundamental and Applied Toxicology* 6: 44–52.

[13] Dinse, G.E. and Lagakos, S.W. (1983): Regression analysis of tumor prevalence data. *The Journal of the Royal Statistical Society, Series C* 32: 236–248.

[14] Lin, K.K. and Reschke, M.F. (1987): The use of the logistic model in space motion sickness prediction. *Aviation, Space, and Environmental Medicine*, August: A9–A15.

[15] Armitage, P. (1955): Tests for linear trends in proportions and frequencies. *Biometrics* 11: 375–386.

[16] Armitage, P. (1971): *Statistical Methods in Medical Research*. John Wiley & Sons Inc., New York.

[17] Bailer, A. and Portier, C. (1988): Effects of treatment-induced mortality on tests for carcinogenicity in small samples. *Biometrics* 44: 417–431.

[18] Bieler, G.S. and Williams, R.L. (1993): Ratio estimates, the delta method, and quantal response tests for increased carcinogenicity. *Biometrics* 49: 793–801.

[19] Mantel, N. and Haenszel, W. (1959): Statistical aspects of the analysis of data from retrospective studies of disease. *Journal of National Cancer Research* 22: 719–748.

[20] Ali, M.W. (1990): Exact versus asymptotic tests of trend of tumor prevalence in tumorigenicity experiments: A comparison of P-values for small frequency of tumors. *Drug Information Journal* 24: 727–737

[21] Mantel, N. (1980): Assessing laboratory evidence for neoplastic activity. *Biometrics* 36: 381–399.

[22] Ali, M.W. (1990b): A comparison of power between exact and approximate tests of trend of tumor prevalence when tumor rates are low. *Proceedings of the Biopharmaceutical Section of the American Statistical Association*, American Statistical Association, Alexandria, VA, pp. 66–71.

[23] Hayashi, M., Yoshimura, I., Sofuni, T., and Ishidate, M. Jr. (1989): A procedure for data analysis of the rodent micronucleus test involving a historical control. *Environmental and Molecular Mutagenesis* 13: 347–356.

[24] Louis, T.A. (1981): Confidence intervals for a binomial parameter after observing no successes. *The American Statisticians* 35(3): 154.

[25] Blyth, C.R. (1986): Approximate binomial confidence limits. *Journal of American Statistical Association* 81: 843–855.

[26] Vollset, S.E. (1993): Confidence intervals for binomial proportion. *Statistics in Medicine* 12: 809–824.

[27] Jovanovic, B.D. and Viana, M.A.G. (1996): Upper confidence bounds for binomial probability in safety evaluation. *Proceedings of the Biopharmaceutical Section of the American Statistical Association*, American Statistical Association, Alexandria, VA, pp. 140–144.

[28] Jovanovic, B.D. and Levy, P.S. (1997): A look at the rule of three. *The American Statistician* 51(2): 137–139.

[29] Lee, P.M. (1997): *Bayesian Statistics: An Introduction*, 2nd edn. Arnold, London.

[30] Ibrahim J.G. and Ryan L.M. (1996): Use of historical controls in time-adjusted trend tests for carcinogenicity. *Biometrics* 52: 1478–1485.

[31] Tarone, R.E. (1982): The use of historical control information in testing for a trend in proportions. *Biometrics* 38: 215–220.

[32] National Cancer Institute (1977): Bioassay of nitrilotriacetic acid (NTA) and nitrilotriacetic acid trisodium salt, monohydrate (Na_3NTA-H_2O) for possible carcinogenicity. Technical report no. 6; National Cancer Institute, Bethesda, MD.

[33] Rosenthal, R. and Rubin, D.B. (1984): Multiple contrast and ordered Bonferroni procedure. *Journal of Educational Psychology* 76: 1028–1034.

[34] Lehman, E.L. and Romano, J.P. (2005): *Testing Statistical Hypotheses*. Springer-Verlag, New York.

[35] Haseman, J.K. (1983): A reexamination of false-positive rates for carcinogenesis studies. *Fundamental and Applied Toxicology* 3: 334–339.

[36] Lin, K.K. and Rahman, M.A. (1998): Overall false positive rates in tests for linear trend in tumor incidence in animal carcinogenicity studies of new drugs. *Journal of Pharmaceutical Statistics* 8(1): 1–22 (discussion).

[37] Dunson, D.B., Haseman, J.K., van Birgelen, A.P.J.M., Staiewicz, S., and Tennant, R.W. (2000): Statistical analysis of skin tumor data from Tg.AC mouse assays. *Toxicological Sciences* 55: 293–302.

[38] Haseman, J.K. (1985): Issues in carcinogenicity testing: dose selection. *Fundamental and Applied Toxicology* 5: 66–78.

[39] Chu, K.C., Cueto, C., and Ward, J.M. (1981): Factors in the evaluation of 200 National Cancer Institute carcinogen bioassays. *Journal of Toxicology and Environmental Health* 8: 251–280.

[40] McConnell, E.E., Solleveld, H.A., Swenberg, J.A., and Boorman, G.A. (1986): Guidelines for combining neoplasms for evaluation of rodent carcinogenesis studies. *Journal of National Cancer Institute* 76: 283–289.

[41] Haseman, J.K. (1984): Statistical issues in the design, analysis and interpretation of animal carcinogenicity studies. *Environmental Health Perspective* 58: 385–392.

Further Readings

Ames, B.N. and Gold, L.S. (1990): Too many rodent carcinogens: Mitogenesis increases mutagenesis. *Science* 240: 970–971.

Bickis, M. and Krewski, D. (1989): Statistical issues in the analysis of the long-term carcinogenicity bioassay in small rodents: An empirical evaluation of statistical decision rules. *Fundamental and Applied Toxicology* 12: 202–221.

Brown, C.C. and Fears, T.R. (1981): Exact significance levels for multiple binomial testing with application to carcinogenicity screens. *Biometrics* 37: 763–774.

Charles River Company (undated): Spontaneous Neoplastic Lesions in the Crl:CD BR Rat, Wilmington, MA. (Information Complied by P.L. Lang and included in the class notes of Comparative Pathology, T.P. O'Neill, FDA/CDER Staff College).

Charles River Company (1987): Spontaneous Neoplastic Lesions in the Crl:CD-1 (ICR) BR Mouse, Wilmington, MA. (Information Complied by P.L. Lang and included in the class notes of Comparative Pathology, T.P. O'Neill, FDA/CDER Staff College).

Charles River Company (1989): Spontaneous Neoplastic Lesions in the B6C3F1/CrlBR Mouse, Wilmington, MA. (Information Complied by P.L. Lang and included in the class notes of Comparative Pathology, T.P. O'Neill, FDA/CDER Staff College).

Charles River Company (1990): Spontaneous Neoplastic Lesions in the CDF (F-344)/CrlBR Rat, Wilmington, MA. (Information Complied by P.L. Lang and included in the class notes of Comparative Pathology, T.P. O'Neill, FDA/CDER Staff College).

Chen, J.J. and Gaylor, D.W. (1987): The upper percentiles of the distribution of the logrank statistics for small numbers of tumors. Unpublished report; National Center for Toxicological Research, FDA.

Chen, J.J., Lin, K.K., Huque, M.F., and Arani, R.B. (2000): Weighted P-value for animal carcinogenicity trend test. *Biometrics* 56: 586–592.

Cochran, W. (1954): Some methods for strengthening the common χ^2 tests. *Biometrics* 10: 417–451.

Cohen, S.M. and Ellwein, L.B. (1990): Cell proliferation in carcinogenesis. *Science* 249: 1007–1011.

Cox, D.R. (1959): The analysis of exponentially distributed life-times with two types of failures. *Journal of Royal Statistical Society, Series B*, 21: 411–421.

Dinse, G.E. (1994): A comparison of tumor incidence analyses applicable in single-sacrifice animal experiments. *Statistics in Medicine* 13: 689–708.

Fairweather, W.R. (1988): Statistical considerations in tumorigenicity study review (abstract). Presented at the Drug Information Association Meeting in Toronto, Canada, July 12, 1988.

Fairweather, W.R., Bhattacharyya, A., Ceuppens, P.P., Heimann, G., Hothorn, L.A., Kodell, R.L., Lin, K.K., et al. (1998): Biostatistical methodology in carcinogenicity studies. *Drug Information Journal* 32: 401–421.

Farrar, D.B. and Crump, K.S. (1988): Exact statistical tests for any carcinogenic effect in animal bioassays. *Fundamental and Applied Toxicology* 11: 652–663.

Farrar, D.B. and Crump, K.S. (1990): Exact statistical tests for any carcinogenic effect in animal bioassays. II. Age-adjusted tests. *Fundamental and Applied Toxicology* 15: 710–721.

Fears, T.R. and Tarone, R.E. (1977): Response to use of statistics when examining lifetime studies in rodents to detect carcinogenicity. *Journal of Toxicology and Environmental Health* 3: 627–632.

Fears, T.R., Tarone, R.E., and Chu, K.C. (1977): False-positive and false-negative rates for carcinogenicity screens. *Cancer Research* 37: 1941–1945.

Food and Drug Administration, U.S. Department of Health and Human Services (1987): *Guideline for the Format and Content of the Nonclinical/Pharmacology/Toxicology Section of An Application*. FDA, Rockville, MD.

Gart, J.J., Chu, K.C., and Tarone, R.E. (1979): Statistical issues in interpretation of chronic bioassays for carcinogenicity. *Journal of National Cancer Institute* 62: 957–974.

Gart, J.J. and Tarone, R.E. (1987): On the efficiency of age-adjusted tests in animal carcinogenicity experiments. *Biometrics* 43: 235–244.

Gaylor, D.W. and Hoel, D.G. (1981): Statistical analysis of carcinogenesis data from chronic animal studies. *Carcinogens in Industry and the Environment*, J.M. Sontag, ed. Marcel Dekker, New York.

Goldberg, K.M. (1985): An algorithm for computing an exact trend test for multiple $2 \times K$ contingency tables. Paper Presented at Symposium on Long-Term Animal Carcinogenicity Studies.

Hardisty, J.F. and Eustis, S.L. (1990): Toxicological pathology: A critical stage in study interpretation. *Progress in Predictive Toxicology*, D.B. Clayson, I.C. Munro, P. Shubik, and J.A. Swenberg, eds. Elsevier Science Publisher B.V., Biomedical Division, New York.

Haseman, J.K. (1977): Response to use of statistics when examining lifetime studies in rodents to detect carcinogenicity. *Journal of Toxicology and Environmental Health* 3: 633–636.

Haseman, J.K. (1990): Use of statistical decision rules for evaluating laboratory animal carcinogenicity studies. *Fundamental and Applied Toxicology* 14: 637–648.

Haseman, J.K., Huff, J., and Boorman, G.A. (1984): Use of historical control data in carcinogenicity studies in rodents. *Toxicologic Pathology* 12: 126–135.

Haseman, J.K., Huff, J., Rao, G.N., and Eustis, S.L. (1989): Sources of variability in rodent carcinogenicity studies. *Fundamental and Applied Toxicology* 12: 793–804.

Haseman, J.K., Winbush, J.S., and O'Donnell, M.W. (1986): Use of dual control groups to estimate false positive rates in laboratory animal carcinogenicity studies. *Fundamental and Applied Toxicology* 7: 573–584.

Heimann, G. and Neuhaus, G. (1998): Permutational distribution of the log-rank statistic under random censorship with applications to carcinogenicity assays. *Biometrics* 54: 168–184.

Heyse, J.F. and Rom, D. (1988): Adjusting for multiplicity of statistical tests in the analysis of carcinogenicity studies. *Biometrical Journal* 30: 883–896.

Hoel, D.G. and Walburg, H.E. (1972): Statistical analysis of survival experiments. *Journal of the National Cancer Institute* 49: 361–372.

Holm, S. (1979): A simple sequentially rejective multiple test procedure. *Scandinavian Journal of Statistics* 6: 65–70.

ICH (1995): S1C Dose Selection for Carcinogenicity Studies of Pharmaceuticals: ICH—S1C.

ICH (1998): S1B testing for carcinogenicity of pharmaceuticals. ICH—S1B; *Federal Register*; vol. 63: 8983–8986, 1998. Sun J (1999): On the use of historical control data for trend test in carcinogenicity studies. *Biometrics* 55(4): 1273–1276.

Kodell, R.L., Haskin, M.G., Shaw, G.W., and Gaylor, D.W. (1983): CHRONIC: A SAS procedure for statistical analysis of carcinogenesis studies. *Journal of Statistical Computation Simulation* 16: 287–310.

Kuritz, S.J., Landis, J.R., and Koch, G.G. (1988): A general overview of Mantel-Haenszel methods: Applications and recent developments. *Annual Review Of Public Health* 9: 123–160.

Lin, K.K. (1988): Peto prevalence method versus regression methods in analyzing incidental tumor data from animal carcinogenicity experiments: An empirical study. *Proceedings of the Biopharmaceutical Section of the American Statistical Association*, New Orleans, LA, pp. 95–100.

Lin, K.K. (1989): Methods of statistical analysis of animal tumorigenicity studies. *Proceedings of the Biopharmaceutical Section of the American Statistical Association*, Alexandria, VA, pp. 142–147.

Lin, K.K. (1995): A regulatory perspective on statistical methods for analyzing new drug carcinogenicity study data. *Bio/Pharm Quarterly* 1(2): 18–20.

Lin, K.K. (1997): Control of overall false positive rates in animal carcinogenicity studies of pharmaceuticals. Presented at 1997 FDA Forum on Regulatory Sciences, December 8–9, 1997, Bethesda, MD.

Lin, K.K. (2000): Carcinogenicity studies of pharmaceuticals. *Encyclopedia of Biopharmaceutical Statistics*, S.C. Chow, ed. Marcel Dekker, New York, pp. 88–103.

Lin, K.K. and Ali, M.W. (2006): Statistical review and evaluation of animal carcinogenicity studies. *Statistics in the Pharmaceutical Industry*, C.R. Buncher and J.Y. Tsay, eds., 3rd edn. Marcel Dekker Inc., New York.

Lin, K.K. and Rahman, M.A. (1998b): False positive rates in tests for trend and differences in tumor incidence in animal carcinogenicity studies of pharmaceuticals under ICH Guidance S1B. Unpublished report, Division of Biometrics 2, Center for Drug Evaluation and Research, Food and Drug Administration.

Mancuso, J.Y., Hongshik, A., Chen, J.J., and Mancuso, J.P. (2002): Age-adjusted exact trend tests in the event of rare occurrences. *Biometrics* 58: 403–412.

National Technical Information Service, U.S. Department of Commerce (1990): Studies/ Chronic, Data Formats for Chronic/Oncogenicity Rodent Bioassays; PB90–213885, Springfield, VA.

Office of the Federal Register (1985): Chemical carcinogens: A review of the science and its associated principles. Part II, Office of Science and Technology Policy, *Federal Register* 47–58. (Note: The paper was also published with the same title and authorized by U.S. Interagency Staff Group on Carcinogens in Environmental Health Perspectives, 67, 201–282).

Salsburg, D.S. (1977): Use of statistics when examining lifetime studies in rodents to detect carcinogenicity. *Journal of Toxicology and Environmental Health* 3: 611–628.

Salsburg, D.S. (1983): The lifetime feeding study in mice and rats—an examination of its validity as a bioassay for human carcinogens. *Fundamental and Applied Toxicology* 3: 63–67. Tarone, R.E. (1990): A modified Bonferroni method for discrete data. *Biometrics* 46: 515–522.

U.S. Department of Health and Human Services (1999): *Guidance for Industry: Providing Regulatory Submissions in Electronic Formats—NDAs.* Center for Drug Evaluation and Research, Food and Drug Administration.

U.S. Department of Health and Human Services (2001): *Guidance for Industry: Statistical Aspects of the Design, Analysis, and Interpretation of Chronic Rodent Carcinogenicity Studies of Pharmaceuticals.* Center for Drug Evaluation and Research, Food and Drug Administration.

Westfall, P.H. (1985): Simultaneous small-sample multivariate Bernoulli confidence intervals. *Biometrics* 41: 1001–1013.

Westfall, P.H. and Young, S.S. (1989): P value adjustments for multiple tests in multivariate binomial models. *Journal of American Statistical Association* 84: 780–786.

Woodruff, R.S. (1971): A simple method for approximating the variance of a complicated estimate. *Journal of the American Statistical Association* 66: 411–414.

Appendix 21.A

Format for Submission of Data of 2 Year Carcinogenicity Studies as well as Transgenic Mouse Studies Using All Except the TgAC Mouse Models (Data Format Table on Page 7 (Appendix 1) of the Associated Document Study Data Specifications)

	Tumor Dataset for Statistical Analysis[a,b] (tumor.xpt)			
Variable	**Label**	**Type**	**Codes**	**Comments**
STUDYNUM	Study number	char		c
ANIMLNUM	Animal number	char		a,c
SPECIES	Animal species	char	M = mouse R = rat	
SEX	Sex	char	M = male F = female	
DOSEGP	Dose group	num	Use 0, 1, 2, 3, 4,... in ascending order from control. Provide the dosing for each group.	
DTHSACTM	Time in days to death or sacrifice	num		
DTHSACST	Death or sacrifice status	num	1 = Natural death or moribund sacrifice 2 = Terminal sacrifice 3 = Planned intermittent sacrifice 4 = Accidental death	
ANIMLEXM	Animal microscopic examination code	num	0 = No tissues were examined 1 = At least one tissue was examined	
TUMORCOD	Tumor type code	char		c,d
TUMORNAM	Tumor name	char		c,d
ORGANCOD	Organ/tissue code	char		c,e

(continued)

Tumor Dataset For Statistical Analysis[a,b] (tumor.xpt)				
Variable	Label	Type	Codes	Comments
ORGANNAM	Organ/tissue name	char		[c,e]
DETECTTM	Time in days of detection of tumor	num		
MALIGNST	Malignancy status	num	1 = Malignant 2 = Benign 3 = Undetermined	[d]
DEATHCAU	Cause of death	num	1 = Tumor caused death 2 = Tumor did not cause death 3 = Undetermined	[d]
ORGANEXM	Organ/Tissue microscopic examination code	num	1 = Organ/Tissue was examined and was usable 2 = Organ/Tissue was examined but was not usable (e.g., autolyzed tissue) 3 = Organ/Tissue was not examined	

[a] Each animal in the study should have at least one record even if it does not have a tumor.

[b] Additional variables, as appropriate, can be added to the bottom of this dataset.

[c] ANIMLNUM is limited to no more than 12 characters; ORGANCOD and TUMORCOD are limited to no more than 8 characters; ORGANNAM and TUMORNAM should be as concise as possible.

[d] A missing value should be given for the variable MALIGNST, DEATHCAU, TUMORNAM, and TUMORCOD when the organ is unusable or not examined.

[e] Do not include a record for an organ that was usable and no tumor was found on examination. A record should be included for organs with a tumor, organs found unusable, and organs not examined.

APPENDIX 21.B: Sample tumor data species. Rat sex: Male.

STUDY	ANIMNUM	SPECIES	SEX	DSDTHMODE	DSDTHDAY	ATNUM	TUMNUM	TUMOR		ORGAN		ORGTUMDAY	MALIGN	DEATH	MAXTUM
4285	1032	R	M	0	733	2	1	816	fibroma	1840	subcutaneous tissue	625	2	2	1
4285	1021	R	M	0	733	2	1	856	fibrosarcoma	1840	subcutaneous tissue	700	1	2	1
4285	1333	R	M	3	318	1	1	856	fibrosarcoma	1840	subcutaneous tissue	282	1	1	1
4285	1014	R	M	0	730	2	1	819	lipoma	1840	subcutaneous tissue	730	2	2	1
4285	1224	R	M	2	694	1	1	819	lipoma	1840	subcutaneous tissue	430	2	2	1
4285	1441	R	M	4	682	1	1	819	lipoma	1840	subcutaneous tissue	427	2	2	1
4285	1029	R	M	0	589	1	1	2137	sarcoma, NOS	1840	subcutaneous tissue	563	1	1	1
4285	1016	R	M	0	730	2	1	856	fibrosarcoma	1890	tail	726	1	2	1
4285	1003	R	M	0	729	2	1	808	interstitial cell tumor	1440	testis	729	2	2	1
4285	1013	R	M	0	694	1	1	808	interstitial cell tumor	1440	testis	694	2	2	1
4285	1020	R	M	0	729	2	1	808	interstitial cell tumor	1440	testis	729	2	2	1

4285	1021	R	M	0	733	2	1	808	interstitial cell tumor	1440	testis	733	2	2	1
4285	1053	R	M	0	734	2	1	808	interstitial cell tumor	1440	testis	734	2	2	1
4285	1203	R	M	2	693	1	1	808	interstitial cell tumor	1440	testis	693	2	2	1
4285	1417	R	M	4	730	2	1	808	interstitial cell tumor	1440	testis	730	2	2	1
4285	1420	R	M	4	730	2	1	808	interstitial cell tumor	1440	testis	730	2	2	1
4285	1422	R	M	4	596	1	1	808	interstitial cell tumor	1440	testis	596	2	2	1
4285	1438	R	M	4	733	2	1	808	interstitial cell tumor	1440	testis	733	2	2	1
4285	1440	R	M	4	733	2	1	808	interstitial cell tumor	1440	testis	733	2	2	1
4285	1452	R	M	4	734	2	1	808	interstitial cell tumor	1440	testis	734	2	2	1
4285	1454	R	M	4	734	2	1	808	interstitial cell tumor	1440	testis	734	2	2	1
4285	1313	R	M	3	669	1	1	844	mesothelioma	1440	testis	669	1	1	1
4285	1208	R	M	2	697	1	1	961	C-cell adenoma	1640	thyroid gland	·	·	·	2
4285	1343	R	M	3	523	1	1	961	C-cell adenoma	1640	thyroid gland	·	·	·	2
4285	1015	R	M	0	618	1	1	961	C-cell adenoma	1640	thyroid gland	618	2	2	1
4285	1016	R	M	0	730	2	1	961	C-cell adenoma	1640	thyroid gland	730	2	2	1
4285	1019	R	M	0	730	2	1	961	C-cell adenoma	1640	thyroid gland	730	2	2	1
4285	1035	R	M	0	733	2	1	961	C-cell adenoma	1640	thyroid gland	733	2	2	1
4285	1224	R	M	2	694	1	1	961	C-cell adenoma	1640	thyroid gland	694	2	2	1
4285	1229	R	M	2	717	1	1	961	C-cell adenoma	1640	thyroid gland	717	2	2	1
4285	1245	R	M	2	668	1	1	961	C-cell adenoma	1640	thyroid gland	668	2	2	1

· · ·

Appendix 21.C

Format for Submission of Data of Carcinogenicity Studies Using Tg.AC Transgenic Mice

Sample Tg.AC mouse bioassay data number of papillomas, by study weeks.

Group	Gender	Animal No.	Tumor Site	1	2	3	...	26	27
2	M	16	SOA	0	0	1	...	19	19
			NSOA	0	0	0	...	0	0
			A	0	0	0	...	0	0
			B	0	0	0	...	0	0
			C	0	0	0	...	0	0
			D	0	0	0	...	0	0
			E	0	0	0	...	0	0
			F	0	0	0	...	0	0
		17	SOA	0	0	0	...	0	0
			NSOA	0	0	0	...	0	0
			A	0	0	0	...	0	0
			B	0	0	0	...	0	0
			C	0	0	0	...	0	0
			D	0	0	0	...	0	0
			e	0	0	0	...	0	0
			f	0	0	0	...	0	0
...	...	19	SOA	0	0	1	...	4	5
			NSOA	0	0	0	...	0	0
			a	0	0	0	...	0	0
			b	0	0	0	...	0	0
			c	0	0	0	...	0	0
			d	0	0	0	...	0	0
			e	0	0	0	...	0	0
			f	0	0	0	...	0	0

Note: SOA, site of application; NSOA, nonsite of application; a, mouth; b, genital area; c, scrotal; d, vaginal; e, anal; d, abdominal.

Chapter 22

Design and Analysis of Time-to-Tumor Response in Animal Studies: A Bayesian Perspective

Steve Thomson and Karl K. Lin

Contents

22.1   Introduction

As opposed to simple data description, statistical inference involves drawing conclusions about a data-generating process based on the implications of probability models for observed events. Parameters are certain key descriptors or indices of these models, and are almost always unobservable. Inferential statistics then is basically the process of drawing conclusions about these parameters based on the observed data. In carcinogenicity analyses the key parameter is almost always related to the

551

probability of developing a tumor as a function of increasing drug dose. Sometimes it will also involve other covariates like gender or baseline weight, or, for combination drugs, mixtures of drug doses.

A critical concept in all probability models is that of the probability density (mathematically one would describe this as the Radon–Nikodym derivative with respect to some dominating measure) of the random variable that represents the potentially observed values. The sum of the values of the density, or more generally its integral, over the values within a specified set of values defines the probability that the random variable takes a value within the set. In a typical model, the distribution is indexed by some parameter or parameters which, in this chapter, are generally denoted by θ. The θ may denote a single value or a vector of parameter values. The differences should be clear from the context. When this probability function or density is considered as a function of the parameters it is called a likelihood. Thus for a density $f(y|\theta)$ and a specific value y of Y, the function $L(\theta|y) = f(y|\theta)$ is also a likelihood function of θ. A commonly expressed caveat is it that, given the observed value of Y, the likelihood provides a measure of how "relatively likely" is any particular value of θ.

The so-called likelihood principle in statistics is that all of the information from the sample about the parameters is contained in the likelihood function. Thus for those who agree with this principle, all analyses should be based on the likelihood. Birnbaum showed that this principle is a consequence of sufficiency and a simple conditionality argument. However, not all statisticians agree with this principle (for an extensive discussion with comments, see Berger and Wolpert [1]).

Suppose we write Pr(A) as the probability of an event A, and Pr($A|B$) as the probability of event A given that event B occurred. The latter are called conditional probabilities. Bayes' rule or Bayes theorem is just a way of relating conditional probabilities. Suppose H is some event of interest with H^c its complement, i.e., anything other than H, so that the probability of H^c is $1 - \text{Pr}(H)$. Suppose that D is some other, usually observed, event, then, in the simplest possible case of Bayes rule we have

$$\text{Pr}(H|D) = \frac{\text{Pr}(D|H)\text{Pr}(H)}{\text{Pr}(D|H)\text{Pr}(H) + \text{Pr}(D|H^c)\text{Pr}(H^c)}.$$

This simple observation is the basis of Bayesian analysis in statistics.

Currently there seem to be three main approaches to statistical inference, which might be labeled as frequentist, "likelihoodist," or Bayesian. Actually, most statisticians move from one approach to another as convenient. Frequentist methods (as were emphasized in Chapter 21 [2]) take the parameters as fixed and model the distribution of responses. One then indirectly assesses the implications of the model by comparing the observed statistics to the distribution of responses. However, the a priori nature of this derivation implies that values that were not observed affect conclusions. This leads to the often noted observation that many frequentist techniques depend as much or more on what did not happen as they do on what did happen. Since many of these frequentist techniques depend upon values that did not occur in the sample, they violate the likelihood principle. Statistics that are basically frequentist in derivation but do follow the likelihood principle are sometimes called Likelihoodist.

Bayesian techniques also start with a likelihood $L(\theta|y)$. In a Bayesian framework initial knowledge about a parameter θ is expressed as a probability distribution for θ, i.e., a "prior" density $\pi(\theta)$. This is meant to represent the probability of that the parameter occurs in various regions of the possible parameter space. Then, by Bayes rule, the distribution of θ given the data, i.e., the so-called posterior distribution of θ, has a density (again, mathematically relative to some dominating measure) proportional to $f(y|\theta)\,\pi(\theta)$. This often is written as something like $f(\theta|y)$. The normalizing constant for this density is $\int f(y|\theta)\,\pi(\theta)\,d\theta$, where the $d\theta$ denotes the appropriate dominating measure (e.g., counting measure for discrete random variables, Lebesgue measure for continuous random variables, etc.). Bayes' original contribution was the application of this theorem for a binary random variable with essentially a uniform prior on the proportion of "successes" (e.g., Fienberg [3]). Alternatively, Bayes rule applied to inference can be summarized in the expression:

$$\Pr(\text{parameter}|\text{data}) \propto \Pr(\text{data}|\text{parameter}) * \Pr(\text{parameter}).$$

Frequentist and likelihoodist methods start by defining a summary statistic for the parameters analyzed. The random behavior of the statistic is assessed. Then the statistic or statistics are evaluated at the sample data, and the observed value of the statistic is compared to theoretical values derived from the random behavior of the statistic. Thus, one way to summarize the differences in statistical approaches is to note that frequentist and likelihoodist methods take data as variable and condition on fixed, unobserved parameters. Bayesian methods take parameters as variable and condition on the fixed, observed data to derive the posterior distribution of the parameters. It is notable that the commonly used "*p*-value" measures the probability that a statistic is at or "more extreme" than the observed value from the sample. Thus the *p*-value depends upon values that were not observed, i.e., the more extreme values, and hence the *p*-value approach to hypothesis testing violates the likelihood principle.

Once a likelihood and a prior is specified, the Bayesian machinery is automatic. Given actual data, the analysis of a parameter is usually based on its marginal distribution, integrating out the effect of other parameters from the posterior distribution. Unlike standard frequentist analysis, the approach to both fixed and random parameters is the same. Both are basically treated as random, although random parameters usually have higher order, hierarchical parameters. In a Bayesian approach, as further data are added, today's posterior distribution of the parameters becomes tomorrow's prior distribution.

Spiegelhalter et al. [4], in a very readable text on medical applications define four schools of Bayesian analysis characterized by, as they describe it, increasing "purity" of Bayesian thought:

1. In the *empirical Bayes* approach data are used to estimate the prior, usually by estimating the parameters of the prior, and plugging these estimated values into the estimand, usually using a maximum likelihood or other estimation method (e.g., see [5]).

2. The *reference Bayes* approach attempts to use noninformative or "objective" priors, where the effect of the prior is supposedly small. The idea of a noninformative prior is a prior that does not closely determine the outcome. The reference Bayes approach is described in detail in Bernardo and Smith [6]. As they discuss, truly noninformative priors may not be attainable, but it does seem that one often can derive roughly noninformative priors.

3. The *proper Bayes* approach uses informative priors to summarize appropriate prior knowledge, either through historical models or elicitation of expert opinion.

4. The *decision-theoretic* or "full" Bayes approach uses loss functions to define the utility of decisions. Bayes rules then maximize expected utility over the prior parameter distribution. Application of this approach seems to be rare in biostatistics.

A key notion in Bayesian analysis is that of exchangeability. Consider a sequence of random variables $Y_1, Y_2, \ldots, Y_n$. If these are stochastically independent, each with density $f(y_i|\theta)$, the joint density of the sequence is $\prod f(y_i|\theta)$. Since the joint density is just the product of the individual densities, any permutation of the order of the random variables leads to exactly the same density. Exchangeability of the sequence $Y_1, Y_2, \ldots, Y_n$ is a generalization of this notion, where the joint density of the sequence is the same for each permutation of the subscripts. That is, if $p(1)$, $p(2), \ldots, p(n)$ represents any permutation of the subscripts $1, 2, \ldots, n$, and for each such permutation π, the joint distribution of $Y_1, Y_2, \ldots, Y_n$ is the same as that of $Y_{p(1)}, Y_{p(2)}, \ldots, Y_{p(n)}$, then the sequence is said to be exchangeable. Suppose as a thought experiment that we can consider this as a part of an infinite sequence of random variables, where each finite subsequence is exchangeable. Then we say the sequence is infinitely exchangeable.

Suppose a random variable Y_i takes values of only 0 or 1, where the probability of a 1 is denoted by some θ, so the probability of a 0 for that variable is $1 - \theta$. Thus the density (with respect to counting measure on 0 and 1) is the Bernoulli distribution:

$$f(y|\theta_i) = \theta_i^y (1 - \theta_i)^{1-y}.$$

For an infinite exchangeable sequence of Bernoulli random variables $Y_1, Y_2, \ldots,$ $Y_n, \ldots$ de Finetti (e.g., see Bernardo and Smith [6]) showed that there was a distribution $Q(\theta)$, with density $q(\theta)$, such that the joint distribution of $Y_1, Y_2, \ldots, Y_n$ could be written as

$$f(y_1, y_2, \ldots, y_n) = \int \prod \theta^{y_i} (1 - \theta)^{1-y_i} q(\theta) d\theta.$$

Going from right to left, this is quite expected, and just involves a standard conditioning argument. The astonishing thing about this is that if one can consider these as finite subsequences of an infinitely exchangeable sequence, we necessarily have a distribution on θ which can be identified as a prior distribution, i.e., right to left. Perhaps equally astonishing is that this theorem generalizes to general densities. Thus, basically, exchangeability in a block of random variables indexed by a certain parameter implies the existence of a prior distribution on that parameter. However, it should be noted that this only applies if there is an infinite sequence of exchangeable random variables. In most circumstances it would seem to be an easy thought experiment to just consider the observed finite collection of exchangeable random variables as part of an infinite collection of potential random variables, and thus de Finetti's results would apply.

22.2 Design of Rodent Carcinogenicity Studies

Many factors determine the adequacy of an animal carcinogenicity study, including the species and strain of the animals, sample size, dose selection, method of allocation of animals, route of administration, animal care and diet, caging, drug stability, and study duration. To assess the impact of the dose, it is generally assumed that a tumor response at a high dose with a relatively small number of animals would imply an observable tumor response at a lower dose in a larger study. Then the existence of such a signal in the animal species is used as evidence of a carcinogenicity risk in humans. To detect a clear signal, the general goal of such a study should be to maximize animal exposure by testing at some maximum tolerated doses (i.e., the MTD). Details of the design of carcinogenicity studies are given in the Food and Drug Administration (FDA) Draft Guidance [7] and, with more details on the actual analysis, in the Rahman and Lin chapter in this book [2], as well as in Lin [8].

An important statistical consideration is that a sufficient number of animals should remain in a study for the full duration of treatment to ensure a chance of detecting whether or not there are any carcinogenic effects. For analyses of standard two year rodent studies with nontransgenic animals, mice or rats, it has been recommended that each dose and concurrent control group contain at least 50–60 animals of each sex. Interim sacrifices may be useful to detect onset of not immediately fatal tumors. If there are any interim sacrifices it is usually recommended that the count of the animals should be increased by the number of animals scheduled for interim sacrifices.

With standard laboratory rodents, animals are usually exposed to the test substance for essentially their entire normal life span, generally 24 months for rats and roughly the same for mice. With transgenic mouse models, the study length is usually much less. Early mortality losses, even if unavoidable, may render a study uninformative, leaving too few animals living long enough to represent adequate exposure to the chemical, so it is important that the doses be high enough to induce tumors, but not so high that toxic effects have strong detrimental effect on survival.

The simplest endpoint is just the observed proportion of animals with the tumor by the end of the study. However, this has a potential flaw in that differences in mortality could reduce the number of animals at risk of developing the tumor, and thus reduce the crude incidence proportion of animals with tumors. For example, if any dose group, particularly the high dose group, exceeds the maximally tolerated dose, a number of animals may die prior to tumor onset, and thus may not be at risk of developing tumors.

In general, when approaching any statistical experimental design, one is interested in the effect of specified values of parameters of the data-generating process on the outcome of the experiment. Such values determine treatment effect, mortality effects, food consumption, animal weights, etc. Assessing the effect of specified parameters is exactly what is done in a typical frequentist analysis of a statistical problem. In particular, one particular type of this analysis is a power analysis where one computes the probability of detecting an effect for certain specified parameters. That is, from the point of view of any particular collection of postulated parameter values, a frequentist analysis of the possible outcomes seems to be appropriate. Although there are some who would not completely agree, (for example, see Stangl and Berry [9] or Berry [10]), it is a personal opinion that design of experiments is basically a frequentist exercise. However, when assessing a design, there are a number of Bayesian measures that may be incorporated into the basically frequentist analysis of such experiments. One such Bayesian approach that might be useful would be to specify priors for some parameters, instead of just some specified values. These priors may be on nuisance parameters in which one is not particularly interested, or be a way to summarize information in priors on critical parameters. For example, if one has a fairly sure grasp on the behavior of the distribution of likely values of any nuisance parameters it would make sense to assess the marginal distribution behavior of estimators where one integrates over the distribution of the nuisance parameters.

Because of the complexity of the analysis the operating characteristics of the procedure should be assessed by using simulation. For example, one could postulate data-generating processes corresponding to a high tumor rate, a moderate rate, and a low rate. One could then generate samples corresponding to these conditions and then assess the rate of correct decisions. For somewhat different problems than typical carcinogenicity analyses, this approach is discussed in Ref. [11]

These studies are usually conducted at the request of regulators, whose agreement on the exact design of the studies is normally required. Analyses are usually conducted separately by gender. A Bayesian analysis of a clinical study may have some advantages in terms of incorporating prior information and arguably has a more natural interpretation of results than frequentist or likelihoodist methods. However, it will be important to get the agreement of regulators prior to running a study whose analysis will be based such methodology. Again, see the preceding chapter for discussion and further references for details on the design of these studies.

22.3   Bayesian Estimation and Hypothesis Testing

22.3.1   Bayes Estimates, Quadratic Loss versus Absolute Loss

Once a probability model is chosen, one can specify appropriate prior distributions for the parameters. As noted in the introduction, these lead to the posterior distribution $f(\theta|y)$. Reasonable point estimates of θ, written here as $\theta(y)$, are based on summary features of $f(\theta|y)$. Three natural summaries are the mode, median, and mean of the values of the posterior distribution. The mode of the posterior distribution is the value with the highest density or probability, i.e., for the posterior of θ:

$$\theta_{Mode}(y) = \arg \max f(\theta|y).$$

The median of the posterior is a value such that the posterior probability of being at or below the value as well as at or above the value is at least 0.5, i.e., it satisfies the posterior probability relation:

$$\text{Pr}_\theta|_x(\theta \geq \theta_{Median}(y)) \geq 0.5 \text{ and } \text{Pr}_\theta|_x(\theta < \theta_{Median}(y)) \geq 0.5.$$

The mean is the expected value of a random variable following the posterior probability distribution. That is, for a discrete posterior defined on $\theta_1, \theta_2, \ldots, \theta_n$:

$$\theta_{Mean}(y) = \sum \theta_i f(\theta_i|y),$$

and more generally:

$$\theta_{Mean}(y) = \int \theta f(\theta|y) d\theta.$$

Optimality in estimation requires some measure of appropriateness, and usually is based on some form of a loss function, where increasing distance of the estimator $\theta(y)$ from the "true" parameter θ is denoted by increasing loss. One loss function is the absolute loss, where the loss is the absolute value of the difference, i.e., loss $= |\theta(y) - \theta|$. Another is quadratic loss, i.e., loss $= (\theta(y) - \theta)^2$. The expected posterior loss for each of these is just the expected loss weighted by the posterior distribution:

$$\int |\theta(y) - \theta| f(\theta|y) d\theta \quad \text{or} \quad \int (\theta(y) - \theta)^2 f(\theta|y) d\theta.$$

These are called the Bayes risk of the estimator, and are associated with the specific loss function used. An optimal estimator of θ is the estimator than minimizes the posterior expected loss, i.e., the Bayes risk. This is generally the posterior median for absolute loss and the posterior mean for quadratic loss.

A subset of the parameter space whose posterior probability is $1 - \alpha$ is said to be a $100(1 - \alpha)\%$ credible set for the true value of θ. That is, S is an interval or set, such that $1 - \alpha = \int_S f(\theta|y) d\theta$. When such credible sets are intervals they are often called interval estimators. The region with the smallest volume or area is called the highest posterior density credible region or interval. The usual credible intervals provided by the most software are based on the percentiles of the posterior distribution. For example if $P_{\alpha/2}$ is the $100 \, \alpha/2\%$ percentile of the distribution and $P_{1-\alpha/2}$ is the $100(1 - \alpha/2)\%$ percentile, then $[P_{\alpha/2}, P_{1-\alpha/2}]$ is a $100(1 - \alpha)\%$ credible interval, i.e.,

$$\text{Pr}[P_{\alpha/2} < \theta < P_{1-\alpha/2}] = 1 - \alpha \text{ (or with discrete probabilities } \geq 1 - \alpha).$$

22.3.2   General Decision Theory

More generally Bayesian methods are easily adapted to defining rules into an action space, listing various possible "actions" that could be done on the basis of the data. As above, one can define a loss function on the basis the action space and derive Bayes rules. While this formulation may be of use in general decision, its use in the analysis of carcinogenicity studies seems to be limited.

22.3.3   Bayes Factors versus Posterior Probabilities

A problem of great interest is the assessment of whether or not a certain statement about the parameters in a statistical model is supported by the data. Frequentists often cast such questions in the framework of hypothesis testing, i.e., as a question "is the specified parameter 0 (or some other specified value)?", and test the corresponding null hypothesis. The significance levels or "p-values" associated with testing these null hypotheses are used to assess the strength of evidence against the null hypothesis (i.e., small p-values imply rejection of the null hypothesis). Bayesians have several similar measures. One of the more popular measures is the "Bayes factor" of a hypothesis. Suppose we have distinct possible hypotheses numbering 1 to k, and denoted by H_k, with at least one H_k true, but when it applies, none of the other hypotheses are true. Writing Y for the observed data, and following Bayes rule, we can write $\Pr(Y|H_k)$ as the marginal likelihood of the data for the model H_k. It is obtained averaging over the parameters, η, left free in the hypothesis H_k:

$$\Pr(Y|H_k) = \int \Pr(Y|H_k,\eta)d\eta.$$

By Bayes rule, for hypotheses H_k, $k = 0, 1$,

$$\Pr(H_k|Y) = \frac{\Pr(Y|H_k)\Pr(H_k)}{\Pr(Y|H_0)\Pr(H_0) + \Pr(Y|H_1)\Pr(H_1)}.$$

So, that,

$$\frac{\Pr(H_1|Y)}{\Pr(H_0|Y)} = \frac{\Pr(Y|H_1)}{\Pr(Y|H_0)}\frac{\Pr(H_1)}{\Pr(H_0)}.$$

The term $\Pr(Y|H_1)/\Pr(Y|H_0)$ is the so-called Bayes factor of H_1 over H_0. It represents the amount the prior odds of H_1 over H_0 is moved by the observed data to the posterior odds H_1 over H_0 (or perhaps more explicitly the change in the prior odds for the model denoted by H_1 over the model denoted by H_0 to the corresponding posterior odds).

Pooling two of the original categories together, Kass and Raferty [12] cite Jeffrey's original scale for interpreting the Bayes factor:

Bayes Factor	Strength of Evidence in Favor of H_0 over H_1
1 to 3.2	"Not worth more than a bare mention"
3.2 to 10	Substantial
10 to 32	Strong
32 to 100	Very strong
>100	Decisive

Kass and Raftery further propose the following alternative guidelines for interpreting Bayes factors:

Bayes Factor	Strength of Evidence in Favor of H_0 over H_1
1 to 3	"Not worth more than a bare mention"
3 to 20	Positive
20 to 150	Strong
>150	Very strong

An alternative is to use posterior probabilities. For example, when one of a number of possible models or hypotheses is assumed to be true we can compute the posterior probability of the hypotheses as

$$\Pr(H_k|Y) = \frac{\Pr(Y|H_k)\Pr(H_k)}{\sum_i \Pr(Y|H_i)\Pr(H_i)}.$$

Then an appropriate decision would be to choose the model or hypothesis with the highest posterior probability.

For a likelihood $f(y|\theta)$ with parameters θ, the deviance is defined as

$$D(\theta) = -2\log\left(f(y|\theta)\right).$$

So, for example, the deviance for $y_i \sim \text{Binomial}(n_i, \theta_i)$, for $i = 1, \ldots, n$. is computed as $D(\theta) = -2\sum(y_i\log\theta_i + (n_i - y_i)\log(1 - \theta_i) + \log(n_i/y_i))$. The latter term is free of the parameters and often dropped. In frequentist analyses, the deviance is often used as a measure of fit, where models with smaller deviance have better fit.

Akaike [13] introduced the first of a number of so-called information measures of fit for various models. The Akaike information criterion (AIC) is defined as the AIC $= \max_\theta D(\theta) + 2k = -2\log\max_\theta f(y,\theta) + 2k$, where k is the number of parameters.

Note that most standard statistical distributions are so-called exponential distributions, i.e., they have a distribution that can be expressed as

$$f(y|\theta) = \exp\left(\theta^t T(y) - b(\theta)\right),$$

as θ ranges over the natural parameter space Θ, a subset of the r dimensional real numbers. Assuming that the sample is from an exponential family likelihood and that the parameter distribution can be modeled as a mixture with components defined on linear manifolds, Schwarz [14] used Baye's rule to determine that the most probable posterior model would asymptotically tend to satisfy a very similar criterion to the AIC. This often called the Bayesian information criterion (BIC) or the Schwarz information criterion (SIC). The $\mathrm{BIC}(\theta) = \max_\theta D(\theta) + k \log n = -2 \log \max_\theta f(y, \theta) + k \log n$, where k is the number of parameters and n is the sample size.

The AIC and the BIC depend upon a count of the number of parameters as penalty for complicated models. When lower-level parameters depend upon higher-level parameters as in random effects models or hierarchical models the exact count of these parameters is not necessarily clear. For example, consider the simplest possible hierarchical model. Suppose we have k samples with n_k observations per sample, with $y_{ij} \sim \mathrm{Normal}(\mu_i, \sigma^2)$, $i = 1, \ldots k, j = 1, \ldots, n_k$, with prior $\mu_i \sim \mathrm{Normal}$ (μ_0, τ^2), where σ^2, τ^2 are fixed. As $\tau^2 \to 0$, the actual number of μ_i parameters effectively goes to 1. As the τ^2 increases the effective number of parameters goes to k. So it seems to be sensible to consider the effective number of parameters as somewhere between those two bounds.

The deviance information criterion (DIC), introduced by Spiegelhalter et al. [15], is an information measure similar to the AIC and BIC, particularly oriented toward hierarchical models. The expected deviance $E_\theta(D(\theta))$ could be used as a measure of model fit, where increasing expected deviance implies increasingly worse fit. An estimate of the effective number of parameters of the model, or perhaps a better name, the "complexity" of the model, can be estimated as $p_D = E_\theta(D(\theta)) - D(E(\theta))$, where that latter term comes from inserting the posterior expectation of θ into the deviance. The larger is p_D, the easier it is for the model to fit the data. Then the DIC can be defined as $\mathrm{DIC} = p_D = D(E(\theta)) + 2p_D$.

An alternative way of viewing the DIC is, roughly, with $D(\theta)$ denoting the usual deviance, $\mathrm{DIC} \approx E(D(\theta)) + 1/2(\mathrm{Var}(D(\theta)))$. For good models we would want the deviance and the variance to be as small as possible. Thus, again, models with smaller DIC should be preferred to models with larger DIC. Models are penalized both by the value of $E_\theta(D(\theta))$, which favors a good fit, but also (in common with AIC and BIC) by an estimate of the number of parameters, p_D. Since $E_\theta(D(\theta))$ will decrease as the number of parameters in a model increases, the p_D term compensates for this effect by favoring models with a smaller number of parameters.

At least one advantage of the DIC over other information criteria for Bayesian model selection is that the DIC is easily calculated from the samples generated by a Markov chain Monte Carlo (MCMC) simulation. Both the AIC and BIC require calculating the likelihood at its maximum over θ, which is not readily available from the MCMC simulation. But to calculate the DIC, we compute $E_\theta(D(\theta))$ the average of $D(\theta)$ over the samples of θ, and $D(E(\theta))$ as the deviance evaluated at the average of the samples of θ. However, the DIC does depend upon the parameterization of the model, and can differ, apparently sometimes dramatically, for functionally equivalent models.

The DIC can be automatically computed for most statistical models analyzed using the WinBUGS program [16,17]. The other information criteria are provided by some standard software (e.g., several SAS procedures [18]).

22.4 Strengths and Weaknesses of the Bayesian Approach

Given a statistical model of a certain data generating process, indexed by some parameters, virtually all statistical analyses of the parameters will attempt to provide some sort of nominally optimal or at least adequate estimate of the parameters (i.e., estimation) or an assessment of the viability of certain hypotheses about the process (i.e., hypothesis testing). In almost all statistical analyses, the end user also wants a measure of the appropriateness of the estimate or assessment of the hypothesis.

There may be a number of reasons for choosing a Bayesian approach to the analysis of a statistical problem. One could argue that probability is a natural measure of ignorance about parameters in any model. That is, prior ignorance about a parameter is naturally expressed as a probability distribution on the parameter, namely the prior distribution. That measure of ignorance can be updated by the information in the statistical model via Bayes theorem, giving a distribution reflecting updated knowledge of the data conditional upon the observed data in the model. It would be possible to argue that this is a schematic of the traditional scientific process.

Several possible comparisons of frequentist and Bayesian methods follow:

1. Interpretation of estimates:

   For estimation using a frequentist analysis, this usually entails either a measure of the variance of the estimator or an interval estimator. Both the estimator and its variance estimate are derived from the theoretical distribution using the probability model. In the frequentist approach one then actually computes the values of the estimator and its variance by inserting the observed sample values. Once the sample is drawn and the values are actually entered into the estimator, it is no longer possible to make any probabilistic claim about the resulting estimate. All one can say is that the observed value is one of a number of values that may have occurred. For example, frequentist $100*(1 - \alpha)\%$ confidence intervals are defined so that if the model is true, and the exact process that generated the data is repeated, about $100*(1 - \alpha)\%$ of these intervals would contain the true parameter value. However, a given collection of observed data will define one specific confidence interval. What is the probability that this computed confidence interval contains the true parameter value? The parameter takes a fixed value. Once the data are given they are also fixed. So the computed interval is also fixed from the data. Thus the only reasonable answer to this question is either 1 or 0, depending upon whether or not the parameter is actually in the interval or not. One could argue that this denies the whole point of the exercise!

The corresponding Bayesian interval is a $100*(1 - \alpha)\%$ so-called credible interval. This is a subset of the parameter space on which the posterior probability, conditional on the observed data, that the parameter takes a value in the interval is $(1 - \alpha)$. Since this is a probability assessment, unlike the frequentist confidence interval, if the model, including the prior, is true, the probability that the parameter takes a value in the interval is $1 - \alpha$. It would seem that the Bayesian credible interval is thus a more interpretable interval estimate of the parameter than the similar confidence interval. In some circumstances the Bayesian credible interval and the usual confidence interval may coincide, but even in those circumstances, it would seem to be hard to argue that the Bayesian interval is not more interpretable. Similarly we can assess the posterior probability that an actual Bayesian estimate of the parameter is in any particular interval or satisfies any particular criteria. The best we can claim for a frequentist estimator is a description of its potential behavior prior to drawing the sample, not the probability that an actual estimate occurs in some interval or satisfies some criterion. Thus there seems to be a reasonable argument that when faced with actual data, the Bayesian procedures seem to be much more interpretable.

2. Concerns about the prior distribution:

The so-called posterior distribution of a parameter denoted θ has a density proportional to the product $f(y|\theta) \, \pi(\theta)$, the original likelihood times the prior. Thus, even if the likelihood is relatively large in some region, the prior can down weight the observed values in the likelihood so that the posterior probability that the parameter is in the region possibly implied by the data can be relatively small. This sensitivity to the prior is probably the most commonly raised objection to Bayesian techniques. However, this may be more of an argument for the careful choice of a prior than a reason to reject Bayesian methods. Much the same objection could be made about the likelihood. If it is chosen poorly, with relatively small weight near observed values, one will have poor estimators. The Bayesian approach forces one to separate the decision about an appropriate likelihood from the choice of an appropriate prior reflecting knowledge about the parameter, and possibly could even be interpreted as a point in its favor.

It would seem that in most problems one has some idea of the likely range of values of a parameter. For example, if θ is the proportion of animals with a certain tumor in a standard carcinogen study, the probability that θ is near 0 seems to be a lot higher than the probability that it is near 1. But if one wishes to ignore such knowledge one could place a uniform prior on θ. The problem is more apparent with nominally unbounded parameters, e.g., what is the chance of observing 10,000 papilloma on a typical Tg.AC mouse, or of observing a human whose height is greater than 10 m? One of the strengths of the Bayesian approach is that such insight is readily incorporated into the statistical model. Alternatively, if one does not want to use such prior knowledge, so-called noninformative or objective priors may be useful. Note however, in some sense, "noninformative" is a misnomer since all priors tell some story about the knowledge of the parameters.

3. Consistency with the likelihood principle:

In the introduction above, it was noted that the common p-value approach to hypothesis testing violates the likelihood principle. Similar results are often true in estimation. For example, unbiasedness is an often used criterion to limit the number of estimators in a frequentist analysis, i.e., for data with from a model with density $f(y|\theta)$ we determine an estimator $S(y)$, such that $E(S(y)|\theta) = \theta$. In frequentist analysis a minimum variance unbiased estimator is often considered appropriate. But the variance computation is based on the probability density, usually depending upon possible values that were not observed. Hence the use of unbiased estimators or similar procedures will usually violate the likelihood principle. As noted above, Bayesian procedures automatically satisfy the likelihood principle.

4. Existence of a prior, de Finetti's theorem:

As noted earlier, loosely, a sequence of random variables is said to be exchangeable if each subset has the same probability under permutation of the indices in the sequence. De Finetti's theorem states that a sequence is exchangeable if and only if there is a mixture distribution that functions as a prior distribution on the indexing parameter. This can be used to justify the existence of a prior distribution. Given that one accepts the existence of a prior distribution the Bayesian machinery is virtually automatic.

5. Coherence of estimators:

One way to define coherence is that if condition A is true, and condition A implies condition B, then the evidence for condition B is at least as strong as the evidence for condition A. In the somewhat twisted logic of frequentist hypothesis testing, one tests for rejection, with a smaller p-value providing stronger evidence that the so-called null hypothesis can be rejected. Schervish [19] provides example of when such frequentist p-values are not coherent. That is, he provides examples of when hypothesis A implies hypothesis B, so not-B implies not-A, but with the same data, the p-value for testing the hypothesis that not-A is false, i.e., A is true, is smaller (i.e., more significant) than the corresponding p-value for hypothesis not-B. That is, evidence for B is less strong than evidence for A. By comparison, posterior probabilities are inherently coherent. However, one might further note that Schervish [20] provides examples of Bayes factors that also display a lack of coherence.

6. Rational decision making and the complete class theorem:

As discussed in Bernardo and Smith ([6], pp. 16–45) certain axioms of rational decision making imply a Bayesian approach to making decisions. One can question the appropriateness of these axioms, but they at least seem reasonable. Further, the complete class theorem states that from a decision theoretic point of view Bayes rules almost surely minimize the risk of any procedure. However, it should be noted that this result only applies to a compact parameter space with convex loss. For standard parameters this implies the parameter space is bounded. In practice this is probably not a problem. However, convex loss implies that a discrepancy from the true parameter value a long way from the true value is worse than the same discrepancy close to the true value. For example, to be a further millimeter off when you estimate someone's height as 1000 m is worse than being a millimeter off when you estimate their height to be say 1.8 m. This would seem to be a very debatable condition for a loss function. It would seem to be more appropriate to say that when the discrepancy is very large a little more discrepancy would hardly matter. Thus a more reasonable loss function would seem to be locally convex, but concave for large discrepancies. There does not seem to be a corresponding theorem such a more appealing loss function.

7. Large sample asymptotics:

In parametric problems Bayesian methods generally satisfy large sample optimality conditions, e.g., "best asymptotic normality." Of course other non-Bayesian procedures also generally satisfy such conditions, for example, maximum likelihood estimators (MLEs). However, while they are asymptotically optimal, Bayesian procedures are usually exact. That is, given the likelihood and the prior the Bayesian procedures result in exact specification of estimators and statistics. They do not depend upon asymptotics in increasing sample size. Unlike Bayesian techniques, many frequentist procedures, e.g., MLEs, depend upon asymptotics in increasing sample size for justification, so that one has to assume the sample is sufficiently large for the asymptotics to apply.

8. Stopping rules:

Since most carcinogenicity studies are designed with fixed sample sizes, concerns about when to stop collecting data can be ignored. But for other studies it may be worth noting that from a purely Bayesian point of view, as long as the data-generating process can be assumed to remain the same, data collection can stop at any time. In general, frequentist statistics would have to adjust for the stopping rule, but unless the stopping rule changes the likelihood in some way, Bayesian methods could ignore it.

9. Computational convenience:

While arguably intellectually quite compelling, Bayesian methods are not generally easier to apply than frequentist methods. Many frequentist analyses involve maximizing some function while Bayesian techniques generally require integration of functions over probability densities. Typically, the former is a much easier problem than the latter. Prior to the development of MCMC techniques, many of these integrations were highly difficult or virtually impossible. Even with modern MCMC techniques, computation of these integrals can be challenging, and may require special programming in a language like C or FORTRAN. For many problems, however, general purpose programs like WinBUGS or its derivatives seem to be adequate.

22.5   Methods of Analysis

22.5.1   Statistical Analysis of Mortality Data

One important aspect of the analysis of tumor data is the assessment of animal mortality. Frequentist analysis often starts with nonparametric assessments as say in

Kaplan–Meier and Nelson–Aalen estimates of survival, with logrank or Wilcoxon or other tests of differences in the survival curves. Considering that a Bayesian analysis requires prior probability distributions on all parameters it may appear that a Bayesian nonparametric analysis is an oxymoron. The general Bayesian approach to nonparametric problems usually involves a prior distribution on the space of probability measures, and is mathematically beyond the scope of this chapter. See Chapter 3 of Ibrahim et al. [21] for an initial review of this methodology, or for a more general introduction Schervish [22]. There are a number of related papers in the literature (e.g., [23,24], etc.)

However, some models can be fit using standard Bayesian software like WinBUGS. A general approach to right censored data can be summarized as follows:

Let $S(t)$ be the survival function, i.e., with T the random variable denoting survival time, it is the probability of survival past time t, to the event labeled "failure,"

$$S(t) = \Pr(T > t).$$

Write $f(t)$ as the density of T. So $f(t) = (d/dt)(1 - S(t))$. The so-called instantaneous hazard function is $h(t) = f(t)/S(t)$ and represents the rate of failure at time t given survival to time t. The so-called cumulative hazard is computed as

$$H(t_i) = \int_0^{t_i} h(u)du.$$

So $f(t) = h(t) S(t)$. Also $\log(S(t)) = -H(t)$, so $S(t) = e^{-H(t)}$. Then $f(t) = h(t)e^{-H(t)}$.

Cox (see [21]) proposed a simple model to adjust the hazard for covariates, denoted x. Namely, this is to define the specific hazard for an animal as $h(t)\exp(x_i'\varphi)$, $h(t)$ is the baseline hazard holding all covariates at 0. These are called proportional hazards models because of the effect on the hazards, or more generally semiparametric models.

The standard Cox regression form of the proportional hazards model for survival specifies the hazard function:

$$h(t|x) = h_0(t) \exp(x'\beta).$$

For obvious reasons this is often called a proportional hazards model (i.e., proportional across levels of $x'\beta$). It is one of a general class of so-called semiparametric models, since in the frequentist framework no particular restriction is placed on $h_0(t)$, but the exponential term is parameterized. However note that the baseline hazard is partially confounded with the specification of treatment effects (i.e., a multiplicative constant can be moved to either the baseline hazard or the term with covariates). So if there are m different covariate parameters, there are only $m-1$ degrees of freedom for assessing the effects among these covariates. This is not a Bayesian point, but is inherent in the parameterization.

Frequentist analysis of this model uses asymptotics to analyze the linear predictor, ignoring the baseline hazard $h_0(t)$. A Bayesian analysis requires priors on all parameters, including the baseline hazard. Perhaps the simplest Bayesian model would postulate a within interval constant baseline hazard. That is, suppose the time axis can be partitioned as $(a_1 = 0, a_2], (a_2, a_3], \ldots, (a_T, a_{T+1}]$. Assume a constant baseline hazard λ_j for observations in $(a_j, a_{j+1}]$. Thus one needs to specify an appropriate prior for the baseline hazard. Usually one parameterizes this so that the baseline hazard is essentially the hazard of the control group.

Suppose one specifies a model for the event defined as a failure. This could be natural death or perhaps death caused by certain tumor, particularly a rapidly fatal tumor. Other events could cause the animal to drop out of the risk set for the event, in which case it is considered as censored. If the censoring mechanism is stochastically independent of the event mechanism it can be ignored in the likelihood computations.

Suppose we want to compare survival in k different treatment groups. Using so-called dummy coding, we can define, for each treatment group k,

$$\delta_k = \begin{cases} 1 & \text{for the } i\text{th treatment group} \\ 0 & \text{otherwise.} \end{cases}$$

Then at least three possibly relevant models for treatment effect could be defined as follows:

1. Parameterization of a different effect for each treatment with vehicle (with k treatments, not counting vehicle control),

$$x_i'\beta = \beta_0 + \beta_1\delta_1 + \beta_2\delta_2 + \cdots + \beta_k\delta_k.$$

2. Parameterization of a linear effect of measured dose over the k treatment groups with vehicle,

$$x_i'\beta = \beta_0 + \beta_1 \text{ dose (or log dose for a linear effect).}$$

3. Parameterization of no differences in survival across treatment groups with vehicle,

$$x_i'\beta = \beta_0.$$

For each of these models $\exp(\beta_0)$ is confounded with the baseline hazard $h_0(t)$ and is not estimated. In model (1), with this coding, the effect of the difference between treatment group i and the control group is assessed by the β_k.

Let $t_i = $ time to event or censoring and it is in the interval $(a_{j-1}, a_j]$. So the integrated cumulative baseline hazard can be written as

$$H_0(t_i) = e^{x'\beta} \int_0^{t_i} h_0(u)du = e^{x'\beta}\left\{ \sum_{k=1}^{j-1} \lambda_k(a_k - a_{k-1}) + \lambda_j(t_i - a_{j-1}) \right\},$$

with hazard $h_0(t_i) = e^{x'\beta}\lambda_j$.

Then the likelihood for subject i can be written as

$$L_i(\lambda,\beta) \propto \begin{cases} e^{-H_0(t_i)} & \text{if } i\text{th subject is censored at time } t_i, \\ \lambda_j e^{x'\beta} e^{-H_0(t_i)} & \text{if } i\text{th subject fails at time } t_i. \end{cases}$$

Because this looks like a sample of exponential interarrival times it is not surprising that the simple event/no event distributions to seem to correspond to Poisson random variables.

For subject i censored or failed at time t_j, let γ_{ik}

$$= \begin{cases} \lambda_k(a_k - a_{k-1}) & \text{for } t_j > a_k, \\ \lambda_j(t_j - a_{j-1}) & \text{for } a_{j-1} < t_j < a_j, \\ 0 & \text{otherwise.} \end{cases}$$

Then $S(t) = e^{-H(t)} = \prod_{k=1}^{T} \exp(-e^{x'\beta}\gamma_{ik})$. Note that for intervals above a_j, $-e^{x'\beta}\lambda_{ik} = 0$, so $\exp(-e^{x'\beta}\lambda_{ik}) = 1$ and does not contribute to the product. Further, with respect to the model parameters, $(t_j - a_{j-1})$ is constant, and hence can be incorporated in the likelihood for subjects who fail by multiplying λ_j by this difference. Thus, for subject i, the likelihood can also be written as:

$$L_i(\lambda,\beta) \propto \begin{cases} \displaystyle\prod_{k=1}^{T} \exp(-e^{x'\beta}\gamma_{ik}) & \text{if } i\text{th subject is censored at time } t_i, \\ \displaystyle\gamma_{ij}e^{x'\beta}\prod_{k=1}^{T} \exp(-e^{x'\beta}\gamma_{ik}) & \text{if } i\text{th subject fails at time } t_i. \end{cases}$$

Note this corresponds to the likelihood of T-independent Poisson random variables with mean $e^{x'\beta}\lambda_{ik}$ where all responses are zero except at time j with the occurrence of a failure event in the jth interval $(a_{j-1}, a_j]$. This is only a computational convenience but allows estimation of the appropriate parameters using a standard program like WinBUGS (WinBUGS programs for these analyses are included in Appendix). A gamma prior on the λ_j is mathematically convenient (although see Gelman [25]).

The analysis of a large number of other useful survival models from Bayesian point of view, including parametric models like the Weibull, log-normal, or gamma models, as well as other semiparametric models are clearly presented in Ibrahim et al. [21].

Example 1

The following example is meant to illustrate a standard Bayesian approach to assessing these issues. The drug was administered to mice for a period of 2 years. Animals were randomized by weight to five treatment groups of 60 animals per gender, including two nominally identical vehicle controls, and three treatment groups with nominal dose levels at 3, 10, and 30 mg/kg/day, respectively. Unless there are problems in the conduct of the study, any observed differences between the two control groups should be due solely to randomization. So for all actual analysis

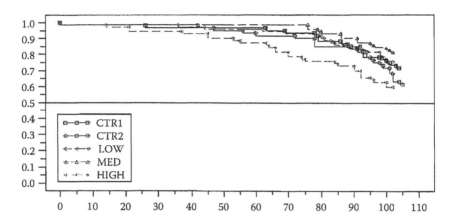

FIGURE 22.1:   Kaplan–Meier estimated survival distributions for Example 1.

the two control groups were pooled. The remaining treatment groups were labeled as low, medium, and high, respectively. Animals were housed individually, with water available on demand. Kaplan–Meier plots of the survival time are displayed in Figure 22.1:

As noted above, at least three possible models are suggested:

1. Parameterization of no differences in survival across treatment groups with vehicle, i.e., constant dose effect) $x_i'\beta = \beta_0$

2. Parameterization of a differential effect over the controls, over the treatment groups, i.e., $x_i'\beta = \beta_0 + \beta_1 * \delta_1 + \beta_2 * \delta_2 + \beta_3 * \delta_3$

3. Parameterization of a linear effect of dose, $x_i'\beta = \beta_0 + \beta_1 *$ dose

This analysis assumes a within interval constant baseline hazard, in days (0, 175], (175, 350], (350, 480], (480, 525], (525, terminal]. Note that for computational reasons it is strongly recommended that intervals be defined so that they each contain events.

These models were analyzed using WinBUGS 1.4.3, and had DICs of 7.065, 10.069, and 8.061, suggesting the model with no differences across treatment groups is the best model i.e., model (1) above seems to be the most appropriate. After 25,000 iterations, with an additional initial 5000 iteration "burn-in," fitting the last two models resulted in the following covariate parameter estimates. Note that model (1) only fits the baseline hazard, and does not involve treatment parameters. Models (2) and (3) resulted in the following parameter estimates (Table 22.1):

When 0 is in the credible interval associated with a parameter, it can be interpreted as suggesting we cannot conclude that the parameter is not 0. That is, the parameter could be 0. For the models above the credible interval for the trend parameter as well

TABLE 22.1: Parameter summaries for Example 1.

	Estimate	95% Credible Interval
Dose groups differ (Model 2)		
Controls vs. high	0.5077	0.7491, 0.924
Controls vs. medium	0.1212	−0.3153, 0.5444
Controls vs. low	−0.0815	−0.5369, 0.3577
Trend (Model 3)		
Slope	0.1779	0.0377, 0.31

as the difference between pooled controls and the maximum dose group excludes zero, while the credible intervals for the difference between the medium dose and the low dose with the pooled controls both contain zero. This suggests that the two former parameters are not zero, while there is no strong evidence that the latter two parameters are not zero. These results differ from the conclusions one would reach with the DIC, since there is evidence of increasing trend in mortality, and a clear difference between the high-dose group and the pooled controls. The inconsistency with the conclusions drawn from the DIC may suggest that the evidence of a trend is not overly strong, while the effects of the differences from controls in the low-dose and medium-dose groups dilutes the measure of overall difference from the pooled controls.

A WinBUGS program for the analysis of heterogeneity in treatment is included in Appendix.

22.5.2 Models for Tumorigenicity

As discussed in Chapter 21, the Bernoulli and binomial probability models are very useful models to represent the presence or absence of a tumor in a fixed size treatment group. To model the occurrence of say y_i tumors out of n_i animals, a binomial distribution is a useful model for tumor counts:

$$f(y_i|\theta, n_i) = \binom{n_i}{y_i} \theta_i^{y_i}(1 - \theta_i)^{1-y_i}$$

for $n_i = 1$, i.e., modeling the outcome of each animal separately, this is just the Bernoulli distribution noted above.

We are interested in the effect of covariates on the θ, for animal carcinogenicity studies, the covariate of primary interest is usually the dose. For such models a transformation of an expression in terms of the covariates into the θ is often used as a means to incorporate the effect of the covariates. Any increasing function, F, of the parameters with a range in 0 to 1, is a potentially useful transform. Note this includes any cumulative distribution function. So if F is any cumulative probability distribution (c.d.f.) function, $F^{-1}(\theta)$ will map the θ into the expression in the covariates. With a linear term $x'\beta$ as the usual expression in the covariates, and with $\Phi(.)$

denoting a standard normal cumulative distribution, the three most popular trans-
forms seem to be

$$\text{The logit transform: } \text{logit}(\theta) = \log[\theta/(1 - \theta)] = x'\beta,$$

$$\text{The probit transform: } \text{probit}(\theta) = \Phi^{-1}(\theta) = x'\beta,$$

$$\text{The complementary log–log transform: } \log[-\log(1 - \theta)] = x'\beta.$$

For most values of θ the logit and the probit provide quite proportionate values, but
the logit transform is computationally somewhat easier to deal with. Both are also
symmetric about 0.5. However the complementary log–log transform is not symmetric about any value (the corresponding c.d.f. is $1 - \exp[-\exp(.)]$).

The primary model for dealing with simple presence or absence of a tumor is the
logit-transformed θ with a Bernoulli or binomial distribution on tumor counts. Note
that for simple success–fail dichotomies, the logit of θ is the log odds of success
versus failure (i.e., not success). So the effect of a parameter can be interpreted as a
measure of relative improvement. However, other so-called link functions of θ are
feasible, and require only a slight modification of the methods summarized below.

22.5.3   Logistic Regression

As discussed in Chapter 21, in many circumstances it is important that time to
death or censoring be included in any tumorigenicity model. This can be modeled
as a function of time of death as say $g(t_i)$ as a function of time for subject i, e.g., a
polynomial expression in time would be $g(\gamma, t_i) = \gamma_1 t_i + \cdots + \gamma_k t_i^k$. With the
dummy effect coding for dose this would lead to a model:

$$\text{logit}(\theta_i) = x_i'\beta + g(\gamma, t_i) = \beta_0 + \beta_1\delta_1 + \beta_2\delta_2 + \cdots + \beta_k\delta_k + \gamma_1 t_i + \cdots + \gamma_k t_i^k.$$

Because of identification problems with such a large number of parameters this is
almost always modeled as linear in time, i.e., $g(\gamma, t_i) = \gamma_1 t_i$. Note this model
assumes that tumor incidence depends upon time in study and treatment group. If
these interact, so there is marked differential mortality across treatment groups this
simple model may no longer apply. In some cases, interaction terms may be
incorporated into the model to adjust for the differential mortality, giving a
model like:

$$\text{logit}(\theta_i) = \beta_0 + \beta_1\delta_1 + \cdots + \beta_k\delta_k + \gamma_1 t_i + \eta_1\delta_1 t_i + \cdots + \eta_k\delta_k t_i,$$

where the $\delta_j t_i$ represents product of the indicator of the jth treatment group with the t_i
time-to-event. However, this model incorporates a number of parameters, and is
often not well identified.

Appropriate default priors for regression parameters might be univariate normal
β_j, γ_1, and $\eta_k \sim N(0, v_k)$ for some appropriate variances $v_\beta, v_\gamma, v_\eta$. To allow for

correlation in the prior distributions one could specify all or some of these to be multivariate normal, with a vector mean 0 and some positive definite matrix Σ as the variance matrix.

One typical application would be a model for the presence or absence of a certain type of tumor. Define a simple logit model for tests of trend and pairwise comparisons. Define θ_{ijk} as the probability of tumor j in animal i in treatment group k. That is, with $j = 1$ to n_t tumors and $i = 1$ to n_s animals, and dose d_k, $j = 1$ to n_d, leaving the experiment at time t_i and subject effect δ_i:

$$\text{logit}(\theta_{ijk}) = \alpha_j + \beta_j d_k + \gamma_j t_i + \delta_i, \quad k = 1, \ldots, n_d, \quad j = 1, \ldots, n_t, \quad i = 1, \ldots, n_s,$$

with random subject effect $\delta_i \sim N(\mu_\delta, \sigma_\delta^2)$. Where $I_{[0]}$ is the point mass distribution at 0, assign model priors:

$$\alpha_j \sim N(\mu_\alpha, \sigma_\alpha^2)$$

$$\beta_j \sim \pi_j I_{[0]} + (1 - \pi_j)N(\mu_\beta, \sigma_\beta^2) \quad \text{for } j = 1, \ldots, n_t.$$

and

$$\pi_j \sim \text{Beta}(a, b),$$

$$\gamma_j \sim N(\mu_g, \sigma_g^2) \quad \text{for } j = 1, \ldots, n_s,$$

σ_α^2, σ_β^2, $\sigma_g^2 \sim$ inverse gamma(c, d), possibly with different c's and d's for each variance.

For tumor j, the posterior distribution of π_j can be interpreted as the probability that the slope for the ith tumor, β_j, is zero.

The model for pairwise comparisons is similar:

$$\text{logit}(\theta_{ijk}) = \alpha_j + \beta_{jk} + \gamma_j t_i + \delta_i, \quad k = 2, \ldots, n_d, \quad j = 1, \ldots, n_t,$$
$$i = 1, \ldots, n_s, \quad \text{with } \beta_{j0} = 0,$$

$$\pi_{jk} \sim \text{Beta}(a, b) \quad \text{for } k = 2, \ldots, n_d,$$

$$\beta_{jk} \sim \pi_{jk} I_{[0]} + (1 - \pi_{jk})N(\mu_{\beta k}, \sigma_{\beta k}^2) \quad \text{for } j = 1, \ldots, n_t, \quad k = 2, \ldots, n_d.$$

Note that with this parameterization, the β_{jk} represent the deviation of treatment effect from the first group, usually controls. Now, for tumor i, the posterior distribution of π_{jk} is the probability that the differential effect of the kth treatment group over the controls is 0, and corresponds to a frequentist test of the hypothesis that the parameter is 0.

Choosing the right a's and b's for the Beta priors and the c's and d's for the inverse gamma prior should lead to reasonably noninformative priors on π and variance parameters. WinBUGS programs implementing these programs are included in the Appendix. As noted previously, Gelman [25] points out that the inverse gamma prior for variances can be very informative, and suggests that the uniform is much better. However, for the cases the authors have attempted, use of the uniform prior on the inverse of variances seems to be fatal for the WinBUGS programs used in the analyses above.

Note the strengths and weaknesses of these simple models, for example, the adjustment for early mortality is linear, where as it seems more appropriate to model the increasing probability in tumors as an exponential process. Still the linear term may be adequate and is used in some frequentist analyses.

Example 2

Again, the frequentist approach to testing the significance of carcinogenicity in the presence of multiplicities is to adjust the type I error rate (i.e., the probability of rejecting a true hypothesis of no differences). The Bayesian approach is less tied to type I error, and assesses the probability of each of the multiple events on the basis of all information in the trial, including other events. The fact that these are conditional on observed data allows one to specify analyses conditional on data based criteria. The criterion used here was that there should be at least one tumor in the high-dose group and one or more tumor in the remaining dose groups. These criteria were selected prior to data inspection.

In this study the drug was administered with the diet. Animals were initially housed together in groups of five. The effect of this housing was analyzed separately, and, at least overall, for female animals, seemed to be negligible, but the method of dose administration and housing may be interpreted as suggesting that effects should be analyzed with explicit subject effects. For the analysis the mixed two-stage/three-stage hierarchical models for tests of trend and pairwise comparisons defined above were used. For testing trend, we use the following priors:

$$\pi_j \sim \text{Beta}(1, 3),$$

$$\gamma_j \sim N(\mu_g, \sigma_g^2) \quad \text{for } j = 1, \ldots, n_t.$$

with $\mu_\delta = \mu_\alpha = \mu_\beta = \mu_g = \mu_s = 0$ and $\sigma_\delta^2 = 100$,

$$\sigma_\alpha^2, \sigma_\beta^2, \sigma_g^2 \sim \text{Inverse gamma } (1,3).$$

For pairwise comparisons of the control to the remaining dose groups we use postulate the prior:

$$\pi_{jk} \sim \text{Beta}(1, 3) \quad \text{for } k = 3, 4.$$

These models were implemented in WinBUGS 1.4.3. Table 22.2 indicates the observed frequency of selected tumors and the estimated probability that the linear dose effect (i.e., slope) is zero, followed by the probability that the differential effect of the high dose over the control effect is zero. The rightmost column is the estimated probability that the differential effect of the medium dose over the control effect is zero.

TABLE 22.2: Selected tumor incidence and Bayesian probabilities that parameter is 0.

Organ	Tumor	cntrl	low	med	high	trend = 0	High vs. Cntrl	Med vs. Cntrl
Adrenal	Phaeochromocytoma	7	1	11	16	0.0000	0.0000	0.0572
	Cortical adenoma	9	0	0	1	0.7769	0.7513	0.6824
Pancreas	Islet cell adenoma	3	0	0	1	0.9681	0.8272	0.8248
Parathyroid	Adenoma	3	2	0	1	0.9786	0.8436	0.8439
Thyroid	C-cell adenoma	12	4	4	5	0.9786	0.8919	0.9045
	C-cell carcinoma	2	1	1	1	0.9552	0.8407	0.8429
Uterus	Adenocarcinoma	3	0	3	11	0.0019	0.00810	0.7644
	Stromal polyp	6	5	5	5	0.9603	0.8023	0.8224
	Leiomyoma	0	0	1	1	0.8876	0.7508	0.7587
	Adenoma	1	0	1	1	0.9406	0.7985	0.8073
Vagina	Benign granular cell	1	1	1	1	0.9501	0.81340	0.8167

Thus, in this particular experiment, there is strong evidence of a trend over dose in phaechromocytoma in the adrenals (probability of 0 difference is less than 0.00005, so probability of a trend is at least 0.99995). Similarly, there is strong evidence that tumor incidence is much higher in the high-dose group than in the pooled controls (probability less than 0.00005). The evidence of a difference in phaechromocytoma between the medium-dose groups and controls is only slightly more debatable (probability of no difference is 0.0572). There is strong evidence of a trend in adenocarcinoma of the uterus (probability of 0 is 0.0019, so the probability of a trend is 0.9981), as well as evidence of a difference between the high-dose group than and controls (probability of 0 is 0.0081).

An example program is included in Appendix.

22.5.4   Incorporating Prior Information

As noted above, in a likelihood based analysis of tumorigenicity, a Bernoulli or binomial likelihood seems to a natural choice. That is, for $Y = y$ occurrences out of n possible tries or animals,

$$f(y|\theta) \text{ proportional to } \theta^y (1 - \theta)^{n-y} \quad \text{for } 0 < \theta < 1,$$

where $y = 0$ or 1, with $n = 1$ for a Bernoulli trial. Bernoulli trials are useful to represent the presence or absence of a tumor within an individual animal. Priors such that the posterior distribution can be interpreted as being in the same family as the original distribution are said to be conjugate. Such priors tend to result in distributions with good numerical properties. For the Bernoulli or binomial models above, if we specify a Beta prior density Beta(a, b), i.e., $\pi(\theta)$ is proportional to $\theta^{a-1}(1 - \theta)^{b-1}$, the posterior density is proportional to $\theta^{y+a-1}(1 - \theta)^{n-y+b-1}$, i.e., another Beta density. This corresponds to the Beta-binomial model discussed in Chapter 21. Figure 21.2 displays a range of these useful prior distributions.

A noninformative prior is supposed to provide no particular restriction on the parameter. The label "noninformative" is actually a misnomer, since any prior does have some effect on the estimation, so that truly noninformative priors do not exist. A better label would be "not very informative," but that does not seem to be commonly used. Other labels are "objective" or "reference" priors. For a Bernoulli or binomial one possible noninformative prior would be a uniform distribution, i.e., a Beta(1, 1) prior. It weights all values of θ between 0 and 1 equally. The problem with this prior is that it is not invariant across transformations of θ. If we want a prior to be noninformative for θ, it would seem to be reasonable that it should be noninformative for a transformed θ. For example if a prior $\pi(\theta) = 1$ over $0 < \theta < 1$, the distribution of say θ^2 would be skewed, and hence informative. Jeffreys proposed a parameterization of the prior that is invariant to transformation, namely suppose we could parameterize with either θ or η, where $\eta = g(\theta)$ for some 1-1 smooth function $g(.)$. Then with $\pi(.)$ denoting the prior in each case, we have $\pi(\eta) = \pi(\theta)|d\theta/d\eta|$. Jeffry's proposed priors are meant to provide the same model distribution for each parameterization. This implies that $\pi(\theta) = (I(\theta))^{1/2}$, where $I(\theta)$ is the Fisher information for θ:

$$I(\theta) = -E\left(\frac{d^2\log f(y|\theta)}{d\theta^2} \middle| \theta\right).$$

For example, for a Binomial random variable distributed as $B(n, \theta)$, the Jeffrey's prior is proportional to $\theta^{-1/2}(1 - \theta)^{-1/2}$ which corresponds to a Beta(0.5, 0.5) distribution. While Jeffrey's priors seem to be adequate to represent noninformative priors in most carcinogenicity studies, they do not always result in proper densities and do not generalize well to multivariate problems. This led Bernardo to propose so-called reference priors. Bernardo's insight (Bernardo and Smith [6]) was to cast the choice of a prior as a density that minimizes the information in a sample. Often no such minimum exits, in which case one uses asymptotic results to define the prior. For simple Bernoulli or binomial models this turns out to coincide with Jeffrey's prior. However, they often will differ (e.g., for negative binomial models).

An early Bayesian approach incorporating the use of historical control groups, as well as an adjustment for multiplicity based on exchangeability, is the model for pairwise comparisons proposed by Meng and Dempster [26], similar to that proposed by Dempster et al. [27]. They consider a situation where the current study has two treatments, a control group and a treatment group. In addition, suppose there are $T - 1$ historical control groups. Following their notation, let θ_{ij} denote the probability of tumor j, $j = 1$ to k, in group i, where $i = 0$ denotes the current study, and $i = 1, \ldots,$ $T - 1$ for M control groups. Starting with the logit transform noted above:

$$\text{logit}(\theta) = \log[\theta/(1 - \theta)] \quad \text{for } 0 < \theta < 1.$$

The response measures are Y_{ij}, namely the number of animals with the jth tumor in the ith dose group out of n_{ij} animals in the dose group. These are modeled as binomial random variables with distribution $B(n_{ij}, \theta_{ij})$, for the $i = 0$ to $T - 1$ control groups as follows:

$$\text{logit}(\theta_{ij}) = b_i + u_j + d_{ij} \quad \text{for } i = 0 \text{ to } T - 1 \text{ control groups},$$

and, for the current treatment group, with $i = T$, as

$$\text{logit}(\theta_{Tj}) = \eta + b_0 + u_j + d_{0j} + t_j \quad \text{for the current treatment group}.$$

Here u_j denotes the mean background rate for tumor j over many experiments, both in the past and in the future, and b_i, for $i = 0$ to $T - 1$ study groups, represents the within study effect common to all tumors, so the $b_i + u_j$ represents the background rate (in controls) and is exchangeable across controls. The exchangeability assumption implies that in terms of knowledge differences in lethality are random. Suppose η is the average treatment effect, d_{ij} denote the deviation from the background rate $b_i + u_j$, and t_j denotes the treatment effect on the jth tumor. Note that this model does not adjust for differences in mortality across treatment groups and essentially assumes equal lethality of tumors.

As is common with these logit models, Meng and Dempster model the b_i, u_j, d_{ij} parameters as normal random variables with mean 0 and variances σ_b^2, σ_u^2, and σ_d^2

$$b_i \sim N(0.0, \sigma_b^2), \quad u_j \sim N(0.0, \sigma_u^2), \quad d_{ij} \sim N(0.0, \sigma_d^2).$$

They propose estimating variance parameters by maximum likelihood or assuming they are a priori fixed, and then approximating the likelihood with a multivariate normal density. They then propose basically a maximum likelihood estimation of the remaining parameters, with Wald statistics to provide estimated credible intervals. However, such models are easily handled using MCMC techniques available in programs like WinBUGS.

Westfall and Soper [28] and Ibrahim et al. [29] provided methods for incorporating historical prior information into time-adjusted dose effects in carcinogenicity studies. Their approach is basically a frequentist survival analysis, but is easily adapted to a fully Bayesian approach. Please see the preceding Chapter 21 [2] for a discussion of these and other techniques.

With normal data the estimated variances have chi-square distributions, which are generalizations of gamma distributions. Conjugate priors are generally numerically attractive, so that if they are sensible, are often used. Since the variance parameter appears in the denominator it is traditional to use inverse gamma priors on the parameters. Gelman [25] notes that these are often quite informative priors and recommends others, including uniform priors. However, this reviewer has had difficulty applying these priors in WinBUGS programs, and they may require special programming in lower-level language like C or FORTRAN.

22.5.5   Multiplicity

In a Bayesian context, one typically analyzes the marginal distribution of parameters. There are several Bayesian approaches to multiple comparisons, beginning with a possible argument that they may not be needed (since conditioning on data, not parameters).

Except for papilloma counts in Tg.AC mice, the usual response measures in these rodent carcinogenicity studies typically involve analysis of a number of different tumors, i.e., multiple endpoints. The actual response variables are usually the presence or absence of the different tumors in certain specified organs or systemically in animals within dose groups. It is possible that future analyses may involve the actual number of detected tumor sites with the organ, but that does not seem to be typical of current carcinogenicity studies, and may require more care in assessing neoplasms than a simple decision about presence or absence.

Most rodent carcinogencity studies involve the observation of a number of different neoplasms by organ combinations. Different toxicologists may identify certain neoplasms differently. Further, they may prefer to combine the neoplasms within some organs and some neoplasms across some organs, with the possibility of different combinations by different toxicologists. Many of them follow some of the recommendations for combinations in McConnell et al. [30]. Even after combining neoplasms and organs there are usually a number of cancers on which treatment effect is to be assessed. This is somewhat different from a standard multiple comparison problem in that the number of comparisons to be done is dependent upon the tumors observed, and to some extent on the toxicologist, and thus the number of comparisons may to some extent be considered as random. There have been a number of approaches recommended for these analyses. Some authors condition on the number of tumors organ combinations observed and treat this as a standard multiple comparison problem. Primarily based on his experience, Haseman [31] proposed rules for judging actual statistical significance based the observed *p*-value for pairwise tests between the high dose treatment group and controls, with different rules for whether or not the tumor is classified as rare or common. Lin and Rahman [32] proposed similar rules for tests of trend in tumorigenicity across treatment doses. Currently Center for Drug Evaluation and Research (CDER) at the FDA tends to follow these Haseman–Lin–Rahman rules to judge statistical significance of tests on tumors. These rules are also described in detail in Chapter 21.

Bayesian approaches to the analysis of parameters typically analyze the marginal distribution of each parameter, integrating out the other parameters. If the tumor organ combinations can be considered to be unrelated, i.e., the presence of one has no effect on the other, it makes sense to analyze the results independently. If the tumor organ combinations are related with clear causal relations, i.e., the presence of one particular tumor is associated with the presence of another, one may model the actual causal relation. Alternatively suppose that it is felt that the probability of one type of tumor is roughly similar to a number of others, although they may be associated in some way. That is, suppose that we want to model a situation where some block of tumors have probabilities that behave roughly similarly, i.e., some are "large," some are "small," but it is not really clear which tumors will have relatively large probabilities and which will have small probabilities. This is just a statement that the tumor incidences within the block of tumors are basically exchangeable, and thus it makes sense to model tumor incidences within the block as exchangeable random variables, and hence the probabilities associated with tumors incidence in this block are naturally represented as having some prior distribution. Presumably knowledge about the tumor will allow one to specify a family of prior distributions.

Depending on the pathologist identifying the neoplasms there are often many tumors with very low incidence. For those neoplasms with only one case, or two or three cases with each case in different treatment groups, or some other small number of cases, testing differences may be pointless, with no test having a chance of being statistically significant. Again a frequentist analysis assesses the sample distribution based on the parameters, so that if one rigidly follows the frequentist paradigm one should adjust the multiple comparisons for such low incidence cases. From a Bayesian point of view this may not be necessary. For example, in the frequentist paradigm parameters are fixed but unknown quantities. To be specific, suppose one has five nominal treatment groups including controls, but after setting up the statistical analysis it is noted that two of these groups are identical controls (this design is not uncommon). Unless there are other trends in the data, any treatment differences between the controls should be due solely to randomization. Thus in the frequentist analysis it would seem to be more appropriate to combine these control groups and thus reduce the number of groups to be compared to four. Again, this seems reasonable because parameters are fixed. Or in another circumstance perhaps all the animals in one dose group die very early. Again, in the frequentist paradigm, it would seem to be reasonable to change the hypotheses being tested, so that for tumorigenicity analyses this treatment group may be ignored.

In the Bayesian paradigm the analysis is based on the distribution of the parameters conditioned on the fixed, observed data. The manner in which we adjust for results has some flexibility. Unlike in the frequentist analysis, deleting the low incidence comparisons, which have insufficient information on which to draw conclusions, would seem to be a defensible approach, quite analogous to the adjustments in testing noted above in the frequentist paradigm. Of course, deleting incident comparisons because they have discouraging results would not be appropriate!

22.5.6   Hierarchical Models

The posterior of a Bayesian model is $f(y|\theta)\,\pi(\theta)$. A hierarchical model is a model where the prior density $\pi(\theta)$ is decomposed into further conditional or prior densities: $\pi(\theta|\theta_2)\,\pi(\theta_2|\theta_3)\ldots\pi(\theta_{n-1}|\theta_n)$, where the parameter θ_i is parameterized by θ_{i+1}. The parameters θ_i are often called something like stage i or level i hyperparameters. Most problems in Bayesian analysis can be cast as hierarchical models. Note that the simple logit model as discussed in Section 22.5.3 is essentially a two-stage hierarchical model.

Since these animals are so highly inbred, with some forms of treatment administration one might expect subject effects to be basically ignorable. Even with subject effects, provided there are sufficient tumors within each organ for identification of parameters it may make sense to analyze tumors nested within organ. For pairwise comparisons, a hierarchical three-stage model for comparisons of a treatment group to control, similar to that proposed in Berry and Berry [33] can be used. The model they propose for the pairwise comparison is basically a logit model with an effect for organ b and tumor j and assumes animals are complete replicates. Instead of parameterizing the coefficients, they parameterize the log odds, i.e., for θ_{bjk} organ b, tumor j, and $k=0$ for control and $k=1$ for treatment they define the logit of a θ_{i0j},

$$\text{logit}(\theta_{bj0}) \sim N(\mu_{bj},\sigma_\gamma^2) \quad \text{for } b=1,\ldots,B \quad \text{and} \quad j=1,\ldots,n_b.$$

Then the primary parameter of interest is $\varphi_{bj}=\text{logit}(\theta_{bj1})-\text{logit}(\theta_{bj0})$.

Berry and Berry propose the mixture prior for φ_{bj}, where $I_{[0]}$ is the point mass distribution at 0:

$$\varphi_{bj} \sim \pi_b I_{[0]} + (1-\pi_b)N(\mu_{\varphi b},\sigma_{\varphi b}^2) \quad \text{for } b=1,\ldots,B \text{ and } j=1,\ldots,n_b.$$

Then for tumor j, π_b is the prior probability of no difference in tumor incidence between treatment and control, and the posterior distribution of this parameter would be particularly useful for the decision about whether or not there is a treatment effect. Note that the $1 - \pi_b$ has been called the posterior inclusion probability. These are probabilities, so a reasonable prior distribution would be a Beta distribution. They further propose normal distributions on mean parameters and inverse gamma priors on variances, and further parameterize these priors, resulting in a three-stage hierarchical model. However, their original model is designed for another application and does not include an adjustment for differential mortality. When incorporating this adjustment in the model above, there seem to have been a number of parameter identification issues that limit its usefulness with a general program like WinBUGS.

So the mixed one- and two-stage models proposed in Section 22.5.3 above may be more appropriate.

22.5.7 Tumor Process Model

Lindsey and Ryan [34] defined a three-state model for a single type of tumor in a specific organ in rodent carcinogenicity studies. They present a tumor process model where animals either are or remain tumor-free, develop a tumor, or die, i.e., in terms of a stochastic processes, an initial state, a transitional state, and an absorbing state. This model was implemented in a Bayesian framework in French and Ibrahim [35] and Dunson and Dinse [36].

All animals are assumed to start the study without tumors, and either die naturally or are sacrificed at the end of the study. The primary events being modeled are tumor onset and death. Tumor onset is not observable, and is hence treated as a latent variable. Time-to-event data are usually modeled in terms of hazard functions. Let Y be the event being modeled, then the hazard function is defined as

$$h(t) = \lim_{\varepsilon \to 0} \Pr(t < Y < t + \varepsilon | Y \geq t)/\varepsilon.$$

Following the model in Lindsey and Ryan, Dunson and Dinse, and French and Ibrahim have the following schematic diagram for tumor incidence (Figure 22.2) (from [35]):

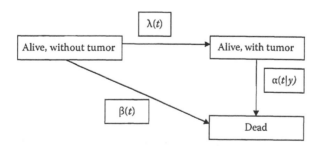

FIGURE 22.2: Process model for tumor incidence. (Taken from French, J.L. and Ibrahim, J.G., *Biometrics*, 58, 906, 2002. With permission.)

In the notation in French and Ibrahim [35], though Dunson and Dinse [36] are quite similar,

let $T_i =$ time to death for animal i,
$O_i =$ time-to-tumor onset,
and $Z_i = \min(T_i, O_i)$.

Thus, for animals that do not develop a tumor $Z_i = T_i$ is observable, and for animals that do develop a tumor X_i is unobservable, and $T_i - Z_i =$ the amount of time the animal was alive with the tumor. Define $\delta_i = 1$ if the animal develops a tumor, 0 otherwise. Define $d_i = 1$ if the animal died a natural death or moribund sacrifice, 0 otherwise (i.e., animal sacrificed).

Then for $t \geq z > 0$, baseline hazards can be defined as follows:

$$\lambda(t) = \lim_{\varepsilon \to 0} \Pr(t < Y < t + \varepsilon, \delta = 1 | Y \geq t)/\varepsilon,$$

$$\beta(t) = \lim_{\varepsilon \to 0} \Pr(t < Y < t + \varepsilon, \delta = 0 | Y \geq t)/\varepsilon,$$

and

$$\alpha(t|y) = \lim_{\varepsilon \to 0} \Pr(t < T < t + \varepsilon | T \geq t, Y = y, \delta = 1)/\varepsilon.$$

For these baseline hazards, for animals $i = 1, \ldots, n$, we have the corresponding subject specific hazards $\lambda_i(t, x_i) = \lambda(t) \exp(x_i'\varphi)$, $\beta_i(t, x_i) = \beta(t) \exp(x_i'\rho)$, and $\alpha_i(t, x_i) = \alpha(t|y) \exp(x_i'\gamma)$. They assume that the baseline hazards of death with and without tumor are proportional, i.e., $\alpha(t|y) = \eta\beta(t) \exp(x_i'\rho)$ with $\eta > 0$.

As they note, by the end of the study all animals are assumed to die of either natural causes (including tumors) or sacrifice. They note that each animal can be classified into one of four groups: sacrificed without tumor (SNT), sacrificed with tumor (SWT), died without tumor (DNT), or died with tumor (SNT). For each animal in each group one has the following contribution to the likelihood:

$$\text{SNT}(\delta = 0, d = 0) \quad \exp\left\{ - \int_0^t [\lambda(u) + \beta(u)]du \right\},$$

$$\text{SWT}(\delta = 1, d = 0) \quad \lambda(x) \exp\left\{ - \int_0^x [\lambda(u) + \beta(u)]du - \eta \int_x^t \beta(u)du \right\},$$

$$\text{DNT}(\delta = 0, d = 1) \quad \beta(t) \exp\left\{ - \int_0^t [\lambda(u) + \beta(u)]du \right\},$$

$$\text{DWT}(\delta = 1, d = 1) \quad \lambda(x)\beta(t)\eta \exp\left\{ - \int_0^x [\lambda(u) + \beta(u)]du - \eta \int_x^t \beta(u)du \right\}$$

Then incorporating the subject specific hazards, we have the contribution of the ith animal to the complete data likelihood, as

$$l_i = (\lambda_i(t_i, x_i))^{\delta i}(\beta_i(t_i, x_i))^{\mathrm{d}i(1-\delta i)}(\alpha_i(t_i, x_i))^{\mathrm{d}i\,\delta i}$$

$$\exp\left\{-\int_0^{xi}[\lambda_i(u, x_i) + \beta(u, x_i)]\mathrm{d}u - \delta_i\int_{xi}^{ti}\alpha_i(u, x_i)\mathrm{d}u\right\}.$$

The authors suggest modeling the baseline hazards for $\lambda(t)$ and $\beta(t)$ as piecewise constant functions on intervals $(a_j, a_{j+1}]$, $j = 1, \ldots T$. Let $\theta' = (\lambda_1, \ldots, \lambda_T, \beta_1, \ldots, \beta_T, \eta)$ be vector of baseline parameters. Let N_t denote the number of animals with tumor onset in the interval $(a_{t-1}, a_t]$, b_t as the number of tumor bearing animals dying of natural causes in $(a_{t-1}, a_t]$, c_t as the number of nontumor bearing animals dying of natural causes in the interval $(a_{t-1}, a_t]$, T_{it}^T is the time the ith animal spends with the tumor in the interval, and T_{it}^{NT} is the time the ith animal spends in the interval without the tumor. Then, reorganizing the responses into the number of events in each of the T intervals, gives the following likelihood:

$$l_{\mathrm{comp}}(\theta, \varphi) = \prod_{t=1}^{T}\left\{\lambda_t^{Ni}\beta_t^{bt+ct}\exp\left[-\lambda_t\sum_i T_{it}^{NT}\exp(x_i^t\psi)\right.\right.$$

$$\left.-\beta_t\sum_i T_{it}^{NT}\exp(x_i^t\rho) - \beta_t\eta\sum_i T_{it}^T\exp(x_i^t(\rho+\gamma))]\right\}$$

$$* \exp\left\{\sum_i x_i^t(\delta_i\psi + d_i\rho + \delta_i d_i\gamma)\right\}\eta^{\sum_t b_t}.$$

The $N_{t,}$, T_{it}^T, and T_{it}^{NT} are not directly observable (although the sum of the latter two is). They treat these as latent variables with parameters to be determined in a hierarchical fashion. As can be seen the models get quite complicated and while they are arguably reasonable models of the tumor generating process, they currently do not seem to have been much used. The interested reader is directed to the papers cited above for details.

22.5.8   Bayesian Version of Dunson's Model for Tg.AC Mice

As noted in Section 21.7, studies using transgenic mice have become an important alternative to classical long term rodent tests. Chapter 21 also includes a discussion of the model proposed in Dunson et al. [37] for the analysis of Tg.AC mice. For each mouse, the data usually consist of a weekly count of the detectable papillomas. To reiterate their model, let Z_{ij} denote the count of skin papillomas on the back of animal i at week j. As noted in their paper, the change in this "tumor burden" is the number of new papillomas minus the number of old papillomas that regress. They define $M_{ij} = \max\{Z_{i1}, \ldots, Z_{ij-1}\}$, the maximum tumor burden for mouse i between weeks 1 and $j - 1$ and $Y_{ij} = M_{ij+1} - M_{ij}$, the maximum tumor increase for mouse

i between weeks $j-1$ and j. With study duration T, in the simplest model, at week j, $t_{ij} = j/T$, the proportion of time animal i remains in the study. For tumor onset the authors suggest a term for each animal, b_i, and as well as a term for dose, d_i.

$$Y_{ij} \sim \text{Poisson}(\mu_{ij})$$

with

$$\mu_{ij} = \begin{cases} \exp{(\beta_1 + (b_i + \gamma_1)t_{ij}d_i)} & \text{if } M_{ij} = 0, \\ \exp{(\beta_2 + \gamma_2 d_i)} & \text{if } M_{ij} > 0. \end{cases}$$

The authors suggest that the dosage of the actual treatment groups should be on a log scale so that $\exp(k \log(\text{dose})) = (\text{dose})^k$ is linear in a power of dose. For the no dose control, $d_i = 0$, and then $\exp(\beta_1)$ models the background rate of appearance of the first papillomas. The probability of detecting the first papilloma should increases with time and dose and is modeled with the term $\exp((b_i + \gamma_1)t_{ij}d_i)$. The term b_i allows for heterogeneity across mice in time to first tumor. The second term in the model corresponds to the development of further tumors, but does not include a term for animal heterogeneity and assumes that the background rate of additional tumors developing is $\exp(\beta_2)$ in the control group. Again, when dose is on a log scale, the rate for additional tumors is also assumed to be linear in a power of dose. As seems traditional for many counting process models, the mouse specific variable b_i is assumed to be normal with mean 0 and variance σ^2.

$$b_i \sim \text{Normal}(0, \sigma^2).$$

Following this convention, Dunson et al. propose the following priors on the parameters:

$$\beta_1 \sim \text{Normal}(m_{01}, v_{01}), \quad \beta_2 \sim \text{Normal}(m_{02}, v_{02}),$$

$$\gamma_1 \sim \text{Normal}(m_{03}, v_{03}), \quad \gamma_2 \sim \text{Normal}(m_{04}, v_{04}),$$

and

$$\sigma^2 \sim \text{Inverse-gamma}(a_{01}, a_{02}).$$

As noted above, for normal random variables data the gamma prior is conjugate to a chi-square distribution, so the inverse gamma is appropriate for the usual normal distribution where one is concerned with inverse of the standard deviation. In their paper, the authors suggest that $m_{01} = m_{02} = m_{03} = m_{04} = 0.0$, $v_{01} = v_{02} = v_{03} = v_{04} = 1000$, and $a_{01} = a_{02} = 0.001$ as providing reasonably non-informative priors.

22.6 Software

A Bayesian analysis of a parameter requires a review of its marginal distribution, i.e., integrating out all other parameters. Such integrations can be quite challenging. It seems that the recent revolution in Bayesian analysis is largely due to the development of better techniques for these performing these integrations, in particular MCMC methods. The basic idea is to construct a Markov chain whose stationary distribution is the posterior one is trying to estimate (e.g., see Gammerman [38] or Robert and Cassella [39]). This can be done using the Metropolis or Metropolis–Hasting's algorithms, where one samples from a proposal distribution to see if the observations can be assumed to be treated as coming from the stationary distribution. However, so-called Gibbs sampling seems to be more common, i.e., assume we are interested in k parameters $\theta_1, \ldots, \theta_k$. Then, writing $\pi(.|.)$ as the appropriate conditional distributions, starting from initial conditions at $i = 1$, and denoting the ith iterate of the kth parameter as θ_k^i and denoting $\sim$ as the operation of sampling we have the standard Gibbs iteration:

$$\theta_1^i \sim \pi(\theta_1 | \theta_2^{i-1}, \ldots, \theta_k^{i-1})$$

$$\theta_2^i \sim \pi(\theta_2 | \theta_1^i, \theta_3^{i-1}, \ldots, \theta_k^{i-1})$$

$$\cdots$$

$$\theta_k^i \sim \pi(\theta_k | \theta_1^i, \ldots, \theta_{k-1}^i).$$

Note that up to normalization this just involves the likelihood times the posterior and is generally easy to implement.

Whether using Metropolis–Hastings or Gibbs sampling, or later developments, the point is that upon convergence you are sampling from the stationary distribution of the Markov chain. The ergodic theorem states that the integral of any function of the parameters is calculated by taking the average of the function evaluated at the values drawn from this stationary distribution. This does require a so-called "burn-in" so that sampled values come from a distribution close to the stationary distribution. Checking convergence to the stationary distribution seems to have been a veritable cottage industry in the 1990s, and is reviewed in the previously cited references. Many of these are available in the so-called Bayesian output analysis (BOA) program.

Many applications of these techniques will require programming with some computer language like C or perhaps the venerable FORTRAN. However some general purpose software is available. WinBUGS (Spiegelhalter et al. [17]) is probably the most well known general purpose program for these Bayesian analyses. The WinBUGS internet site states that: "Bayesian inference Using Gibbs Sampling (BUGS) is a piece of computer software for the Bayesian analysis of complex statistical models using MCMC methods." By default, for unbounded distributions, it starts with metropolis steps and changes to Gibbs sampling. It is currently available for download on the internet at http://www.mrc-bsu.cam.ac.uk/bugs (or search for BUGS or WinBUGS). OpenBUGS is an open source version that is also available. However, all of the various versions of BUGS are very general software, and may have problems fitting some models, particularly if they include some parameters that are close to being not identified. Syntax is basically a subset of R or S-PLUS, and is generally quite easy to use. However, when actually writing the program it is usually easier to modify an existing program. The online WinBUGS manual includes a number of examples that can be useful, as well as references to other related examples and software. Congdon [40–42] includes large menus of various Bayesian analyses with appropriate discussions. For virtually all of them he provides a library on the Web where corresponding WinBUGS programs can be downloaded and are an excellent source for starting an analysis.

The R programming library includes a number of packages for Bayesian analyses. The R2WinBUGS package allows one to run a WinBUGS or OpenBUGS program from within R. The package bayesSurv reviews Bayesian analyses of survival data and seems to include many programs for Bayesian survival analysis corresponding to the techniques described in Ibrahim et al. [21]. As the name indicates, the package MCMCpack includes a number of scripts to execute various MCMC techniques, while BOA and coda are output analysis programs to assess the stationarity results from the MCMC iterations.

SAS (see SAS Institute [18]) is a popular, well supported program character-ized by some very good data handling characteristics. SAS release 9.1 had several experimental procedures that could be downloaded for proportional hazards regression, generalized linear models, and regression. In the successor, SAS 9.2, these have been incorporated in the standard PROCs PHGLM, GENMOD, and REG, respectively. In addition there is a new procedure PROC MCMC that seems to be a general program for analyses using MCMC, and includes numerous features for output analysis to assess the results of the MCMC fitting. However, the authors have not had sufficient experience with the procedure to assess it further.

Appendix: WinBUGS

The following WinBUGS programs were used for the analyses in Examples 1 and 2. They are included for interest, but without any warranty. Note that normal distributions in WinBUGS are parameterized in terms of mean and precision, the inverse of the variance. So an inverse gamma prior on a variance is equivalent to a gamma prior on the precision.

Testing homogeneity in mortality over four parameter groups:

```
model{
  a[1]<-0; a[2]<-300; a[3]<-400; a[4]<-450; a[5]<-500; a[6]<-550
  a[7]<-600; a[8]<-700
  for (i in 1:N) { lin.pred[i] <- beta[1]*equals(dose[i],2)+
      beta[2]*equals(dose[i],3)+beta[3]*equals(dose[i],4)
  for (j in 1:T) {
          d[i,j]<- fail[i]*step(obs.t[i]-a[j])*step(a[j+1]-obs.t[i])
          gamma[i,j] <- (a[j+1]-a[j])*step(obs.t[i] - a[j+1])+
            (obs.t[i]-a[j])*step(a[j+1]-obs.t[i])*step(obs.t[i]-a[j])
          theta[i,j] <- lambda[j] * exp(lin.pred[i])
          d[i,j] ~ dpois(mu[i,j])
          mu[i,j] <- theta[i,j]*gamma[i,j]
                        }
                }
  for ( j in 1:T) {
          mn[j] <- 0.01*j
          r[j] <- 0.001*j*j
          lambda[j] ~ dgamma(mn[j],r[j])
          part[j] <- lambda[j]*(a[j+1]-a[j])
                }
  for (m in 1:3) {
          beta[m] ~ dnorm (0.0, 0.001)
          }
  for ( k in 1:T) {
          sum[k]    <- sum(part[1:k])
          S.high[k]   <- exp( -(exp(beta[3])*sum[k]))
          S.med[k]    <- exp( -(exp(beta[2])*sum[k]))
          S.low[k]    <- exp( -(exp(beta[1])*sum[k]))
          S.veh[k]    <- exp( -(sum[k]))
                }
      }
  inits
```

```
list(beta=c(-.5,0,0.5))
data
list(N=300,T=7)
dose[] obs.t[] fail[]
   1      704    0
   1      255    1
          - data -
   4      645    1
   4      710    0
END
```

Assessing simple trend in tumorigenicity:

nn = no. animals* no.tumors = 300*11, time[] = time on study
fail[j] = occurrence of jth tumor.

```
model{
    for (i in 1:nn) {
       fail[i] ~ dbern(p[i])
       term[i] <- alpha[tmr[i]]+beta[tmr[i]]*(0.3*equals(trt[i],2)+
           equals(trt[i],3)+3*equals(trt[i],4))+gam[tmr[i]]
              *time[i]+
           subj[animl[i]]
       p[i] <-exp(term[i])/(1+exp(term[i]))
              }
    for (j in 1:ns){
       subj[j] ~ dnorm(mur,taur)
              }
    for (k in 1:nt){
       gam[k] ~dnorm(mug,taug)
       alpha[k] ~dnorm(mua,taua)
       z1[k] ~ dbern(pix)
       z2[k] ~ dnorm(mub,taub)
       beta[k] <- z1[k]*z2[k]
       betaeq0[k] <- equals(beta[k],0)
              }
       pix~dbeta(1,1)
       mug~dnorm(mug0,taug0)
       mua~dnorm(mua0,taua0)
       mub~dnorm(mub0,taub0)
       sigb~ dgamma(alpb,betb)
       siga~ dgamma(alpx,betx)
       sigg~dgamma(alpg,betg)
       taub<-1/sigb
       taua<-1/siga
       taug<-1/sigg
              }
inits
list(pix=0.5)
data
list(nn=3300,ns=300, nt=11,
```

```
mub0 = 0, mua0 = 0, mur = 0, mug0 = 0, taub0 = 0.01, taua0 = 0.01,
 taur = 0.01, taug0 = 0.01,
alpb = 4, alpg = 4, alpx = 4, betb = 0.5, betg = 0.5, betx = 0.5),
trt[] animl[] tmr[] time[] fail[]
1        1       1 22.67     0
1        1       2 22.67     1
 . . .
4      300      11 98.67     0
end
```

The pairwise comparisons were performed with simple modifications of this program.

References

[1] Berger, J.O. and Wolpert, R.L. (1988): *The Likelihood Principle*, 2nd edn. Institute of Mathematical Statistics, Hayward, CA (available online).

[2] Rahman, M.A. and Lin, K.K. (2008): Design and analysis of chronic carcinogenicity studies of pharmaceuticals in rodents. In: *Design and Analysis of Clinical Trials with Time-to-Event Endpoints*, K. Peace (ed.). Taylor & Francis, New York.

[3] Fienberg, S.E. (2006): When did Bayesian inference become "Bayesian"? *Bayesian Analysis* 1: 1–40.

[4] Spiegelhalter, D.J., Abrams, K.R., and Myles, J.P. (2004): *Bayesian Approaches to Clinical Trials and Health-Care Evaluation*. Wiley, New York.

[5] Carlin, B.P. and Louis, T.A. (2000): *Bayes and Empirical Bayes Methods for Data Analysis*, 2nd edn. Chapman & Hall, New York.

[6] Bernardo, J.M. and Smith, A.F.M. (2000): *Bayesian Theory*. Wiley, New York.

[7] U.S. Department of Health and Human Services (2001): *Guidance for Industry Statistical Aspects of the Design, Analysis, and Interpretation of Chronic Rodent Carcinogenicity Studies of Pharmaceuticals (DRAFT GUIDANCE)*. Center for Drug Evaluation and Research, Food and Drug Administration. Available at http://www.fda.gov/CDER/GUIDANCE/#Pharmacology/Toxicology

[8] Lin, K.K. and Ali, M.W. (2006): Statistical review and evaluation of animal tumorigenicity studies. In: *Statistics in the Pharmaceutical Industry*, C.R. Buncher and J.Y. Tsay (eds.), 3rd edn. Marcel Dekker, Inc., New York.

[9] Stangl, D.K. and Berry, D.A. (1998): Bayesian statistics in medicine: Where are we and where should we be going? *Sankhya, Series B* 60(Pt.1): 176–195.

[10] Berry, D.A. (2006): Bayesian clinical trials. *Nature Reviews Drug Discovery* 5: 27–36.

[11] U.S. Department of Health and Human Services (2006): *Guidance for the Use of Bayesian Statistics in Medical Device Clinical Trials (Draft Guidance for Industry and FDA Staff)*. Center for Devices and Radiological Health, Food and Drug Administration. Available at http://www.fda.gov/cdrh/osb/guidance/1601.html

[12] Kass, R.E. and Raftery, A.F. (1995): Bayes factors. *Journal of the American Statistical Association* 90(430): 773–795.

[13] Akaike, H. (1973): *Information Theory and an Extension of the Maximum Likelihood Principle*. *Proceedings of 2nd International Symposium on Information Theory*, B. Petrov and F. Csaki (eds.). Akademai Kiado, Budapest, pp. 267–281.

[14] Schwarz, G. (1978): Estimating the dimension of a model. *Annals of Statistics* 6(2): 461–464.

[15] Spiegelhalter, D.J., Best, N.G., Carlin, J.B., and van der Linde, A. (2002): Bayesian measures of model complexity and fit (with discussion). *Journal of the Royal Statistical Society, Series B (Statistical Methodology)* 64(4): 583–639.

[16] Lunn, D.J., Thomas, A., Best, N., and Spiegelhalter, D. (2000): WinBUGS— A Bayesian modelling framework: Concepts, structure, and extensibility. *Statistics and Computing* 10: 325–337.

[17] Spiegelhalter, D.J., Thomas, A., and Best, N.G. (2007): *WinBUGS Version 1.4.3 User Manual*. MRC Biostatistics Unit, Cambridge, U.K.

[18] SAS Institute Inc. (2008): *SAS/STAT® 9.2 User's Guide*. SAS Institute, Cary, NC.

[19] Schervish, M.J. (1996): P values: What they are and what they are not. *American Statistician* 50(3): 203–206.

[20] Schervish, M.J. (1998): Bayes factors: What they are and what they are not. *American Statistician* 52(3): 203–206.

[21] Ibrahim, J.G., Chen, M.-H., and Sinha, D. (2001): *Bayesian Survival Analysis*. Springer Verlag, New York.

[22] Schervish, M.J. (1995): *Theory of Statistics*. Springer Verlag, New York.

[23] Muliere, P. and Walker, S. (1997): A Bayesian non-parametric approach to survival analysis using polya trees. *Scandinavian Journal of Statistics* 24(3): 331–340.

[24] Nieto-Barajas, L.E. and Walker, S. (2004): Bayesian nonparametric survival analysis via Levy driven Markov processes. *Statistica Sinica* 14: 1127–1146.

[25] Gelman, A. (2006): Prior distributions for variance parameters in hierarchical models. *Bayesian Analysis* 1(3): 515–533.

[26] Meng, C.L.Y. and Dempster, A.P. (1987): A Bayesian approach to the multiplicity problem for significance testing with binomial data. *Biometrics* 43(2): 301–311.

[27] Dempster, A.P., Selwyn, M.R., and Weeks, B.J. (1983): Combining historical and randomized controls for assessing trends in proportions. *Journal of the American Statistical Association* 78(382): 221–227.

[28] Westfall, P.H. and Soper, K.A. (2001): Using priors to improve multiple animal carcinogenicity tests. *Journal of the American Statistical Association* 96(455): 827–834.

[29] Ibrahim, J.G., Ryan, L.M., and Chen M.-H. (1998): Use of historical controls to adjust for covariates in trend tests for binary data. *Journal of the American Statistical Association* 93: 1282–1293.

[30] McConnell, E.E., Solleveld, H.A., Swnberg, J.A., and Boorman, G.A. (1986): Guidelines for combining neoplasms for evaluation of rodent carcinogenesis studies. *Journal of the National Cancer Institute* 76: 283–289.

[31] Haseman, J.K. (1983): A reexamination of false-positive rates for carcinogenicity studies. *Fundamental and Applied Toxicology* 3: 334–339.

[32] Lin, K.K. and Rahman, M.A. (1998): Overall false positive rates in tests for linear trend in tumor incidence in animal carcinogenicity studies of new drugs. *Journal of Biopharmaceutical Statistics* 8(1): 1–15.

[33] Berry, S.M. and Berry, D.A. (2004): Accounting for multiplicities in assessing drug safety: A three-level hierarchical mixture models. *Biometrics* 60(2): 418–426.

[34] Lindsey, J.C. and Ryan, L.M. (1993): A three-state multiplicative model for rodent tumorigenicity experiments. *Applied Statistics* 42(2): 283–300.

[35] French J.L. and Ibrahim, J.G. (2002): Bayesian methods for a three-state model for rodent carcinogenicity studies. *Biometrics* 58(4): 906–916.

[36] Dunson, D.B. and Dinse, G.E. (2001): Bayesian incidence analysis of tumorigenicity data. *Applied Statistics* 50(2): 125–141.

[37] Dunson, D.B., Haseman, J.K., van Birgelen, A.P.J.M., Stasiewicz, S., and Tennant, R.W. (2000): Statistical analysis of skin tumor data from Tg.AC mouse bioassays. *Toxicological Sciences* 55: 293–302.

[38] Gamerman, D. and Lopes, H.F. (2006): *Markov Chain Monte Carlo: Stochastic Simulation for Bayesian Inference*, 2nd edn. Chapman & Hall, New York.

[39] Robert, C.P. and Casella, G. (2005): *Monte Carlo Statistical Methods*, 2nd edn. Springer Verlag, New York.

[40] Congdon, P. (2003): *Applied Bayesian Modelling*. Wiley, New York.

[41] Congdon, P. (2005): *Bayesian Models for Categorical Data*. Wiley, New York.

[42] Congdon, P. (2006): *Bayesian Statistical Modelling*, 2nd edn. Wiley, New York.

Index

Milton Keynes UK
Ingram Content Group UK Ltd.
UKHW030901141024
449569UK00025B/1281